FRONTIERS IN NUTRITIONAL SCIENCE

This series of books addresses a wide range of topics in nutritional science. The books are aimed at advanced undergraduate and graduate students, researchers, university teachers, policy makers and nutrition and health professionals. They offer original syntheses of knowledge, providing a fresh perspective on key topics in nutritional science. Each title is written by a single author or by groups of authors who are acknowledged experts in their field. Titles include aspects of molecular, cellular and whole body nutrition and cover humans and wild, captive and domesticated animals. Basic nutritional science, clinical nutrition and public health nutrition are each addressed by titles in the series.

Editor in Chief
P.C. Calder, University of Southampton, UK

Editorial Board
A. Bell, Cornell University, Ithaca, New York, USA
F. Kok, Wageningen University, The Netherlands
A. Lichtenstein, Tufts University, Massachusetts, USA
I. Ortigues-Marty, INRA, Thiex, France
P. Yaqoob, University of Reading, UK
K. Younger, Dublin Institute of Technology, Ireland

Titles available
1. Nutrition and Immune Function
   Edited by P.C. Calder, C.J. Field and H.S. Gill
2. Fetal Nutrition and Adult Disease: Programming of Chronic Disease through Fetal Exposure to Undernutrition
   Edited by S.C. Langley-Evans

FETAL NUTRITION AND ADULT DISEASE

Programming of Chronic Disease through Fetal Exposure to Undernutrition

Edited by

S.C. Langley-Evans

Division of Nutritional Biochemistry, School of Biosciences, University of Nottingham, UK

CABI Publishing
in association with
The Nutrition Society

CABI Publishing is a division of CAB International

CABI Publishing
CAB International
Wallingford
Oxfordshire OX10 8DE
UK

Tel: +44 (0)1491 832111
Fax: +44 (0)1491 833508
E-mail: cabi@cabi.org
Web site: www.cabi-publishing.org

CABI Publishing
875 Massachusetts Avenue
7th Floor
Cambridge, MA 02139
USA

Tel: +1 617 395 4056
Fax: +1 617 354 6875
E-mail: cabi-nao@cabi.org

A catalogue record for this book is available from the British Library, London, UK.

Library of Congress Cataloging-in-Publication Data
Fetal nutrition and adult disease : programming of chronic disease
through fetal exposure to undernutrition / edited by S.C. Langley-Evans.

    p. cm. -- (Frontiers in nutritional science)
Includes index.
    ISBN 0-85199-821-6 (alk paper)
    1. Chronic diseases--Etiology.   2. Fetus--Nutrition.   3. Nutritionally
induced diseases.   I. Langley-Evans, S. C.   II. Title.   III. Series.
RB156.F48 2004
616′.044--dc22

                                                        2003026166

ISBN 0 85199 821 6

Typeset by AMA DataSet Ltd, UK.
Printed and bound in the UK by Biddles Ltd, King's Lynn.

Contents

Contributors   vii

Preface   ix

Part 1: Programming the Fetus

1. **Fetal Programming of Adult Disease: an Overview**   1
   Simon C. Langley-Evans

2. **Nutritional Basis for the Fetal Origins of Adult Disease**   21
   Jane Harding

3. **Intrauterine Hypoxaemia and Cardiovascular Development**   55
   Dino A. Giussani and David S. Gardner

Part 2: Programming Human Disease

4. **Epidemiology of the Fetal Origins of Adult Disease: Cohort Studies of Birthweight and Cardiovascular Disease**   87
   Janet Rich-Edwards

5. **Early-life Origins of Adult Disease: is There Really an Association Between Birthweight and Chronic Disease Risk?** 105
   Rachel Huxley

6. **Experimental Models of Hypertension and Cardiovascular Disease**   129
   Simon C. Langley-Evans

7. **Associations between Fetal and Infant Growth and
    Non-insulin-dependent Diabetes**   157
    Simon C. Langley-Evans

8. **Programming of Diabetes: Experimental Models**   171
    Brigitte Reusens, Luise Kalbe and Claude Remacle

9. **Birthweight and the Development of Overweight and
    Obesity**   195
    Aryeh D. Stein

10. **Maternal Nutrition in Pregnancy and Adiposity in Offspring** 211
    Bernhard H. Breier, Stefan O. Krechowec and Mark H. Vickers

11. **Renal Disease and Fetal Undernutrition**   235
    Lori L. Woods

12. **Perinatal Determinants of Atopic Disease**   259
    Kitaw Demissie, Katherine D. Chung and Bijal A. Balasubramanian

13. **Fetal Programming of Immune Function**   311
    Thomas W. McDade and Christopher W. Kuzawa

Part 3: Biological Basis of Nutritional Programming

14. **Programming in the Pre-implantation Embryo**   333
    Lorraine E. Young, William D. Rees and Kevin D. Sinclair

15. **Endocrine Responses to Fetal Undernutrition: the Growth
    Hormone–Insulin-like Growth Factor Axis**   353
    *Michael E. Symonds, David S. Gardner, Sarah Pearce and Terence
    Stephenson*

16. **Impact of Intrauterine Exposure to Glucocorticoids upon
    Fetal Development and Adult Pathophysiology**   381
    Amanda J. Drake and Jonathan R. Seckl

Index   419

Contributors

Bijal A. Balasubramanian, *Division of Epidemiology, University of Medicine and Dentistry of New Jersey – School of Public Health, 683 Hoes Lane West, 2nd Floor, Room 205, Piscataway, NJ 08854, USA.*

Bernhard H. Breier, *Liggins Institute for Medical Research, Faculty of Medical and Health Sciences, University of Auckland, Private Bag 92019, 2–6 Park Avenue, Grafton, Auckland, New Zealand.*

Katherine D. Chung, *Department of Epidemiology, School of Public Health, University of Medicine and Dentistry of New Jersey, Robert Wood Johnson, 675 Hoes Lane, Piscataway, NJ 08854, USA.*

Kitaw Demissie, *Department of Epidemiology, School of Public Health, University of Medicine and Dentistry of New Jersey, Robert Wood Johnson, 675 Hoes Lane, Piscataway, NJ 08854, USA.*

Amanda J. Drake, *School of Molecular and Clinical Medicine, University of Edinburgh, Molecular Medicine Centre, Western General Hospital, Edinburgh EH4 2XU, UK.*

David S. Gardner, *Academic Division of Child Health, School of Human Development, Queen's Medical Centre, University Hospital, Nottingham NG7 2UH, UK.*

Dino A. Giussani, *Department of Physiology, University of Cambridge, Downing Street, Cambridge, UK.*

Jane Harding, *University of Auckland, Private Bag 92019, Auckland, New Zealand.*

Rachel Huxley, *Heart and Vascular Disease Programme, Institute for International Health, Sydney, NSW 2042, Australia.*

Luise Kalbe, *Laboratoroire de Biologie Cellulaire, Catholic University of Louvain, Place Croix du Sud 5, B-1348, Louvain-la-Neuve, Belgium.*

Stefan O. Krechowec, *Liggins Institute for Medical Research, Faculty of Medical and Health Sciences, University of Auckland, Private Bag 92019, 2–6 Park Avenue, Grafton, Auckland, New Zealand.*

Christopher W. Kuzawa, *Northwestern University, Department of Anthropology, 1810 Hinman Avenue, Evanston, IL 60208-1310, USA.*

Simon C. Langley-Evans, *School of Biosciences, University of Nottingham, Sutton Bonington Campus, Loughborough LE12 5RD, UK.*

Thomas W. McDade, *Northwestern University, Department of Anthropology, 1810 Hinman Avenue, Evanston, IL 60208-1310, USA.*

Sarah Pearce, *Academic Division of Child Health, School of Human Development, Queen's Medical Centre, University Hospital, Nottingham NG7 2UH, UK.*

William D. Rees, *Rowett Research Institute, Greenburn Road, Bucksburn, Aberdeen AB21 9SB, UK.*

Claude Remacle, *Laboratoire de Biologie Cellulaire, Catholic University of Louvain, Place Croix du Sud 5, B-1348, Louvain-la-Neuve, Belgium.*

Brigitte Reusens, *Laboratoire de Biologie Cellulaire, Catholic University of Louvain, Place Croix du Sud 5, B-1348, Louvain-la-Neuve, Belgium.*

Janet Rich-Edwards, *Harvard School of Medicine, Department of Ambulatory Care & Prevention, 113 Brookline Avenue, Boston, MA 02215, USA.*

Jonathan R. Seckl, *School of Molecular and Clinical Medicine, University of Edinburgh, Molecular Medicine Centre, Western General Hospital, Edinburgh EH4 2XU, UK.*

Kevin D. Sinclair, *School of Biosciences, University of Nottingham, Sutton Bonington Campus, Loughborough LE12 5RD, UK.*

Aryeh D. Stein, *Department of International Health, Emory University, Rollins School of Public Health, 1518 Clifton Rd NE – Room 750, Atlanta, GA 30322, USA.*

Terence Stephenson, *Academic Division of Child Health, School of Human Development, Queen's Medical Centre, University Hospital, Nottingham NG7 2UH, UK.*

Michael E. Symonds, *Academic Division of Child Health, School of Human Development, Division of Child Health, E Floor East Block, Queen's Medical Centre, University Hospital, Nottingham NG7 2UH, UK.*

Mark H. Vickers, *Liggins Institute for Medical Research, Faculty of Medical and Health Sciences, University of Auckland, Private Bag 92019, 2–6 Park Avenue, Grafton, Auckland, New Zealand.*

Lori L. Woods, *Division of Nephrology and Hypertension, L463 Oregon Health and Science University, 3181 S.W. Sam Jackson Park Road, Portland, OR 97239-3098, USA.*

Lorraine E. Young, *University of Nottingham, School of Human Development, Division of Obstetrics and Gynaecology, D Floor East Block, Queen's Medical Centre, Nottingham NH7 2UH, UK.*

Preface

For many years adult lifestyle factors have been believed to be the primary cause of major health problems encountered in the westernized nations. Obesity, heart disease and diabetes are known to stem from a sedentary lifestyle associated with a fat- and salt-rich diet. This is not, however, the whole story, and it is becoming clear that the environment that an individual encounters during life in the womb may be equally as important in establishing risk of these diseases. The process through which events *in utero* exert effects that manifest as disease decades later is termed fetal programming.

Interest in the potential for human disease to be programmed by early life events has grown enormously in recent years. The implications for public health, in both the developed and the developing world, have resulted in a number of experimental researchers joining forces with epidemiologists in this field in order to explore the nature of the problem and underlying biological and molecular mechanisms of programming. The level of interest is reflected by the large and successful World Congresses on the Fetal Origins of Adult Disease held in Mumbai and Brighton. The international critical mass of researchers in this field has now prompted the foundation of a new learned society devoted to the study of the fetal origins of adult disease hypothesis.

This book aims to paint a broad picture of current understanding of fetal programming. The volume presents a range of epidemiological data demonstrating links between events in fetal life and the development of cardiovascular disease, non-insulin-dependent diabetes, obesity and disorders of the immune system. These findings are supported by contributions from basic experimental research that aims to test the fetal origins hypothesis and to elucidate the supporting biological principles and activities at the molecular and cellular level.

The book is divided into three parts. 'Programming the fetus' sets out the basic principles of programming and considers the potential contribution of undernutrition and other insults during critical phases of embryonic and fetal development, to abnormal physiology and disease processes in later life. 'Programming human disease' provides the core of the book and shows how suggestive epidemiological evidence for an association between characteristics at birth and later disease is replicated in experimental models. A hypothesis by its very nature requires robust challenges, and, importantly, this part of the book also presents data that question the birthweight–disease association, highlighting the importance of well-designed experimental studies. The final part of the book, 'Biological basis of nutritional programming', sets out current ideas about the inter-relationships of maternal nutrition, placental function and fetal endocrinology, and looks at how early nutrient–gene interactions may exert permanent influences on the health and well-being of an individual.

I would like to give my thanks to all of the authors for their contribution to this book and I beg their forgiveness for my continual nagging about deadlines. I also thank the Series Editor Philip Calder for the opportunity to put this volume together.

Simon Langley-Evans
Editor
January 2004

1 Fetal Programming of Adult Disease: an Overview

SIMON C. LANGLEY-EVANS

School of Biosciences, University of Nottingham, Sutton Bonington Campus, Loughborough LE12 5RD, UK

What is Programming?

This book is concerned with the fetal programming of disease, and examines a new paradigm for considering the aetiology of disease, based upon a range of evidence from human populations and experiments with animal models. Programming is the process through which the environment encountered before birth, or in infancy, shapes the long-term control of tissue physiology and homeostasis. The premise for this book is that such early programming profoundly shapes the profile of health and disease experienced by individuals across their life span. This is an important new concept in the arena of public-health medicine which implies that strategies for the prevention of disease that are targeted towards modifying diet and behaviour among adults will be insufficient to achieve their goals. For much of the population, the roots of disease may go much deeper and lead to intrauterine factors over which we can exert little control.

Although the primary driver for the current interest in this area was the discovery in the 1980s of strong associations between early life events and cardiovascular mortality, the first clues to programming of health and disease were reported much earlier. In 1964, Rose noted that the risk of ischaemic heart disease was almost doubled in individuals who had had siblings that were stillborn or who had died in early infancy. Similarly Forsdahl (1967) found that, among Norwegians, risk of cardiovascular mortality was greatest in areas of the country with a high level of infant mortality in the same generation of individuals. Since then, a large number of studies (Huxley *et al.*, 2002) has suggested that exposure to adverse factors during fetal life or early infancy may predispose, or programme, the individual to suffer specific non-communicable diseases in adult life.

Defining programming

The first attempt to define programming in the area of human biology and health was by Alan Lucas (1991). He described programming as the permanent response of an organism to a stimulus or insult during a critical period of development. In simple terms, this definition suggests that when a fetus or neonate is exposed to an unusual environment during a rapid phase of growth, the resulting adaptive responses may become permanently fixed in place. In terms of health and well-being many years later, the effects of programming may be profound, as irreversible maladaption may result in detriment to organ function or longevity.

In other spheres of interest, programming has been recognized for some time. In crocodilians, sex is determined by a programming process rather than by the existence of sex chromosomes (Deeming and Ferguson, 1989). Crocodile and alligator populations are maintained with a female:male ratio of approximately 7:1 by virtue of the nesting behaviour of mothers. Female crocodilians lay their eggs in raised mounds of earth, within which there is a considerable gradient in temperature. Incubation within a very narrow range of temperatures activates aromatases in the eggs, which generate androgens and promote the development of male embryos (Deeming and Ferguson, 1989). Outside this 1–2°C range of temperature, eggs will develop with female embryos.

Another classical example of programming relates to the psychosocial development of young birds. Konrad Lorenz (1952) used the term 'imprinting' to describe the way in which the first object encountered by newly hatched ducks and geese will be followed as if it was the mother of the birds. This phenomenon is analogous to programming, as the behaviour depends upon exposures during critical periods of development, shortly before and shortly after hatching, and is triggered by clear stimuli, which include the call of mother before hatching and the sight of a moving object.

Demonstration of principle

Laboratory experiments with animal species have demonstrated effectively the principle of programming and its likely impact upon the health of human beings. The treatment of neonatal female rats with a single dose of testosterone, within a narrow window of time in the first week of life, induces profound changes upon subsequent reproductive development, which are not seen if treatment is given later in life (Barraclough, 1961). Testosterone treatment remodels key structures within the hypothalamus and, as a result, the animals are unable to ovulate and the reproductive organs eventually atrophy. Interestingly, the brain develops structures normally observed in male animals, and these females adopt male patterns of behaviour (Ito et al., 1986).

Further examples of this demonstration of principle will be seen later in this book. One noteworthy experiment, however, was reported by Beach et al. (1982), who showed that feeding a zinc-deficient diet in mouse pregnancy had consequences that lasted for three generations. Offspring of zinc-deficient mothers had impaired immune functions as young adults. When these offspring were then mated, it was found that the second-generation offspring shared the same immune impairments of their parents. It was only in the next generation bred from these animals that the effect of the initial nutritional insult was lost.

In evolutionary terms, this concept is almost compatible with the Lamarckian viewpoint (Humphreys, 1996), in which acquired characteristics may be transmitted to subsequent generations. If adaptations to prevailing conditions during fetal development could be transmitted in an epigenetic manner, as suggested by the experiment of Beach *et al.* (1982), and conferred a survival advantage, then this would essentially promote rapid changes in a population through adaptive acquisition of characteristics.

Critical periods of development

Within the generally recognized definition of programming, it is stated that long-term effects of an insult or stimulus will stem only from exposure during a critical period of development. Other authors may refer to these critical periods as 'sensitive' or 'vulnerable' periods. The importance of the critical exposure period during programming is well demonstrated by the example of the effect of testosterone treatment on the female rat neonate above (Barraclough, 1961). If exposure does not fall within the narrow window of sensitivity, then no effect will be observed.

Our current understanding is that critical periods of development are essentially periods of rapid cell division within a tissue. Mammalian cells have the capacity to undergo a limited number of divisions before they reach the point where further replication is impossible, or apoptotic mechanisms leading to cell death are initiated (replicative senescence) (Jennings *et al.*, 2000). In humans, 42 rounds of cell division occur, mainly before birth, and the majority of the organs are fully developed *in utero*. In other species, cell division may occur both before and after birth. If we accept that critical periods of programming relate to periods of cell division, then we would expect that in humans most, if not all, of the critical periods would occur during fetal life. In a less mature animal at birth, such as the rat, we would argue that there are critical periods both before and after birth. This has been demonstrated in relation to the development of the pancreas and programming of long-term glucose metabolism (Snoeck *et al.*, 1990; Dahri *et al.*, 1991; see also Chapter 8, this volume).

Some of the vulnerability to adverse conditions, of the animal undergoing rapid cell division and growth, is illustrated by studies of sheep fetuses. In experiments where maternal undernutrition was imposed in late gestation, the rate of subsequent fetal growth was totally unaffected in the lambs that were previously only slow growing. However, those lambs that were following a rapid growth trajectory *in utero* exhibited a marked reduction in growth rate (Harding *et al.*, 1992).

The same critical periods for programming of later physiology and disease risk will not apply to all the organs within the animal. In humans, some organs undergo early differentiation and growth during early phases of development.

The 6-week embryo, for example, already has a beating, four-chambered heart. The organs that develop early are those that are required in a critical functional sense during fetal life, such as the heart, brain and liver. Other systems that are essentially non-functional, or lack mature characteristics *in utero* (kidney, lung, immune system), undergo rapid growth and development later in gestation, in preparation for delivery.

The timing of fetal exposure to adverse conditions will thus determine the long-term outcome and consequences of that exposure. The fetus caught by famine during early development, should it survive, may thus be prone to heart disease and cognitive delay, whereas the kidney and lung may be totally un-affected. Specific exposure to famine in later gestation may similarly predispose to renal disease without compromising other organs.

Insults and stimuli

Nutrition

Investigations of the impact of fetal programming upon physiology and human health are at a relatively early stage, and the full range of agents or intrauterine scenarios that are able to act as stimuli or insults is not yet known. From the point of view of public health, the role of maternal nutrition appears to be of para-mount importance. In early accounts of the relationship between early-life factors and coronary heart disease in adult life, Barker and others identified maternal nutrition and health as risk factors for either neonatal death or long-term predisposition for disease (Barker *et al.*, 1993). Poor nutrition and health were proposed to 'prejudice the ability of mothers to nourish their babies *in utero* and during infancy'. This assertion is largely based upon a misguided inter-polation of animal experiments into human biology (Fig. 1.1). Low birthweight and altered proportions at birth are linked to variation in nutritional status in domestic animals and in rodents, but the same is not true of humans living in most parts of the world. In contrast to pigs (Widdowson, 1971), sheep (Wallace *et al.*, 1999) and rats (Hastings-Roberts and Zeman, 1977), the growth of the human fetus is remarkably well protected from even major and prolonged perturbation of the diet (Antonov, 1947; Mathews *et al.*, 1999).

In considering the impact of maternal diet in pregnancy upon later health, much of the debate has been focused on inappropriate issues. The 'Barker hypothesis' suggests that maternal undernutrition promotes retardation of fetal growth, which manifests as low weight at birth or disproportion (thinness, or shortness in relation to head circumference) at birth, depending on the timing (Barker, 1994). As low weight at birth and disproportion appear to predict later risk of heart disease and diabetes, the link between maternal diet and disease has been proposed, and is now generally accepted.

However, unlike other species, the growth of the human fetus does not appear to be particularly sensitive to variations in maternal diet (see Chapter 2, this volume). Human fetal growth rates are determined genetically and may be constrained by socio-economic status (which may, to some extent, reflect diet),

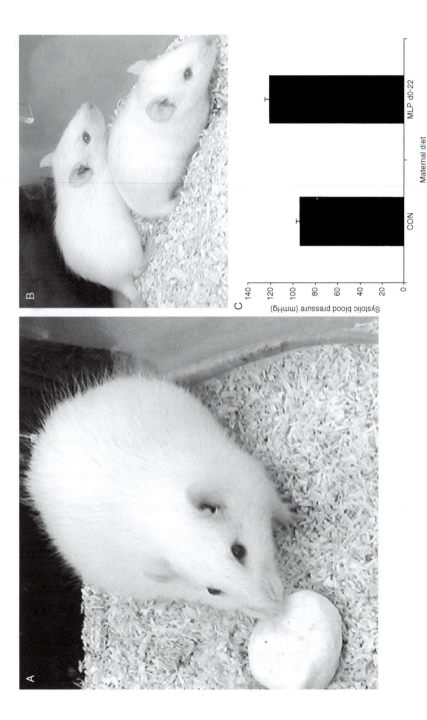

Fig. 1.1. Experimental models of programming. The feeding of experimental diets of reduced protein content to pregnant rats (A) results in offspring that are apparently normal in terms of gross anatomy and general indices of health (B). Programmed changes to cardiovascular and renal physiology mean that such offspring will develop significantly raised blood pressure by the time of weaning (C).

cigarette smoking and maternal size (Campbell, 1991). Although studies of extreme famine situations indicate some impact of undernutrition upon birthweight, the effects are remarkably small (Antonov, 1947; Prentice *et al.*, 1987). In well-nourished populations, such as the UK, there appears to be little evidence that variation in the diet of the population accounts for variation in weight at birth (Doyle *et al.*, 1992; Mathews *et al.*, 1999), although Godfrey *et al.* (1996) reported that high intakes of sucrose in early pregnancy and low intakes of protein in late pregnancy could reduce weight at birth. This effect was very small however, with a maximal change of 217 g in birthweight (average infant weights in the UK are approximately 3500 g). Barker (1994) has stated that a 1 kg reduction in weight at birth is related to an increase in blood pressure of 6 mmHg at age 60. Based on the data of Godfrey *et al.* (1996) the greatest variation in maternal diet in pregnancy will increase later blood pressure by a clinically insignificant 1.3 mmHg.

There is also a lack of evidence to suggest that body proportions at birth are related to maternal nutrient intakes. Examination of maternal diet in early and late gestation revealed that head circumference at birth, ponderal index at birth (a marker of relative thinness) or the ratio of infant weight to placental weight were unrelated to macro- or micronutrient intakes of the mother, after adjustment for socio-economic status and smoking behaviour (Fig. 1.2).

Despite these concerns about the validity of the claim that prenatal undernutrition may programme human disease, there is a strong body of evidence to support the hypothesis. Much of this evidence comes from studies of animals. An ever-increasing body of work shows that exposing the developing rat or sheep fetus to maternal food restriction (global undernutrition), or deficiencies of specific nutrients, results in programmed changes to normal physiology and the initiation of disease processes (Bertram and Hanson, 2001; Langley-Evans, 2001). The time span required to perform adequate studies of human diet in pregnancy in relation to later disease risk largely excludes the possibility of robust epidemiological examination of this issue.

There are, however, two studies that support the concept that maternal undernutrition in pregnant women has consequences for the long-term health of their offspring. Godfrey *et al.* (1994) reported a study of 10–11-year-old Jamaican children whose mothers had undergone nutritional assessment during their pregnancies. Anthropometric markers of undernutrition, including a low triceps skinfold thickness, were found to relate significantly to blood pressure in childhood. It is not clear whether or not these relationships may extend to hypertension and other cardiovascular disease states as the children age. Similarly, the blood pressures of Aberdeen men in their forties could be related to the diets of their mothers, which had been monitored and recorded in some detail by their obstetricians. Here, the consumption of high levels of carbohydrate coupled with low intakes of animal protein during pregnancy appeared predictive of later hypertension in the offspring (Campbell *et al.*, 1996).

It is important to emphasize that although the assertion that undernutrition promotes fetal growth retardation and therefore directly programmes disease risk is plainly incorrect, the direct association between maternal nutritional status and later disease risk has been demonstrated in animal species, and appears to exist

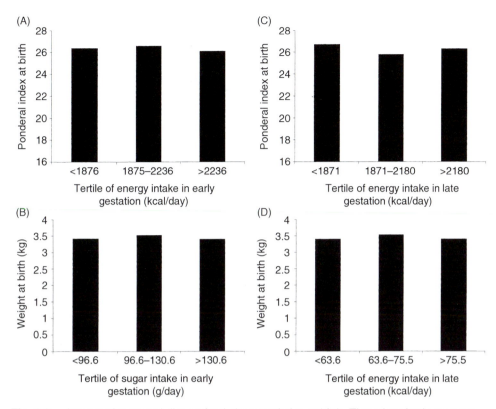

Fig. 1.2. Impact of maternal diet on fetal characteristics at birth. Three hundred pregnant women living in Northampton, UK, had their diets analysed, using 5-day food diaries, between 11 and 15 weeks' gestation (early gestation) and at 32 weeks' gestation (late gestation). Nutrient intakes were used in regression analyses to explore the relationships between fetal characteristics at birth that have been related to later disease risk, and maternal nutritional status. (A) Ponderal index at birth in offspring of women grouped by tertile of energy intake in early gestation. Ponderal index is an index of relative thinness at birth (weight (kg)/length (m)^3). (B) Weight at birth in offspring of women grouped by tertile of sucrose intake in early gestation. (C) Ponderal index at birth in offspring of women grouped by tertile of energy intake in late gestation. (D) Weight at birth in offspring of women grouped by tertile of protein intake in late gestation. None of the relationships were significantly different in univariate analysis or after adjustment for maternal social class, smoking behaviour, height and weight.

independently of changes in fetal growth pattern (Langley-Evans and Nwagwu, 1998). Regarding programmed disease as a consequence of profound fetal injury is overly simplistic, and we should view programming as a subtle and complex metabolic response to nutrient–gene interactions during a period of plasticity. Simple assessments of associations between characteristics at birth that are as crude and multifactorial in origin as birthweight cannot reveal the mechanistic aspects of nutritional programming, or advance our capacity to identify and treat individuals at risk of disease. More robust experimental studies are required.

Environmental agents

In addition to the possibility that marginal intakes of macro- or micronutrients programme the development of the fetus, it is also likely that non-nutrient components of the diet may also exert programming effects. Phyto-oestrogen components of the diet, and oestrogen-like compounds present in the water supply, have been implicated in the aetiology of human reproductive disorders.

Environmental hormone disruptors present in the food chain are substances that lead to endocrine changes in an adult individual or their developing progeny (Toppari and Skakkebaek, 1999). Many of these agents act as hormone agonists, promoting inappropriate stimulation of metabolism, while others have an inhibitory antagonist effect. Examples of the latter would encompass the anti-androgens, which *in utero* would oppose the actions of testosterone and other androgenic hormones that drive the development of the male genitalia and internal reproductive structures. Vinclozolin, a fungicide used in fruit production, is known to have anti-androgenic properties, and studies in rats have shown that prenatal exposure at doses below the legal maximum allowed in human foodstuffs has a pronounced feminizing effect on male pups (Gray *et al.*, 1994). Males exposed to vinclozolin before birth suffered increased prevalence of hypospadias, atrophic sexual organs and even developed vaginal pouches. There is no evidence for these prenatal effects of anti-androgens in humans, but exposures to agents such as vinclozolin are certainly associated with testicular abnormalities in adults (Zober *et al.*, 1995).

Agonists that are associated with reproductive disorders are essentially oestrogen-like compounds. The classical example of this is the drug diethylstilbestrol (DES) which was widely administered to pregnant women between the 1940s and 1970s. DES had adverse effects among exposed male fetuses who developed extensive abnormalities of the exterior and internal reproductive structures. The oestrogen agonist effects of DES on female fetuses were more severe, and the drug promoted vaginal and uterine abnormalities in a high proportion of those exposed in the first 12 weeks of development (Stillman, 1982). At the present time, much of the concern about the impact of oestrogen-like compounds relates to falling male fertility, which has been attributed both to the effects of dietary phyto-oestrogens, and to the appearance of excreted oestrogens (from women using oral contraceptives) entering the water supply (Chapin *et al.*, 1996). Studies of fish caught near sewage outlets have shown increases in the number of intersex individuals, attributed to this contamination (van Aerle *et al.*, 2001).

Although there is no clear evidence that prenatal exposure to endocrine disruptors in humans is related to long-term disorders, there is a suggestive temporal association. Much of our exposure to these agents is related to the use of fertilizers and pesticides in agriculture, the use of oral contraceptives, and the heavy use of plastics in packaging and preparation of food. These exposures increased over the last 50 years of the 20th century and over the same period the incidence of male reproductive disorders such as hypospadia, cryptorchidism and testicular cancers has increased, and average sperm counts have fallen (Auger *et al.*, 1995; Chapin *et al.*, 1996).

Essentially these effects of oestrogen mimics and other endocrine disruptors have a similar impact to the broad array of chemical agents that we regard as teratogens. Teratogens are agents that essentially disrupt the normal processes of tissue differentiation and cause mild–severe organ and tissue malformation. A prime example of this process is the drug thalidomide, which was administered to pregnant women in the 1960s, causing the cessation of limb growth in exposed fetuses (Brent and Holmes, 1988). Perhaps one way of regarding any other programming agent that alters long-term physiology is as a mild teratogen. Many studies have shown that disease processes ascribed to programming are associated with a reduction in the number of functional units within an organ (e.g. kidney and pancreas) and essentially an alteration of organ structure (Snoeck *et al.*, 1990; Langley-Evans *et al.*, 1999).

The putative role of environmental hormone disruptors in determining reproductive abnormalities illustrates the major role of hormone balance and hormone–receptor imbalances in programming of human development and disease. Disruption of the normal androgen or oestrogen environment during critical periods of development has even been invoked as an explanation for variation in human sexual behaviours. The neuroendocrine theory of homosexuality suggests sexual orientation to be influenced by and, in part, determined by exposure of the developing fetus to inappropriate concentrations of androgens (McFadden and Pasanen, 1998). Animal experiments suggest that prenatal exposure to testosterone may determine homosexuality in females, a finding consistent with observations that homosexuality is more prevalent among individuals with congenital adrenal hyperplasia (Ditman *et al.*, 1992).

Hypoxia

Periods of fetal hypoxia may also exert long-term effects upon the developing animal (Moore, 2001). In general the spectrum of effects observed is similar to that noted with nutritional programming. This is in keeping with the viewpoint that much of the programming related to human disease is a response to a signal of physiological stress *in utero*. As described in Chapter 16 of this volume, that signal is likely to be an increase in fetal exposure to the glucocorticoid class of steroid hormones (Langley-Evans, 1997).

Fetal adaptive responses

Programming of the fetus is an adaptive response to the prevailing conditions *in utero*. During programming, the fetus is encountering a hostile environment at a time of maximal vulnerability. In the simplest terms, it must adapt or die. In so far as we view programming as a step towards major disease in adult life, the response to the hostile environment is essentially a maladaption.

This, of course, assumes that the hostile environment that triggered the adaptation is transient and that the conditions encountered in postnatal life are more favourable. Hales has argued that the adaptive responses to undernutrition or other adverse factors during intrauterine life establish a 'thrifty phenotype'

(Hales and Barker, 2001). In the context of the programming of non-insulin-dependent diabetes, for example, a fetus subjected to undernutrition would acquire this thrifty phenotype. Changes in general metabolic activity and, in particular, enhancement of the processing of glucose, enable the fetus to survive the immediate insult. Persistence of these metabolic adaptations to promote thrift, or more efficient use of substrates, is a survival advantage to the individual born into an environment where food is always scarce.

Essentially the thrifty fetus acquires a metabolism that confers a survival advantage by interaction with its mother *in utero*. This advantage increases the probability that the individual will reproduce and, if environmental conditions are unchanged, the next generation may also acquire the metabolic advantage. Over time this will change populations by selecting for individuals whose genes promote an interaction with the environment that manifests as the thrifty phenotype. The population will thus evolve.

The thrifty fetus born into a world of relative plenty, however, is likely to be disadvantaged and to suffer disease due to the enhanced metabolic efficiency. Substrates will be stored readily as excess fat, insulin resistance will develop and the adult will be at high risk for the metabolic syndrome and its related pathologies. This concept is considered in greater detail in Chapter 10 of this book. This maladaptive programming to favour thrifty metabolism can be observed in many populations who undergo a transition from poverty to relative affluence. An example of this is the group of Jewish migrants to Israel from Ethiopia, known as the Falashas (Cohen *et al.*, 1988). This group was moved from a country regularly blighted by famine to an essentially westernized nation. Within 5 years of the migration, rates of non-insulin-dependent diabetes among the Falashas had risen to nearly 18%, which was 30 times greater than the prevalence among Ethiopians living in Ethiopia and twofold greater than in the rest of the Israeli population (Cohen *et al.*, 1988). In the same way, it is believed that the early decades of the 21st century will see an explosion in the prevalence of diabetes and cardiovascular disease on the Indian subcontinent, as the metabolically thrifty population shifts to a more westernized way of living and eating (Robinson, 2001).

Programming and Physiological Function

The concept of functional capacity

All organs and tissues have specialized functions that are reflected by their cellular structures. Within the lung, for example, the alveoli are mainly lined with thin-walled type I epithelial cells that provide a minimal barrier to oxygen diffusion. These cells have low capacity for metabolic functions and are supported by less numerous, but more active, type II epithelial cells, that are larger and less effective facilitators of oxygen exchange. Similarly, the kidney possesses specialized cells that make up the glomeruli and hence the filtration units of the organ. The pancreas contains islets of Langerhans with their specialized β-cells wherein insulin is synthesized.

These various structures, the alveoli, the glomeruli and the islets, with their specialized cell types are responsible for functions that cannot be duplicated by other components. Thus the number of alveoli present in the lung or the number of islets in the pancreas will determine the ability of the organs to function (i.e. perform gaseous exchange, or regulate glucose handling). Each organ thus has a maximum capacity to perform a function, which is determined by the type and number of cells or functional structures that are present. This can be described as a functional capacity.

Figure 1.3 is a schematic representation of how functional capacity varies across the life span. For the majority of organs, a high percentage of the maximal functional capacity is established before birth and the capacity continues to increase to some extent during childhood. The human lung, for example, continues to undergo cell division and lay down new alveoli until the age of 8 years. In the case of some organs, such as the kidney, functional capacity is not increased at all after birth. For some systems there is an extended period of increase postnatally. The deposition of mineral in bone, which is a primary determinant of the ability of bone to perform its function, continues into the third decade of life.

Once maximal functional capacity is achieved, a period of stability will follow, but this may be short-lived and all systems will decline as we age. In the case of the kidney, the functional units are irreplaceable fragile structures and episodes of hypertension, exposure to toxins or hyperglycaemia may all cause loss. Eventually in adult life the functional capacity of an organ may fall below the minimum level that is necessary to maintain healthy function, and disease processes will ensue.

This view of functional capacity may be helpful in considering the role of programming in determining human disease risk. Risk may be increased by an accelerated decline in functional capacity during adult life, and reduced by

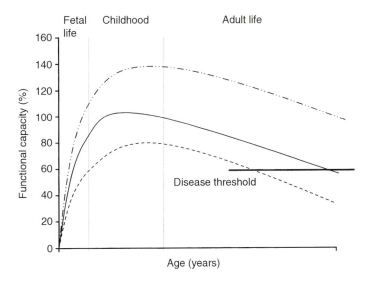

Fig. 1.3. The concept of functional capacity.

factors that slow the rate of decline. Programming factors, however, may modify the attainment of the maximal capacity. For example, the feeding of a restricted diet in pregnancy is known to reduce the number of nephrons present in the rat kidney at birth (Langley-Evans et al., 1999). This reduction of maximal capacity is then associated with an accelerated progression to renal dysfunction (Nwagwu et al., 2000; Marchand et al., 2002). Where programming factors lower the maximal functional capacity, the disease threshold will be achieved sooner (lower line in Fig. 1.3) than would normally be expected (middle line in Fig. 1.3). Conversely, prenatal factors or influences in infancy that have the effect of increasing the maximal functional capacity attained will delay the decline towards the disease threshold and healthy physiological function will be maintained until later in life (upper line in Fig. 1.3).

Programming at the cellular level

The details of the specific mechanisms that underpin the fetal programming of human disease states are likely to be complex and, at the present time, are poorly understood. It is highly likely, however, that the process of programming will follow relatively simple, general principles that involve adaptive changes to either cell numbers, cell types or cellular signalling and responses.

Programmed changes in cell number would be consistent with the concept of programmed changes to functional capacity outlined above. A tissue with fewer cells capable of meeting a specialized function will, by definition, struggle to maintain that function. A clear example of this would be the reduction in pancreatic β-cell numbers that is observed following nutrient restriction during rat pregnancy and lactation (Snoeck et al., 1990), leading to impaired insulin responses to glucose. This mode of programming exemplifies the simplest route through which early insults may establish permanent physiological changes that predispose to disease.

Modification of the array of cell types present within an organ will also modify functional capacity. This is illustrated by the kidneys of rats exposed to maternal undernutrition in fetal life. These animals have kidneys that are of similar overall size to those of animals exposed to a nutritionally adequate diet in utero. However, the total nephron number is significantly reduced (see Chapter 11, this volume). The maintenance of normal tissue mass in the face of a 30% reduction in the number of functional units suggests that the nutritional insult has promoted the development of early cell lines that play no role in the construction of nephrons (Marchand and Langley-Evans, 2001). This model of programming has been compared to the clonal selection of B lymphocyte lines in the maturation of the immune system (Lucas, 1991). The developing embryo consists of many precursor cells with the capacity to follow particular fates, and the imposition of stimuli or insults during critical developmental windows may promote certain lines over others. Kwong et al. (2000) have demonstrated that, in the early rat embryo subjected to protein restriction, there is evidence of an imbalance of cell numbers between the inner cell mass and trophectoderm, which is consistent with this 'clonal selection' viewpoint.

The healthy functioning of organs and tissues depends upon homeostatic mechanisms that are regulated via nervous and hormonal sensing and signalling. These are processes that will be influenced both by changes in the overall number and type of cells that are present within a mature system. It is also possible for programming to exert influences upon these processes through more subtle transformations of cellular functioning. As described earlier in this chapter, in the context of environmental endocrine disruptors, prenatal exposures to hormones and related agents at inappropriate concentrations or inappropriate times during development may have a huge impact upon developing organs and systems. These changes in cell function may be mediated through increases or decreases in concentrations in hormones that are normally present during intrauterine development, through exposure to hormones of either fetal or maternal origin at stages of development when they should not normally be present, or through up-regulation of the expression of hormone receptors, which will effectively increase the biological effect of the prevailing hormone concentration.

The endpoint of all these endocrine shifts will be changes in the expression of a broad range of fetal genes. Even if these changes are short lived, it is likely that the impact of the change in the usual developmental sequence or pattern of gene switching on or off will be profound. There is also considerable interest in whether gene expression could be permanently disturbed and hence exert changes in normal metabolism and cell signalling throughout life. There is a growing body of evidence from animal studies to suggest that this is the case and, in particular, expression of receptors for key hormones appears to be permanently up-regulated by periods of prenatal undernutrition (Bertram *et al.*, 2001; Sahajpal and Ashton, 2003).

Susceptible tissues, targets for programming

In earlier sections of this chapter a number of tissues and organs have been indicated as vulnerable targets for programming. There is very strong evidence, from both animals and humans, that when the fetus is subject to an insult *in utero* the kidneys and the pancreas undergo structural adaptations that result in a predisposition to later disease (Snoeck *et al.*, 1990; Dahri *et al.*, 1991; Hinchcliffe *et al.*, 1992; Langley-Evans *et al.*, 1999; Manalich *et al.*, 2000). As work in this area considers a greater breadth of systems, it is becoming clear that all tissues are programmable by virtue of their plasticity during development. Whenever tissues undergo phases of rapid cell division to increase in size, or undergo phases of differentiation that determine the profile of cells present in the mature structure, then they will be vulnerable to any adverse exposure.

Evidence is available to show that the development of all the major organs can be disturbed by nutritional factors, stress hormones or other factors in fetal life. In the brain, the number of neurons present, and presumably the linkages they form, in early life is perturbed by fluctuations in maternal nutrient intake in pregnancy (Plagemann *et al.*, 2000). Similarly, the functional capacity of the human lung seems to be related to programming influences (Barker *et al.*, 1991), and the structure and compliance of the arteries may be affected likewise (Martyn and Greenwald, 2001). The fetal rat liver alters the zonation of metabolism between different regions following exposure to maternal undernutrition (Ozanne and Hales, 1999). In both animals and humans, it appears that there are complex interactions between genetics, diet in postnatal life and programming factors, in determining later bone mineral content and osteoporotic fracture risk (Gale *et al.*, 2001; Mehta *et al.*, 2002). Although yet to be convincingly demonstrated, it is expected that the gastrointestinal tract, the reproductive organs, adipose tissue and muscle will exhibit the same range of developmental sensitivities.

Contribution to disease risk

The concept set out in this chapter is shown schematically in Fig. 1.4. Essentially, the way in which we have traditionally viewed risk of non-infectious disease has been transformed by the addition of programming influences to the equation. If we regard disease risk within a population as being normally distributed, then most people will, by definition, carry a near-average risk, with lesser proportions having either significantly lower than average, or significantly higher than average risk. Until relatively recently it had been believed that each individual's risk was determined by a genetic component modified by the interaction with adult environment. The latter comprises lifestyle factors such as diet, smoking

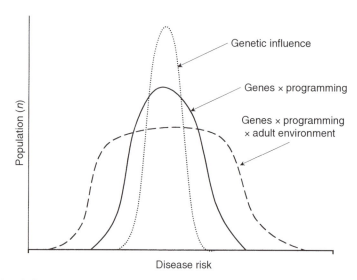

Fig. 1.4. Influences upon disease risk. If we assume that the prevalence of risk factors for any non-communicable disease are normally distributed in a population, the overall distribution will be a compound determined by the interaction between genes, programming influences and adult environmental factors.

habit, alcohol consumption and physical activity levels, of which diet may be the most important. We can now factor in prenatal factors, or a programmed risk component, to produce the overall distribution of risk in the population. Thus those at lowest risk may be those with genetic protection against disease coupled to ideal conditions during development and a healthy adult lifestyle. Those at greatest risk will combine a genetic predisposition to disease with adverse conditions in fetal life and a poor adult diet and sedentary lifestyle. The individual's response to components of the adult diet is thus determined by much more than immediate nutrient–gene inter-actions, and represents a programming–nutrient–gene triad of interactions (Fig. 1.5).

The overall impact of each of the three contributions to total risk is difficult to estimate and generalizations are impossible. Obviously, there are numerous examples of catastrophic single-gene defects that have an effect that overrides the contribution of both programming and adult lifestyle. However, it is evident that programming stimuli might also have the capacity to override the influence of genes. Studies of the spontaneously hypertensive rat, which carries a genetic predisposition to high blood pressure, indicate that cross-fostering to a normotensive mother can prevent the development of the adult hypertensive syndrome (Cierpial and McCarty, 1991). This appears to be a postnatal programming of blood pressure control systems attributable to either diet in lactation or behavioural stimuli (Cierpial and McCarty, 1987). It is also obvious that adult lifestyle factors leading to obesity will have profound effects on health and disease risk that can overcome both genetic and programming influences.

Evidence that Programming is a Determinant of Human Disease Risk

Work by other authors in this book will deal with the detailed evidence that programming during fetal and/or neonatal life contributes to an individual's, or population's, risk for major non-communicable diseases. In brief, however, the now very large body of evidence may be summarized under two headings:

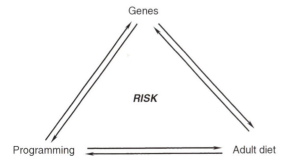

Fig. 1.5. Programming and the determination of disease risk.

Epidemiological studies

The springboard for current investigations into the fetal programming of adult disease came from ecological and cohort studies that reported associations between, first, high infant mortality rates and, secondly, low weight at birth and later cardiovascular disease (Barker *et al.*, 1993; Barker, 1994). Over the past decade a significant body of epidemiological evidence has been obtained suggesting that the environment encountered in fetal life determines risk of major disease in adulthood. Individuals of low weight at birth have up to twofold greater risk of coronary heart disease and up to eightfold greater risk of diabetes later in life (see Chapters 4 and 7, this volume). Similarly, variations in proportions at birth appear predictive of later disease. Diabetes, hypertension and coronary heart disease associate with thinness at birth. Hypertension and atopic conditions are predicted by shortness in relation to head circumference (Barker, 1994).

Studies of young adult men exposed to intrauterine famine during the Dutch Hunger Winter of 1944 indicate that obesity may also be determined, in part, through nutritional programming (Ravelli *et al.*, 1976; see also Chapter 9, this volume). Men who were exposed to maternal undernutrition in early to mid-gestation were twice as likely to become obese by the age of 19 than men born after the famine. Men who were exposed to fetal undernutrition in late gestation had a lower risk of obesity. Similarly, Law *et al.* (1992) noted that waist–hip ratio, an indicator of how body fat is distributed, was negatively related to weight at birth. This suggests that abdominal fatness is programmed before birth. This has enormous consequences in terms of risk of developing the metabolic syndrome and its associated disease sequelae.

Experimental studies

The hypothesis is that maternal nutrition during pregnancy is the main factor responsible for this programming of adult disease. The time span between fetal exposure to nutritional deficits and adult disease endpoints, and the difficulties of reliably studying the nutritional status of free-living individuals, preclude the completion of adequate epidemiological studies to properly evaluate the existence and nature of programming influences upon human health. Although very robust meta-analyses have cast some doubt on the validity of the association between birthweight and human disease endpoints (Huxley *et al.*, 2002; see also Chapter 5, this volume), a large number of animal models have demonstrated that exposure to even relatively mild restriction of specific nutrients in the maternal diet can exert important long-term effects upon cardiovascular (Chapter 6, this volume) and renal (Chapter 11, this volume) health, upon body composition and obesity (Chapter 10, this volume) and upon glucose metabolism (Chapter 8, this volume). Studies of this nature allow for invasive measurements and are now being used to evaluate the role of nutrient–gene interactions and materno-fetal endocrine signalling in the programming of physiological function and disease processes.

References

Antonov, A.N. (1947) Children born during the siege of Leningrad in 1942. *Journal of Pediatrics* 30, 250–259.

Auger, J.R., Kuntsmann, J.M., Cyglik, F. and Jouannet, P. (1995) Decline in semen quality among fertile men in Paris during the past 20 years. *New England Journal of Medicine* 332, 281–285.

Barker, D.J.P. (1994) *Mothers, Babies and Disease in Later Life*. BMJ Publishing Group, London.

Barker, D.J.P., Godfrey, K.M., Fall, C., Osmond, C., Winter, P.D. and Shaheen, S.O. (1991) Relation of birthweight and childhood respiratory infection to adult lung-function and death from chronic obstructive airways disease. *British Medical Journal* 303, 671–675.

Barker, D.J.P., Gluckman, P.D., Godfrey, K.M., Harding, J.E., Owens, J.A. and Robinson, J.S. (1993) Fetal nutrition and cardiovascular disease in adult life. *Lancet* 341, 938–941.

Barraclough, C.A. (1961) Production of anovulatory, sterile rats by single injections of testosterone proprionate. *Endocrinology* 68, 62–67.

Beach, R.S., Gershwin, M.E. and Hurley, L.S. (1982) Gestational zinc deprivation in mice: persistence of immunodeficiency for three generations. *Science* 218, 469–471.

Bertram, C.E. and Hanson, M.A. (2001) Animal models and programming of the metabolic syndrome. *British Medical Bulletin* 60, 103–121.

Bertram, C., Trowern, A.R., Copin, N., Jackson, A.A. and Whorwood, C.B. (2001) The maternal diet during pregnancy programs altered expression of the glucocorticoid receptor and type 2 11 beta-hydroxysteroid dehydrogenase: Potential molecular mechanisms underlying the programming of hypertension *in utero*. *Endocrinology* 142, 2841–2853.

Brent, R.L. and Holmes, L.B. (1988) Clinical and basic science lessons from the thalidomide tragedy – what have we learned about the causes of limb defects? *Teratology* 38, 241–251.

Campbell, D.M. (1991) Maternal and fetal nutrition. In: McClaren, D.S. *et al.* (eds) *Textbook of Paediatric Nutrition*. Churchill Livingstone, London, pp. 3–20.

Campbell, D.M., Hall, M.H., Barker, D.J.P., Cross, J., Shiell, A.W. and Godfrey, K.M. (1996) Diet in pregnancy and the offspring's blood pressure 40 years later. *British Journal of Obstetrics and Gynaecology* 103, 273–280.

Chapin, R.E., Stevens, J.T., Hughes, C.L., Kelce, W.R., Hess, R.A. and Daston, G.P. (1996) Endocrine modulation of reproduction. *Fundamental and Applied Toxicology* 29, 1–17.

Cierpial, M.A. and McCarty, R.A. (1987) Preweaning behavioural development in spontaneously hypertensive, borderline hypertensive and Wistar–Kyoto normotensive rats. *Developmental Psychobiology* 20, 57–69.

Cierpial, M.A. and McCarty, R.A. (1991) Adult blood pressure reduction in spontaneously hypertensive rats reared by normotensive Sprague–Dawley mothers. *Behavioral and Neural Biology* 56, 262–270.

Cohen, M.P., Stern, E., Rusecki, Y. and Ziedler, A. (1988) The high prevalence of diabetes in young Ethiopian migrants to Israel. *Diabetes* 37, 824–828.

Dahri, S., Snoeck, A., Reusens-Billen, B., Remacle, C. and Hoet, J.J. (1991) Islet function in offspring of mothers on low protein diet during gestation. *Diabetes* 40, 115–120.

Deeming, D.C. and Ferguson, M.W.J. (1989) The mechanism of temperature dependent sex determination in crocodilians: a hypothesis. *American Zoologist* 29, 973–985.

Ditman, R.W., Kappes, M.E. and Kappes, M.H. (1992) Sexual behaviour in adolescent and adult females with congenital adrenal hyperplasia. *Psychoneuroendocrinology* 17, 153–170.

Doyle, W., Wynn, A.H.A., Crawford, M.A. and Wynn, S.W. (1992) Nutritional counselling and supplementation in the second and third trimester of pregnancy: a study in a London population. *Journal of Nutrition and Medicine* 3, 249–256.

Forsdahl, S. (1967) Are poor living conditions in childhood and adolescence an important risk factor for arteriosclerotic heart disease? *British Journal of Preventative and Social Medicine* 31, 91–95.

Gale, C.R., Martyn, C.N., Kellingray, S., Eastell, R. and Cooper, C. (2001) Intrauterine programming of adult body composition. *Journal of Clinical Endocrinology and Metabolism* 86, 267–272.

Godfrey, K.M., Forrester, T., Barker, D.J.P., Jackson, A.A., Landman, J.P., Hall, J.St E., Cox, V. and Osmond, C. (1994) The relation of maternal nutritional status during pregnancy to blood pressure in childhood. *British Journal of Obstetrics and Gynaecology* 101, 398–403.

Godfrey, K.M., Robinson, S., Barker, D.J.P., Osmond, C. and Cox, V. (1996) Maternal nutrition in early and late pregnancy in relation to placental and fetal growth. *British Medical Journal* 312, 410–414.

Gray, L.E., Ostby, J.S. and Kelce, W.R. (1994) Developmental effects of an environmental antiandrogen: the fungicide vinclozolin alters sexual differentiation in the male rat. *Toxicology and Applied Pharmacology* 129, 46–52.

Hales, C.N. and Barker, D.J.P. (2001) The thrifty phenotype hypothesis. *British Medical Bulletin* 60, 5–20.

Harding, J., Liu, L., Evans, P., Oliver, M. and Gluckman, P. (1992) Intrauterine feeding of the growth retarded fetus – can we help? *Early Human Development* 29, 193–197.

Hastings-Roberts, M.M. and Zeman, F.J. (1977) Effects of protein deficiency, pair-feeding, or diet supplementation on maternal, fetal and placental growth in rats. *Journal of Nutrition* 107, 973–982.

Hinchcliffe, S.A., Lynch, M.R.J., Sargent, P.H., Howard, C.V. and van Zelzen, D. (1992) The effect of intrauterine growth retardation on the development of renal nephrons. *British Journal of Obstetrics and Gynaecology* 99, 296–301.

Humphreys, J. (1996) Lamarck and the general theory of evolution. *Journal of Biological Education* 30, 295–303.

Huxley, R., Neil, A. and Collins, R. (2002) Unravelling the fetal origins hypothesis: is there really an inverse association between birth weight and subsequent blood pressure? *Lancet* 360, 659–665.

Ito, S., Murakami, S., Yamamouchi, K. and Arai, Y. (1986) Perinatal androgen exposure decreases the size of the sexually dimorphic preoptic nucleus in the rat. *Proceedings of the Japanese Academy Series B* 62, 408–411.

Jennings, B.J., Ozanne, S.E. and Hales, C.N. (2000) Nutrition, oxidative damage, telomere shortening and cellular senescence: individual or connected agents of aging? *Molecular Genetics and Metabolism* 71, 32–42.

Kwong, W.Y., Wild, A.E., Roberts, P., Willis, A.C. and Fleming, T.P. (2000) Maternal undernutrition during the preimplantation period of rat development causes blastocyst abnormalities and programming of postnatal hypertension. *Development* 127, 4195–4202.

Langley-Evans, S.C. (1997) Intrauterine programming of hypertension by glucocorticoids. *Life Science* 60, 1213–1221.

Langley-Evans, S.C. (2001) Fetal programming of cardiovascular function through exposure to maternal undernutrition. *Proceedings of the Nutrition Society* 60, 505–513.

Langley-Evans, S.C. and Nwagwu, M. (1998) Impaired growth and increased activities of glucocorticoid sensitive enzyme activities in tissues of rat fetuses exposed to maternal low protein diets. *Life Science* 63, 605–615.

Langley-Evans, S.C., Welham, S.J.M. and Jackson, A.A. (1999) Fetal exposure to a maternal low protein diet impairs nephrogenesis and promotes hypertension in the rat. *Life Sciences* 64, 965–974

Law, C.M., Barker, D.J.P., Osmond, C., Fall, C.H.D. and Simmonds, S.J. (1992) Early growth and abdominal fatness in adult life. *Journal of Epidemiology and Community Health* 46, 184–186.

Lorenz, K. (1952) *King Solomons Ring*. Cromwell, New York.

Lucas, A. (1991) Programming by early nutrition in man. In: Bock, G.R. and Whelan, J. (eds) *The Childhood Environment and Adult Disease*. John Wiley & Sons, Chichester, UK, pp. 38–55.

Manalich, R., Reye, L., Herrera, M., Melendi, C. and Fundora, I. (2000) Relationship between weight at birth and the number and size of renal glomeruli in humans: a histomorphometric study. *Kidney International* 58, 770–773.

Marchand, M.C. and Langley-Evans, S.C. (2001) Intrauterine programming of nephron number: the fetal flaw revisited. *Journal of Nephrology* 14, 327–331.

Marchand, M.C., Dunn, R., Aihie-Sayer, A., Cooper, C. and Langley-Evans, S.C. (2002) Evidence of increased age-related renal injury in rats exposed to maternal low protein diets *in utero*. *Proceedings of the Nutrition Society* 61, 131A.

Martyn, C.N. and Greenwald, S.E. (2001) A hypothesis about a mechanism for the programming of blood pressure and vascular disease in early life. *Clinical and Experimental Pharmacology and Physiology* 28, 948–951.

Mathews, F., Yudkin, P. and Neil, A. (1999) Influence of maternal nutrition on outcome of pregnancy: prospective cohort study. *British Medical Journal* 319, 339–343.

McFadden, D. and Pasanen, E. (1998) Comparisons of the auditory systems of heterosexuals: click evoked otoacoustic emissions. *Proceedings of the National Academy of Sciences* 95, 2709–2713.

Mehta, G., Roach, H.I., Langley-Evans, S.C., Reading, I., Oreffo, R.O.C., Aihie-Sayer, A., Clarke, A.M.P. and Cooper, C. (2002) Intrauterine exposure to a maternal low protein diet reduces adult bone mass and alters growth plate morphology. *Calcified Tissue International* 71, 493–498.

Moore, L.G. (2001) Human genetic adaptation to high altitude. *High Altitude Medicine and Biology* 2, 257–279.

Nwagwu, M.O., Cook, A. and Langley-Evans, S.C. (2000) Evidence of progressive deterioration of renal function in rats exposed to a maternal low protein diet *in utero*. *British Journal of Nutrition* 83, 79–85.

Ozanne, S.E. and Hales, C.N. (1999) The long-term consequences of intra-uterine protein malnutrition for glucose metabolism. *Proceedings of the Nutrition Society* 58, 615–619.

Plagemann, A., Harder, T., Rake, A., Melchior, K., Rohde, W. and Dorner, G. (2000) Hypothalamic nuclei are malformed in weanling offspring of low protein malnourished rat dams. *Journal of Nutrition* 130, 2582–2589.

Prentice, A.M., Cole, T.J., Foord, F.A., Lamb, W.H. and Whitehead, R.G. (1987) Increased birthweight after prenatal dietary supplementation of rural African women. *American Journal of Clinical Nutrition* 46, 912–925.

Ravelli, G., Stein, Z. and Susser, M.W. (1976) Obesity in young men after famine exposure in utero and in early infancy. *New England Journal of Medicine* 295, 349–353.

Robinson, R. (2001) The fetal origins of adult disease – no longer just a hypothesis and may be critically important in South Asia. *British Medical Journal* 322, 375–376.

Rose, G. (1964) Familial patterns in ischaemic heart disease. *British Journal of Preventative and Social Medicine* 18, 75–80.

Sahajpal, V. and Ashton, N. (2003) Renal function and AT_1 receptor expression in young rats following intrauterine exposure to a maternal low protein diet. *Clinical Science* 104, 607–614.

Snoeck, A., Remacle, C., Reussens, B. and Hoet, J.J. (1990) Effect of a low protein diet during pregnancy on the fetal rat endocrine pancreas. *Biology of the Neonate* 57, 107–118.

Stillman, R.J. (1982) *In utero* exposure to diethylstilbestrol: adverse effects on the reproductive tract and reproductive performance in male and female offspring. *American Journal of Obstetrics and Gynecology* 142, 905–921.

Toppari, J. and Skakkebaek, N.E. (1999) Environmental hormone disruptors and their potential impact during development. In: O'Brien, P.M.S., Wheeler, T. and Barker, D.J.P. (eds) *Fetal Programming: Influences on Development of Disease in Later Life.* RCOG Press, London, pp. 195–204.

van Aerle, R., Nolan, M., Jobling, S., Christiansen, L.B., Sumpter, J.P. and Tyler, C.R. (2001) Sexual disruption in a second species of wild cyprinid fish (the gudgeon, *Gobio gobio*) in United Kingdom freshwaters. *Environmental Toxicology and Chemistry* 20, 2841–2847.

Wallace, J.M., Bourke, D.A. and Aitken, R.P. (1999) Nutrition and fetal growth: paradoxical effects in the overnourished adolescent sheep. *Journal of Reproduction and Fertility* 54 (suppl.), 385–399.

Widdowson, E.M. (1971) Intra-uterine growth retardation in the pig. *Biology of the Neonate* 19, 329–340.

Zober, A., Hoffman, G. and Ott, M.G. (1995) Study of morbidity of personnel with potential exposure to vinclozolin. *Occupational Environmental Medicine* 52, 233–241.

2 Nutritional Basis for the Fetal Origins of Adult Disease

JANE HARDING

University of Auckland, Private Bag 92019, Auckland, New Zealand

Introduction

The existence of a relationship between size at birth and disease risk in later life is now widely accepted. Babies with reduced birthweight have an increased risk of coronary heart disease, non-insulin-dependent diabetes and stroke, and also of their risk factors, hypertension, dyslipidaemia and impaired glucose tolerance (Barker, 1998). These relationships are seen across the birthweight range and across many different populations (Huxley *et al.*, 2000).

The biological basis of these relationships has been attributed to programming. This term, although widely and often inappropriately used, refers to a well-established biological phenomenon whereby an insult or stimulus at a critical period of development results in permanent changes in structure or function. There are many common and classical examples of this biological phenomenon (see Chapter 1, this volume). Since all of these examples involve stimuli or insults during early development, the programming phenomenon as the basis of the relationship between size at birth and later disease risk is both biologically plausible and compatible with the epidemiological observations. This is not to say, however, that small size at birth is critical to the relationship between a programming insult and postnatal disease risk. As will be discussed in more detail below, it is at least as feasible, and in fact perhaps more likely, that programming phenomena acting during fetal life may alter both size at birth and postnatal disease risk through parallel but non-causal pathway mechanisms.

In the field of the fetal origins of adult disease, the question then arises as to the nature of the key programming stimuli. A number of programming stimuli have been proposed, and perhaps the most substantial body of experimental data supports that of prenatal glucocorticoid exposure (Seckl, 2001). This will be discussed elsewhere in this book (Chapter 16). The proposal to be discussed in this chapter is that nutrition is also a key programming stimulus in fetal life. While other chapters will address various aspects of nutrition in detail, the aim of this chapter is to provide an overview of some principles that might be helpful in understanding the relationships between nutrition, size at birth and later disease risk.

Nutrition as a Programming Stimulus

Limitation of nutrient supply to the growing fetus was proposed as a key programming stimulus very early in the story of the fetal origins hypothesis (Barker, 1992). This proposal was later modified to suggest that the programming stimulus arose when nutritional supply to the fetus was inadequate for fetal demand (Barker, 1998). This minor modification took into account some of the more confusing aspects of the epidemiological and physiological observations, as discussed below. However, despite many apparently contradictory studies, the hypothesis that nutrition can be a programming stimulus, and indeed perhaps may be the major programming stimulus, arises largely from three lines of evidence as described in the following sections.

Animal studies

From the time of the first reported epidemiological observations of a relationship between size at birth and later disease risk, growth physiologists have attempted to reproduce such observations in experimental animals. Small size at birth can be induced in a number of ways in experimental animals, but most easily and simply by inducing varying degrees of maternal undernutrition. From the first, therefore, maternal undernutrition was in widespread use in animal experiments investigating the effects of reduced birth size on postnatal physiology. Such experiments rapidly bore fruit, with the demonstration that lowering the protein content of the diet in pregnant rats resulted not only in reduced birthweight but also in increased blood pressure (Langley and Jackson, 1994) and impaired glucose tolerance (Desai et al., 1995) in their adult offspring. Such experiments were readily replicated, showed a dose–response effect, and rapidly convinced many doubters that such an apparently implausible relationship as that reported between birthweight and postnatal disease risk in humans may indeed have a biological basis.

Similar experiments have now been undertaken in guinea-pigs (Persson and Jansson, 1992; Kind et al., 2003) and sheep (Hoet and Hanson, 1999; Oliver et al., 2001a,b, 2002). Thus there can be no doubt that, in a number of animal species, restriction of maternal nutrition can lead both to reduced size at birth and also to permanent changes in postnatal physiology. Hence there is clear experimental evidence for the hypothesis that nutrition may be a key programming stimulus.

Human evidence

Clear-cut data on the relationship between maternal nutrition during pregnancy, size at birth and postnatal disease risk are extremely difficult to obtain for human populations. Some of these difficulties are discussed below. However, there are some limited data that are becoming increasingly convincing. The first are those related to the outcome of the Dutch Hunger Winter. This involved a 5-month period at the end of the Second World War, when a part of the previously well-nourished population of The Netherlands was exposed to severe famine. Since the famine was of limited duration and abrupt in both onset and relief, it has been possible, by following up the infants born to women exposed to the famine, to determine the relationship between maternal famine exposure, size at birth and later disease risk. These studies are ongoing, but those completed to date have shown that severe maternal famine can result in altered postnatal disease risk in the offspring. Babies exposed to famine at different times during gestation had altered birthweight (Lumey *et al.*, 1993) and, as adults, had an increased risk of glucose intolerance (A.C. Ravelli *et al.*, 1998), obesity (G.-P. Ravelli *et al.*, 1976; A.C. Ravelli *et al.*, 1999), an atherogenic lipid profile (Roseboom *et al.*, 2000a), altered coagulation profile (Roseboom *et al.*, 2000b) and perhaps increased risk of coronary heart disease (Roseboom *et al.*, 2000c). Interestingly, these relationships were not confined to famine exposure in late gestation, nor were they confined to babies of lower birthweight. The issues of the timing of the undernutrition and of the dissociation from effects on birth-weight will be discussed later. Suffice it to say for now that these pseudo-experiments as the result of the atrocities of war have provided perhaps the best evidence to date that maternal undernutrition may function as a programming stimulus for postnatal disease risk in humans.

Biological plausibility

The third line of evidence supporting the hypothesis that nutrition can be a key programming stimulus arises essentially from its biological plausibility. It has been estimated that only perhaps 15% of variation in birthweight in humans may be due to genetic influences (Polani, 1974) while the majority is related to aspects of maternal size and body composition. Early cross-breeding experiments between large and small parents of the same species confirmed the importance of maternal size rather than genetic origin in determining size at birth (Walton and Hammond, 1938). Such experiments have been replicated in many species and by embryo transplant experiments to exclude parent-of-origin effects (Snow, 1989; Allen *et al.*, 2002). In human pregnancy after assisted fertilization techniques, size at birth is also related to the size of the host mother rather than that of the egg donor (Brooks *et al.*, 1995), again confirming the critical role of the mother in the regulation of fetal growth.

This normal limitation of fetal growth in late gestation, such that size at birth is related to maternal phenotype, reflects a phenomenon called maternal constraint. Maternal constraint reflects the limitation imposed by capacity of the mother to supply nutrients to her fetus. The major regulator of fetal growth in the late gestation mammalian fetus is thus nutrient supply. Since nutrient supply is the major regulator of size at birth, and size at birth relates to postnatal growth and function, there is clear plausibility for the thesis that nutrition before birth is a key programming stimulus.

Some of the experimental details lying behind this apparently straight-forward thesis are now discussed in more detail.

Nutritional Regulation of Fetal Growth

Fetal growth is regulated in a fundamentally different way from postnatal growth (Table 2.1). In postnatal life, growth is largely regulated by the child's genetic heritage, with the best predictor in childhood of ultimate adult height being mid-parental height. Provided minimal nutritional and emotional requirements are met, this genetic determination of fetal growth is mediated via the child's endocrine status, most notably that of the somatotrophic (growth hormone (GH)/insulin-like growth factor (IGF)) axis. However, in fetal life, genetics are thought to contribute only a small amount to regulation of fetal growth. Fetal nutrition appears to be the major regulator of fetal growth, and fetal endocrine status, particularly that of the insulin and the somatotrophic axes, primarily mediates the effects of nutrition rather than the effects of genetic heritage.

Nutrition of the fetus

Despite extensive data in experimental animals showing that maternal undernutrition results in reduced size at birth, it has been widely believed that maternal nutrition has little effect on the growth of the baby in human pregnancy. Nevertheless there is clear evidence that women with chronic under-nutrition have an increased risk of having small babies (Kramer, 1987). It has

Table 2.1. Differences between the major regulators of growth before and after birth.

	Fetal growth	Postnatal growth
	Normally constrained by maternal factors	Normally to genetic potential
Genetic influences	Small	Dominant
Nutrition	Limited especially in late gestation	Permissive
	May be limited by placental function	
Endocrine regulation		
Growth hormone (GH)	Minimal effect	Dominant
IGF-1	Important, regulated by nutrition	Important, regulated by GH
Insulin	Important, regulated by nutrition	Permissive, regulated by nutrition

IGF-I, insulin-like growth factor-I.

also been shown that in an apparently well-nourished developed population, as many of 32% mothers delivering otherwise unexplained small-for-gestational-age babies have evidence of an eating disorder before and/or during pregnancy (Conti *et al.*, 1998). Thus even in generally well-nourished populations, overall maternal nutrient intake can influence the size of the baby.

The most clear-cut evidence of the effects of severe maternal undernutrition only during pregnancy, as opposed to before as well as during pregnancy, derives from the studies of the Dutch famine. These studies show that in a previously well-nourished population, severe famine in late gestation results in a decrease in mean birthweight (Lumey *et al.*, 1993).

In contrast, numerous clinical trials of nutritional supplementation during pregnancy in women with varying degrees of chronic malnutrition have resulted in only very small changes in birthweight (weighted mean difference +25 g). This is the case even in those populations most likely to benefit, i.e. chronically undernourished women receiving balanced protein calorie supplementation (weighted mean difference +24 g) (Kramer, 2002a). However, the risk of giving birth to an infant that is small for gestational age is substantially reduced in these studies (odds ratio 0.64, 95% confidence intervals 0.53–0.78) (Kramer, 2002a), suggesting that some babies may benefit much more than others from maternal supplementation. How might these findings be compatible with the earlier assertion that nutrition is the major regulator of fetal growth in late gestation?

Perhaps the most critical point is the recognition of the distinction between maternal nutrition and fetal nutrition. The fetus lives at the end of a long 'supply line', whereby the supply of nutrients to the fetus, rather than to the mother, determines fetal growth (Fig. 2.1). Thus the nutrients available to the fetus depend not only on maternal dietary intake but also on her metabolic and endocrine profile regulating the circulating nutrients in her blood which are potentially available to the fetus. These nutrients are then transported to the placenta, determined in part by the uterine blood flow, and across the placenta, regulated in part by placental size and function (see below). Finally, nutrients are taken up into the fetus, regulated by both umbilical blood flow and by fetal endocrine status.

This whole series of coordinated and interconnected steps contributes to the potentially large differences between maternal nutrition and fetal nutrition. Many common causes of impaired fetal growth in developed communities act by impairing various steps along the fetal supply line. Thus fetal nutrition, and

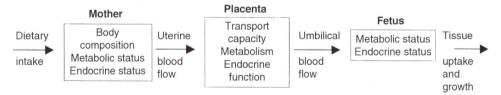

Fig. 2.1. The fetal supply line. Multiple factors at each step along the supply line will determine the ultimate effect of any change in maternal nutrition on fetal nutrition and hence on fetal growth.

hence fetal growth, can be severely impaired if uterine blood flow is reduced, such as by maternal pre-eclampsia, despite good levels of maternal nutrient intake. Similarly, quite marked limitation of maternal nutrient intake may have little effect on fetal nutrition, and hence on fetal growth, if the maternal endocrine status, blood flow and placental transfer capacity combine to provide a very efficient supply of these nutrients to the fetus.

The mechanisms by which fetal nutrition, in turn, regulates fetal growth are multiple and are touched on here only briefly. First, nutrition may regulate the function of the supply line, and particularly placental structure and function (see below). Secondly, the major endocrine and paracrine regulators of growth in the fetus are themselves regulated by fetal nutrition. Fetal growth can be seen as mediated by the balance of the major anabolic and catabolic hormones in the fetus (Table 2.2). The major anabolic hormones, particularly insulin and the IGFs, stimulate the uptake of glucose and amino acids into fetal tissues (Fowden and Hay, 1988; Harding *et al.*, 1994; Liu *et al.*, 1994), while thyroid hormones regulate oxygen uptake (Fowden and Silver, 1995). However, increased supplies of these hormones, provided experimentally in the absence of increased nutrient supply, do not result in increased overall growth of the fetus (Fowden *et al.*, 1989; Lok *et al.*, 1996). Rather, the levels of these hormones are themselves regulated by nutrient supply, and particularly that of glucose, amino acids and oxygen (Oliver *et al.*, 1993, 1996).

This linking of fetal growth to nutrient supply by the regulation of fetal endocrine status provides an efficient mechanism to prevent overgrowth of the fetus. Teleologically, the fetus must not grow so big that fetal nutrient demand exceeds the maternal capacity to provide nutrients, nor so big that it exceeds maternal capacity eventually to deliver the baby. Hence the normal phenomenon of maternal constraint operates via limitation of fetal growth according to the maternal capacity to deliver nutrients. This limitation is, at least in part, via the nutritional regulation of the fetal endocrine mediators of fetal growth.

Fetal substrates

The major metabolic substrates of the late gestation mammalian fetus are glucose, lactate and amino acids. This appears to be true in all species studied to

Table 2.2. Some major endocrine and paracrine regulators of fetal growth in late gestation.

Anabolic	Catabolic
Insulin	Glucocorticoids
IGFs	Catecholamines
Thyroid hormone	Inflammatory cytokines
Epidermal growth factor	
Other growth factors (e.g. fibroblast growth factor)	
Transforming growth factor β	

IGFs, insulin-like growth factors.

date, although the proportions vary in different species and at different times in gestation. Other substrates may also contribute to a small degree in some species (Fowden, 1994; Harding and Gluckman, 2001). For example, the human fetus in late gestation largely uses glucose as its major oxidative substrate. Species with large amounts of adipose tissue at birth, such as the guinea-pig and human newborn, also derive some oxidative metabolic substrate from free fatty acids which readily cross the placenta. This placental transfer does not occur in other commonly studied laboratory species.

Despite these similarities in the major fetal substrates, there are important species differences in both maternal and fetal metabolism that must be understood in order to interpret the likely effect of altered nutrition on the fetus in different species. A few examples of this are given below.

First, maternal metabolism varies between species. The common species used for studies of fetal growth, metabolism and endocrinology is the sheep. This is because the fetal sheep is large, has a prolonged gestation and tolerates intrauterine surgery and instrumentation without premature delivery. However, the sheep is a ruminant. That is to say, circulating glucose in the mother is not derived from the diet. Rather, the maternal dietary substrates are fermented in the rumen, releasing gluconeogenic substrates, largely short-chain fatty acids and amino acids, which are then used by the maternal liver to synthesize glucose. This results in potentially large fluctuations in circulating maternal glucose concentrations, depending on maternal eating pattern. Thus undernutrition of the pregnant ewe results in direct undernutrition of her fetus, because maternal blood glucose concentrations fall, leading to reduced glucose supply to the fetus. The immediate effect of maternal undernutrition on the fetus is likely to be much smaller in human pregnancy, where glucose is derived from the diet as well as being synthesized by the maternal liver. Limited maternal nutrition therefore results in much smaller decreases in maternal blood glucose in the pregnant human than in the sheep, and hence fetal glucose supply is better maintained during maternal undernutrition in human pregnancy.

Secondly, placental function varies between species, both in terms of placental metabolism and substrate transfer capacity. Maternal undernutrition in many species results in the generation of ketones from fatty acids in the maternal liver. These may substitute for glucose as a metabolic substrate for maternal tissues. In sheep, ketones cross the placenta to the fetus in only small amounts (Miodovnik *et al.*, 1982). Rather, they are taken up by the placenta (Thorstensen *et al.*, 1995), apparently substituting for glucose in placental oxidative metabolism to maintain placental lactate production, while sparing glucose supply for the fetus. In contrast, the human placenta is permeable to ketones and fatty acids (Paterson *et al.*, 1967; Saleh *et al.*, 1989), which are then available to fetal tissues. The fetal brain has been shown to take up ketones preferentially as a metabolic substrate (Adam *et al.*, 1975). Again, this potentially spares glucose for other tissues. Thus, in the sheep, maternal undernutrition results in altered fetal substrate uptake, with reduced glucose uptake, increased amino acid oxidation and maintenance of lactate supply via placental ketone metabolism (Harding and Gluckman, 2001). In the human, maternal undernutrition results in better maintenance of fetal glucose supply and the availability of ketones as an alternative substrate for the fetal brain. Thus apparently similar nutritional insults can result in very different fetal metabolic responses in different species.

Thirdly, differing growth rate and body composition in fetuses of different species will place different demands on the available nutrient supply (Harding, 2001). Thus a small animal with a short gestation, such as the guinea-pig, has fetuses with a relatively high growth rate in late gestation (68 g/kg/day) compared with larger species with a longer gestation, such as the human (15 g/kg/day) or horse (9 g/kg/day) (Fowden, 1994). Such small fetuses must allocate a larger proportion of their total energy consumption for growth (76% versus 43% in human or 17% in horse fetuses). Restriction of nutrient supply would therefore be predicted to have a much greater effect on fetal growth in these small species than it would in a larger species with a relatively smaller demand.

Similarly, species such as the guinea-pig and human infant have a much higher proportion of body fat at birth than many other commonly studied species (12 and 16%, respectively, versus 2% in the horse) (Fowden, 1994). Fat has a very high energy density, and therefore a given rate of fat tissue acquisition will require a higher energy input than other tissues. Thus, once again, these species must allocate a larger proportion of available energy supply for tissue growth. Restriction of nutrient supply would therefore be predicted to have greater effect on fetal fat deposition in these species than in those that are leaner at birth.

Fetal growth trajectory

The epidemiological studies have related size at birth, generally as reflected in birthweight, to subsequent disease risk. Size at birth is generally accepted as reflecting an integrated sum of the processes involved in regulating fetal growth. While this may well be true, it is also critical to recognize that birthweight is not the same as fetal growth, and that very different intrauterine growth patterns may result in very similar birth phenotypes.

We have shown in sheep that fetal growth trajectory is set very early in pregnancy (Harding, 1997a). Ewes that were undernourished from 60 days before until 30 days after conception, and subsequently well nourished for the remainder of pregnancy, had fetuses with a slow growth trajectory in late gestation. When examined at 125 days' gestation these fetuses were of normal weight and length compared to well-nourished controls (term = 145 days) (Harding, 1997b). When allowed to deliver spontaneously, such fetuses also had normal birthweight, although their girth was reduced (Hawkins *et al.*, 2000a). Furthermore, these slowly growing fetuses were able to continue their slow growth trajectory in the face of a 10-day period of severe maternal undernutrition in late gestation, whereas rapidly growing fetuses of periconceptually well-nourished ewes slowed their growth in the face of late gestation undernutrition (Harding, 1997b). Once again, the effect of each of these changes in growth, both in the periconception period and in response to late undernutrition, did not result in altered weight or length of the fetus close to term. However, it did result in different fetal body composition. Ten days of maternal undernutrition in late gestation increased the size of the fetal heart and kidneys. Periconception undernutrition alone also increased fetal heart size. The combination of both periconception plus later undernutrition reduced brain size, while late undernutrition in a previously well-nourished fetus reduced lung size (Harding, 1997b; Harding and Gluckman, 2001).

These studies demonstrate some of the complexities of the interaction between nutrition, different fetal growth trajectories and size at birth. First, growth trajectory may be set very early in pregnancy. This is consistent with other experimental data (see below), and also with the finding in human pregnancy that fetuses that were already small on ultrasound in the first trimester had a high risk of being born small (Smith *et al.*, 1998). Secondly, patterns of early growth may determine later responses to subsequent nutritional insults. These effects would be extremely difficult to detect in human pregnancy. Thirdly, weight and length at birth reflect very little of the variation in growth trajectory during pregnancy.

Finally, the effect of different growth trajectories on postnatal growth, body composition and pathophysiology has yet to be determined. We have shown that sheep undernourished for 20 days in late gestation have reduced size at birth and, despite rapid postnatal catch-up growth, have altered body composition, but not body weight, as adults (Oliver *et al.*, 2001b). Despite this altered phenotype, they do not have perturbations in glucose tolerance or hypothalamo–pituitary–adrenal (HPA) axis function in adulthood (Oliver *et al.*, 2002; Bloomfield *et al.*, 2003a). In contrast, we found that sheep undernourished for only 10 days in late gestation have normal size at birth but show postnatal perturbation in glucose tolerance and HPA axis function. Interestingly, the changes in glucose tolerance were related to size at birth rather than nutrition group, while the changes in HPA axis function were related to nutrition group, and hence to growth trajectory before birth, rather than to size at birth.

These findings provide some interesting clues as to the possible causal relationships between maternal nutrition, size at birth and later disease risk. Given the dissociation already described between maternal nutrition and fetal nutrition, and between fetal growth and size at birth, a direct causal relationship, as initially proposed, seems most unlikely (Fig. 2.2). Rather, our findings suggest that there are likely to be multiple different pathways by which nutrition before birth may act as a programming stimulus for later disease risk. Changes in maternal nutrition may or may not alter fetal nutrition. In turn, altered fetal nutrition is likely to alter fetal growth trajectory, but may or may not alter size at birth. Structure and function of different organ systems, and thus different possible postnatal disease risks, are likely to be affected differently by each of these perturbations. If this schema is correct, then both the search for a single programming stimulus or critical period, and the search for a simple relationship between maternal nutrition and postnatal disease risk, are equally doomed to failure.

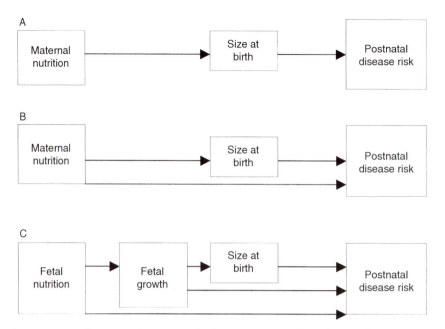

Fig. 2.2.   Possible causal pathways in the nutritional origins of adult disease.
(A) Simple causal relationship. Maternal nutrition determines size at birth, which in
turn determines postnatal disease risk. It is clear that this model no longer fits the
available experimental data. (B) Indirect relationship. Maternal nutrition determines
both size at birth and postnatal disease risk. In this model, programming of postnatal
disease risk can occur without perturbation of size at birth, consistent with some of
the experimental data. (C) Multiple pathways. Fetal nutrition, rather than maternal
nutrition, is the underlying programming stimulus. This determines postnatal
disease risk either directly, or indirectly via fetal growth trajectory, with or without
perturbation of size at birth. Recent experimental data suggest a model of at least
this complexity.

Body proportions

It is widely assumed that nutritional insults at various times in gestation result
in different patterns of fetal growth and different body proportions at birth.
In particular, the presumption has been that fetal nutrient limitation in late
gestation, particularly in the last trimester, results in fetuses that, at birth, have
asymmetrical body proportions, with relative preservation of head growth and
reduced body weight, particularly fat mass. In contrast, symmetrically small
babies are thought to have experienced a nutritional insult from early in
pregnancy, resulting in proportionate reduction in body weight, length and head
circumference (Barker *et al.*, 1995; Dennison *et al.*, 1997). Many widely used
texts describe these two different patterns of fetal growth restriction as having
different causes, providing different clinical problems and warranting different
management. However, more careful study of body proportions across large
human datasets has failed to distinguish these two different populations of
growth-restricted babies (Kramer *et al.*, 1989). Rather, there appears to be a

continuum of alteration in fetal growth and body proportions, consistent with a continuum of altered growth trajectories as described above.

Furthermore, there are few experimental data to support the concept of different timings of nutritional insult resulting in different fetal growth patterns. Indeed, in sheep, it is fetuses exposed to maternal undernutrition from early or mid-pregnancy through to term that have reduced ponderal index (i.e. are thin), whereas fetuses exposed to maternal undernutrition only in early or mid-pregnancy have an increased ponderal index (Owens *et al.*, 1996).

There is also a widespread, but somewhat simplistic, perception that the major mechanism by which nutrient limitation to the fetus results in impaired fetal growth is by simple limitation of substrate supply for tissue synthesis. While this may undoubtedly be true, particularly for some micronutrients (see below), it is by no means apparent from the available experimental data that this is the only phenomenon. For example, it is now clear that maternal undernutrition in the first half of pregnancy, during which time embryonic and fetal nutrient requirements are tiny and most unlikely to exceed supply, still results in per-turbed growth of the fetus. Maternal protein restriction in pigs results in reduced fetal weight and length at mid-gestation, although protein requirements at this time must be trivial relative to uterine supply (Pond *et al.*, 1991). Similarly, we have shown in sheep that maternal undernutrition either around the time of conception or in late gestation, for a defined period, may result in an increase rather than decrease in the size of the fetal heart, liver and kidneys (Harding, 1997b; Harding and Gluckman, 2001). Limited nutrient supply for tissue growth cannot simply explain an increase in organ size in this way. However, the mechanisms by which these changes occur are by no means clear.

One commonly proposed mechanism for the observed altered body proportions is that the fetus with asymmetrical growth restriction and relative preservation of head size has been hypoxic *in utero*. The hypothesis here is that hypoxaemia results in altered distribution of cardiac output with relative preservation of brain blood supply, and thus allows continued growth of the fetal brain at the expense of the periphery, particularly muscle and viscera (see Chapter 3, this volume). There is no doubt that such redistribution of cardiac output does occur during fetal hypoxaemia (Thornburg and Morton, 1994). Furthermore, there is good evidence that this does happen in some growth-restricted human fetuses, and that the redistribution of cardiac output can be reversed by administration of supplemental oxygen (Arduini *et al.*, 1988; Meyenburg *et al.*, 1991). However, it is also clear that hypoxaemia occurs only late in the process of fetal growth restriction, and that many fetuses with impaired fetal growth are not hypoxaemic *in utero* (Nicolaides *et al.*, 1989). Furthermore, relative preservation of head size is also seen in fetal sheep after maternal undernutrition, when the fetuses are clearly documented not to be hypoxaemic (Harding, 1997a). Indeed, if anything, there is an increase in fetal oxygenation during maternal undernutrition because reduced fetal growth results in reduced oxygen demand (Harding and Gluckman, 2001). Thus hypoxaemia alone cannot explain 'head sparing' in many situations.

There are a number of other mechanisms by which altered body proportions may occur in response to limited fetal nutrient supply. As already discussed, the uptake of glucose and amino acids into fetal tissues is, in part, regulated by fetal insulin and IGF concentrations. However, some tissues are able to take up glucose in the absence of insulin; most notably the brain and the liver. Thus reduced fetal glucose supply will result in reduced circulating fetal insulin levels and reduced glucose uptake into insulin-sensitive tissues such as muscle. However, glucose uptake into the brain will be maintained, potentially preserving brain growth at the expense of peripheral tissues.

Similarly, as already described, maternal undernutrition in humans results in increased supply of ketones that cross the placenta (Saleh *et al.*, 1989). Ketones are taken up preferentially by the fetal brain (Adam *et al.*, 1975; Harding and Evans, 1991). Once again, brain growth may therefore be maintained in the face of limited glucose supply, in this case by substitution of alternative substrates. Similarly, lactate is taken up preferentially by the fetal heart (Fisher *et al.*, 1980) for use as an oxidative fuel, and, at least in sheep, maternal undernutrition results in relative preservation of fetal lactate supply (Harding and Gluckman, 2001). Thus growth of the fetal heart may also be maintained by substrate substitution, even in the face of limited glucose supply.

To summarize, while there is no doubt that hypoxaemia may contribute to altered distribution of cardiac output, and hence altered body proportions, in some growth-restricted fetuses, there are many other, potentially more complex, mechanisms whereby altered body proportions may result from limited substrate supply. These mechanisms are likely to vary between species and with timing and duration of the nutritional insult.

Nutritional Regulation of Placental Function

The placenta forms perhaps the most complex and critical part of the fetal supply line. There are a number of ways in which the placenta might influence fetal nutrition and hence fetal growth. In turn, many of these mechanisms are themselves influenced by nutrient supply, providing an additional layer of complexity in our understanding of the possible role of nutrition as a programming influence.

Nutritional regulation of placental growth

There are many reports of a relationship between placental size and long-term risk, particularly of hypertension and coronary heart disease (Godfrey, 2002). In most studies, the relationship is with fetal–placental weight ratio, i.e. fetal growth relative to that of the placenta, rather than with absolute placental weight. A change in this ratio therefore suggests a mismatch between fetal and placental growth. The reported relationships are also quite variable, with both high and low ratios being associated with increased disease risk, and even relationships of a U-shape being reported (Martyn *et al.*, 1996).

Some of the difficulties in understanding these varying, and often conflicting, reports are in part because the factors that regulate placental growth are poorly understood. First, placental weight is a rather gross measure of the complexities of placental function. Secondly, as described above, there are marked species differences that need to be kept in mind. The pattern of changes in fetal–placental weight ratios with gestation are different in different species. For example, in sheep, placental weight reaches its maximum in mid-pregnancy and then declines again towards term, at the same time as fetal weight is increasing rapidly (Barcroft, 1946). In contrast, in the human placenta, weight continues to increase up until term, albeit at a much slower rate than that of the fetus. Despite these differences in growth pattern, all species show ongoing placental maturation in late gestation, with increasing placental structural changes resulting in increased surface area and potential transport capacity as fetal demand is increasing rapidly towards term.

In general, prolonged maternal undernutrition during pregnancy in experimental animals results in reduced weight of both the fetus and placenta, and an increase in the fetal–placental weight ratio, suggesting greater placental efficiency and/or preservation of fetal growth relative to that of the placenta. However, maternal undernutrition in early pregnancy, or a change in nutrition in mid-pregnancy, can result in increased placental weight (Faichney and White, 1987; Kelly and Newnham, 1990; Kelly, 1992; Heasman et al., 1998). Similarly, in adolescent sheep, a high plane of nutrition throughout pregnancy results in reduced size of the placenta and the fetus, apparently because available nutrients are used to support growth of the mother at the expense of the conceptus (Wallace et al., 2001). However, if maternal food intake is reduced from 50 days' gestation, placental weight and lamb birthweight are increased (Wallace et al., 1999). These findings raise interesting questions about how placental growth is regulated very early in pregnancy 'in anticipation' of increased fetal demand later in gestation. These animal findings also parallel human studies. One study in an apparently well-nourished population found that low carbohydrate intake in early pregnancy, particularly when associated with high protein intake in late pregnancy, resulted in an increased placental weight relative to that of the fetus at birth (Godfrey et al., 1996). Similarly, women who were exposed to famine in early pregnancy during the Dutch Hunger Winter and who subsequently were well nourished had increased placental weight at term (Lumey, 1998).

Changes in placental weight are also a poor measure of placental structure, and hence potential transport capacity. Guinea-pigs subjected to undernutrition before and during pregnancy have reduced placental weight. However, their placentas also show reduced exchange surface area and mean barrier thickness for diffusion (Roberts et al., 2001). Thus the impairment of placental transport capacity is likely to be even greater than the change in gross placental weight would suggest. Similar findings have been reported in sheep after changes in maternal nutrition in mid-gestation, which resulted in increased placental size, suggesting that the apparent compensation for nutrient limitation may be less than predicted on the basis of placental weight alone (Robinson et al., 1994).

Oxygenation also appears to be important in the regulation of placental growth. In human pregnancy maternal anaemia is associated with increased placental–fetal weight ratio (Lao and Wong, 1997). Both anaemia and hypoxia also alter the structure of the placenta, and particularly vascular development (Burton et al., 1996; Kadyrov et al., 1998). Since the placenta receives a large proportion of fetal cardiac output, placental vascular resistance has a major influence on fetal cardiac load and hence on long-term cardiovascular development (Thornburg, 2001). Thus changes in the placental vascular structure induced by altered nutrition and oxygen supply may contribute an explanatory link between fetal nutrition, postnatal cardiovascular function and disease risk.

Placental transport capacity

Nutrients required by the fetus cross the placenta by several different mechanisms. Many important small molecules, such as oxygen, cross the placenta by simple diffusion down a concentration gradient. The rate of diffusion is therefore determined by blood flow, placental surface area and barrier thickness. As already described, these in turn may be influenced by maternal nutrition, especially in early pregnancy.

Other critical fetal macronutrients cross the placenta by carrier-mediated mechanisms. The major fetal oxidative substrate, glucose, crosses the placenta by facilitated diffusion using the glucose transporters (GLUTs). The concentrations of the GLUTs vary on both the maternal and fetal sides of the placental barrier. We have previously shown in rats that maternal undernutrition in early, but not late, pregnancy results in increased placental expression of GLUT 1 throughout pregnancy (Gluckman et al., 1996). We have also found that both acute hyper- and hypoglycaemia increase the expression of GLUT 1 and GLUT 3 in the sheep placenta (Currie and Bassett, unpublished). In human placental syncytial cells in culture, glucose transporter activity is inversely related to extracellular glucose concentrations (Illsley et al., 1998).

Another major group of essential fetal substrates, amino acids, crosses the placenta by active transport using a number of amino acid transporters. Evidence for nutritional regulation of these transporters is still evolving (Battaglia and Regnault, 2001). However, the placentas of human intrauterine growth-restricted fetuses have reduced expression and activity of a number of amino acid transporters (Mahendran et al., 1993; Sibley et al., 1997). The reduction in sodium-dependent system A transporter activity in human placentas is also proportional to the severity of the growth restriction (Glazier et al., 1997).

Placental metabolism

The placenta may markedly influence fetal nutrition by its own metabolic processes. This occurs in several ways. First, the placenta is a highly metabolically active organ, consuming at least half of the available glucose and oxygen delivered via the utero-placental circulation in late-gestation sheep (Owens et al., 1987a,b). When the delivery of nutrients is reduced by acute maternal undernutrition in sheep, glucose consumption by the placenta is decreased, sparing glucose for fetal consumption (Harding and Gluckman, 2001). When placental size, and hence fetal growth, is restricted by limited placental implantation sites (carunclectomy), there is also a redistribution of nutrients between the fetus and placenta, with the placenta now receiving proportionately less glucose and oxygen than the fetus (Owens *et al.*, 1989). However, if the supply of nutrients to the placenta is reduced, by decreasing uterine blood flow, placental glucose consumption may be maintained at the expense of the fetus by placental uptake of glucose from the fetal rather than from the maternal circulation (Gu *et al.*, 1987). Thus, under some circumstances, the need to maintain placental metabolic demand may compromise nutrient supply to the fetus. Similarly, in fetal growth restriction induced by carunclectomy in sheep, the placenta may take up amino acids from the fetal circulation to maintain placental metabolic demand at the expense of the fetus (Owens *et al.*, 1989). This observation may explain the clinical observations of fetal wasting in late gestation in some growth-restricted human fetuses (Divon *et al.*, 1986).

The second mechanism that contributes to placental metabolic regulation of fetal nutrition is that placental metabolism itself provides some important fetal nutrients. One of the key fetal substrates, lactate, is produced in the placenta, largely from glucose of both maternal and fetal origin (Gu *et al.*, 1987). Lactate may be a key fetal nutrient, in part, because it does not readily cross the placenta out of the fetal circulation. Hence, even when supply of glucose from the mother is reduced, ongoing lactate production by the placenta maintains a substrate that is specifically available in the fetal circulation. Similarly, the placenta takes up branched-chain amino acids from the maternal circulation and produces the related keto acids for release to the fetus, again maintaining a supply of potential oxidative substrates in the fetal circulation (Smeaton *et al.*, 1989).

Placental metabolism is also required to provide key nutrients to the fetus by a series of complex, and as yet poorly understood, series of feto-placental metabolic interactions (Battaglia and Regnault, 2001). For example, there is a glutamine–glutamate cycle in the feto-placental unit (Chung *et al.*, 1998). Glutamine is taken up by the fetus from the placenta in large amounts. The fetal liver then deaminates this glutamine to glutamate, which is, in turn, taken up and oxidized in large amounts by the placenta (Vaughn *et al.*, 1995). The function of this cycle is not clearly defined, but glutamine synthesis may provide a mechanism for placental transfer of ammonia nitrogen to the fetus for disposal as urea (Faichney, 1981). There is some evidence that fetal capacity for urea synthesis is impaired in growth-restricted human neonates (Boehm *et al.*, 1991; van Goudoever *et al.*, 1995). It has also been proposed that placental glutamate oxidation may be important for placental steroidogenesis and for purine synthesis, and hence may contribute to the regulation of fetal growth (Makarewicz and Swierczynski, 1988; Battaglia and Regnault, 2001).

Similarly, there is a feto-placental serine–glycine cycle (Chung *et al.*, 1998). Neither serine nor glycine crosses the placenta from the mother in large amounts. Rather, most is synthesized within the feto-placental unit (Moores *et al.*, 1993). Serine is converted to glycine in the placenta and glycine is converted to serine in the fetal liver (Cetin *et al.*, 1991, 1992). The net result of this cycle, and particularly the placental synthesis of glycine from serine, is the directing of the β carbon of serine into synthetic reactions requiring activated single-carbon units, such as nucleotide synthesis and DNA methylation (Chung *et al.*, 1998). These placental metabolic pathways may interact (Fig. 2.3), becoming critically important in the regulation of cell division and gene activation, essential for normal growth. It should also be noted that this cycle depends on folate cofactors (*see* below). Thus there are a number of mechanisms by which placental function is regulated by nutritional status, and the placenta, in turn, contributes to the regulation of fetal nutrition.

Placental endocrinology

The placenta may also have a major influence on fetal nutrition via its contribution to the regulation of maternal and fetal endocrine status. In both humans and sheep, the placenta produces large amounts of placental lactogen and growth hormone. Both hormones have an important influence on maternal metabolism, contributing to the insulin resistance of pregnancy and thus increasing the availability of glucose and fatty acids in the maternal circulation potentially available for the fetus and fetal growth (Gluckman, 1995). They may also contribute to the regulation of fetal nutrient supply via their effects on maternal

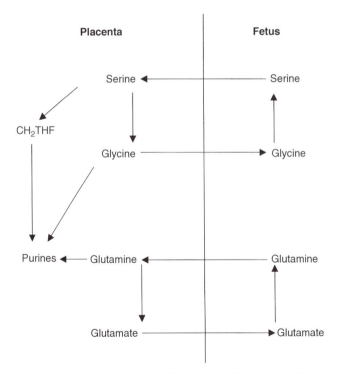

Fig. 2.3. Diagram of some feto-placental interactions in amino acid metabolism, and their possible contribution to placental purine synthesis. CH$_2$THF, methylene tetrahydrofolate.

appetite. Recombinant placental lactogen enhances appetite in young lambs (Min et al., 1996), while GH administration reduces food intake in pregnant sheep (Oliver, unpublished observations).

In addition, GH contributes to the regulation of nutrient partitioning between mother and fetus (Palmer et al., 1996). In undernourished rats, GH administration increases maternal weight gain but inhibits fetal growth (Chiang and Nicoll, 1991), apparently because available nutrients are directed towards maternal tissues at the expense of fetal growth. However, in well-nourished mothers, GH treatment increases fetal weight in both rats (Sara and Lazarus, 1975) and sheep (Blanchard et al., 1991; Jenkinson et al., 1999). In turn, both GH and placental lactogen secretion are regulated by nutrition, with maternal undernutrition inducing a prompt rise in concentrations of both GH (Bauer et al., 1995) and placental lactogen (Oliver et al., 1992) in fetal sheep.

Placental endocrine function may, in turn, contribute to regulation of placental transport capacity. Maternal GH administration for 10 days in sheep results in increased placental transfer capacity for simple diffusion (Harding et al., 1997). Both maternal and fetal IGF-I concentrations also appear to regulate placental function. Short-term maternal IGF-I infusion increases placental uptake of glucose and amino acids (Liu et al., 1994), while fetal IGF-I infusion increases their transfer from placenta to fetus (Harding et al., 1994). Again, both maternal and fetal IGF-I concentrations are regulated by glucose and insulin supply (Oliver et al., 1993, 1996). In turn, the placenta also contributes to the regulation of fetal endocrine status, taking up IGF-I from the circulation when concentrations are high, and secreting IGF-I into the fetus when concentrations are low (Iwamoto et al., 1992). In these several different ways, nutritional supply to the mother and to the fetus are tightly linked with placental function and fetal growth.

Maternal Nutrition and Fetal Programming

It is generally accepted that women's total macronutrient and energy intake during pregnancy has little effect on birthweight. As referred to above, energy supplements result in little change in birthweight, even in undernourished populations (Kramer, 2002a). It has been proposed that this may be because the minimum level of nutrients required to support fetal growth is really quite low, and that above this minimal level, pregnant women can adapt to a wide variety of food intake with minimal or no effect on the birthweight of their baby (Lechtig et al., 1975).

However, this does not mean that maternal diet has no programming effect on the fetus. Rather, the balance of protein and energy intake may be critical. Careful review shows that those studies involving nutritional supplement during pregnancy, where a high proportion of the supplemental calories are derived from protein, may actually decrease birthweight (weighted mean difference −58 g) (Kramer, 2002b). This is consistent with other findings that the balance of macronutrients in the maternal diet may have longer-term effects on their offspring. Women consuming a low-carbohydrate diet in early pregnancy, and particularly when associated with a high-protein diet in late pregnancy, have, on average, smaller, thinner babies with smaller placentas (Godfrey *et al.*, 1996, 1997). Similarly, high protein intake during pregnancy, unless balanced by a high carbohydrate intake, has been associated with reduced birthweight and placental weight, and with increased blood pressure and impaired pancreatic function in the adult offspring (Campbell *et al.*, 1996; Shiell *et al.*, 2000). Interestingly, data from the Dutch Hunger Winter demonstrated no relationship between famine exposure and later blood pressure, but there was an association between raised adult blood pressure and maternal consumption of rations of low protein density (Roseboom *et al.*, 2001a).

Fetal nutritional status may also be more affected by maternal body composition before and in early pregnancy than by maternal dietary intake during pregnancy. Maternal body composition, particularly fat deposits, may influence the balance of circulating nutrients in the mother, for example by determining the balance of circulating glucose versus fatty acids concentrations and the availability of ketones during fasting (see above). Jamaican women who were light and thin in early pregnancy tended to have smaller babies (Thame *et al.*, 1997). Reduced skinfold thickness in early pregnancy, in both Jamaican and British women, was also associated with elevated blood pressure in their 11-year-old offspring (Godfrey *et al.*, 1994; Clark *et al.*, 1998). Indian women of low body weight during pregnancy had offspring with increased risk of coronary heart disease (Stein *et al.*, 1996).

There is growing evidence that micronutrients may be at least as important as macronutrients in determining size at birth and postnatal disease risk. There is much work to be done in this area, and only a few examples are given here. The likely role of individual amino acids has been referred to above. Glycine is a conditionally essential amino acid in the fetus. It is required for synthesis of many critical proteins required for the growing fetus, such as collagen, haem, creatine and nucleic acids (Jackson, 1991). These proteins represent end pathways for glycine use, in that the nitrogen in these proteins is not recycled, and thus the demand for glycine is high during rapid growth. There is evidence that many apparently well-nourished women are only marginally glycine sufficient during pregnancy, and many more may be frankly glycine insufficient in chronically poorly nourished populations (Jackson *et al.*, 1997). Furthermore, a diet high in methionine may aggravate glycine deficiency, as glycine is diverted to detoxify the excess methionine (Meakins *et al.*, 1998). Rats given a low-protein diet during pregnancy have offspring with increased blood pressure as adults (Langley and Jackson, 1994). Supplementing the low-protein maternal diet in pregnancy with glycine alone prevents the postnatal hypertension (Jackson *et al.*, 2002), providing strong evidence that glycine supply itself may be a critical programming influence.

The metabolic pathways for glycine in the fetus and the feto-placental glycine–serine cycle involve folate-dependent cofactors. Inadequate folate intake thus limits the capacity of the feto-placental unit to synthesize these amino acids (Narkewicz *et al.*, 2002). The active form of folic acid, tetrahydrofolate (THF), is also an essential cofactor in many reactions requiring transfer of methyl groups. Conversion of serine to glycine generates methylene THF (see above), which can be used for the synthesis of purines and pyrimidines for DNA. Hence folate availability is central to tissue growth.

Alternatively, methylene THF can be reduced to methyl THF, which is used for methylation of homocysteine to regenerate methionine (Fig. 2.4). It has been suggested that one mechanism by which maternal protein restriction during pregnancy in rats leads to long-term changes in blood pressure and glucose tolerance in the offspring is via perturbation of this methylation pathway, by functional increase in demand for methyl THF (Rees, 2002). In human populations, mutations in the genes encoding key enzymes in the synthesis of methyl THF are common (Frosst *et al.*, 1995) and are associated both with pregnancy complications, including miscarriage and hypertension, and low birthweight (Girling and De Swiet, 1998; Obwegser *et al.*, 1999), and also with the increased risk of cardiovascular disease in adult life (Ma *et al.*, 1996). Folate supplements may reduce the risk of pre-eclampsia and fetal growth restriction by improving methionine generation from homocysteine (Leeda *et al.*, 1998). Folate supplements may also prevent some birth defects, such as neural tube defects, apparently at least in part by the same mechanism (Czeizel, 2000; Rees, 2002). Of interest, therefore, are recent findings, in a chronically undernourished

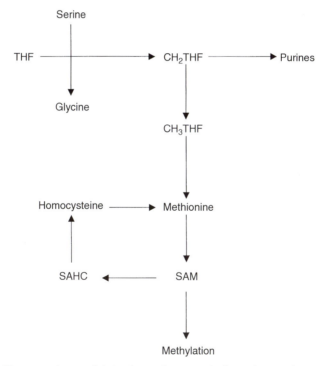

Fig. 2.4. Diagram of some folate-dependent metabolic pathways that are likely to be important for purine synthesis, hence tissue growth and DNA methylation, hence gene expression. THF, tetrahydrofolate; CH_2THF, methylene tetrahydrofolate; CH_3THF, methyl tetrahydrofolate; SAM, *S*-adenosyl methionine; SAHC, *S*-adenosyl homocysteine.

Indian population, that size at birth is most strongly associated with folate status and with intakes of foods rich in micronutrients, such as vegetables and fruits (Rao *et al.*, 2001).

In turn, methionine generated from the interaction of methyl THF and homocysteine is used for synthesis of S-adenosyl methionine (SAM). SAM is the methyl donor for more than 100 different transmethylation reactions, including methylation of DNA and proteins, phospholipid synthesis and neurotransmitter synthesis (Chiang *et al.*, 1996). Methylation of DNA is critical for normal embryonic development and for epigenetic modification of gene expression, e.g. imprinting. Gene knock-out mice unable to synthesize methyl THF have very high plasma homocysteine levels, low levels of SAM, and show global hypomethylation of DNA (Chen *et al.*, 2001). In contrast, methylation of DNA is increased in the fetal liver after maternal low-protein diet in rats (Rees *et al.*, 2000).

These metabolic pathways point to possible mechanisms whereby maternal dietary intake, particularly of glycine and folate, may interact with the maternal genetic background to influence both fetal growth and long-term disease risk. Maternal diet may also influence fetal gene expression via similar pathways. Genetically identical mice may have different coat colours, depending on the coat colour of the mother (Morgan *et al.*, 1999). These effects are epigenetic phenomena, whereby coat colour is determined by the inherited pattern of methylation and hence activation of the genes controlling coat colour. Importantly, the degree of methylation, and hence gene expression and coat colour, can be altered by feeding the mother a diet high in methyl donors during pregnancy (Wolff *et al.*, 1998). There seems little doubt that many more such examples of the nutritional regulation of gene expression will become apparent in the future.

Another specific amino acid potentially important as a micronutrient for programming phenomena is taurine. Taurine is essential for many aspects of cell function, and particularly for the development of the pancreatic β-cell (Sturman, 1993). Rats fed a low-protein diet in pregnancy have offspring with impaired pancreatic β-cell function. Supplementary taurine provided to these β-cells in culture does not reverse this impairment. However, supplementing the maternal diet with taurine during pregnancy restores pancreatic β-cell function in the offspring (Cherif *et al.*, 1998). Furthermore, we have shown in sheep that maternal undernutrition in early pregnancy results in altered function of the fetal pancreatic β-cells in late pregnancy (Oliver *et al.*, 2001a). This is associated with elevated circulating taurine concentrations in both mother and fetus, suggesting that a specific perturbation in metabolism of this amino acid may underlie the pancreatic dysfunction.

Micronutrients other than amino acids may also be important in programming phenomena. Even in developed countries, many women do not consume the recommended amounts of many micronutrients during pregnancy (Schofield *et al.*, 1989; Rogers and Emmett, 1998). In a British study of maternal diet in the first trimester of pregnancy, intake of thiamin, niacin, riboflavin, magnesium, phosphorus, iron and vitamin C were more important than total energy or protein intake in predicting size at birth (Doyle *et al.*, 1989). In another similar study, maternal intake of vitamin C in early pregnancy was independently predictive of both placental weight and birthweight (Mathews *et al.*, 1999). There have been few long-term studies of maternal mineral intake in relationship to postnatal outcome of their offspring. However, follow-up of participants in randomized clinical trials of maternal supplements during pregnancy offers much scope for such investigations. To date there is one report of a study of calcium supplementation during pregnancy. This resulted in lower blood pressure of the offspring, despite having no effect on birthweight (Belizan *et al.*, 1997). Further trials are awaited with interest.

Timing of Nutritional Effects on Fetal Programming

Most experimental work regarding the effect of manipulating maternal nutrition on disease risk of the offspring has involved maternal nutritional manipulation, either throughout pregnancy or in late gestation. However, a growing number of experiments point to the importance of timing of a nutritional insult in determining its long-term effects. Nutritional manipulations at different times in pregnancy have different effects on birth size, as already discussed, but are also likely to have different effects on different organ systems and hence on disease risks.

Data in humans regarding the timing of nutritional effects are limited. Reference has already been made to the interaction between carbohydrate intake in early pregnancy and protein intake in late pregnancy with regard to both size at birth and postnatal outcome (Godfrey *et al.*, 1994, 1996; Campbell *et al.*, 1996; Shiell *et al.*, 2000). Similarly, data from the Dutch famine, which provides the clearest evidence regarding the timing of nutritional influences in human pregnancy, have suggested that exposure to famine in late gestation results in offspring with an increased risk of glucose intolerance. However, exposure in early pregnancy is associated with increased risk of hyperlipidaemia, and perhaps coronary heart disease (Roseboom *et al.*, 2001b).

The link between nutritional insult in late pregnancy and later pancreatic dysfunction is consistent with the rat data, where a low-protein diet during pregnancy results in offspring with glucose intolerance (Dahri *et al.*, 1991). Exposure to the low-protein diet in only the first part of pregnancy has no such effect, whereas exposure to the low-protein diet in late pregnancy also results in offspring with glucose intolerance (Alvarez *et al.*, 1997). It is likely that this relates to perturbation of the development of pancreatic β-cells in late gestation (Petrik *et al.*, 1999).

However, there is an increasing body of evidence suggesting that nutritional effects in early pregnancy may be critical in programming later disease risk. This is particularly important because effects in early pregnancy may have minimal or no effect on size at birth, making these relationships difficult to detect. In sheep, mild maternal undernutrition in the first half of pregnancy results in offspring with altered HPA axis and cardiovascular function (Hawkins *et al.*, 1999, 2000b) and elevated blood pressure after birth (Hawkins *et al.*, 1997). Similarly, mild maternal undernutrition before and for only the first 7 days after mating results in perturbed HPA axis function of the fetus in late pregnancy (Edwards and McMillen, 2002). Dexamethasone administration for 48 h at 27 days' gestation, but not at 64 days' gestation, results in offspring with increased cardiac output and elevated blood pressure in adult life (Dodic *et al.*, 1999) but does not perturb glucose tolerance (Gatford *et al.*, 2000) or HPA axis function (Dodic *et al.*, 2002). Once again, these data suggest not only the importance of early nutrition but also of different programming mechanisms for different organ systems and subsequent predisposition to hypertension and glucose intolerance, respectively.

Recent data suggest that the period immediately around the time of conception may be critically important in the programming of some aspects of postnatal function. In rats, a low-protein diet continued only during the period up to implantation (4 days of a 21-day rat pregnancy) results in hypertension of the offspring (Kwong *et al.*, 2000). These studies also point to some possible mechanisms for this effect, in that this very short period of nutritional insult alters allocation of the blastocyst cells to the inner and outer cell mass which will eventually give rise to the fetus and placenta, respectively. Thus the number of the cells in the blastocyst appears to be determined by nutritional signals before implantation. These experiments also suggest that cell cycle length is altered in the developing blastocyst, potentially altering the number of cells available for allocation to different organs later in development. These effects are similar to those induced by progesterone administration in sheep, where exposure to progesterone for only 3 days, beginning on the day of mating, results in altered numbers of blastomeres allocated to the inner and outer cell mass and to altered fetal and placental size in mid-gestation (Kleemann *et al.*, 2001). This is true even when unexposed embryos are transplanted into progesterone-exposed ewes, suggesting that the signal is derived from the maternal environment, presumably via oviductal and uterine secretions, rather than from direct exposure of the embryo itself to progesterone.

Our own data suggest that, in sheep, events very early in pregnancy are critical to many aspects of fetal development. Ewes undernourished from 60 days before to 30 days after mating have fetuses which have an altered growth trajectory in late gestation (Harding, 1997b) and are born thin but not light (Hawkins *et al.*, 2000a). These fetuses have altered pancreatic β-cell function in late gestation (Oliver *et al.*, 2001a) and altered metabolic and endocrine function (Oliver *et al.*, 2000). They have accelerated maturation of the fetal HPA axis, and some deliver early (Bloomfield *et al.*, 2003b). These findings all point to critical effects of nutritional signals on development before any of the relevant organ systems, which will later be involved in disease risk, have developed. Our finding that there was a delay in the rise of maternal progesterone concentrations in undernourished ewes points to a possible signalling mechanism being altered endocrine function of the placenta (Bloomfield, unpublished). Altered maternal taurine and serine concentrations also suggest that altered maternal adaptation to pregnancy may contribute to these signals (Oliver *et al.*, 2001a; van Zijl *et al.*, 2002). Thus much work is required to refine further the critical period for some of these perturbations, the signals involved and their subsequent effects on postnatal physiology. If, indeed, nutrition in the period around the time of conception, or possibly even before conception, is critical, then much future work will need to focus on public health interventions to achieve good nutritional status of women and girls before pregnancy begins.

Conclusions

The epidemiological evidence for associations between size at birth and disease risk in adult life has been widely accepted. These associations are thought to be due to programming events in fetal life, resulting both in altered size at birth and in altered structure and function, leading to postnatal disease risk. There is a substantial body of evidence from animal experiments, and growing evidence in humans, that nutrition can be a key programming stimulus. Nutrition alters fetal and placental growth, and metabolic and endocrine status both before and after birth. However, the effects of a given nutritional stimulus or insult will vary with the species, timing in gestation and the balance of other macro- and micronutrients available to the fetus. Maternal nutrition may bear little relationship to fetal nutrition, and fetal growth may or may not be reflected in size at birth. Furthermore, nutritional effects may result in altered postnatal function without apparent effect on fetal growth. Despite the large amount of work still required to clarify these relationships, it is clear that nutrition before birth can be a key programming stimulus for postnatal disease risk. Nutrition may well be the basis for the fetal origins of adult disease.

References

Adam, P.A.J., Raiha, N., Rahiala, E.-L. and Kekomaki, M. (1975) Oxidation of glucose and D-β-OH-butyrate by the early human fetal brain. *Acta Paediatrica Scandinavica* 64, 17–24.

Allen, W.R., Wilsher, S., Turnbull, C., Stewart, F., Ousey, J., Rossdale, P.D. and Fowden, A.L. (2002) Influence of maternal size on placental, fetal and postnatal growth in the horse. I. Development *in utero. Reproduction* 123, 445–453.

Alvarez, C., Martin, M.A., Goya, L., Bertin, E., Portha, B. and Pascual-Leone, A.M. (1997) Contrasted impact of maternal rat food restriction on the fetal endocrine pancreas. *Endocrinology* 138, 2267–2273.

Arduini, D., Rizzo, G., Mancuso, S. and Romanini, C. (1988) Short-term effects of maternal oxygen administration on blood flow velocity waveforms in healthy and growth-retarded fetuses. *American Journal of Obstetrics and Gynecology* 159, 1077–1080.

Barcroft, J. (1946) *Researches on Prenatal Life*. Blackwell Scientific Publications, Oxford, UK.

Barker, D.J.P. (1992) The fetal origins of adult hypertension. *Journal of Hypertension* 10, S39–S44.

Barker, D.J.P. (1998) *Mothers, Babies and Health in Later Life*. Churchill Livingstone, Edinburgh, UK.

Barker, D.J.P., Martyn, C.N., Osmond, C. and Weild, G.A. (1995) Abnormal liver growth *in utero* and death from coronary heart disease. *British Medical Journal* 310, 704.

Battaglia, F.C. and Regnault, T.R.H. (2001) Placental transport and metabolism of amino acids. *Placenta* 22, 145–161.

Bauer, M.K., Breier, B.H., Harding, J.E., Veldhuis, J.D. and Gluckman, P.D. (1995) The fetal somatotropic axis during long term maternal undernutrition in sheep: evidence for nutritional regulation *in utero*. *Endocrinology* 136, 1250–1257.

Belizan, J.M., Villar, J., Bergel, E., del Pino, A., Di Fulvio, S., Galliano, S.V. and Kattan, C. (1997) Long term effect of calcium supplementation during pregnancy on the blood pressure of offspring: follow up of a randomised controlled trial. *British Medical Journal* 315, 281–285.

Blanchard, M.M., Goodyer, C.G., Charrier, J., Kann, G., Garcia Villar, R., Bousquet-Melou, A., Toutain, P.L. and Barenton, B. (1991) GRF treatment of late pregnant ewes alters maternal and fetal somatotropic axis activity. *American Journal of Physiology* 260, E575–E580.

Bloomfield, F.H., Oliver, M.H., Giannoulias, C.D., Gluckman, P.D., Harding, J.E. and Challis, J.R.G. (2003a) Brief undernutrition in late-gestation sheep programmes the HPA axis in adult offspring. *Endocrinology*, 144, 2933–2940.

Bloomfield, F.H., Oliver, M.H., Hawkins, P., Campbell, M., Phillips, D.J., Breier, B.H., Gluckman, P.D., Challis, J.R.G. and Harding, J.E. (2003b) A periconceptual nutritional origin for non-infectious preterm birth. *Science* 300, 606.

Boehm, G., Gedlu, E., Muller, M.D., Beyreiss, K. and Raiha, N.C.R. (1991) Postnatal development of urea- and ammonia-excretion in urine of very-low-birth-weight infants small for gestational age. *Acta Paediatrica Hungarica* 13, 31–45.

Brooks, A.A., Johnson, M.R., Steer, P.J., Pawson, M.E. and Abdalla, H.I. (1995) Birth weight: nature or nurture? *Early Human Development* 42, 29–35.

Burton, G.J., Reshetnikova, O.S., Milovanov, A.P. and Teleshova, O.V. (1996) Stereological evaluation of vascular adaptations in human placental villi to differing forms of hypoxic stress. *Placenta* 17, 49–55.

Campbell, D.M., Hall, M.H., Barker, D.J., Cross, J., Shiell, A.W. and Godfrey, K.M. (1996) Diet in pregnancy and the offspring's blood pressure 40 years later. *British Journal of Obstetrics and Gynaecology* 103, 273–280.

Cetin, I., Fennessey, P.V., Quick, A.N., Marconi, A.M., Meschia, G., Battaglia, F.C. and Sparks, J.W. (1991) Glycine turnover and oxidation, hepatic serine synthesis from glycine in fetal lambs. *American Journal of Physiology* 260, E371–E378.

Cetin, I., Fennessey, P.V., Sparks, J.W., Meschia, G. and Battaglia, F.C. (1992) Fetal serine fluxes across fetal liver, hindlimb, and placenta in late gestation. *American Journal of Physiology* 263, E786–E793.

Chen, Z., Karaplis, A.C., Ackerman, S.L., Pogribny, I.P., Melnyk, S., Lussier-Cacan, S., Chen, M.F., Pai, A., John, S.W.M., Smith, R.S., Bottiglieri, T., Bagley, P., Selhub, J., Rudnicki, M.A., James, S.J. and Rozen, R. (2001) Mice deficient in methylenetetrahydrofolate reductase exhibit hyperhomocysteinemia and decreased methylation capacity, with neuropathology and aortic lipid deposition. *Human Molecular Genetics* 10, 433–443.

Cherif, H., Reusens, B., Ahn, M.T., Hoet, J.J. and Remacle, C. (1998) Effects of taurine on the insulin secretion of rat fetal islets from dams fed a low-protein diet. *Journal of Endocrinology* 159, 341–348.

Chiang, M.H. and Nicoll, C.S. (1991) Administration of growth hormone to pregnant rats on a reduced diet inhibits growth of their fetuses. *Endocrinology* 129, 2491–2495.

Chiang, P.K., Gordon, R.K., Tal, J., Zeng, G.C., Doctor, B.P., Pardhasaradhi, K. and McCann, P.P. (1996) S-Adenosylmethionine and methylation. *FASEB Journal* 10, 471–480.

Chung, M., Teng, C., Timmerman, M., Meschia, G. and Battaglia, F.C. (1998) Production and utilization of amino acids by ovine placenta *in vivo*. *American Journal of Physiology* 274, E13–E22.

Clark, P.M., Atton, C., Law, C.M., Shiell, A., Godfrey, K. and Barker, D.J.P. (1998) Weight gain in pregnancy, triceps skinfold thickness, and blood pressure in offspring. *Obstetrics and Gynecology* 91, 103–107.

Conti, J., Abraham, S. and Taylor, A. (1998) Eating behavior and pregnancy outcome. *Journal of Psychosomatic Research* 44, 465–477.

Czeizel, A.E. (2000) Primary prevention of neural-tube defects and some other major congenital abnormalities: recommendations for the appropriate use of folic acid during pregnancy. *Paediatric Drugs* 2, 437–449.

Dahri, S., Snoek, A., Reusens-Billen, B., Remacle, C. and Hoet, J.J. (1991) Islet function in offspring of mothers on low-protein diet during gestation. *Diabetes* 40(suppl. 2), 115–120.

Dennison, E., Fall, C., Cooper, C. and Barker, D. (1997) Prenatal factors influencing long-term outcome. *Hormone Research* 48(suppl. 1), 25–29.

Desai, M., Crowther, N.J., Ozanne, E., Lucas, A. and Hales, C.N. (1995) Adult glucose and lipid metabolism may be programmed during fetal life. *Biochemical Society Transactions* 23, 331–335.

Divon, M.Y., Chamberlain, P.F., Sipos, L., Manning, F.A. and Platt, L.D. (1986) Identification of the small for gestational age fetus with the use of gestation age-independent indices of fetal growth. *American Journal of Obstetrics and Gynecology* 155, 1197–1201.

Dodic, M., Peers, A., Coghlan, J.P., May, C.N., Lumbers, E., Yu, Z.Y. and Wintour, E.M. (1999) Altered cardiovascular haemodynamics and baroreceptor–heart rate reflex in adult sheep after prenatal exposure to dexamethasone. *Clinical Science* 97, 103–109.

Dodic, M., Peers, A., Moritz, K., Hantzis, V. and Wintour, E.M. (2002) No evidence for HPA reset in adult sheep with high blood pressure due to short prenatal exposure to dexamethasone. *American Journal of Physiology* 282, R343–R350.

Doyle, W., Crawford, M.A., Wynn, A.H. and Wynn, S.W. (1989) Maternal nutrient intake and birthweight. *Journal of Nutrition and Dietetics* 2, 415–422.

Edwards, L.J. and McMillen, I.C. (2002) Impact of maternal undernutrition during the periconceptual period, fetal number, and fetal sex on the development of the hypothalamo–pituitary–adrenal axis in sheep during late gestation. *Biology of Reproduction* 66, 1562–1569.

Faichney, G.J. (1981) Amino acid utilisation by the foetal lamb. *Proceedings of the Nutrition Society* 6, 48–53.

Faichney, G.J. and White, G.A. (1987) Effects of maternal nutritional status on fetal and placental growth and on fetal urea synthesis in sheep. *Australian Journal of Biological Science* 40, 365–377.

Fisher, D.J., Heymann, M.A. and Rudolph, A.M. (1980) Myocardial oxygen and carbohydrate consumption in fetal lambs *in utero* and in adult sheep. *American Journal of Physiology* 238, H399–H405.

Fowden, A.L. (1994) Fetal metabolism and energy balance. In: Thorburn, G.D. and Harding, R. (eds) *Textbook of Fetal Physiology*. Oxford University Press, Oxford, UK, pp. 70–82.

Fowden, A.L. and Hay, W.W. (1988) The effects of pancreatectomy on the rates of glucose utilization, oxidation and production in the sheep fetus. *Quarterly Journal of Experimental Physiology* 73, 973–984.

Fowden, A.L. and Silver, M. (1995) The effects of thyroid hormones on oxygen and glucose metabolism in the sheep fetus during late gestation. *Journal of Physiology* 482, 203–213.

Fowden, A.L., Hughes, P. and Comline, R.S. (1989) The effects of insulin on the growth rate of the sheep fetus during late gestation. *Quarterly Journal of Experimental Physiology* 74, 703–714.

Frosst, P., Blom, H.J., Milos, R., Goyette, P., Sheppard, C.A., Matthews, R.G., Boers, G.J.H., den Heiher, M., Kluijtmans, L.A.J., van der Heuvel, L.P. and Rozen, R. (1995) A candidate genetic risk factor for vascular disease: a common mutation in methylenetetrahydrofolate reductase. *Nature Genetics* 10, 111–113.

Gatford, K.L., Wintour, E.M., De Blasio, M.J., Owens, J.A. and Dodic, M. (2000) Differential timing for programming of glucose homoeostasis, sensitivity to insulin and blood pressure by *in utero* exposure to dexamethasone in sheep. *Clinical Science* 98, 553–560.

Girling, J. and de Swiet, M. (1998) Inherited thrombophilia and pregnancy. *Current Opinion in Obstetrics and Gynecology* 10, 135–144.

Glazier, J.D., Cetin, I., Perugino, G., Ronzoni, S., Grey, A.M., Mahendran, D., Marconi, A.M., Pardi, G. and Sibley, C.P. (1997) Association between the activity of the system A amino transporter in the microvillous plasma membrane of the human placenta and severity of fetal compromise in intrauterine growth restriction. *Pediatric Research* 42, 514–519.

Gluckman, P.D. (1995) The endocrine regulation of fetal growth in late gestation: the role of insulin-like growth factors. *Journal of Clinical Endocrinology and Metabolism* 80, 1047–1050.

Gluckman, P.D., Cutfield, W., Harding, J.E., Milner, D., Jensen, E., Woodall, S., Gallaher, B., Bauer, M. and Breier, B.H. (1996) Metabolic consequences of intrauterine growth retardation. *Acta Paediatrica Scandinavica Suppl.* 417, 3–6.

Godfrey, K.M. (2002) The role of the placenta in fetal programming – a review. *Placenta* 23, S20–S27.

Godfrey, K.M., Forrester, T., Barker, D.J.P., Jackson, A.A., Landman, J.P., Hall, J.S., Cox, V. and Osmond, C. (1994) Maternal nutritional status in pregnancy and blood pressure in childhood. *British Journal of Obstetrics and Gynaecology* 101, 398–403.

Godfrey, K., Robinson, S., Barker, D.J.P., Osmond, C. and Cox, V. (1996) Maternal nutrition in early and late pregnancy in relation to placental and fetal growth. *British Medical Journal* 312, 410–414.

Godfrey, K.M., Barker, D.J.P., Robinson, S. and Osmond, C. (1997) Maternal birthweight and diet in pregnancy in relation to the infant's thinness at birth. *British Journal of Obstetrics and Gynaecology* 104, 663–667.

Gu, W., Jones, C.T. and Harding, J.E. (1987) Metabolism of glucose by fetus and placenta of sheep. The effects of normal fluctuations in uterine blood flow. *Journal of Developmental Physiology* 9, 369–389.

Harding, J.E. (1997a) Prior growth rate determines the fetal growth response to acute maternal undernutrition in fetal sheep of late gestation. *Prenatal and Neonatal Medicine* 2, 300–309.

Harding, J.E. (1997b) Periconceptual nutrition determines the fetal growth response to acute maternal undernutrition in fetal sheep of late gestation. *Prenatal and Neonatal Medicine* 2, 310–319.

Harding, J.E. (2001) The nutritional basis of the fetal origins of adult disease. *International Journal of Epidemiology* 30, 15–23.

Harding, J.E. and Evans, P.C. (1991) β-Hydroxybutyrate is an alternative substrate for the fetal sheep brain. *Journal of Developmental Physiology* 16, 293–299.

Harding, J.E. and Gluckman, P.D. (2001) Growth, metabolic and endocrine adaptations to fetal undernutrition. In: Barker, D.J.P. (ed.) *Fetal Origins of Cardiovascular*

Disease and Lung Disease. Lung Biology in Health and Disease. Marcel Dekkar, New York, pp. 181–197.

Harding, J.E., Liu, L., Evans, P.C. and Gluckman, P.D. (1994) Insulin-like growth factor 1 alters feto-placental protein and carbohydrate metabolism in fetal sheep. *Endocrinology* 134, 1509–1514.

Harding, J.E., Evans, P.C. and Gluckman, P.D. (1997) Maternal growth hormone treatment increases placental diffusion capacity but not fetal or placental growth in sheep. *Endocrinology* 138, 5352–5358.

Hawkins, P., Crowe, C., Clader, N.A., Saito, T., Ozaki, T., Stratford, L.L., Noakes, D.E. and Hanson, M.A. (1997) Cardiovascular development in late gestation fetal sheep and young lambs following modest maternal nutrient restriction in early gestation. *Journal of Physiology* 505, 18P.

Hawkins, P., Steyn, C., McGarrigle, H.H., Saito, T., Ozaki, T., Stratford, L.L., Noakes, D.E. and Hanson, M.A. (1999) Effect of maternal nutrient restriction in early gestation on development of the hypothalamic–pituitary–adrenal axis in fetal sheep at 0.8–0.9 of gestation. *Journal of Endocrinology* 163, 553–561.

Hawkins, P., Oliver, M.H., Gluckman, P.D. and Harding, J.E. (2000a) Periconceptual maternal undernutrition alters fetal growth and length of gestation in sheep. *Proceedings of the Fourth Annual Congress of the Perinatal Society of Australia and New Zealand.* The Perinatal Society of Australia and New Zealand, Parramatta, Australia, p. 43

Hawkins, P., Steyn, C., Ozaki, T., Saito, T., Noakes, D.E. and Hanson, M.A. (2000b) Effect of maternal undernutrition in early gestation on ovine fetal blood pressure and cardiovascular reflexes. *American Journal of Physiology* 279, R340–R348.

Heasman, L., Clarke, L., Firth, K., Stephenson, T. and Symonds, M.E. (1998) Influence of restricted maternal nutrition in early to mid gestation on placental and fetal development at term in sheep. *Pediatric Research* 44, 546–551.

Hoet, J.J. and Hanson, M.A. (1999) Intrauterine nutrition: Its importance during critical periods for cardiovascular and endocrine development. *Journal of Physiology* 514, 617–627.

Huxley, R.R., Shiell, A.W. and Law, C.M. (2000) The role of size at birth and postnatal catch-up growth in determining systolic blood pressure: a systematic review of the literature. *Journal of Hypertension* 18, 815–831.

Illsley, N.P., Sellers, M.C. and Wright, R.L. (1998) Glycaemic regulation of glucose transporter expression and activity in the human placenta. *Placenta* 19, 517–524.

Iwamoto, H.S., Murray, M.A. and Chernausek, S.D. (1992) Effects of acute hypoxemia on insulin-like growth factors and their binding proteins in fetal sheep. *American Journal of Physiology* 263, E1151–E1156.

Jackson, A.A. (1991) The glycine story. *European Journal of Clinical Nutrition* 45, 59–65.

Jackson, A.A., Persaud, C., Werkmeister, G., McClelland, I.S., Badaloo, A. and Forrester, T. (1997) Comparison of urinary 5-L-oxoproline (L-pyroglutamate) during normal pregnancy in women in England and Jamaica. *British Journal of Nutrition* 77, 183–196.

Jackson, A.A., Dunn, R.L., Marchand, M.C. and Langley-Evans, S.C. (2002) Increased systolic blood pressure in rats induced by maternal low-protein diet is reversed by dietary supplementation with glycine. *Clinical Science* 103, 633–639.

Jenkinson, C.M., Min, S.H., MacKenzie, D.D., McCutcheon, S.N., Breier, B.H. and Gluckman, P.D. (1999) Placental development and fetal growth in growth hormone-treated ewes. *Growth Hormone and IGF Research* 9, 11–17.

Kadyrov, M., Kosanke, G., Kingdom, J. and Kaufmann, P. (1998) Increased fetoplacental angiogenesis during first trimester in anaemic women. *Lancet* 352, 1747–1749.

Kelly, R.W. (1992) Nutrition and placental development. *Proceedings of the Nutrition Society of Australia* 17, 203–211.

Kelly, R.W. and Newnham, J.P. (1990) Nutrition of the pregnant ewe. In: Oldham, C.M., Martin, G.B. and Purvis, I.W. (eds) *Reproductive Physiology of Merino Sheep. Concepts and Consequences*. School of Agriculture (Animal Science) The University of Western Australia, pp. 161–168.

Kind, K.L., Clifton, P.M., Grant, P.A., Owens, P.C., Sohlstrom, A., Roberts, C.T., Robinson, J.S. and Owens, J.A. (2003) Effect of maternal feed restriction during pregnancy on glucose tolerance in the adult guinea pig. *American Journal of Physiology* 284, R140–R152.

Kleemann, D.O., Walker, S.K., Hartwich, K.M., Fong, L., Seamark, R.F., Robinson, J.S. and Owens, J.A. (2001) Fetoplacental growth in sheep administered progesterone during the first three days of pregnancy. *Placenta* 22, 14–23.

Kramer, M.S. (1987) Determinants of low birth weight: methodological assessment and meta-analysis. *Bulletin of the World Health Organization* 65, 663–737.

Kramer, M.S. (2002a) Balanced protein/energy supplementation in pregnancy. *Cochrane Database of Systematic Reviews*.

Kramer, M.S. (2002b) High protein supplementation in pregnancy. *Cochrane Database of Systematic Reviews*.

Kramer, M.S., McLean, F.H., Olivier, M., Willis, D.M. and Usher, R.H. (1989) Body proportionality and head and length'sparing' in growth-retarded neonates: a critical reappraisal. *Pediatrics* 84, 717–723.

Kwong, W.Y., Wild, A.E., Roberts, P., Willis, A.C. and Fleming, T.P. (2000) Maternal undernutrition during the preimplantation period of rat development causes blastocyst abnormalities and programming of postnatal hypertension. *Development* 127, 4195–4202.

Langley, S.C. and Jackson, A.A. (1994) Increased systolic blood pressure in adult rats induced by fetal exposure to maternal low protein diets. *Clinical Science* 86, 217–222.

Lao, T.T. and Wong, W.M. (1997) Placental ratio – its relationship with mild maternal anaemia. *Placenta* 18, 593–596.

Lechtig, A., Yarbrough, C., Delgado, H., Habicht, J.P., Martorell, R. and Klein, R.E. (1975) Influence of maternal nutrition on birth weight. *American Journal of Clinical Nutrition* 28, 1223–1233.

Leeda, M., Riyazi, N., de Vries, J.I., Jakobs, C., van Geijn, H.P. and Dekker, G.A. (1998) Effects of folic acid and vitamin B6 supplementation on women with hyperhomocysteinemia and a history of pre-eclampsia or fetal growth restriction. *American Journal of Obstetrics and Gynecology* 179, 135–139.

Liu, L., Harding, J.E., Evans, P.C. and Gluckman, P.D. (1994) Maternal insulin-like growth factor-I infusion alters feto-placental carbohydrate and protein metabolism in pregnant sheep. *Endocrinology* 135, 895–900.

Lok, F., Owens, J.A., Mundy, L., Robinson, J.S. and Owens, P.C. (1996) Insulin-like growth factor I promotes growth selectively in fetal sheep in late gestation. *American Journal of Physiology* 270, R1148–R1155.

Lumey, L.H. (1998) Compensatory placental growth after restricted maternal nutrition in early pregnancy. *Placenta* 19, 105–111.

Lumey, L.H., Ravelli, A.C., Wiessing, L.G., Koppe, J.G., Treffers, P.E. and Stein, Z.A. (1993) The Dutch famine birth cohort study: design, validation of exposure, and selected characteristics of subjects after 43 years follow up. *Paediatrics and Perinatal Epidemiology* 7, 354–367.

Ma, J., Stampfer, M.J., Hennekens, C.H., Frosst, P., Selhub, J., Horsford, J., Malinow, M.R., Willett, W.C. and Rozen, R. (1996) Methylenetetrahydrofolate reductase polymorphism, plasma folate, homocysteine, and risk of myocardial infaction in US physicians. *Circulation* 94, 2410–2416.

Mahendran, D., Donnai, P., Glazier, J.D., D'Souza, S.W., Boyd, R.D.H. and Sibley, C.P. (1993) Amino acid (system A) transporter activity in microvillous membrane vesicles from the placentas of appropriate and small for gestational age babies. *Pediatric Research* 34, 661–665.

Makarewicz, W. and Swierczynski, J. (1988) Phosphate-dependent glutaminase in the human term placental mitochondria. *Biochemical Medicine and Metabolic Biology* 39, 273–278.

Martyn, C.N., Barker, D.J. and Osmond, C. (1996) Mothers' pelvic size, fetal growth, and death from stroke and coronary heart disease in men in the UK. *Lancet* 348, 1264–1268.

Mathews, F., Yudkin, P. and Neil, A. (1999) Influence of maternal nutrition on outcome of pregnancy: prospective cohort study. British Medical Journal 319, 339–343.

Meakins, T.S., Persaud, C. and Jackson, A.A. (1998) Dietary supplementation with L-methonine impairs the utilization of urea-nitrogen and increases 5-L-oxoprolinuria in normal women consuming a low protein diet. *Journal of Nutrition* 128, 720–727.

Meyenburg, M., Bartnicki, J. and Saling, E. (1991) The effect of maternal oxygen administration on fetal and maternal blood flow values using Doppler ultrasonography. Journal of Perinatal Medicine 19, 185–190.

Min, S.H., MacKenzie, D.D.S., Breier, B.H., McCutcheon, S.N. and Gluckman, P.D. (1996) Growth promoting effects of ovine placental lactogen (oPL) in young lambs: Comparison with bovine growth hormone provides evidence for a distinct effect of oPL and food intake. *Growth Regulation* 6, 144–151.

Miodovnik, M., Lavin, J.P., Harrington, D.J., Leung, L.S., Seeds, A.E. and Clark, K.E. (1982) Effect of maternal ketoacidemia on the pregnant ewe and the fetus. *American Journal of Obstetrics and Gynecology* 144, 585–593.

Moores, R.R., Rietberg, C.C., Battaglia, F.C., Fennessey, P.V. and Meschia, G. (1993) Metabolism and transport of maternal serine by the ovine placenta: Glycine production and absence of serine transport into the fetus. *Pediatric Research* 33, 590–594.

Morgan, H.D., Sutherland, H.G., Martin, D.I. and Whitelaw, E. (1999) Epigenetic inheritance at the agouti locus in the mouse. *Nature Genetics* 23, 314–318.

Narkewicz, M.R., Jones, G., Thompson, H., Kolhouse, F. and Fennessey, P.V. (2002) Folate cofactors regulate serine metabolism in fetal ovine hepatocytes. *Pediatric Research* 52, 589–594.

Nicolaides, K.H., Economides, D.L. and Soothill, P.W. (1989) Blood gases, pH and lactate in appropriate- and small-for-gestational-age fetuses. *American Journal of Obstetrics and Gynecology* 161, 996–1001.

Obwegser, R., Hohlagschwandtner, M. and Sinzinger, H. (1999) Homocysteine – a pathophysiological cornerstone in obstetrical and gynaecological disorders? *Human Reproduction Update* 5, 64–72.

Oliver, M.H., Harding, J.E., Breier, B.H., Evans, P.C. and Gluckman, P.D. (1992) The nutritional regulation of circulating placental lactogen in fetal sheep. *Pediatric Research* 31, 520–523.

Oliver, M.H., Harding, J.E., Breier, B.H., Evans, P.C. and Gluckman, P.D. (1993) Glucose but not a mixed amino acid infusion regulates plasma insulin-like growth factor-I concentrations in fetal sheep. *Pediatric Research* 34, 62–65.

Oliver, M.H., Harding, J.E., Breier, B.H. and Gluckman, P.D. (1996) Fetal insulin-like growth factor (IGF)-I and IGF-II are regulated differently by glucose or insulin in the sheep fetus. *Reproduction, Fertility and Development* 8, 167–172.

Oliver, M.H., Hawkins, P., Gluckman, P.D. and Harding, J.E. (2000) Undernutrition in the periconceptual period influences metabolic responses of fetal sheep to maternal fasting in late gestation. *Proceedings of the Fourth Annual Congress of the Perinatal Society of Australia and New Zealand*. The Perinatal Society of Australia and New Zealand, Parramatta, Australia, p. 92.

Oliver, M.H., Hawkins, P., Breier, B.H., van Zijl, P.L., Sargison, S.A. and Harding, J.E. (2001a) Maternal undernutrition during the periconceptual period increases plasma taurine levels and insulin response to glucose but not arginine in the late gestation fetal sheep. *Endocrinology* 142, 4576–4579.

Oliver, M.H., Harding, J.E. and Gluckman, P.D. (2001b) Duration of maternal undernutrition in late gestation determines the reversibility of intrauterine growth restriction in sheep. *Prenatal and Neonatal Medicine* 6, 271–279.

Oliver, M.H., Breier, B.H., Gluckman, P.D. and Harding, J.E. (2002) Birthweight rather than maternal nutrition influences glucose tolerance, blood pressure and IGF-1 levels in sheep. *Pediatric Research* 52, 516–524.

Owens, J.A., Falconer, J. and Robinson, J.S. (1987a) Effect of restriction of placental growth on oxygen delivery to and consumption by the pregnant uterus and fetus. *Journal of Developmental Physiology* 9, 137–150.

Owens, J.A., Falconer, J. and Robinson, J.S. (1987b) Effect of restriction of placental growth on fetal and utero-placental metabolism. *Journal of Developmental Physiology* 9, 225–238.

Owens, J.A., Owens, P.C. and Robinson, J.S. (1989) Experimental fetal growth retardation: metabolic and endocrine aspects. In: Gluckman, P.D., Johnston, B. and Nathanielsz, P.W. (eds) *Advances in Fetal Physiology: Reviews in Honor of G.C. Liggins*. Perinatology Press, Ithaca, New York, pp. 263–286.

Owens, J.A., Kind, K., Sohlstrom, A., Owens, P.C. and Robinson, J.S. (1996) *Nutritional Programming of Fetal and Placental Phenotype and Later Outcomes: Lessons from the Sheep and Guinea-pig*. Frontiers in Maternal, Fetal and Neonatal Health. Programming for a Life-time of Health., Cornell University, Ithaca, New York.

Palmer, R.M., Thom, A. and Flint, D.J. (1996) Repartitioning of maternal muscle protein towards the foetus induced by a polyclonal antiserum to rat GH. *Journal of Endocrinology* 151, 395–400.

Paterson, P., Sheath, J., Taft, P. and Wood, C. (1967) Maternal and foetal ketone concentrations in plasma and urine. *Lancet* 1, 862–865.

Persson, E. and Jansson, T. (1992) Low birth weight is associated with elevated adult blood pressure in the chronically catheterised guinea pig. *Acta Physiologica Scandinavica* 145, 195–196.

Petrik, J., Reusens, B., Arany, E., Remacle, C., Coelho, C., Hoet, J.J. and Hill, D.J. (1999) A low protein diet alters the balance of islet cell replication and apoptosis in the fetal and neonatal rat and is associated with a reduced pancreatic expression of insulin-like growth factor-II. *Endocrinology* 140, 4861–4873.

Polani, P.E. (1974) Chromosomal and other genetic influences on birth weight variation. In: Elliot, K. and Knight, J. (eds) *Size at Birth*. Elsevier-Excerpta Medica-North Holland, Amsterdam, pp. 127–159.

Pond, W.G., Maurer, R.R. and Klindt, J. (1991) Fetal organ response to maternal protein deprivation during pregnancy in swine. *Journal of Nutrition* 121, 504–509.

Rao, S., Yajnik, C.S., Kanade, A., Fall, C.H.D., Margetts, B.M., Jackson, A.A., Shier, R., Joshi, S., Rege, S., Lubree, H. and Desai, B. (2001) Intake of micronutrient-rich foods in rural Indian mothers is associated with the size of their babies at birth: Pune maternal nutrition study. *Journal of Nutrition* 131, 1217–1224.

Ravelli, A.C., van der Meulen, J.H., Michels, R.P., Osmond, C., Barker, D.J., Hales, C.N. and Bleker, O.P. (1998) Glucose tolerance in adults after prenatal exposure to famine. *Lancet* 351, 173–177.

Ravelli, A.C., van der Meulen, J.H., Osmond, C., Barker, D.J. and Bleker, O.P. (1999) Obesity at the age of 50 y in men and women exposed to famine prenatally. *American Journal of Clinical Nutrition* 70, 811–816.

Ravelli, G.-P., Stein, Z.A. and Susser, M.W. (1976) Obesity in young men after famine exposure in utero and early infancy. *New England Journal of Medicine* 295, 349–353.

Rees, W.D. (2002) Manipulating the sulfur amino acid content of the early diet and its implications for long-term health. *Proceedings of the Nutrition Society* 61, 71–77.

Rees, W.D., Hay, S.M., Brown, D.S., Antipatis, C. and Palmer, R.M. (2000) Maternal protein deficiency causes hypermethylation of DNA in the livers of rat fetuses. *Journal of Nutrition* 130, 1821–1826.

Roberts, C.T., Sohlstrom, A., Kind, K.L., Earl, R.A., Khong, T.Y., Robinson, J.S., Owens, P.C. and Owens, J.A. (2001) Maternal food restriction reduces the exchange surface area and increases the barrier thickness of the placenta in the guinea-pig. *Placenta* 22, 177–185.

Robinson, J.S., Owens, J.A., De Barro, T., Lok, F. and Chidzanja, S. (1994) Maternal nutrition and fetal growth. In: Ward, R.H.T., Smith, S.K. and Donnai, D. (eds) *Early Fetal Growth and Development*. RCOG Press, London, pp. 317–329.

Rogers, I. and Emmett, P. (1998) Diet during pregnancy in a population of pregnant women in South West England. ALSPAC Study Team. Avon Longitudinal Study of Pregnancy and Childhood. *European Journal of Clinical Nutrition* 52, 246–250.

Roseboom, T.J., van der Meulen, J.H., Osmond, C., Barker, D.J.P., Ravelli, A.C. and Bleker, O.P. (2000a) Plasma lipid profiles in adults after prenatal exposure to the Dutch famine. *American Journal of Clinical Nutrition* 72, 1101–1106.

Roseboom, T.J., van der Meulen, J.H., Ravelli, A.C., Osmond, C., Barker, D.J.P. and Bleker, O.P. (2000b) Plasma fibrinogen and factor VII concentrations in adults after prenatal exposure to famine. *British Journal of Haematology* 111, 112–117.

Roseboom, T.J., van der Meulen, J.H., Osmond, C., Barker, D.J., Ravelli, A.C., Schroeder-Tanka, J.M., van Montfrans, G.A., Michels, R.P. and Bleker, O.P. (2000c) Coronary heart disease after prenatal exposure to the Dutch famine, 1944–45. *Heart* 84, 595–598.

Roseboom, T.J., van der Meulen, J.H., van Montfrans, G.A., Ravelli, A.C., Osmond, C., Barker, D.J.P. and Bleker, O.P. (2001a) Maternal nutrition during gestation and adult blood pressure. *Journal of Hypertension*, 19, 29–34.

Roseboom, T.J., van der Meulen, J.H., Ravelli, A.C., Osmond, C., Barker, D.J.P. and Bleker, O.P. (2001b) Effects of prenatal exposure to the Dutch famine on adult disease in later life: an overview. *Molecular and Cellular Endocrinology* 185, 93–98.

Saleh, A.K., Al-Muhtaseb, N., Gumaa, K.A. and Shaker, M.S. (1989) Maternal, amniotic fluid and cord blood metabolic profile in normal pregnancy and gestational diabetics during recurrent withholding of food. *Hormone and Metabolic Research* 21, 507–513.

Sara, V.R. and Lazarus, L. (1975) Maternal growth hormone and growth and function. *Developmental Psychobiology* 8, 489–502.

Schofield, C., Stewart, J. and Wheeler, E. (1989) The diets of pregnant and post-pregnant women in different social groups in London and Edinburgh: calcium, iron, retinol, ascorbic acid and folic acid. *British Journal of Nutrition* 62, 363–377.

Seckl, J.R. (2001) Glucocorticoid programming of the fetus; adult phenotypes and molecular mechanisms. *Molecular and Cellular Endocrinology* 185, 61–71.

Shiell, A.W., Campbell, D.M., Hall, M.H. and Barker, D.J. (2000) Diet in late pregnancy and glucose–insulin metabolism of the offspring 40 years later. *British Journal of Obstetrics and Gynaecology* 107, 890–895.

Sibley, C., Glazier, J.D. and D'Souza, S. (1997) Placental transporter activity and expression in relation to fetal growth. *Experimental Physiology* 82, 389–402.

Smeaton, T.C., Owens, J.A., Kind, K.L. and Robinson, J.S. (1989) The placenta releases branched-chain keto acids into the umbilical and uterine cirulations in the pregnant sheep. *Journal of Developmental Physiology* 12, 95–99.

Smith, G.C.S., Malcolm, M.D., Smith, F.S., McNay, M.B. and Fleming, J.E.E. (1998) First-trimester growth and the risk of low birth weight. *New England Journal of Medicine* 339, 1817–1822.

Snow, M.H.L. (1989) Effect of genome on size at birth. In: Sharp, F., Fraser, R.B. and Milner, R.D.G. (eds) *Fetal Growth*. Royal College of Obstetricians and Gynaecologists, London, pp. 3–12.

Stein, C.E., Fall, C.H., Kumaran, K., Osmond, C., Cox, V. and Barker, D.J.P. (1996) Fetal growth and coronary heart disease in South India. *Lancet* 348, 1269–1273.

Sturman, J.A. (1993) Taurine in development. *Physiological Reviews* 73, 119–147.

Thame, M., Wilks, R.J., McFarlane-Anderson, N., Bennett, F.I. and Forrester, T.E. (1997) Relationship between maternal nutritional status and infant's weight and body proportions at birth. *European Journal of Clinical Nutrition* 51, 134–138.

Thornburg, K.L. (2001) Physiological development of the cardiovascular system *in utero*. In: Barker, D.J. (ed.) *Fetal Origins of Cardiovascular and Lung Disease. Lung Biology in Health and Disease*, Vol. 15. Marcel Dekker, New York, pp. 97–139.

Thornburg, K.L. and Morton, M.J. (1994) Development of the cardiovascular system. In: Thorburn, G.D. and Harding, R. (eds) *Textbook of Fetal Physiology*. Oxford University Press, Oxford, UK, pp. 95–130.

Thorstensen, E.B., Harding, J.E. and Evans, P.C. (1995) β-Hydroxybutyrate may be a placental substrate during undernutrition. *New Zealand and Australian Perinatal Societies' Annual Scientific Meeting, Auckland, New Zealand*, A158.

Van Goudoever, J.B., Sulkers, E.J., Halliday, D., Degenhart, H.J., Carnielli, V.P., Wattimena, J.L. and Sauer, P.J. (1995) Whole-body protein turnover in preterm appropriate for gestational age and small for gestational age infants: Comparison of [^{15}N]glycine and [1–^{13}C]leucine administered simultaneously. *Pediatric Research* 37, 381–388.

van Zijl, P.L., Oliver, M.H. and Harding, J.E. (2002) Periconceptual undernutrition in sheep leads to longterm changes in maternal amino acid concentrations. *Perinatal Society of Australia and New Zealand 6th Annual Congress and Federation of the Asia and Oceania Perinatal Societies' 12th Congress, Christchurch, New Zealand*, p. 191.

Vaughn, P.R., Lobo, C., Battaglia, F.C., Fennessey, P.V., Wilkening, R.B. and Meschia, G. (1995) Glutamine–glutamate exchange between placenta and fetal liver. *American Journal of Physiology* 268, E705–E711.

Wallace, J.M., Bourke, D.A., Aitken, R.P. and Cruikshank, M.A. (1999) Switching maternal nutrient intake at the end of the first trimester has profound effects on placental development and fetal growth in adolescent ewes carrying singleton fetuses. *Biology of Reproduction* 61, 101–110.

Wallace, J., Bourke, D., Da Silva, P. and Aitken, R. (2001) Nutrient partitioning during adolescent pregnancy. *Reproduction* 122, 347–357.

Walton, A. and Hammond, J. (1938) The maternal effects on growth and conformation in Shire horse–Shetland pony crosses. *Proceedings of the Royal Society of London – Series B: Biological Sciences* 125, 311–335.

Wolff, G.L., Kodell, R.L., Moore, S.R. and Cooney, C.A. (1998) Maternal epigenetics and methyl supplements affect agouti gene expression in A^{vy}/a mice. *FASEB Journal* 12, 949–957.

3 Intrauterine Hypoxaemia and Cardiovascular Development

DINO A. GIUSSANI[1],* AND DAVID S. GARDNER[2]

[1]Department of Physiology, University of Cambridge, Downing Street, Cambridge, UK; [2]Academic Division of Child Health, School of Human Development, Queen's Medical Centre, University Hospital, Nottingham NG7 2UH, UK

The Fetal Cardiovascular Response to Acute Hypoxaemia

One of the most common challenges that a fetus faces during gestation is an episode of oxygen deprivation or acute hypoxaemia. In simple terms, the fetal cardiovascular defence against acute hypoxaemia is represented by three changes: changes in heart rate, changes in arterial blood pressure and changes in the distribution of the fetal cardiac output to the various organs. These are survival adaptations that ensure the maintenance of normal oxidative metabolism and critical organ functions. The pattern and magnitude of the fetal heart, blood pressure and circulatory defence responses to acute hypoxaemia are dependent on the stage of gestation at which the challenge occurs and, consequently, the maturity of the mechanisms that mediate them. Traditionally, the fetal cardiovascular responses to acute hypoxaemia have been studied in the late gestation sheep fetus, i.e. past 120 days out of a 145–150-day term for most ovine breeds. However, a few studies have concentrated on the fetal cardiovascular responses to an episode of oxygen deprivation earlier in gestation and also as the fetus approaches term, just prior to birth (Boddy *et al.*, 1974; Iwamoto *et al.*, 1989; Fletcher, 2001; Gunn *et al.*, 2001).

Fetal heart and blood pressure responses to acute hypoxaemia

In the fetus, the ventricles beat in parallel as opposed to in series, since the double circulation through the lungs is not yet established. As a result, in the fetal period, the cardiac output is usually referred to as the combined ventricular output. When the immature sheep fetus is exposed to a 1 h episode of acute

---

* Fellow of the Lister Institute for Preventive Medicine.

hypoxaemia (reducing its P_aO_2 from a baseline of approximately 24 mmHg to
c. 13 mmHg) between 80 and 100 days of gestation, there is either no
change (< 90 days) or an increase (< 100 days) in fetal heart rate, and fetal
blood pressure usually remains unaltered from baseline (Boddy et al., 1974;
Iwamoto et al., 1989). The absence of a hypertensive response to acute hypoxaemia in the young sheep fetus may be related to a decrease in the combined
ventricular output. Although heart rate can sometimes increase, the reduced
stroke volume usually favours a fall in ventricular output (Iwamoto et al., 1989).
In contrast, an episode of acute hypoxaemia of similar magnitude and duration
in fetuses older than approximately 120 days of gestation invariably induces
a transient fall in fetal heart rate and a gradual increase in fetal arterial blood
pressure (Boddy et al., 1974; Cohn et al., 1974; Iwamoto et al., 1989; Giussani
et al., 1994a). The mature fetal bradycardic response to episodes of reduced
oxygenation has also been shown in the human fetus during acute hypoxaemia
secondary to uterine contractions during the actual processes of labour and
delivery (Beard and Rivers, 1979). Bradycardia during reduced oxygenation
also occurs in fetuses of other species, such as the rhesus monkey (Jackson et al.,
1987), cat, guinea-pig, rabbit (Rosen and Kjellmer, 1975; Javorka et al., 1978),
llama (Llanos et al., 1995; Giussani et al., 1996; Giussani et al., 1999a), dog
(Monheit et al., 1988), seal (Liggins et al., 1980), and even in embryonic chicks
(Tazawa, 1981; Mulder et al., 1998) and alligators (Warburton et al., 1995) in
late incubation.

Fetal circulatory response to acute hypoxaemia

In similar fashion to the fetal heart and blood pressure responses, the distribution
of the combined ventricular output during episodes of acute hypoxaemia
of equivalent magnitude and duration also differs between the early- and
late-gestation sheep fetus.

   Using the microsphere technique, it has been shown that prior to 110 days
of gestational age, there are no changes in vascular resistance or blood flow in
the fetal carcass (taken to mean muscle and skin of the limbs and trunk), but
reduced vascular resistance, thereby allowing increased blood flow in the cerebral, myocardial and adrenal circulations (Boddy et al., 1974; Cohn et al., 1974;
Iwamoto et al., 1989). In contrast, at gestational ages greater than 110 days, a
similar degree of fetal hypoxaemia leads to pronounced vasoconstriction in the
carcass, the gastrointestinal tract, the spleen, the kidney and the lungs, shunting
blood flow away from the peripheral circulations towards the cerebral, myocardial and adrenal vascular beds (Cohn et al., 1974; Sheldon et al., 1979;
Jensen and Berger, 1993). Importantly, studies by Jensen and colleagues
(Jensen et al., 1987) have provided evidence that the amount of oxygen
delivered to peripheral organs determines the amount of oxygen consumed by
these organs. Therefore, during a shortage of oxygen supply, peripheral vasoconstrictor responses reduce oxygen delivery to, and consumption by, peripheral
tissues, ensuring the maintenance of oxidative metabolism in central organs.
However, during periods of moderate hypoxaemia, the cerebral circulation of

the fetus does not autoregulate. Thus, during moderate hypoxaemic conditions, there is a linear relationship between arterial blood pressure and cerebral blood flow in the range of blood pressures over which autoregulation is normally demonstrated (Purves and James, 1969).

During acute hypoxaemia there is also a redistribution of blood flow within the fetal brain, as the increase in blood flow to the brainstem is greater than that seen in other regions (Carter and Gu, 1988; Richardson *et al.*, 1989). This redistribution of blood flow within the brain is an obvious survival mechanism *in utero*, permitting neuronal activity to be maintained in important control centres in the fetal brainstem. Myocardial blood flow is also linearly related to the reciprocal of P_aO_2 (partial pressure of oxygen in arterial blood), permitting the fetus to maintain a constant oxygen delivery to, and oxygen consumption by, the myocardium during normal oxygenation and hypoxaemia (Peeters *et al.*, 1979; Rudolph, 1984). When the fetal P_aO_2 is reduced by c. 50%, myocardial blood flow is increased two- to threefold to maintain myocardial oxygen delivery (Cohn *et al.*, 1974; Sheldon *et al.*, 1979). During basal conditions, adrenal medullary flow is twice as high as adrenal cortical blood flow, and during acute hypoxaemia, the increment from baseline within the two areas appears to be similar (Jensen and Berger, 1991).

Using transit-time flowmetry, the redistribution of the fetal combined ventricular output can also be indexed by a fall in carotid vascular resistance, which increases carotid blood flow, and an increase in femoral vascular resistance, which decreases femoral blood flow (Giussani *et al.*, 1993) (Fig. 3.1). The femoral vasoconstriction also aids the shunting of blood flow away from peripheral circulations, promoting the redistribution of oxygenated blood towards hypoxia-sensitive organs.

As with the fetal heart rate response to lack of oxygen, the redistribution of the combined ventricular output during episodes of acute hypoxaemia has also been demonstrated in the human and non-human primate fetus, fetuses of other mammalian species, and in non-mammalian animals, such as in the avian and reptile embryos. Studies of the distribution of the combined ventricular output in the non-human primate fetus are usually complicated by the additional effects of local anaesthesia, and there are few studies of blood flow distribution under basal conditions (Behrman and Lees, 1971; Paton *et al.*, 1973), and even fewer during acute hypoxaemia (Paton *et al.*, 1973; Jackson *et al.*, 1987). However, the scant studies of fetal rhesus monkeys (Jackson *et al.*, 1987) and fetal baboons (Paton *et al.*, 1973) report a redistribution of the combined ventricular output in favour of the cerebral and myocardial circulations at the expense of peripheral circulations, such as the lung. Recent studies in the chicken embryo suggest it to be a novel model for the study of fetal cardiovascular regulation under adverse conditions as, unlike other species, the direct effects of hypoxaemia on fetal physiology can be assessed in the absence of a functional placenta and thus the concomitant perturbations in fetal nutrient supply and maternal or placental hormones. Mulder *et al.* (1998) reported a significant redistribution of the combined ventricular output during acute hypoxaemia in the chick embryo after 13 days out of a 21-day incubation period. During hypoxaemia, the fractions of the combined ventricular output directed to the

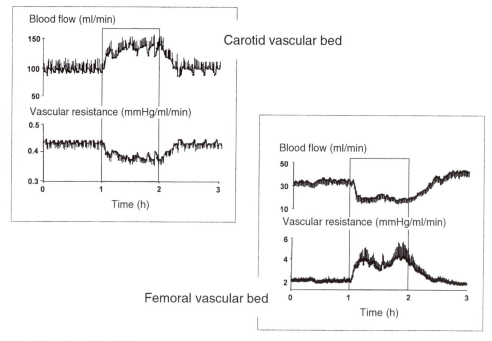

Fig. 3.1. Carotid and femoral haemodynamic changes during acute hypoxaemia in the sheep fetus. Values represent the mean ± SEM calculated every minute for eight fetal sheep at 125–130 days of gestation. Note that the carotid vascular bed undergoes vasodilatation during acute hypoxaemia, as indexed by a fall in carotid vascular resistance and an increase in carotid blood flow. In marked contrast, the femoral vascular bed undergoes vasoconstriction, aiding the redistribution of blood flow away from peripheral circulations.

embryonic heart and brain increased at the expense of the intestine, liver, yolk-sac and carcass.

In human obstetric practice, fetal hypoxaemia secondary to impaired placental perfusion is associated with non-invasive Doppler evidence of redistribution in the fetal arterial circulation. This results in the 'brain-sparing effect', represented by falls in indices of impedance and resistance and an increase in the blood velocity in the common carotid and middle cerebral arteries, and reductions in blood velocities to the umbilical artery and descending aorta resulting from increases in impedance and resistance in those circulations (Bilardo *et al.*, 1988; Vyas *et al.*, 1990). Therefore, typically in obstetric medicine, an increase in the ratio of the resistance indices in central circulations (ascending aorta, carotid artery or middle cerebral artery) to those in peripheral circulations (descending aorta, umbilical, internal iliac or femoral arteries) is representative of redistribution of the fetal combined ventricular output in favour of the brain at the expense of the fetal trunk (Akalin-Sel and Campbell, 1992).

Umbilico-hepatic blood flow patterns and preferential streaming

The umbilical venous return supplies the fetus with oxygen and nutrients, and therefore the distribution of this flow has important consequences for oxygen and glucose delivery to the upper body organs during basal and hypoxaemic conditions. Early studies by Barclay *et al.* in 1939 and Rudolph and Heymann in 1967 showed that the umbilical venous blood, which is rich in oxygen as it comes directly from the placenta, is conducted to the inferior vena cava, where it is joined by the hepatic portal vein. From here, branches are provided to the left and right lobes of the liver, but blood flows principally through the ductus venosus, which connects the umbilical vein and the inferior vena cava. By injecting radionuclide-labelled microspheres into the tributaries of the portal and umbilical veins, Edelstone *et al.* (1978) measured the blood supply to the liver from different sources. They reported that under basal conditions 75–85% of hepatic blood flow is derived from the umbilical vein and only *c.* 3–4% of total liver blood flow is supplied by the hepatic artery, which provides blood to both lobes. The remaining flow, conducted to the right lobe of the liver, is derived from the portal vein. This hepatic shunt therefore permits the well-oxygenated umbilical venous blood to preferentially bypass the hepatic microcirculation.

During episodes of acute hypoxaemia, an increase in vascular resistance of the umbilical veins and the hepatic vasculature occurs, causing a pronounced fall in liver blood flow, which is characterized by a greater flow in the right than the left hepatic lobe (Bristow *et al.*, 1983). While constriction of the umbilical veins distends and recruits vessels in the placenta, thereby increasing the surface area for gaseous exchange (Edelstone, 1980), constriction of the hepatic vasculature enhances the shunting of blood flow through the ductus venosus, thus improving delivery of umbilical venous blood to the upper organs. In addition to facilitating oxygen delivery, preferential shunting patterns in the fetal circulation also result in higher concentrations in the ascending aortic blood of metabolic substrates, the most important of which is glucose (Charlton and Johengen, 1984).

When considering the overall change in umbilical blood flow in response to acute hypoxaemia, the scientific literature is scant and contradictory, reporting that umbilical blood flow is either maintained (Cohn *et al.*, 1974; Edelstone, 1980), increased (Goodwin, 1968), or even reduced (Dilts *et al.*, 1969) during the period of fetal oxygen deprivation. These contradictory reports are largely due to either point measurements of umbilical blood flow taken at varying periods following the onset of adverse intrauterine conditions, as with radio-active microspheres (Cohn *et al.*, 1974; Edelstone, 1980), or to measurement of umbilical flow in the exteriorized sheep fetus, with additional effects of anaesthesia (Dilts *et al.*, 1969). Clinically, indirect measurements of umbilical blood flow in human pregnancy, obtained by Doppler flow velocimetry, have also shown either an increase in the umbilical artery pulsatility index (PI), signifying an increase in umbilical vascular resistance (Muijsers *et al.*, 1990), or no significant change in the umbilical artery PI during episodes of hypoxaemia (Morrow *et al.*, 1990).

The haemodynamic responses of the umbilical vascular bed to an episode of acute stress in the fetus may not only change with time following the onset of the stress, but they may also be affected by anaesthesia. Further investigation of continuous, direct measurement of umbilical blood flow during basal and stressful intrauterine conditions is therefore a high priority. While most perinatologists accept that umbilical flow is remarkably constant and unresponsive to a variety of stresses, including fetal hypoxaemia, recent studies by Gardner *et al.* (2001a) have reported that continuous measurements of umbilical blood flow by an implanted Transonic flow probe around an umbilical artery within the fetal abdomen in chronically instrumented, unanaesthetized fetal sheep preparations show important changes in the umbilical circulation during hypoxaemic conditions. Minute-by-minute analyses revealed that there was a transient decrease in umbilical vascular conductance at the onset of hypoxaemia. Shortly after, however, a significant increase in umbilical blood flow occurred, which remained elevated for the duration of the hypoxaemic challenge (Fig. 3.2).

Mechanisms of the Fetal Cardiovascular Responses to Acute Hypoxaemia

Both the fetal heart and fetal circulation are under extensive intrinsic (local) and extrinsic (neural and endocrine) control. Historically, the chronological development of knowledge about mechanisms mediating the fetal heart and circulatory responses to acute hypoxaemia has shed information on neural, then endocrine and, finally, local pathways. Therefore it seems appropriate to discuss them in that order.

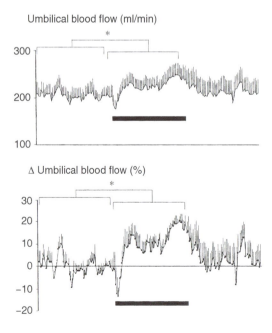

Fig. 3.2. Umbilical blood flow responses to acute hypoxaemia. The figure shows the umbilical haemodynamic response, represented by absolute values for mean umbilical blood flow and per cent changes from baseline of mean umbilical blood flow, during the acute hypoxaemia protocol in seven fetal sheep at *c.* 130 days of gestation. Cardiovascular data were averaged each minute during a baseline period (1 h normoxia), 1 h of hypoxaemia (bar) and 1 h of recovery. Significant differences are: *, $P < 0.05$, baseline versus hypoxaemia. (Modified from Gardner *et al.*, 2001a.)

Neural afferent and efferent control of fetal cardiovascular responses to acute hypoxaemia

It is now well established that carotid sinus nerve section alone abolishes the fetal bradycardia and the initial elevations in femoral vascular resistance and in perfusion pressure, but not the increase in carotid blood flow, observed in intact fetuses at the onset of acute hypoxaemia (Giussani *et al.*, 1993) (Fig. 3.3). These effects of carotid sinus nerve section were attributed to interruption of carotid chemoreflex, rather than baroreflex, signals, due to the relative timings of the fetal bradycardia and hypertensive responses to acute hypoxaemia: in the intact fetuses the initial episode of bradycardia occurred prior to any significant elevation in fetal arterial blood pressure (Giussani *et al.*, 1993). In agreement with this, Blanco *et al.* (1983) reported that after transection of the fetal spinal cord at L_1–L_2, acute hypoxaemia failed to elicit a significant elevation in arterial pressure, even though the initial fetal bradycardic response still occurred. Confirmation of this was achieved by Bartelds *et al.* (1993), who injected sodium cyanide into the caudal vena cava of fetuses in which the carotid or aortic bodies had been denervated. The injection was found to elicit bradycardia in the aortic-, but not carotid-, denervated fetuses. Taken together, the data from these studies demonstrate the importance of the fetal carotid chemoreceptors in initiating fetal heart rate and peripheral vasoconstrictor responses to acute hypoxaemia. Accordingly, fetal carotid sinus nerve section has been shown not only to abolish the initial rise in fetal femoral vascular resistance, but also to abolish the initial renal (Green *et al.*, 1997) and pulmonary (Moore and Hanson, 1991) vasoconstrictor responses to acute hypoxaemia in the sheep fetus at 0.8–0.9 of gestation.

Several studies have demonstrated the importance of chemoreflex-mediated changes in cardiac sympathetic and parasympathetic chronotropic drive in mediating the fetal heart rate responses at the onset of acute hypoxaemia. Establishment of sympathetic innervation of the fetal heart is known to occur between 85 and 100 days in the sheep (Lebowitz *et al.*, 1972), with chronotropic and inotropic responsiveness to isoprenaline being present as early as 60 (Nuwayhid *et al.*, 1975) and 90 (Rawashdeh *et al.*, 1988) days, respectively. Therefore, prior to *c.* 120 days, the relative influence of cholinergic mechanisms is less than later in gestation, and the balance of cholinergic and adrenergic inputs is such that there is no fetal bradycardia during hypoxaemia (Boddy *et al.*, 1974; Iwamoto *et al.*, 1989). However, in fetuses older than 120 days, fetal bradycardia at the onset of acute hypoxaemia is produced by carotid chemoreflex-mediated increases in efferent vagal activity (Giussani *et al.*, 1993, 1994a), resulting in relative dominance of cholinergic over adrenergic stimulation of the pacemaker centres of the heart (Fig. 3.4). Accordingly, the initial fetal bradycardia during an episode of acute hypoxaemia is abolished by carotid sinus nerve section (Bartelds *et al.*, 1993; Giussani *et al.*, 1993), vagotomy (Boddy *et al.*, 1974) or muscarinic acetylcholine receptor blockade using atropine (Cohn *et al.*, 1974; Parer, 1984; Giussani *et al.*, 1993). In addition, during very severe episodes of acute hypoxaemia, a component of the fetal bradycardia may be attributed to a direct depressive effect of tissue hypoxia in the myocardium (Lumbers *et al.*, 1986).

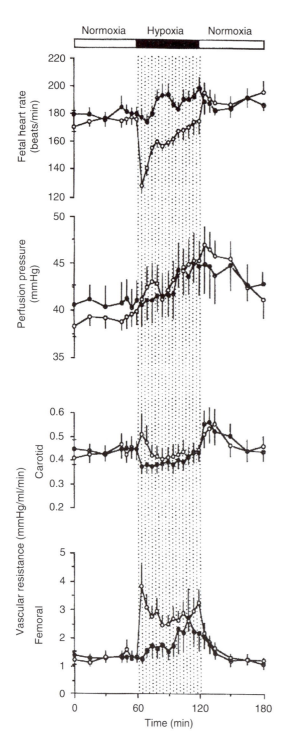

Fig. 3.3. Fetal heart rate, perfusion (arterial–venous) pressure and vascular resistance in the carotid and femoral vascular beds in intact (○) and carotid sinus-denervated (●) sheep fetuses during a 1 h episode of acute hypoxaemia (shaded area) at 118–125 days of gestation. Values are mean + SEM. (Taken from Giussani *et al.*, 1993.)

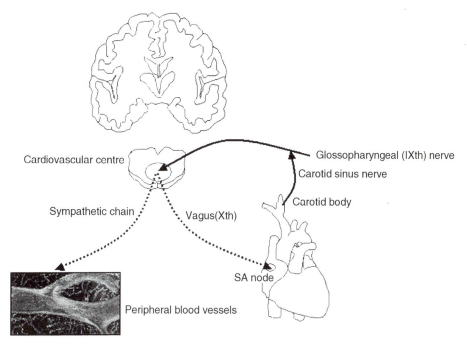

Fig. 3.4. Carotid chemoreflex pathways in the fetus. Diagrammatic representation of the fetal carotid chemoreflex showing the principal afferent (solid lines) and efferent (dashed lines) pathways controlling cardiac and peripheral vasomotor responses during acute hypoxaemia.

Fetal chemoreflexes are also important in initiating peripheral vasoconstriction during acute hypoxaemia (Giussani *et al.*, 1993). In response to an episode of acute hypoxaemia, carotid chemoreflexes activate the sympathetic nervous system, resulting in increases in peripheral vascular tone (Fig. 3.4). This includes femoral vasoconstriction, which is mediated by α-adrenergic efferents (Reuss *et al.*, 1982; Giussani *et al.*, 1993) and which is used as an index of the redistribution of blood flow away from the peripheral vasculature (Okamura *et al.*, 1992; Giussani *et al.*, 1996). Several lines of experimental evidence emphasize the importance of intact sympathetic nervous system efferents in mediating redistribution of the fetal cardiovascular output (CVO) and increasing peripheral vascular tone during acute stress. Dawes (1968) demonstrated that sectioning of the sciatic nerves abolished the normal asphyxia-induced fall in femoral blood flow present in intact fetuses. More recently, it has been shown that the increment in fetal femoral vascular resistance during acute hypoxaemia is attenuated with carotid sinus nerve section or fetal treatment with phentolamine, whereas combination of both interventions invariably leads to fetal death (Giussani *et al.*, 1993).

In sympathetic nerve terminals, noradrenaline is co-localized with neuropeptide Y (NPY) (Allen *et al.*, 1983), and this peptide may be co-released with noradrenaline, depending on the frequency and pattern of nerve stimulation

(Bloom et al., 1988). In the adult, NPY is known to have a wide variety of actions; however, one of its earliest actions described in the literature is of potent and long-lasting vasoconstriction, either via a direct effect on NPY-Y$_1$ receptors in peripheral circulations or by potentiation of the vasopressor effects of constrictor agents, such as catecholamines (Edvinsson et al., 1984). Recent evidence suggests that sympathetic release of NPY may also contribute to the peripheral vasoconstrictor response to episodes of acute oxygen deprivation in the fetus, particularly during severe hypoxaemic conditions (Fletcher et al., 2000; Sanhueza et al., 2003).

Endocrine control of fetal cardiovascular responses to acute hypoxaemia

Once the fetal cardiovascular responses to acute hypoxaemia have been initiated by activation of fetal chemoreflex pathways, maintenance, modification or reversal of these responses may then occur, with the subsequent release of humoral agents into the fetal circulation. These include the secretion of vasoconstrictor hormones (e.g. catecholamines, arginine vasopressin and angiotensin II) to reinforce the peripheral vasoconstriction and redistribution of the fetal CVO, as well as other humoral agents (e.g. catecholamines and cortisol) that promote changes in fetal metabolism to enhance survival during the period of reduced oxygen availability (Giussani et al., 1994a; Hooper, 1995).

During the last third of gestation, episodes of acute hypoxaemia elicit increases in ovine fetal plasma noradrenaline and adrenaline concentrations (Jones and Robinson, 1975). Levels of both noradrenaline and adrenaline have been shown to be increased significantly by 5 min of hypoxaemia, and show strong inverse exponential correlation with the P_aO_2 achieved (Cohen et al., 1982). The fetal adrenal gland has been shown to be the source of most of the elevation in both fetal plasma adrenaline and noradrenaline concentrations during acute hypoxaemia (Jones et al., 1988), as chemical adrenal demedullation using acid formalin completely abolished the hypoxaemia-induced rise in fetal plasma adrenaline concentrations and reduced the noradrenaline response to 10% of normal, indicating that the adrenal medulla is the principal source of the increase in circulating catecholamines during hypoxaemia in fetal sheep. This is supported by direct measurements of fetal adrenal output of catecholamines during hypoxaemia, using a method in the sheep fetus based on the 'adrenal clamp' technique first developed by Edwards and colleagues for use in the conscious calf (Edwards et al., 1974; Hardy et al., 1974). A prompt adrenal secretion of adrenaline and noradrenaline was demonstrated in the ovine fetus at the onset of the challenge (Cohen et al., 1984). In those elegant studies, changes in peripheral plasma catecholamines were usually, although not always, quantitatively equivalent to those measured directly in the adrenal effluent.

The increase in circulating catecholamines in the sheep fetus during acute hypoxaemia has important functional consequences. The restoration of fetal heart rate towards basal levels as the episode of acute hypoxaemia progresses has been attributed to an increase in cardiac β-adrenoceptor stimulation (Court et al., 1984). Therefore, β-adrenoceptor antagonism with propranolol augments fetal bradycardia, decreases the CVO and reduces myocardial blood flow during acute hypoxaemia (Court *et al.*, 1984). The increase in circulating catecholamine concentrations may also maintain or augment the redistribution of the fetal CVO during acute hypoxaemia. For example, α-adrenoceptor blockade with phentolamine has been shown to attenuate the peripheral vasoconstriction that occurs throughout the duration of hypoxaemia (Giussani *et al.*, 1993).

Plasma concentrations of arginine vasopressin (AVP) and angiotensin II increase in the ovine fetus during episodes of acute hypoxaemia (Alexander *et al.*, 1974; Broughton Pipkin *et al.*, 1974; Rurak, 1978; Robillard *et al.*, 1981; Wood *et al.*, 1990; Raff *et al.*, 1991; Giussani *et al.*, 1994b; Green *et al.*, 1998; Gardner *et al.*, 2002a). The release of both peptides during acute hypoxaemia has been shown to be independent of aortic or carotid chemo- and baroreceptors (Giussani *et al.*, 1994b; Green *et al.*, 1998), and may be augmented by concurrent hypercapnia and acidosis (Wood *et al.*, 1990; Raff *et al.*, 1991; Gardner *et al.*, 2002a). Although the fetal sheep is relatively unresponsive to AVP at less than 100 days (Wiriyathian *et al.*, 1983), exogenously administered AVP has dose-dependent effects on fetal heart rate and arterial blood pressure after 120 days (Rurak, 1978; Tomita *et al.*, 1985). The AVP-evoked hypertension has been shown to be mediated by V_1-receptors (Ervin *et al.*, 1992). The bradycardia associated with AVP infusion is not entirely attributable to baroreflexes, since some AVP-induced reduction in fetal heart rate persists even with hexamethonium treatment (Iwamoto *et al.*, 1979).

The fetal and umbilico-placental vasculatures are known to be responsive to exogenously administered angiotensin II (Iwamoto and Rudolph, 1981; Rosenfeld, 2001). Infusions of angiotensin II, to produce circulating levels similar to those measured following haemorrhage in fetal sheep, produce fetal hypertension and increases in heart rate, CVO, myocardial flow and vascular resistance values in the gastrointestinal, renal, thyroid and umbilico-placental circulations (Iwamoto and Rudolph, 1981). Angiotensin II is known to be important in maintaining basal arterial blood pressure and vascular tone during the last third of gestation, and it has been shown that blockade of angiotensin II production (Forhead *et al.*, 2000), or action (Iwamoto and Rudolph, 1979), results in a reduction in basal arterial blood pressure and umbilico-placental perfusion.

Paracrine control of fetal cardiovascular responses to acute hypoxaemia

Local modulators of chemoreflex, endocrine and vascular function may also play an important role in the control of the fetal cardiovascular responses to acute hypoxaemia (Tenney, 1990; Katusic and Shepherd, 1991; Shepherd and Katusic, 1991). These include agents such as adenosine, nitric oxide (NO), prostacyclin (PGI_2), histamine and bradykinin, endothelin-1, oxygen-derived free-radicals, prostaglandin H_2 and thromboxane A_2 (Katusic and Shepherd, 1991; Shepherd and Katusic, 1991). A number of these agents may influence cardiovascular responses to acute hypoxaemia in the fetus by acting at the vascular endothelium, and also by modulating chemoreflex and endocrine functions. For example, the purine nucleoside, adenosine, has been implicated in regulating carotid body function during hypoxia in adult animals. First, it is known that the carotid body expresses the adenosine A_{2a} receptor gene (Kaelin-Lang et al., 1998). Secondly, adenosine has been reported to increase carotid body chemoreceptor fibre activity in the cat (McQueen and Ribeiro, 1986). Thirdly, increased carotid body afferent discharge as a result of hypoxia can be attenuated by adenosine receptor antagonists (McQueen and Ribeiro, 1986). Finally, the stimulatory effects of adenosine on ventilation (Monteiro and Ribeiro, 1987) appear to be mediated within the carotid body. In the fetus, Koos et al. (1995) reported that treatment of fetal sheep with the non-selective adenosine receptor antagonist, 8-(p-sulphophenyl)-theophylline (8-SPT), prevented fetal bradycardia during acute hypoxaemia in a manner similar to bilateral section of the carotid sinus nerves (Bartelds et al., 1993; Giussani et al. 1993). However, the contribution of adenosine to chemoreflex (neural) or chemoreflex-independent (non-neural) mechanisms mediating the redistribution of cardiac output during acute hypoxaemia in the sheep fetus remained unknown.

One recent study (Giussani et al., 2001a) confirmed that fetal treatment with the same adenosine receptor antagonist, 8-SPT, attenuated fetal bradycardia and the increase in fetal arterial blood pressure during acute hypoxaemia, and reported that adenosine receptor antagonism also markedly attenuated the fetal femoral vasoconstrictor response to acute hypoxaemia. Since fetal bradycardia and the initial increase in femoral vascular resistance during acute hypoxaemia are known to be part of the same carotid chemoreflex (Giussani et al., 1993), these findings provide further strong support for the hypothesis that adenosine mediates cardiovascular responses triggered by the carotid body in the fetus. However, in our study, fetal treatment with 8-SPT not only markedly attenuated the initial increase in femoral vascular resistance following the onset of acute hypoxaemia, but substantially reduced femoral vasoconstriction throughout the hypoxaemic challenge. The findings of that study therefore suggested that adenosine may, in addition, contribute to non-chemoreflex (endocrine and local) mechanisms mediating the redistribution of the combined ventricular output during acute hypoxaemia in the late-gestation sheep fetus. Further data showed that fetal treatment with 8-SPT prevented the increase in fetal plasma adrenaline and markedly reduced the increase in fetal plasma noradrenaline throughout the acute hypoxaemic challenge (Giussani et al., 2001a). The combined data therefore suggest that fetal treatment with 8-SPT abolishes the initial femoral vasoconstriction by preventing the actions of carotid body reflexes, and may attenuate sustained vasoconstriction during acute hypoxaemia by reducing the effects of vasoconstrictors which are released into the fetal circulations by chemoreflex-independent mechanisms, such as the release of adrenal medullary catecholamines by the direct actions of hypoxia.

Another example of a local modulator influencing chemoreflex, endocrine and vascular function is nitric oxide (NO). In the fetus, the role of NO in the maintenance of basal blood flow in a number of circulations is well established (van Bel et al., 1995; Green et al., 1996; Harris et al., 2001). However, its role in mediating the cardiovascular response to acute hypoxaemia in the fetus is not well understood. Two previous studies have reported that treatment of the sheep fetus with the NO-synthase inhibitor N^G-nitro-L-arginine methyl ester (L-NAME) tended to augment the peripheral vasoconstrictor response to acute hypoxaemia (Green *et al.*, 1996; Harris *et al.*, 2001). However, fetal treatment with L-NAME alone caused generalized vasoconstriction and a pronounced increase in arterial blood pressure, altering basal cardiovascular function even prior to the onset of acute hypoxaemia (Green *et al.*, 1996; Harris *et al.*, 2001). Therefore, in both those studies changes in peripheral vasoconstrictor function during acute hypoxaemia were evaluated from a substantially elevated vasoconstrictor baseline, possibly diluting the effect of hypoxia-induced increases in NO.

In order to assess the contribution of NO to the cardiovascular response during acute hypoxaemia without altering basal cardiovascular function, we have applied the NO clamp technique to the fetus (Morrison *et al.*, 2003). The technique, which was developed to study adrenal function in the adult animal, combines treatment of the animal with L-NAME and the NO donor, sodium nitroprusside (NP) (Hanna and Edwards, 1998). In contrast to treatment with L-NAME alone, combined treatment with L-NAME and NP prevents generalized vasoconstriction and pronounced hypertension, not only maintaining basal cardiovascular function, but also permitting blockade of the *de novo* synthesis of NO during acute hypoxaemia, while compensating for the tonic production of the gas. The results of that study showed that fetal exposure to acute hypoxaemia during treatment with the NO clamp leads to significant enhancement of the peripheral vasoconstrictor response, increased sensitivity of chemoreflex function and greater increments in plasma catecholamine and blood glucose and lactate concentrations (Morrison *et al.*, 2003). These results confirm that, in the fetus, hypoxaemia-induced increases in NO offset the peripheral vasoconstrictor response to acute hypoxaemia (Green *et al.*, 1996; Harris *et al.*, 2001) and these findings have been extended to suggest that NO-induced opposition of peripheral vasoconstrictor function may result, in part, from the inhibitory actions of NO at the levels of the carotid chemoreflex and/or the adrenal medulla. Enhanced chemoreflex function and increments in plasma catecholamine concentrations may also contribute to the enhanced metabolic responses to acute hypoxaemia during fetal treatment with the NO clamp (Morrison *et al.*, 2003).

Modulation of the Fetal Cardiovascular Response to Acute Hypoxia by Irreversible Adverse Intrauterine Conditions: Acute-on-chronic Hypoxia

Although it is established that the fetus can successfully withstand a single, acute hypoxaemic challenge during gestation, little is known about what effects prevailing adverse intrauterine conditions might have on these adaptive mechanisms. This is particularly important since there is increasing clinical evidence to suggest that prolonged hypoxaemia *in utero* accompanies fetal growth retardation (Nicolaides *et al.*, 1989), and that antenatal hypoxaemia may predispose the fetus to birth asphyxia, with subsequent neurodevelopmental handicap

(Creasy and Resnik, 1981). Previous studies that have addressed the effects of prevailing adverse intrauterine conditions on the fetal cardiovascular response to acute hypoxaemia have induced adverse intrauterine conditions experimentally, either by reduction in placental size (carunclectomy) (Robinson et al., 1979), by occlusion of uterine blood flow with a balloon catheter (Block et al., 1984), or by embolization of the umbilico-placental (Block et al., 1989) or utero-placental (Block et al., 1990) circulations. In addition, a series of studies has investigated the fetal cardiovascular responses to acute hypoxaemia in the fetal llama, a species genetically adapted to the chronic hypobaric hypoxia of life at high altitude (Llanos et al., 1995; Giussani et al., 1996, 1999a).

It is recognized that chronic hypoxaemia in the fetus rarely occurs in isolation, and that, in complicated pregnancies, it is most often accompanied by concurrent acidaemia and/or hypoglycaemia (Nicolaides et al., 1989). However, the partial contributions of each of these adverse intrauterine conditions on the subsequent capacity of the fetus to respond to a further acute episode of hypoxaemia are little understood. A comprehensive study by Gardner et al. (2002a) reported that prevailing and independently occurring sustained hypoxaemia, acidaemia or hypoglycaemia alter the cardiovascular responses to a further episode of acute hypoxaemia in fetal sheep during late gestation (Figs 3.5 and 3.6). Alterations in the cardiovascular responses to acute hypoxaemia in all spontaneously compromised fetuses included enhanced pressor and femoral vasoconstrictor responses, which were associated with greater circulating concentrations of plasma noradrenaline and vasopressin. However, only fetuses with prevailing hypoxaemia had significantly elevated basal concentrations of noradrenaline and enhanced chemoreflex function during acute hypoxaemia.

The series of studies by Block et al. (1984, 1989, 1990) reported that fetuses compromised in utero exhibited a basal redistribution of blood flow toward the brain, heart and adrenal glands, and that this basal circulatory compensation was accentuated during an episode of superimposed acute hypoxaemia. The presence of developing acidaemia with hypoxaemia further exaggerated the circulatory compensation during superimposed acute hypoxaemia. These findings are in agreement with those reported by Gardner et al. (2002a) as the increase in peripheral vascular resistance was significantly enhanced during acute hypoxaemia in all groups of compromised fetuses (Fig. 3.6). Further, the enhanced femoral vasoconstrictor response to acute hypoxaemia was associated with marked elevations in plasma catecholamines and vasopressin in all groups of compromised fetuses (Gardner et al., 2002a). The increase in plasma vasopressin during acute hypoxaemia was greatest in the spontaneously acidaemic fetuses, and partial correlation analysis revealed that changes in fetal pH_a rather than P_aO_2, and in fetal plasma vasopressin rather than total plasma catecholamines, during acute hypoxaemia appeared to be the greater determinants of fetal femoral vasoconstriction (Gardner et al., 2002a). In this regard, it is of interest to note that: (i) the llama fetus has enhanced femoral vasoconstrictor and plasma catecholamine, vasopressin and NPY responses to acute hypoxaemia relative to control sheep fetuses at comparable stages of gestation (Giussani et al., 1994a, 1996, 1999a,b; Llanos et al., 1995); (ii) chronic hypoxia for most of the incubation promotes an increase in sympathetic nerve density in

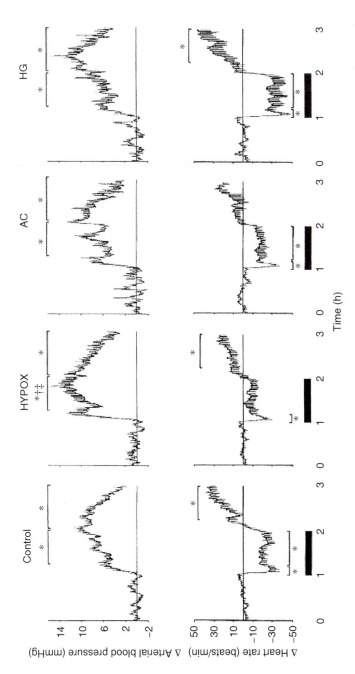

Fig. 3.5. Acute-on-chronic hypoxaemia: fetal arterial blood pressure and heart rate responses. Data represent absolute changes from baseline for mean arterial blood pressure and heart rate during acute hypoxaemia in control ($n = 14$) and spontaneously hypoxaemic (HYPOX; $n = 8$), spontaneously acidaemic (AC; $n = 5$) or spontaneously hypoglycaemic (HG; $n = 6$) fetuses. Values are means ± SEM of cardiovascular data (1 min average) for a baseline period (1 h normoxia), 1 h of hypoxaemia (box) and 1 h of recovery. Statistical differences are: *, $P < 0.05$ normoxia versus early (first 15 min) or late (last 45 min) hypoxaemia or recovery; †, $P < 0.05$ control versus HYPOX fetuses; ‡, $P < 0.05$ HYPOX versus HG fetuses. (Taken from Gardner *et al.*, 2002a.)

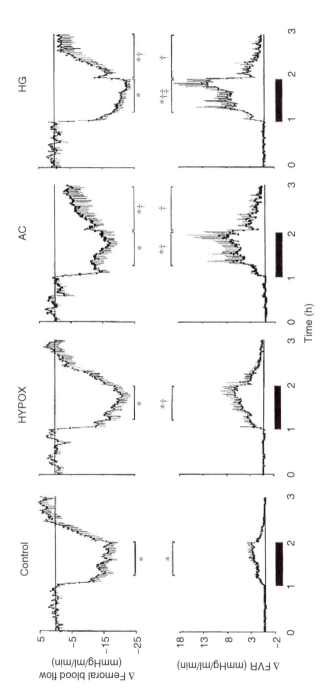

Fig. 3.6. Acute-on-chronic hypoxaemia: fetal femoral blood flow and vascular resistance responses. Data represent absolute changes from baseline for mean fetal femoral blood flow and vascular resistance (FVR) during acute hypoxaemia in control ($n = 14$) and HYPOX ($n = 8$) or AC ($n = 5$) or HG ($n = 6$) fetuses. Values are means ± SEM of cardiovascular data (1 min average) for a baseline period (1 h normoxia), 1 h of hypoxaemia (box) and 1 h of recovery. Statistical differences are: *, $P < 0.05$ normoxia versus early (first 15 min) or late (last 45 min) hypoxaemia or recovery; †, $P < 0.05$ control versus spontaneously compromised (HYPOX or AC or HG) fetuses; ‡, $P < 0.05$ HG versus HYPOX fetuses. (Taken from Gardner et al., 2002a.)

the chick embryo (Ruijtenbeek *et al.*, 2000); and (iii) both llama fetuses (Giussani *et al.*, 1999a) and chronically hypoxaemic, growth-retarded fetal sheep (Block *et al.*, 1989) have a greater dependence on α-adrenergic mechanisms to survive episodes of acute hypoxaemia than control fetal sheep. Taken together, past findings suggest that irreversible adverse intrauterine conditions may enhance the capacity of the compromised fetus to redistribute blood flow away from the periphery to serve hypoxia-sensitive circulations, and that the exact mechanisms recruited to mediate this enhanced response will depend on the interplay between prevailing hypoxaemia, acidaemia or hypoglycaemia in complicated pregnancies.

Modulation of the Fetal Cardiovascular Response to Acute Hypoxia by Reversible Adverse Intrauterine Conditions: Acute-after-chronic Hypoxia

One important paradox in obstetric practice is that the incidence of perinatal morbidity arising from birth hypoxia or asphyxia has remained high, despite the marked improvements in the management of labour in recent years (Hall, 1989). Perinatal mortality in these circumstances may therefore reflect an undiagnosed antenatal compromise rather than the conditions encountered during labour *per se*. One possibility is that fetal exposure to adverse intrauterine conditions before labour may result in attenuation rather than enhancement of cardiovascular defence mechanisms, rendering the fetus more susceptible to the relatively mild or acute hypoxia/asphyxia of uncomplicated labour and delivery. This implies that acute-on-chronic hypoxia and acute-after-chronic hypoxia may have differential effects on the fetal cardiovascular system.

While acute-on-chronic hypoxia may model an irreversible adverse condition, which can therefore be diagnosed in clinical practice, acute-after-chronic hypoxia may model labour or an acute challenge following a reversible period of adversity, which, because of its transient nature, has remained undiagnosed. A common form of reversible adverse intrauterine conditions is compression of the umbilical cord, which has been reported to occur at an incidence of $\geq 40\%$ in human pregnancies (Clapp *et al.*, 1988, 2000; Hall, 1989), either resulting from nuchal cord (Clapp *et al.*, 2000), torsion of the umbilicus during gestation (Rayburn *et al.*, 1981), oligohydramnios (Leveno *et al.*, 1984) or compression during the actual processes of labour and delivery (Wheeler and Greene, 1975). Despite this, little is known about the effects of fetal exposure to compression of the umbilical cord upon the fetal cardiovascular capacity to respond to a subsequent episode of acute hypoxaemia.

Using a computerized system, a recent study (Gardner *et al.*, 2001b) addressed how temporary reversible compression of the umbilical cord may alter the capacity of the fetal cardiovascular system to withstand subsequent acute hypoxia, of the type that may occur during labour and delivery. The umbilical cord of fetal sheep was compressed to reduce umbilical blood flow by a programmed 30% from baseline, for 3 days between 125 and 128 days of gestation (Gardner *et al.*, 2002b). At 128 days the umbilical occluder was deflated to allow umbilical blood flow to return to basal conditions. Following full recovery from cord compression, the fetuses were then subjected to an acute episode of hypoxaemia, between 2 and 7 days after the end of cord compression. The cardiovascular, endocrine and local mechanisms mediating their defence response to acute hypoxaemia were compared with those in appropriate sham-compressed fetuses. During partial umbilical cord compression, fetuses developed mild asphyxia, which was characterized by significant falls in pH_a, P_aO_2 and per cent saturation of haemoglobin, and an increase in arterial P_aCO_2. After 1 day of recovery from cord compression, values for all these variables had returned to basal conditions. When acute hypoxaemia was induced 2–7 days after the end of cord compression, sham-compressed fetuses responded to the challenge with the three classical responses: transient bradycardia, an increase in arterial blood pressure and a redistribution of the combined ventricular output away from the peripheral circulations, indexed in this instance by a pronounced increase in femoral vascular resistance. In marked contrast, while the cardiac response to acute hypoxaemia in cord-compressed fetuses was not affected, the pressor response was diminished because these fetuses had almost lost their capacity to constrict the femoral vascular bed (Fig. 3.7) (Gardner *et al.*, 2002b). Fetal exposure to a period of reversible adverse intrauterine conditions markedly attenuated the peripheral vasoconstrictor response to subsequent acute hypoxaemia. The clinical implication of this finding is that adverse antenatal compromise may render the fetus less able to redistribute its blood flow and, hence, make it more susceptible to subsequent acute challenges, such as those imposed by relatively uncomplicated labour and delivery. This finding may explain, at least in part, why perinatal morbidity arising from birth hypoxia or asphyxia has not been affected by the marked improvements in obstetric practice and the management of labour in recent years (Rosenfeld *et al.*, 1996). Physiologically, it is of interest to determine which mechanisms, normally mediating fetal peripheral vasoconstriction, are being affected by prior compression of the umbilical cord.

Gardner *et al.* (2002b) addressed the possibility that short-term compression of the umbilical cord diminished fetal peripheral vasoconstrictor responses to subsequent acute hypoxaemia because of reduced secretion of vasoconstrictor hormones during acute hypoxaemia and/or reduced responsiveness of the fetal peripheral circulations to constrictor agents. Cord-compressed fetuses had enhanced concentrations of catecholamines during acute hypoxaemia and greater femoral vasopressor responses to increasing bolus doses of exogenous phenylephrine, relative to sham-control fetuses. However, when cord-compressed fetuses were subjected to acute hypoxaemia during the nitric oxide clamp, the femoral vasoconstrictor response was completely restored, and, in some instances, markedly enhanced (Fig. 3.8) (Gardner *et al.*, 2002b). These data suggest that attenuation of the peripheral vasoconstrictor response to acute hypoxaemia in cord-compressed fetuses is not due to either reduced release of catecholamines into the fetal circulation or to reduced sensitivity of the peripheral vasculature to adrenergic agonists. However, in fetuses previously compromised by a reversible period of umbilical cord compression, the balance between vasodilator and vasoconstrictor influences on the peripheral circulations is shifted, resulting in an up-regulation of vasodilator activity, in particular nitric oxide. Whether increased nitric oxide activity reflects local up-regulation in

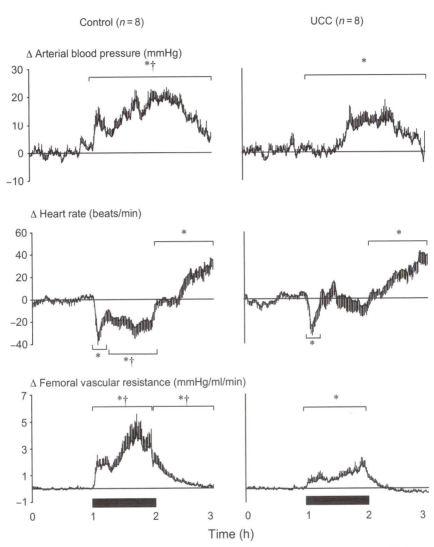

Fig. 3.7. Acute-after-chronic hypoxaemia: fetal cardiovascular responses. Values are means ± SEM of cardiovascular data for control fetuses and for fetuses that had been exposed to a 3-day partial compression of the umbilical cord using the computerized system (UCC). Data are averaged over each minute during a baseline period (1 h normoxia), 1 h of hypoxia (bar) and 1 h of recovery. Acute hypoxaemia was induced in all fetuses by reducing maternal fraction of inspired oxygen (F_iO_2), during which saline was infused intravenously at a rate of 0.25 ml/min. Statistical differences are; *, $P < 0.05$, baseline versus hypoxia or recovery; †, sham-control versus UCC fetuses. (Taken from Gardner *et al.*, 2002b.)

the endothelium of peripheral circulations (Zheng *et al.*, 2000) and/or enhanced production of nitric oxide-dependent vasodilator factors, such as adenosine (Read *et al.*, 1993), oestrogen (Rosenfeld *et al.*, 1996) and/or adrenomedullin (Di Iorio *et al.*, 1998), in the placental and/or fetal circulations remains to be determined.

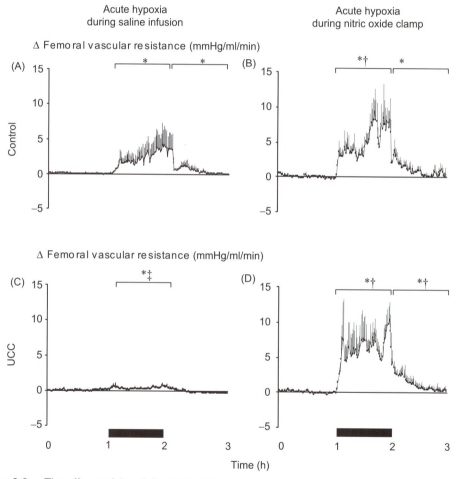

Fig. 3.8.   The effects of the nitric oxide clamp on the femoral vasoconstrictor response to acute hypoxaemia in control and compromised fetuses. Values are means ± SEM for the change from baseline in femoral vascular resistance in control fetuses during saline infusion (A, *n* = 8) and during treatment with the nitric oxide clamp (B, *n* = 6); and cord-compressed (UCC) fetuses during saline infusion (C, *n* = 8) and during treatment with the nitric oxide clamp (D, *n* = 6). Shaded box indicates period of treatment. Statistical differences are: *, *P* < 0.05 baseline versus hypoxia or recovery; †, *P* < 0.05 saline versus nitric oxide clamp; ‡, *P* < 0.05 sham-control versus UCC fetuses. (Taken from Gardner *et al.*, 2002b.)

Chronic Hypoxia During Development, Fetal Growth and Programming of Cardiovascular Disease

The compelling evidence linking small size at birth with later cardiovascular disease, obtained from epidemiological studies of human populations of more than seven countries (Barker, 1998), has renewed and amplified a clinical and scientific interest into the determinants of fetal growth, birthweight and cardio-vascular development and function before and after birth. As early as the 1950s, Penrose (1954) highlighted that the greatest determinant of birthweight was the quality of the intrauterine environment, being twice as great a determinant of fetal growth as the maternal or fetal genotype. Of course, one of the great qualifiers of the fetal intrauterine environment is the maternal nutritional status during pregnancy. As such, the reciprocal association between low birthweight and increased risk of high blood pressure in adulthood, as first described by Barker (1998), has literally exploded a new field of research investigating the effects of materno-fetal nutrition on fetal growth, birthweight and subsequent cardiovascular disease. However, the fetus also nourishes itself with oxygen, and, in contrast to the international effort assessing the effects of maternal nutrition on early development, the effects of materno-fetal oxygen deprivation on fetal growth, birthweight and subsequent cardiovascular disease have been little addressed.

The most common form of materno-fetal hypoxia is pregnancy at high altitude, and in recent studies we have asked whether high altitude is a greater determinant than maternal nutritional status of intrauterine growth retardation, low birthweight, and increased infant mortality. And, if so, whether the chronic fetal hypoxia of pregnancy at high altitude, independent of the maternal nutritional status, can alone programme fetal origins of adult disease. These questions have been addressed in Bolivia, as this country is geographically and socio-economically unique. Bolivia lies in the heart of South America and it is split by the Andean cordillera into areas of very high altitude to the west of the country (4000 m), and sea-level areas where the east of the country spans into the Brazilian Amazon. Facilitating the study design, the two largest cities, and therefore the most populated, with approximately 2 million inhabitants each, are La Paz (4000 m) and Santa Cruz (400 m). Bolivia is also socio-economically unique as both La Paz and Santa Cruz are made up of striking divergent populations economically (Mapa de pobreza, 1995). In Third World countries, and especially in Bolivia, there is an unsurprisingly strong relationship between socio-economic status and nutritional status (Post et al., 1994; Tellez et al., 1994). Joining strengths with Barker, a recent study investigated whether the intrauterine growth retardation observed in the high-altitude regions of Bolivia was primarily due to intrauterine hypoxia or due to the maternal socio-economic nutritional status (Giussani et al., 2001b). Birthweight records were obtained from term pregnancies in La Paz and Santa Cruz, especially from obstetric hospitals selectively attended by wealthy or impoverished mothers. Plots of the cumulative frequency distribution across all birthweights gathered revealed a pronounced shift to the left in the curve of babies from high altitude than from low altitude, despite similarly high maternal economic status

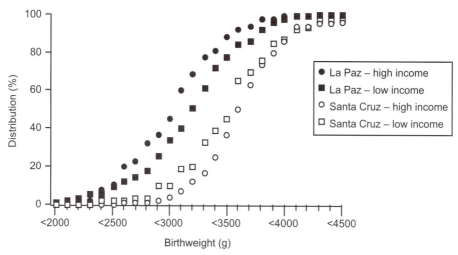

Fig. 3.9. The effects of high altitude versus socio-economic status on birthweight. The curves represent the cumulative frequency distribution across all birthweights in term babies born from mothers of opposing economic status in La Paz (4000 m) and in Santa Cruz (400 m), in Bolivia. (Modified from Giussani *et al.*, 2001b.)

(Fig. 3.9). Interestingly, when lowland babies born from mothers with high or low economic status were compared, a shift to the left in birthweight occurred in low- versus high-income pregnancies; however, this shift was not as pronounced as the effect of high altitude on birthweight alone. Additional data also showed that highland babies from poor families did not have the greatest leftward shift of the relationship as one would have expected. Rather, these babies were actually heavier than highland babies born from families with a high socio-economic status. The apparent conundrum is easily explained by assessing the ancestry of the families. In our study, the low socio-economic group of La Paz contained a high percentage (92%) of women from Amerindian origin, with Aymara indian paternal and maternal surnames (Giussani *et al.*, 2001b). In contrast, the high socio-economic group of La Paz contained a high European admixture. These findings are reminiscent of the observations of Zamudio *et al.* (1993) and Haas *et al.* (1977), who suggested that fetal growth retardation at altitude is correlated with the duration of high-altitude residence, independent of maternal nutrition: the longest-resident population experiencing the least decline and the shortest-residence groups demonstrating the most reduction in birthweight. Accordingly, reductions in birthweight at elevations greater than 3000 m above sea level are greatest in Colorado, intermediate in Andeans and least in Tibetans (Zamudio *et al.*, 1993). Thus, women from high-altitude residence ancestry, such as the Tibetans (Zamudio *et al.*, 1993) and the Aymaras (Haas *et al.*, 1977) give birth to heavier babies than women from low-altitude residence ancestry, such as Han women in China and women from European or mestizo ancestry in South America.

   While such studies suggest that development under the chronic hypoxia of pregnancy at high altitude alone, independent of maternal economic–nutritional status, leads to fetal growth retardation, and that high-altitude residence ancestry may develop a protection against the effects of high altitude on fetal growth, it remains to be elucidated whether hypoxia-induced reductions in birthweight are associated with increased health risks after birth, and whether this risk is different in native and foreign highlanders. Preliminary data suggest that the rates of infant mortality, within the first year of newborn life, are positively correlated with altitude, increasing at a rate of c. 8 deaths per 1000 m increase, and that this relationship is also independent of the maternal socio-economic status. However, the negligible number of studies, in which arterial blood pressure was measured in residents rather than climbers at high altitude, report conflicting results, suggesting either a higher incidence of hypertension in the inhabitants of high-altitude regions of Saudi Arabia (Khalid et al., 1994) or lower resting blood pressure in Peruvian highlanders (Ruiz and Penaloza, 1977). These inconsistencies may again be related to the high-altitude residence ancestry of the individuals being studied.

Summary and Perspectives

The first line of fetal defence to an episode of acute oxygen deprivation, of the magnitude that may occur during labour and delivery, is the cardiovascular system. The fetal cardiovascular defence responses to an episode of acute hypoxaemia include transient bradycardia, an increase in arterial blood pressure, and a redistribution of the fetal combined ventricular output in favour of the adrenal glands, the heart and the brain at the expense of perfusion to the peripheral circulations. The fetal bradycardia and peripheral vasoconstriction at the onset of acute hypoxaemia are triggered by a carotid chemoreflex. The magnitude of the peripheral vasoconstrictor response to acute hypoxaemia will depend on the balance between the release of vasoconstrictor hormones, such as catecholamines and vasopressin, and the modulation of the response by local agents, such as adenosine and nitric oxide.

Recent evidence suggests that adverse intrauterine conditions will modify the capacity of the fetal cardiovascular system to withstand an episode of acute hypoxaemia. However, modifications of the fetal cardiovascular defence to acute hypoxaemia differ markedly if the episode of acute hypoxaemia occurs during adverse intrauterine conditions, as opposed to after the period of adversity. While acute-on-chronic hypoxia enhances the fetal peripheral vasoconstrictor response, acute-after-chronic hypoxia almost suppresses the fetal vasoconstrictor capacity. Suppression of fetal peripheral vasoconstrictor responses to acute hypoxaemia following a period of intrauterine adversity may weaken the redistribution of the fetal cardiac output, thereby rendering the fetal brain more susceptible to birth asphyxia and subsequent neurodevelopmental handicap. Additional evidence suggests that acute-after-chronic hypoxia increases the gain of both sympathetic and nitrergic influences on the fetal peripheral vasculature. However, the enhancement of nitric oxide activity outweighs the increased sympathetic activity, completely masking the peripheral vasoconstriction. The source of the enhanced nitric oxide activity under these circumstances is unknown at present. However, if the source of enhanced nitric oxide activity is the placenta, it is plausible that once this source is lost following delivery, the individual will be born with a hyper-reactive sympathetic system.

Studies at high altitude addressing the question of whether chronic fetal hypoxia during development, independent of the maternal nutritional status, can alone promote low birthweight and programme fetal origins of adult cardiovascular disease, have suggested that fetal exposure to hypoxia, rather than maternal undernutrition, has a greater impact on low birthweight. The intrauterine growth retardation resulting from the chronic hypoxia of pregnancy at high altitude is asymmetric, indicating sustained peripheral vasoconstriction, which shunts blood flow away from the peripheral circulations to spare the brain. The mechanisms mediating this persistent redistribution of the cardiac output in the human fetus under these conditions is unknown at present, but may involve changes in the gain of chemoreflex, endocrine and local influences on the fetal circulation. Additional data from studies at high altitude suggest that high-altitude residence ancestry may develop a protection against the effects of hypoxia on fetal development, and, thereby, against risk of developing cardio-vascular disease at adulthood. This final point re-emphasizes the need for future epidemiological studies relating low birthweight with postnatal cardiovascular dysfunction at altitude to differentiate between native and foreign populations of the highlands.

References

Akalin-Sel, T. and Campbell, S. (1992) Understanding the pathophysiology of intra-uterine growth retardation: the role of the 'lower limb reflex' in redistribution of blood flow. *European Journal of Obstetrics, Gynecology, and Reproductive Biology*, 46(2–3), 79–86.

Alexander, D.P., Bashore, R.A., Britton, H.G. and Forsling, M.L. (1974) Maternal and fetal arginine vasopressin in the chronically catheterised sheep. *Biology of the Neonate* 25, 242–248.

Allen, J.M., Adrian, T.E., Polak, J.M. and Bloom, S.R. (1983) Neuropeptide Y (NPY): in the adrenal gland. *Journal of the Autonomic Nervous System* 9, 559–563.

Barclay, A.E., Barcroft, J., Barron, D.H. and Franklin, K. (1939) A radiographic demonstration of the circulation through the heart in the adult and in the fetus and the identification of the ductus arteriosus. *British Journal of Radiology* 12, 595.

Barker, D.J.P. (1998) *Mothers, Babies, and Disease in Later Life*. Churchill Livingstone, Edinburgh, UK.

Bartelds, B., van Bel, F., Teitel, D.F. and Rudolph, A.M. (1993) Carotid, not aortic, chemoreceptors mediate the fetal cardiovascular response to acute hypoxemia in lambs. *Pediatric Research* 34, 51–55.

Beard, R.W. and Rivers, R.P. (1979) Fetal asphyxia in labour. *Lancet* 2(8152), 1117–1119.

Behrman, R.E. and Lees, M.H. (1971) Organ blood flows of the fetal, newborn and adult rhesus monkey: a comparative study. *Biology of the Neonate* 18(5), 330–340.

Bilardo, C.M., Campbell, S. and Nicolaides, K.H. (1988) Mean blood velocities and flow impedance in the fetal descending thoracic aortic and common carotid artery in normal pregnancy. *Pregnancy and Early Human Development* 18(2–3), 213–221.

Blanco, C.E., Dawes, G.S. and Walker, D.W. (1983) Effect of hypoxia on polysynaptic hind-limb reflexes of unanaesthetized fetal and new-born lambs. *Journal of Physiology* 339, 453–466.

Block, B., Llanos, A. and Creasy, R. (1984) Responses of the growth-retarded fetus to acute hypoxemia. *American Journal of Obstetrics and Gynecology* 148, 878–885.

Block, B., Schlafer, D., Wentworth, R., Kreitzer, L. and Nathanielsz, P. (1989) Intrauterine growth retardation and the circulatory responses to acute hypoxemia in fetal sheep. *American Journal of Obstetrics and Gynaecology* 161, 1576–1579.

Block, B., Schlafer, D., Wentworth, R., Kreitzer, L. and Nathanielsz, P. (1990) Intrauterine asphyxia and the breakdown of physiologic circulatory compensation in fetal sheep. *American Journal of Obstetrics and Gynecology* 162, 1325–1331.

Bloom, S.R., Edwards, A.V. and Jones, C.T. (1988) The adrenal contribution to the neuroendocrine responses to splanchnic nerve stimulation in conscious calves. *Journal of Physiology* 397, 513–526.

Boddy, K., Dawes, G.S., Fisher, R., Pinter, S. and Robinson, J.S. (1974) Foetal respiratory movements, electrocortical and cardiovascular responses to hypoxemia and hypercapnia in sheep. *Journal of Physiology* 243, 599–618.

Bristow, J., Rudolph, A.M., Itskovitz, J. and Barnes, R (1983) Hepatic oxygen and glucose metabolism in the fetal lamb Response to hypoxia. *Journal of Clinical Investigation* 71, 1047–1061.

Broughton Pipkin, F., Lumbers, E.R. and Mott, J.C. (1974) Factors influencing plasma renin and angiotensin II in the conscious pregnant ewe and its foetus. *Journal of Physiology* 243, 619–636.

Carter, A.M. and Gu, W. (1988) Cerebral blood flow in the fetal guinea-pig. *Journal of Developmental Physiology* 10(2), 123–129.

Charlton, V. and Johengen, M. (1984) Nutrient and waste product concentration differences in upper and lower body arteries of fetal sheep. *Journal of Developmental Physiology* 6(5), 431–437.

Clapp, J.F., Peress, N.S., Wesley, M. and Mann, L.I. (1988) Brain damage after intermittent partial cord occlusion in the chronically instrumented fetal lamb. *American Journal of Obstetrics and Gynecology* 159, 504–509.

Clapp, J.F., Stepanchek, W., Lopez, B. and Schmidt, S. (2000) Antenatal nuchal cord: prevalence and associated findings. *Journal of the Society for Gynaecological Investigation* 7(1), 136.

Cohen, W.R., Piasecki, G.J. and Jackson, B.T. (1982) Plasma catecholamines during hypoxemia in fetal lamb. *American Journal of Physiology* 243, R520–R525.

Cohen, W.R., Piasecki, G.J., Cohn, H.E., Young, J.B. and Jackson, B.T. (1984) Adrenal secretion of catecholamines during hypoxemia in fetal lambs. *Endocrinology* 114, 383–390.

Cohn, H.E., Sacks, E.J., Heymann, M.A. and Rudolph, A.M. (1974) Cardiovascular responses to hypoxemia and acidemia in fetal lambs. *American Journal of Obstetrics and Gynecology* 120, 817–824.

Court, D.J., Parer, J.T., Block, B.S. and Llanos, A.J. (1984) Effects of beta-adrenergic blockade on blood flow distribution during hypoxaemia in fetal sheep. *Journal of Developmental Physiology* 6, 349–358.

Creasy, R.K. and Resnik, R. (1981) Intrauterine fetal growth retardation. In: Milunsky, A., Friedman, E.A. and Gluck, L. (eds) *Advances in Perinatal Medicine*, Vol. 4. Plenum Book Medical Company, New York.

Dawes, G.S. (1968) *Fetal and Neonatal Physiology*. Yearbook Medical Publishers, Chicago, Illinois.

Di Iorio, R., Marinoni, E. and Cosmi, E.V. (1998) New peptides, hormones and parturition. *Gynecological Endocrinology* 12, 429–434.

Dilts, P.V., Brinkman, C.R., Kirschbaum, T.H. and Assali, N.S. (1969) Uterine and systemic haemodynamic interrelationships and their response to hypoxia. *American Journal of Obstetrics and Gynecology* 103, 138–157.

Edelstone, D.I. (1980) Regulation of blood flow through the ductus venosus. *Journal of Developmental Physiology* 2, 219–238.

Edelstone, D.I., Rudolph, A.M. and Heymann, M.A. (1978) Liver and ductus venosus blood flows in fetal lambs *in utero*. *Circulation Research* 42, 426–433.

Edvinsson, L., Ekblad, E., Hakanson, A. and Wahlestedt, C. (1984) Neuropeptide Y potentiates the effect of various vasoconstrictor agents on rabbit blood vessels. *British Journal of Pharmacology* 83, 519–525.

Edwards, A.V., Hardy, R.N. and Malinowska, K.W. (1974) The effects of infusions of synthetic adrenocorticotrophin in the conscious calf. *Journal of Physiology* 239(3), 477–498.

Ervin, M.G., Ross, M.G., Leake, R.D. and Fisher, D.A. (1992) V_1- and V_2-receptor contributions to ovine fetal renal and cardiovascular responses to vasopressin. *American Journal of Physiology* 262, R636–R643.

Fletcher, A.J.W.F. (2001) Glucocorticoids and acute hypoxaemia in fetal sheep: cardiovascular, endocrine and metabolic responses. PhD thesis, University of Cambridge, Cambridge, UK.

Fletcher, A.J.W., Edwards, C.M.B., Gardner, D.S., Fowden, A.L. and Giussani, D.A. (2000) Neuropeptide Y in the sheep fetus: effects of acute hypoxemia and dexamethasone during late gestation. *Endocrinology* 141(11), 3976–3982.

Forhead, A.J., Broughton Pipkin, F. and Fowden, A.L. (2000) Effect of cortisol on blood pressure and the renin–angiotensin system in fetal sheep during late gestation. *Journal of Physiology* 526(1), 167–176.

Gardner, D.S., Powlson, A.S. and Giussani, D.A. (2001a) An *in vivo* nitric oxide clamp to investigate the influence of nitric oxide on continuous umbilical blood flow during acute hypoxaemia in the sheep fetus. *Journal of Physiology* 537(2), 587–596.

Gardner, D.S., Fletcher, A.J.W., Swann, M., Fowden, A.L. and Giussani, D.A. (2001b) A novel method for controlled, long term compression of the umbilical cord in fetal sheep. *Journal of Physiology* 535(1), 217–229.

Gardner, D.S., Fletcher, A.J., Bloomfield, M.R., Fowden, A.L. and Giussani, D.A. (2002a) Effects of prevailing hypoxaemia, acidaemia or hypoglycaemia upon the cardiovascular, endocrine and metabolic responses to acute hypoxaemia in the ovine fetus. *Journal of Physiology* 540(1), 351–366.

Gardner, D.S., Fowden, A.L. and Giussani, D.A. (2002b) Adverse intrauterine conditions diminish the fetal defense to acute hypoxia by increasing nitric oxide activity. *Circulation* 106, 2278–2283.

Giussani, D.A., Spencer, J.A., Moore, P.J., Bennet, L. and Hanson, M.A. (1993) Afferent and efferent components of the cardiovascular reflex responses to acute hypoxia in term fetal sheep. *Journal of Physiology* 461, 431–449.

Giussani, D.A., Spencer, J.A. and Hanson, M.A. (1994a) Fetal cardiovascular reflex responses to hypoxaemia. *Fetal and Maternal Medicine Review* 6, 17–37.

Giussani, D.A., McGarrigle, H.H.G., Spencer, J.A.D., Moore, P.J., Bennet, L. and Hanson, M.A. (1994b) Effect of carotid denervation on plasma vasopressin levels during acute hypoxia in the late-gestation sheep fetus. *Journal of Physiology* 477, 81–87.

Giussani, D.A., Riquelme, R.A., Moraga, F.A., McGarrigle, H.H., Gaete, C.R., Sanhueza, E.M., Hanson, M.A. and Llanos, A.J. (1996) Chemoreflex and endocrine components of cardiovascular responses to acute hypoxemia in the llama fetus. *American Journal of Physiology* 271, R73–R83.

Giussani, D.A., Riquelme, R.A., Sanhueza, E.M., Hanson, M.A., Blanco, C.E. and Llanos, A.J. (1999a) Adrenergic and vasopressinergic contributions to the cardiovascular response to acute hypoxaemia in the llama fetus. *Journal of Physiology* 515(1), pp. 233–241.

Giussani, D.A., Riquelme, R.A., Hanson, M.A., Blanco, C.E., Edwards, C.M.B. and Llanos, A.J. (1999b) Pronounced increase in plasma neuropeptide Y (NPY): during acute hypoxemia in the llama fetus during late gestation. *Journal of the Society for Gynaecological Investigication* 6(1), 106A.

Giussani, D.A., Gardner, D.S., Cox, D.R. and Fletcher, A.J.W. (2001a) Purinergic contribution to the circulatory, metabolic and adrenergic responses to acute hypoxemia in fetal sheep. *American Journal of Physiology* 280, R678–R688.

Giussani, D.A., Phillips, P.S., Anstee, S. and Barker, D.J. (2001b) Effects of altitude versus economic status on birth weight and body shape at birth. *Pediatric Research* 49(4), 490–494.

Goodwin, J.W. (1968) The impact of the umbilical circulation on the fetus. *American Journal of Obstetrics and Gynecology* 100, 461–471.

Green, L.R., Bennet, L. and Hanson, M.A. (1996) The role of nitric oxide synthesis in cardiovascular responses to acute hypoxia in the late gestation sheep fetus. *Journal of Physiology* 497, 271–277.

Green, L.R., Bennet, L., Robson, S. and Hanson, M.A. (1997) The role of carotid chemoreceptors in the effects of hypoxia on renal blood flow in the late gestation sheep fetus. *Experimental Physiology* 82, 183–192.

Green, L.R., McGarrigle, H.H., Bennet, L. and Hanson, M.A. (1998) Angiotensin II and cardiovascular chemoreflex responses to acute hypoxia in late gestation fetal sheep. *Journal of Physiology* 507, 857–867.

Gunn, A.J., Quaedackers, J.S., Guan, J., Heineman, E. and Bennet, L. (2001) The premature fetus: not as defenseless as we thought, but still paradoxically vulnerable? *Developmental Neuroscience* 23(3), 175–179.

Haas, J.D., Baker, P.T. and Hunt, E.E. (1977) The effects of high altitude on body size and composition of the newborn infant in Southern Peru. *Human Biology* 49(4), 611–628.

Hall, D.M. (1989) Birth asphyxia and cerebral palsy. *British Medical Journal* 299, 279–282.

Hanna, S.J. and Edwards, A.V. (1998) The role of nitric oxide in the control of protein secretion in the parotid gland of anaesthetized sheep. *Experimental Physiology* 83, 533–544.

Hardy, R.N., Silver, M., Addison, K., Malinowska, K.W. and Edwards, A.V. (1974) The response of the adrenal gland to hypoglycaemia in the conscious calf. *Experientia* 30(7), 819–820.

Harris, A.P., Helou, S., Gleason, C.A., Traystman, R.J. and Koehler, R.C. (2001) Fetal cerebral and peripheral circulatory responses to hypoxia after nitric oxide synthase inhibition. *American Journal of Physiology* 281, R381–R390.

Hooper, S.B. (1995) Fetal metabolic responses to hypoxia. *Reproduction, Fertility, and Development* 7, 527–538.

Iwamoto, H.S. and Rudolph, A.M. (1979) Effects of endogenous angiotensin II on the fetal circulation. *Journal of Developmental Physiology* 1, 283–293.

Iwamoto, H.S. and Rudolph, A.M. (1981) Effects of angiotensin II on the blood flow and its distribution in fetal lambs. *Circulation Research* 48, 183–189.

Iwamoto, H.S., Rudolph, A.M., Keil, L.C. and Heymann, M.A. (1979) Hemodynamic responses of the sheep fetus to vasopressin infusion. *Circulation Research* 44, 430–436.

Iwamoto, H.S., Kaufman, T., Keil, L.C. and Rudolph, A.M. (1989) Responses to acute hypoxemia in fetal sheep at 0.6–0.7 gestation. *American Journal of Physiology* 256, H613–H620.

Jackson, B.T., Piasecki, G.J. and Novy, M.J. (1987) Fetal responses to altered maternal oxygenation in rhesus monkey. *American Journal of Physiology* 252(1), R94–R101.

Javorka, K., Tomori, Z. and Pullmann, R. (1978) Effect of inderal on heart rate changes in rabbit and guinea pig foetuses during hypoxia [author's transl.]. *Bratislav Medical Journal* 69(4), 450–457.

Jensen, A. and Berger, R. (1991) Fetal circulatory responses to oxygen lack. *Journal of Developmental Physiology* 16(4), 181–207.

Jensen, A. and Berger, R. (1993) Regional distribution of cardiac output. In: Hanson, M.A., Spencer, J.A.D. and Rodeck, C.H. (eds) *Fetus and Neonate – Physiology and Clinical Applications*: Vol. 1, *The Circulation*. Cambridge University Press, Cambridge, UK, pp. 23–74.

Jensen, A., Hohmann, M. and Kunzel, W. (1987) Dynamic changes in organ blood flow and oxygen consumption during acute asphyxia in fetal sheep. *Journal of Developmental Physiology* 9, 543–559.

Jones, C.T. and Robinson, R.O. (1975) Plasma catecholamines in foetal and adult sheep. *Journal of Physiology* 248, 15–33.

Jones, C.T., Roebuck, M.M., Walker, D.W. and Johnston, B.M. (1988) The role of the adrenal medulla and peripheral sympathetic nerves in the physiological responses of the fetal sheep to hypoxia. *Journal of Developmental Physiology* 10, 17–36.

Kaelin-Lang, A., Lauterburg, T. and Burgunder, J.M. (1998) Expression of adenosine A2a receptor gene in rat dorsal root and autonomic ganglia. *Neuroscience Letters* 246(1), 21–24.

Katusic, Z.S. and Shepherd, J.T. (1991) Endothelium-derived vasoactive factors: II Endothelium-dependent contraction. *Hypertension* 18, III86–III92.

Khalid, M.E., Ali, M.E., Ahmed, E.K. and Elkarib, A.O. (1994) Pattern of blood pressures among high and low altitude residents of southern Saudi Arabia. *Journal of Human Hypertension* 8(10), 765–769.

Koos, B.J., Chau, A. and Ogunyemi, D. (1995) Adenosine mediates metabolic and cardiovascular responses to hypoxia in fetal sheep. *Journal of Physiology* 488, 761–766.

Lebowitz, E.A., Novick, J.S. and Rudolph, A.M. (1972) Development of myocardial sympathetic innervation in the fetal lamb. *Pediatric Research* 6, 887–893.

Leveno, K.J., Quirk, J.G. Jr, Cunningham, F.G., Nelson, S.D., Santo-Ramos, R., Toofanian, A. and Depalma, R.T. (1984) Prolonged pregnancy: 1 Observations concerning the causes of fetal distress. *American Journal of Obstetrics and Gynecology* 150(1), 465–473.

Liggins, G.C., Qvist, J., Hochachka, P.W., Murphy, B.J., Creasy, R.K., Schneider, R.C., Snider, M.T. and Zapol, W.M. (1980) Fetal cardiovascular and metabolic responses to simulated diving in the Weddell seal. *Journal of Applied Physiology* 49(3), 424–430.

Llanos, A.J., Riquelme, R.A., Moraga, F.A., Cabello, G. and Parer, J.T. (1995) Cardiovascular responses to graded degrees of hypoxaemia in the llama fetus. *Reproduction, Fertility, and Development* 7(3), 549–552.

Lumbers, E.R., McCloskey, D.I., Potter, E.K. and Courtice, G.P. (1986) Cardiac vagal action during hypoxia in adult and fetal sheep. *Journal of the Autonomic Nervous System* 16, 23–34.

Mapa de pobreza (1995) *Una guía para la acción social*, 2nd edn. Ministerio de desarrollo humano, República de Bolivia.

McQueen, D.S. and Ribeiro, J.A. (1986) Pharmacological characterization of the receptor involved in chemoexcitation induced by adenosine. *British Journal of Pharmacology* 88, 615–620.

Monheit, A.G., Stone, M.L. and Abitbol, M.M. (1988) Fetal heart rate and transcutaneous monitoring during experimentally induced hypoxia in the fetal dog. *Pediatric Research* 23(6), 548–552.

Monteiro, E.C. and Ribeiro, J.A. (1987) Ventilatory effects of adenosine mediated by carotid body chemoreceptors in the rat. *Naunyn-Schmiedeberg's Arch Pharmacol* 335, 143–148.

Moore, P.J. and Hanson, M.A. (1991) The role of peripheral chemoreceptors in the rapid response of the pulmonary vasculature of the late gestation sheep fetus to changes in P_aO_2. *Journal of Developmental Physiology* 16, 133–138.

Morrison, S., Fletcher, A.J.W., Gardner, D.S. and Giussani, D.A. (2003) Enhanced nitric oxide activity offsets peripheral vasoconstriction during acute hypoxaemia via chemoreflex and adrenomedullary actions. *Journal of Physiology* 547, 283–291.

Morrow, R.J., Adamson, S.L., Bull, S.B. and Ritchie, J.W. (1990) Acute hypoxemia does not affect the umbilical artery flow velocity waveform in fetal sheep. *Obstetrics and Gynecology* 75(4), 590–593.

Muijsers, G.J., Hasaart, T.H., Ruissen, C.J., Van Huisseling, H., Peeters, L.L.H. and De Haan, J. (1990) The response of the umbilical and femoral artery pulsatility indices in fetal sheep to progressively reduced uteroplacental blood flow. *Journal of Developmental Physiology* 13(4), 215–221.

Mulder, A.L., van Golde, J.C., Prinzen, F.W. and Blanco, C.E. (1998) Cardiac output distribution in response to hypoxia in the chick embryo in the second half of the incubation time. *Journal of Physiology* 508, 281–287

Nicolaides, K.H., Economides, M.D. and Soothill, P.W. (1989) Blood gases, pH and lactate in appropriate- and small-for-gestational-age fetuses. *American Journal of Obstetrics and Gynecology* 161, 996–1001.

Nuwayhid, B., Brinkman, C.R. III, Su, C., Bevan, J.A. and Assali, N.S. (1975) Development of autonomic control of fetal circulation. *American Journal of Physiology* 228, 337–344.

Okamura, K., Shintaku, Y., Watanabe, T., Tanigawara, S., Endo, H., Akagi, K. and Yajima, A. (1992) Femoral artery blood flow monitoring has distinct advantages for examining redistribution of blood flow in fetal acidosis. *Journal of Perinatal Medicine* 20, 215–222.

Parer, J.T. (1984) The effect of atropine on heart rate and oxygen consumption of the hypoxic fetus. *American Journal of Obstetrics and Gynecology* 148, 1118–1122.

Paton, J.B., Fisher, D.E., Peterson, E.N., DeLannoy, C.W. and Behrman, R.E. (1973) Cardiac output and organ blood flows in the baboon fetus. *Biology of the Neonate* 22(1), 50–57.

Peeters, L.L., Sheldon, R.E., Jones, M.D. Jr, Makowski, E.L. and Meschia, G. (1979) Blood flow to fetal organs as a function of arterial oxygen content. *American Journal of Obstetrics and Gynecology* 135, 637–646.

Penrose, L.S. (1954) Some recent trends in human genetics. *Cardiologia* 6 (suppl.), 521–529.

Post, G.B., Lujan, C., San-Miguel, J.L. and Kemper, H.C. (1994) The nutritional intake of Bolivian boys. The relation between altitude and socioeconomic status. *International Journal of Sports Medicine* 15(suppl. 2), S100–S105.

Purves, M.J. and James, I.M. (1969) Observations on the control of cerebral blood flow in the sheep fetus and newborn lamb. *Circulation Research* 25(6), 651–667.

Raff, H., Kane, C.W. and Wood, C.E. (1991) Arginine vasopressin responses to hypoxia and hypercapnia in late-gestation fetal sheep. *American Journal of Physiology* 260, R1077–R1081.

Rawashdeh, N.M., Rose, J.C. and Ray, N.D. (1988) Differential maturation of beta-adrenoceptor-mediated responses in the lamb fetus. *American Journal of Physiology* 255, R794–R798.

Rayburn, W.F., Beynen, A. and Brinkman, D.L. (1981) Umbilical cord length and intrapartum complications. *Obstetrics and Gynecology* 57(4), 450–452.

Read, M.A., Boura, A.L. and Walters, W.A. (1993) Vascular actions of purines in the foetal circulation of the human placenta. *British Journal of Pharmacology* 110, 454–460.

Reuss, M.L., Parer, J.T., Harris, J.L. and Krueger, T.R. (1982) Hemodynamic effects of alpha-adrenergic blockade during hypoxia in fetal sheep. *American Journal of Obstetrics and Gynecology* 142, 410–415.

Richardson, B.S., Carmichael, L., Homan, J., Tanswell, K. and Webster, A.C. (1989) Regional blood flow change in the lamb during the perinatal period. *American Journal of Obstetrics and Gynecology* 160(4), 919–925.

Robillard, J.E., Weitzman, R.E., Burmeister, L. and Smith, F.G. Jr (1981) Developmental aspects of the renal response to hypoxemia in the lamb fetus. *Circulation Research* 48, 128–138.

Robinson, J.S., Kingston, E.J., Jones, C.T. and Thorburn, G.D. (1979) Studies on experimental growth retardation in sheep: The effect of removal of endometrial caruncles on fetal size and metabolism. *Journal of Developmental Physiology* 1, 379–398.

Rosen, K.G. and Kjellmer, I. (1975) Changes in the fetal heart rate and ECG during hypoxia. *Acta Physiologica Scandinavica* 93(1), 59–66.

Rosenfeld, C.R. (2001) Mechanisms regulating angiotensin II responsiveness by the uteroplacental circulation. *American Journal of Physiology, Regulatory, Integrative and Comparative Physiology* 281(4), R1025–R1040.

Rosenfeld, C.R., Cox, B.E. and Roy, T. (1996) Nitric oxide contributes to estrogen-induced vasodilation of the ovine uterine circulation. *Journal of Clinical Investigation* 98, 2158–2166.

Rudolph, A.M. (1984) The fetal circulation and its response to stress. *Journal of Developmental Physiology* 6, 11–19.

Rudolph, A.M. and Heymann, M.A. (1967) The circulation of the fetus *in utero*. *Circulation Research* 21, 163.

Ruijtenbeek, K., Le Noble, F.A., Janssen, G.M., Kessels, C.G., Fazzi, G.E. and Blanco, C.E. (2000) Chronic hypoxia stimulates periarterial sympathetic nerve development in chicken embryo. *Circulation* 102(23), 2892–2897.

Ruiz, L. and Penaloza, D. (1977) Altitude and hypertension. *Mayo Clinic Proceedings* 52(7), 442–445.

Rurak, D.W. (1978) Plasma vasopressin levels during hypoxaemia and the cardiovascular effects of exogenous vasopressin in foetal and adult sheep. *Journal of Physiology* 277, 341–357.

Sanhueza, E.M., Johansen-Bibby, A.A., Fletcher, A.J., Riquelme, R.A., Daniels, A.J., Seron-Ferre, M., Gaete, C.R., Carrasco, J.E., Llanos, A.J. and Giussani, D.A. (2003)

The role of neuropeptide Y in the ovine fetal cardiovascular response to reduced oxygenation. *Journal of Physiology* 546(3), 891–901.

Sheldon, R.E., Peeters, L.L., Jones, M.D. Jr, Makowski, E.L. and Meschia, G. (1979) Redistribution of cardiac output and oxygen delivery in the hypoxemic fetal lamb. *American Journal of Obstetrics and Gynecology* 135(8), 1071–1078.

Shepherd, J.T. and Katusic, Z.S. (1991) Endothelium-derived vasoactive factors: I Endothelium-dependent relaxation. *Hypertension* 18, III-76–III-85.

Tazawa, H. (1981) Effect of O_2 and CO_2 in N_2, He, and SF6 on chick embryo blood pressure and heart rate. *Journal of Applied Physiology* 51(4), 1017–1022.

Tellez, W., Sam-Miguel, J.L., Rodriguez, A., Chavez, M., Lujan, C. and Quintela, A. (1994) Circulating proteins and iron status in blood as indicators of the nutritional status of 10- to 12-year-old Bolivian boys. *International Journal of Sports Medicine* 15(suppl. 2), S79–S83.

Tenney, S.M. (1990) Hypoxic vasorelaxation. *News in Physiological Science* 5, 40.

Tomita, H., Brace, R.A., Cheung, C.Y. and Longo, L.D. (1985) Vasopressin dose–response effects on fetal vascular pressures, heart rate, and blood volume. *American Journal of Physiology* 249, H974–H980.

van Bel, F., Sola, A., Roman, C. and Rudolph, A.M. (1995) Role of nitric oxide in the regulation of the cerebral circulation in the lamb fetus during normoxemia and hypoxemia. *Biology of the Neonate* 68, 200–210.

Vyas, S., Nicolaides, K.H. and Campbell, S. (1990) Doppler examination of the middle cerebral artery in anemic fetuses. *American Journal of Obstetrics and Gynecology* 162(4), 1066–1068.

Warburton, S.J., Hastings, D. and Wang, T. (1995) Responses to chronic hypoxia in embryonic alligators. *Journal of Experimental Zoology* 273(1), 44–50.

Wheeler, T. and Greene, K. (1975) Fetal heart rate monitoring during breech labour. *British Journal of Obstetrics and Gynaecology* 82(3), 208–214.

Wiriyathian, S., Porter, J.C., Naden, R.P. and Rosenfeld, C.R. (1983) Cardiovascular effects and clearance of arginine vasopressin in the fetal lamb. *American Journal of Physiology* 245, E24–E31.

Wood, C.E., Kane, C. and Raff, H. (1990) Peripheral chemoreceptor control of fetal renin responses to hypoxia and hypercapnia. *Circulation Research* 67, 722–732.

Zamudio, S., Droma, T., Norkyel, K.Y., Acharya, G., Zamudio, J.A., Nirmeyer, S.N. and Moore, L.G. (1993) Protection from intrauterine growth retardation in Tibetans at high altitude. *American Journal of Physiology: Anthropology* 91, 215–224.

Zheng, J., Li, Y., Weiss, A.R., Bird, I.M. and Magness, R.R. (2000) Expression of endothelial and inducible nitric oxide synthases and nitric oxide production in ovine placental and uterine tissues during late pregnancy. *Placenta* 21, 516–524.

4 Epidemiology of the Fetal Origins of Adult Disease: Cohort Studies of Birthweight and Cardiovascular Disease

JANET RICH-EDWARDS

Harvard School of Medicine, Department of Ambulatory Care and Prevention, 113 Brookline Avenue, Boston, MA 02215, USA

Introduction

The question of whether, and how, the fetal environment 'programmes' the risk of adult cardiovascular disease has provoked a lively, and still evolving, debate among epidemiologists. Experimental evidence reviewed elsewhere in this volume demonstrates unequivocal evidence that manipulation of fetal environment can change adult phenotype and alter cardiovascular disease risk, among species ranging from rats to alligators to sheep (Deeming and Ferguson, 1989; Langley-Evans *et al.*, 1996; Dodic *et al.*, 2002; Kind *et al.*, 2002). In some cases, experimental induction of the phenotype of a first generation will alter phenotype in second and even third generations, demonstrating non-genetic transmission of phenotype across generations (Dahri *et al.*, 1995; Francis *et al.*, 1999; Roseboom *et al.*, 2000). Despite this proof of principle, comparable evidence of programming of cardiovascular disease in human pregnancy has been elusive. For obvious ethical reasons, experimental data on human pregnancy are scarce. Inferences regarding human fetal programming must be drawn largely from observational data, which suffer from three major limitations: environmental exposures are not randomly assigned, there are decades between fetal exposure and manifest cardiovascular disease, and it is logistically difficult to obtain repeated measures of body size and potential environmental confounders between conception and death among human populations.

To examine evidence of fetal origins of coronary heart disease and stroke, we are left with the difficult task of interpreting inherently tangled observational data from large cohorts of mature adults, falling back on imperfectly measured proxies of fetal environment: birthweight, gestational age, exposure to famine, gestational weight gain and the like. The epidemiologist may envy the clarity of the experimentalist's task. However, the data available from observational studies are essential, as they provide the only human data available. Cautiously interpreted, these data are the best evidence we have at hand to judge the importance and applicability of public health interventions aimed at reducing cardiovascular disease by changing the fetal environment.

This chapter will review the observational cohort studies that relate birthweight to adult cardiovascular disease endpoints, including coronary heart disease and stroke. It will not review the much larger literature on birth size and cardiovascular risk factors, which is reviewed by Rachel Huxley in this volume (Chapter 5). Although there are scattered, and often inconsistent, reports that birth length, ponderal index, chest and head circumferences and maternal pelvic size are associated with cardiovascular disease (CVD) or its risk factors (Barker, 1998), this chapter will focus on birthweight as the most consistently reported measure of newborn anthropometry.

Epidemiological Studies of Birthweight and Cardiovascular Disease

Ecological and migrant studies

The original studies that launched the 'fetal origins hypothesis' were ecological or geographical observations that geographic regions with high infant mortality suffered high cardiovascular mortality 50–70 years later (Forsdahl, 1977; Williams et al., 1979; Barker and Osmond, 1986, 1987). In particular, historical neonatal mortality (mortality in the first month of life) was a strong predictor of current-day risk of stroke, while both neonatal and postneonatal mortality predicted current-day coronary heart disease (CHD) risk (Barker and Osmond, 1986).

These correlation studies prompted speculation that poor conditions in infancy programmed adult cardiovascular disease. However, such studies relied on data about groups of people rather than individuals. As such, they could not establish that the infants with the poorest living conditions were the same individuals who went on to suffer cardiovascular disease. Furthermore, such studies lacked information on potential confounders, such as cigarette smoking, which might have explained associations of high infant mortality with later cardiovascular mortality. Finally, it was impossible to pinpoint the timing of the proposed environmental insult. It was possible, even likely, that those born into poverty remained disadvantaged throughout adolescence and into maturity (Bartley et al., 1994). After all, present infant mortality rates are also positively related to present cardiovascular disease rates (Williams et al., 1979). These ecological data permitted several competing hypotheses. Cardiovascular risk could arise due to factors in the fetal and infant environment, or from an interaction between infant poverty and more affluent adolescent conditions, or because those born poor remained trapped in poverty throughout their lives (Williams et al., 1979; Leon and Ben-Shlomo, 1997). To clarify this issue, one study reported that the association of historic infant mortality with current cardiovascular mortality was greatly attenuated by adjustment for current-day regional socio-economic status, casting doubt on the unique importance of early life environment, other than to launch a pattern of lifelong deprivation (Ben-Shlomo and Davey-Smith, 1991).

Another way to pinpoint the timing of environmental exposure is to study people who move from one environment to another, whether migrating between geographic regions or travelling up or down the ladder of socio-economic position. Such movement provides a naturally occurring (but not randomized) experiment that permits comparison of early and later environment (Elford and Ben-Shlomo, 1997). Several studies have examined whether an individual's risk of CVD is more closely related to the environment at birth or to the environment encountered in later life. These studies have shown that migrants tend to 'acquire' the cardiovascular risk of the countries to which they migrate (Stenhouse and McCall, 1970; Marmot *et al.*, 1975; Alfredsson *et al.*, 1982). Some studies have also been able to evaluate the extent to which migrants retain the cardiovascular risk of their birthplace. For example, three studies have examined CVD rates among migrants within England, Wales and Scotland, where there is a strong geographical gradient in risk of CVD, with higher rates in the north. All three studies concluded that risk of CVD is more associated with region of adult residence than with region of birth. However, two of the three studies also detected independent associations of CVD risk with region of birth (Elford *et al.*, 1989; Osmond *et al.*, 1990; Strachan *et al.*, 1995). Studies of social mobility also reveal that poor social conditions in early life independently predict cardiovascular risk in adulthood, although the strongest prediction is provided by consideration of social position throughout life (Davey-Smith, 1997).

While such migrant studies are useful in identifying critical windows of cardiovascular vulnerability to environmental exposure, they have two major limitations. Migrants and socially mobile individuals may be selectively healthier (or unhealthier) than those in their homelands, leading the unwary investigator or reader to mistake a process of social/health selection for an impact of environmental change. These studies also tend to provide only general indications of early environment; broad exposures such as 'born in East Anglia' or 'social class III' do little to narrow the list of putative agents of fetal or early life programming.

Clearly, the hypotheses raised in these early ecological studies needed to be tested in cohorts of individuals. However, the difficulties of obtaining data on the prenatal and childhood environment of adults now 60 or 70 years old seemed nearly insurmountable. In the absence of direct measurements of prenatal environment, birthweight was chosen as a correlate of infant mortality and a stand-in for fetal conditions. This choice of birthweight as a proxy for individual exposure enabled the first individual-level follow-up studies examining whether birthweight was correlated with adult cardiovascular morbidity and mortality. The cohort studies that examined birthweight as a predictor of cardiovascular disease events are summarized in Table 4.1, where estimates of the strength of associations between birthweight and cardiovascular disease are provided.

Table 4.1. Cohort studies of the association of birthweight with cardiovascular disease endpoints.

Reference	Cohort	Endpoint	Crude or age-adjusted change in risk of endpoint per kg increase in birthweight[a]	BMI-adjusted or stratified change in risk of endpoint per kg increase in birthweight[a]
Barker et al. (1989)	5654 men in Hertfordshire	CHD mortality	Decrease (NS)	NA
Osmond et al. (1993)	5585 women and 10,141 men in Hertfordshire	CVD mortality	Men: decrease ($P < 0.005$); approx. 16% decrease/kg Women: decrease ($P = 0.04$); approx. 18% decrease/kg	NA
Martyn et al. (1996)	13,249 men in Hertfordshire and Sheffield	CVD mortality	CHD: decrease ($P < 0.05$); 23% decrease/kg Stroke: decrease ($P < 0.05$); 28% decrease/kg	NA
Eriksson et al. (1994)	855 men in Gothenburg, Sweden	CHD events	Increase ($P = 0.05$)	NA
Frankel et al. (1996a,b)	1258 men in Caerphilly	CHD events	Decrease ($P = 0.02$); approx. 23% decrease/kg (Frankel et al., 1996a)	Decrease ($P = 0.01$), only with high adult BMI (Frankel et al., 1996b)
Rich-Edwards et al. (1997; 2003)	70,297 female US nurses	CVD events	CHD: 15% decrease/kg ($P = 0.0008$) Stroke: 15% decrease/kg ($P = 0.004$)	CHD: 17% decrease/kg ($P < 0.0001$) Stroke: 16% decrease/kg ($P = 0.001$)
Leon et al. (1998)	14,611 births in Uppsala, Sweden	CVD mortality	Men: CHD: 23% decrease/kg ($P < 0.05$) Stroke: 29% decrease/kg (NS) Women: CHD: 17% decrease/kg (NS) Stroke: 16% decrease/kg (NS)	NA
Koupilova et al. (1999)	1334 men in Uppsala, Sweden (subset of Leon et al., 1998)	CVD mortality	CHD: 26% decrease/kg (NS) Stroke: 53% decrease/kg ($P < 0.05$)	CHD: 31% decrease/kg ($P < 0.05$) Stroke: 53% decrease/kg stroke ($P < 0.05$)

Study	Population	Outcome	Estimate	Comments
Forsen et al. (1999)	3447 women in Helsinki	CHD events	Decrease (P = 0.08 adjusted for gestation length); approx. 14% decrease/kg	NA
Forsen et al. (1997); Eriksson et al. (1999)	3641 men in Helsinki	CHD mortality	Decrease (P = 0.05 adjusted for gestation length); approx. 9% decrease/kg	NA
Eriksson et al. (2000)	3639 men in Helsinki	Stroke events	Decrease (P = 0.03); approx. 18% decrease/kg	NA
Eriksson et al. (2001)	4630 men in Helsinki (new sample)	CHD events	Decrease (P = 0.006); approx. 29% decrease/kg	Thinness at birth associated with increased risk only among those with higher BMI in childhood
Gunnarsdottir et al. (2002)	2399 men and 2376 women in Reykjavik	CHD events in high birthweight population	Men: Decrease (P = 0.10); approx. 17% decrease/kg Women: U-shaped association; excluding 4 kg+: approx. 28% decrease/kg; including 4 kg+: approx. 10% decrease/kg	Adjustment did not change results

[a]Many papers did not present estimates of the change in CVD risk per unit birthweight (lb or kg). Where odds ratios (OR) were presented per lb birthweight, they were translated into estimates per kg birthweight [exp(ln OR/0.454)]. Where estimates are qualified as 'Approx.', they have been approximated by comparing disease frequencies or crude estimates of association presented in the original paper for the low : high birthweight categories. For example, Frankel et al. (1996a) presented age-adjusted CHD incidence as 13.6, 10.6, 12.3 and 8.1 across ascending quartiles of birthweight. It was assumed that the range of birthweights in the study was 2 kg, and they calculated the odds ratio of CHD per kg birthweight as exp[(ln(8.1/13.6))/2] = 0.77, or a 23% decrease in CHD risk per kg increase in birthweight. In cases where an estimate in the highest or lowest category was inconsistent with the general trend across birthweight categories, it was averaged with the adjacent category, to avoid undue influence of using only highest and lowest categories to estimate trend. The reader should treat these estimates with a great deal of caution, as they may be quite different from continuous estimates of the association drawn through all points in the birthweight range.

CHD, coronary heart disease; CVD, cardiovascular disease; BMI, body mass index; NA, not applicable; NS, not significant.

Cohort studies

The original studies of birthweight and coronary heart disease by Barker and colleagues at the Medical Research Council (MRC) unit in Southampton made clever use of health visitor records from 1911 to 1930 in Hertfordshire and Sheffield, England (Barker et al., 1989; Osmond et al., 1993). Attempts were made to trace all singleton births for whom birthweight and weight at 1 year had been recorded by midwives and health visitors. Barker's team successfully traced 68% of the cohort that had infant and childhood weight measures, or 43% of the original cohort of 36,944 births. Adult mortality status and cause of death were determined by record linkage to a national mortality registry. Standardized mortality ratios for cardiovascular disease fell with increasing birthweight for both women (183 deaths; $P = 0.04$) and men (1172 deaths; $P < 0.005$) (Osmond et al., 1993). Compared to infants weighing 8–8.5 lb (3.6–3.8 kg) at birth, low birthweight (< 5.5 lb (< 2.5 kg)) infants had roughly 30–40% higher risk of mortality from coronary heart disease. These risks dropped consistently with increasing birthweight, until the largest group of infants, weighing 10 lb (4.5 kg) or more, at which point cardiovascular risk increased slightly. As adult social class was known only for those who had died, it was not possible to adjust for social position; however, there was no apparent association between birthweight and social class of those who had died. Further follow-up of the men in Hertfordshire and Sheffield permitted examination of coronary heart disease and stroke separately. The MRC team reported a 12% (95% confidence interval, 1–22%) decrease in risk of stroke mortality and 10% decrease in risk of CHD mortality (6–14%) per pound increase in birthweight among men (230 stroke deaths and 1409 CHD deaths) (Martyn et al., 1996).

Other teams of epidemiologists rushed to replicate these findings, and to include studies with more detailed data on adult lifestyle factors and socio-economic conditions that might explain the statistical association of birthweight with CVD. With the exception of a relatively small cohort ($n = 855$) of men in Gothenburg, Sweden born in 1913 (among whom risk of coronary heart disease increased with increasing birthweight) (Eriksson et al., 1994), investigators almost unanimously confirmed the inverse association of birthweight with CVD observed first in Hertfordshire and Sheffield.

Frankel and colleagues examined a group of 1258 men from Caerphilly, South Wales, who were able to report their own birthweight (45% of an original cohort of 2818) (Frankel et al., 1996a). Age-adjusted incident fatal and non-fatal CHD dropped with increasing quartile of birthweight (137 events; $P = 0.01$). Adjustment for adult behavioural, nutritional and socio-economic factors made no material difference to the inverse association of birthweight with CHD risk. Surprisingly, control for the presumed intermediate variables of cholesterol, fibrinogen, systolic blood pressure and lung function slightly strengthened the birthweight–CHD association. The inverse association of birthweight with CHD risk was statistically significant with and without adjustment for height and adult adiposity (although somewhat stronger with adjustment for adult body size). Stratification by adult body mass index (BMI) revealed that the inverse associa-tion of birthweight with CHD was significant only among obese men, implying an interaction between small size at birth and adiposity later in life (Frankel *et al.*, 1996b). This study was the first to demonstrate that adult social position and life-style did not explain the inverse association of birthweight with CHD incidence.

In the USA, Rich-Edwards and colleagues examined associations of birth-weight and non-fatal cardiovascular disease events among 70,297 female nurses who reported their own birthweight (58% of the original cohort of 121,700) (Rich-Edwards *et al.*, 1997). Among full-term singletons, the age-adjusted risks of cardiovascular disease fell consistently with increasing birthweight, for both coronary heart disease (889 cases; $P = 0.11$) and stroke (364 cases; $P = 0.003$). Adjustment for adult BMI somewhat strengthened the inverse asso-ciations, revealing an 11% (95% confidence interval, 0–19%) reduction in risk of CHD and a 23% (11–17%) reduction in risk of stroke for every kilogram increase in birthweight. Inverse associations with birthweight were evident for both ischaemic ($P = 0.008$) and haemorrhagic ($P = 0.02$) stroke. The addition of eight more years of follow-up to this cohort tripled the number of cardiovascular events that were observed in the original study, and led to the more precise age-adjusted estimates of cardiovascular risk associated with a kilogram increase in birthweight, of 0.85 (95% confidence interval, 0.78–0.94) for CHD, and 0.85 (0.77–0.95) for stroke, or 15% reductions in risk for every kilogram increase in birthweight (unpublished data). Like the Caerphilly study, adjustment for hypertension, hypercholesterolaemia, and diabetes only slightly affected the risk estimates. This study confirmed that the birthweight associations were present among women, were robust to adjustment for childhood social class and adult lifestyle, and were present for both haemorrhagic and ischaemic stroke subtypes.

The ideal study would follow a complete cohort from birth to maturity, accounting for the fate of each newborn. The studies in the UK and the USA suffered either from incomplete tracing of a defined birth cohort or did not repre-sent a defined birth cohort (cohorts assembled in adulthood only rarely represent follow-up of a definable group of infants). The failure of these studies to account for all members of a specified birth cohort laid these studies open to charges of selection bias, the suspicion that the observed associations of birthweight with adult disease were an artefact of selective follow-up (although no plausible selection mechanism was proposed to account for such results). In this storm of criticism, Leon and colleagues published the results of an almost complete follow-up of births in an Uppsala hospital from 1915 to 1929 (Leon *et al.*, 1998). The existence of national personal identity numbers allowed the investigators to link birth records to mortality records and census data on socio-economic status. Like the previous studies, the Uppsala study reported reduced mortality from coronary heart disease and stroke with increasing birthweight. While the risk reductions associated with a kilogram increase in birthweight were consistent in direction and magnitude for coronary heart disease (23% for men and 17% for women) and stroke (29% for men and 16% for women), they were statistically significant only for coronary heart disease among men. Adjustment for socio-economic position at birth and in adulthood had little impact on the CHD association among men. A later sub-study of 1334 men who had undergone standardized medical examinations at age 50 and age 60 showed somewhat stronger inverse associations of birthweight with CHD and stroke, which were not explained by measured adult BMI or by blood pressure (Koupilova *et al.*, 1999). Birthweight adjusted for gestational age had a much stronger association with CHD than did birthweight, leading the investigators to surmise that fetal growth rate was more important than gestational length in determining future cardiovascular risk.

Subsequently, Forsen, Eriksson, Barker and colleagues traced 93% of the 7281 people born between 1924 and 1933 in Helsinki University Central Hospital who also had Helsinki school records and remained resident in Finland until national identification numbers were assigned in 1971 (Forsen *et al.*, 1997, 1999; Eriksson *et al.*, 1999, 2000). In both men and women, birthweight had an inverse, if not consistently dose–response, association with CHD that lacked statistical significance: 310 CHD deaths among men, $P = 0.05$ with adjustment for gestation length (Eriksson *et al.*, 1999); 297 CHD events among women, $P = 0.08$ with adjustment for gestation length (Forsen *et al.*, 1999). Stroke events were also inversely associated with birthweight among men (331 cases; $P = 0.03$) (Eriksson *et al.*, 2000). As in the Nurses' Health Study, birthweight was inversely associated with both haemorrhagic and thrombotic strokes, although these associations did not reach statistical significance. The highest risk of CHD death occurred among men with a low ponderal index at birth who had a high BMI in childhood (Eriksson *et al.*, 1999).

Eriksson and colleagues drew a new sample of births from Helsinki University Hospital from 1933 to 1944, for whom serial measurements of height and weight from birth to age 12 years had been recorded (Eriksson *et al.*, 2001). In this cohort of 4630 men, there was a very strong inverse association of birthweight with CHD events (357 cases; $P = 0.006$), which was evident among both term and preterm births. Although the association of birthweight with CHD was not further elaborated in this study, a low ponderal index (kg/m^3) at birth was associated with future CHD risk, particularly among boys who grew to a larger BMI during childhood. The results of this study, which had ample information on childhood growth, are discussed further below.

The most recent study to report on birthweight and adult coronary heart disease obtained birth record data for 4828 (78%) of 6120 participants in the Reykjavik Study of the Icelandic Heart Association from 1967 to 1997 (Gunnarsdottir *et al.*, 2002). The Icelandic population tends toward high birthweight (only 1% of the cohort weighed < 2500 g while 26% weighed more than 4250 g at birth). Even in this higher birthweight range, there was a consistent inverse association of birthweight with coronary heart disease among men, although it did not reach statistical significance (440 cases; $P = 0.10$). Among women there was a reverse J-shaped association, with an upturn in CHD risk at 4000 g (134 cases; $P = 0.11$ for linear trend). Adjustment for adult BMI made no difference to these estimates.

Altogether, there are 13 published studies from eight populations that provide information on the associations between birthweight and cardiovascular disease events. With one exception (the smallest study) (Eriksson *et al.*, 1994), inverse associations were observed between birthweight and CVD. Eight of the 13 studies reported at least one statistically significant inverse association of birthweight with cardiovascular disease. The magnitude and statistical strength of these findings can be compared in Table 4.1. Better estimates of the change in coronary heart disease risk per kilogram change in birthweight are forthcoming in a meta-analysis by Huxley and colleagues.

Critics did not fail to point out the potential flaws of each of these studies, ranging from incomplete follow-up of whole birth cohorts, use of self-reported birthweight, limitation to fatal or non-fatal disease endpoints, failure to adjust for childhood and/or adult socio-economic status, and failure to account for adult lifestyle risk factors, such as smoking (Paneth and Susser, 1995; Kramer and Joseph, 1996). While no single study is perfect, as a group, they have collectively dispelled these criticisms. For example, the Swedish study was able to follow a complete birth cohort (Leon *et al.*, 1998). The UK, Swedish and Finnish studies were based on birth records, and were able to account for socio-economic status at various life junctures (Barker *et al.*, 1989; Forsen *et al.*, 1997; Leon *et al.*, 1998). The US and Swedish studies controlled for such adult lifestyle factors as cigarette smoking, diet and family history (Rich-Edwards *et al.*, 1997; Leon *et al.*, 1998). Through all these tribulations, the association between birthweight and adult cardiovascular disease is remarkably consistent and robust.

Taken as a group, the epidemiological cohort studies of birthweight and CVD tend to show:

- Approximately 40% lower risk of cardiovascular disease for the largest, compared to the smallest infants. A 1 kg increase in birthweight is associated with approximately a 20% decrease in risk of CVD (see Table 4.1).
- Generally stronger inverse associations of birthweight with cerebrovascular disease than with coronary heart disease. Haemorrhagic stroke and thrombotic stroke are each associated with birthweight (Rich-Edwards *et al.*, 1997; Eriksson *et al.*, 2000).
- Studies that adjusted for cardiovascular risk factors, such as blood pressure, diabetes, family history, respiratory function, cholesterol or fibrinogen levels, found that these factors did not explain the association of birthweight with cardiovascular disease (Frankel *et al.*, 1996a; Rich-Edwards *et al.*, 1997; Koupilova *et al.*, 1999).
- Associations of birthweight with cardiovascular disease are generally strengthened by adjustment for gestational age, implicating fetal growth, rather than length of gestation, as the predictor of CVD. However, data on gestational age are notoriously error-prone, and were undoubtedly quite inaccurate in the first half of the 20th century, before modern concern with preterm birth and the advent of ultrasound dating. This may have precluded detection of associations between gestation length and risk of adult disease. More data are needed on the possible association of gestational duration with future CVD risk.
- Almost all the studies reported crude or age-adjusted inverse associations between birthweight and adult cardiovascular events that were at or near statistical significance. Nevertheless, two studies found that adjustment for adult BMI somewhat strengthened the associations between birthweight and coronary heart disease (Rich-Edwards *et al.*, 1997; Koupilova *et al.*, 1999).

- In some studies, macrosomic infants (> 4000 g) appear to have a slightly elevated risk of adult coronary heart disease (but not stroke) compared to average-size infants (Osmond *et al.*, 1993; Leon *et al.*, 1998; Gunnarsdottir *et al.*, 2002). After accounting for their tendency to a larger body size in adulthood, they may have similar, or even lower risk of CHD, compared to average-size counterparts (Rich-Edwards *et al.*, 1997).
- Some, but not all (Koupilova *et al.*, 1999), studies report an interaction between birthweight and weight in childhood (Eriksson *et al.*, 2001) or body mass index in adulthood (Frankel *et al.*, 1996b), with stronger birthweight associations among the heaviest individuals.

Thus, there is a consistently observed inverse association between birthweight and CVD. However, establishment of a consistent statistical association is only the first hurdle that a hypothesis must pass. The interpretation of the association is a surprisingly complex matter.

Is it Birthweight, or is it Postnatal Growth?

The greatest epidemiological challenge to the fetal origins hypothesis relates to the interrelation of fetal and postnatal growth patterns. The interpretation of birthweight, with or without adjustment for adult body size, is a subject of considerable debate and confusion. The confusion centres around disentangling the presumed opposing effects of prenatal and postnatal weight gain.

Weight at birth and weight in adulthood are modestly correlated, for both environmental and genetic reasons. Fetal growth is jointly determined by maternal body size, placental function, growth factors, infection, maternal nutrition and the fetal genome (Tanner, 1990). After birth, genes and environment continue to interact to determine growth. Body size generally tracks from birth to adulthood. Larger infants, on average, become larger adults. However, the rate of growth in infancy (weight centile crossing) may be inversely related to fetal growth, due to the phenomena of 'catch-up' and 'catch-down' growth in infancy (Ong *et al.*, 2000). In the first years of life, 'catch-up' growth may reflect liberation from 'maternal constraint' of fetal growth, while the less frequently observed 'catch-down' growth may indicate rebound from 'maternal promotion', perhaps due to a hyperglycaemic uterine environment.

This complex relationship between size at birth and adult size presents real analytic and interpretational problems, rendered more difficult by the presumed opposite, and probably interacting, relationship of early and late growth with cardiovascular endpoints. While weight gain in early life certainly represents growth in height as well as increases in muscle mass and adiposity, weight gain in adulthood generally represents gains in adiposity. The only firm anchor in this debate is the well-established, direct dose–response association of adult BMI with cardiovascular risk. Adult adiposity is a strong risk factor for cardiovascular disease, especially coronary heart disease (Manson *et al.*, 1990). In the face of this incontrovertible fact, the interpretation of the inverse dose–response association between birthweight and CVD risk becomes problematic, and multiple interpretations are possible.

In several, but not all, studies, stratification by childhood or adult BMI reveals that the highest risk of coronary heart disease occurs in those born at low birthweight who grow to be large adults (Frankel *et al.*, 1996b; Koupilova *et al.*, 1999; Eriksson *et al.*, 2001), in contrast to the lower risk among those who track large or small their whole lives. There are at least three alternative interpretations of this pattern:

1. Rapid weight gain among those born small (perhaps indicating catch-up growth) indicates *in utero* growth restriction or maternal constraint, marking those whose fetal environment was poor, and thus most likely to have been prenatally 'programmed'. In this scenario, fetal programming is thought to be a more or less permanent physiological adaptation to poor fetal environment that is largely unmodified by postnatal environment.

2. Rapid weight gain between birth and adulthood confers risk, above and beyond that associated with either birthweight or attained adult BMI. In other words, a steep road to adult obesity is worse than a level path, regardless of start point. In this scenario, it is the rate of postnatal growth, rather than the absolute starting or ending body size, that is thought to increase cardiovascular disease risk.

3. Constrained prenatal growth truly interacts with rapid postnatal growth, such that those habituated to a poor *in utero* environment have higher disease risk when glutted with a rich postnatal environment (the thrifty phenotype argument). In this scenario, rapid growth is a risk factor only for those born small, as it represents postnatal nutritional overload of an individual pre-programmed for a lean postnatal environment. This is fetal programming with postnatal modification.

These alternative hypotheses are not mutually exclusive, indeed, it seems likely that some features of newborns have been immutably 'set' *in utero*, whether by genes or environment, and that these traits are modified by postnatal environment. It is important to sort out these patterns, because they imply different public health and medical interventions. Most studies offer little insight into which of these mechanisms explains the higher risk observed among those born small and who grow large. The only way out of this conundrum is to isolate the impact of different periods of growth by using serial measurements of weight and height. A few studies have had such data.

Cohort studies with childhood growth data

The first studies to examine weight at birth and in childhood were the original studies in Hertfordshire and Sheffield, which had recorded weights at 1 year as well as at birth. For men, weight at age 1 year was inversely associated with CHD mortality, much as birthweight had been (Barker *et al.*, 1989; Osmond *et al.*, 1993). CHD mortality was highest among males who had low weights at birth and at age 1 year. Among women, this pattern was absent (Osmond *et al.*, 1993). These were the first studies to examine whether the implications of low birthweight were dependent upon growth in infancy.

An important dataset with which to analyse the question of postnatal growth was assembled by Eriksson *et al.* (2001). A sample of 4630 men born at Helsinki University Hospital from 1934 to 1944 was traced through voluntary child welfare clinics, at which they had an average of nine measurings of height and weight in their first year, and nine more measurings until age 12 years. Hospital admission and mortality data were collected from national registries; 357 men had been hospitalized for, or died from, coronary heart disease.

Birthweight was strongly inversely associated with risk of CHD. Compared to boys born weighing more than 4000 g, low birthweight infants (≤ 2500 g) had 3.6 times the risk of CHD, while those born weighing between 2500 and 4000 g had twice the risk of CHD of the largest boys ($P = 0.006$ for the trend in risk across birthweight categories). At 1 year of age, boys who were small in height or weight were at increased risk of future cardiovascular disease; there was a strong graded inverse association of BMI at age 1 year with future cardiovascular disease risk ($P = 0.0004$). The increased risk with small size at age 1 year was evident, regardless of size at birth. When included in the same model, one standard deviation higher birthweight had a hazard ratio of 0.94 (0.83–1.06) and one standard deviation higher weight at age 1 year had a hazard ratio of 0.84 (0.75–0.94).

However, some investigators have argued that adjustment of one weight for a later weight complicates the interpretation of the weight coefficients, as any impact of actual weight *gain* between the two time-points would be shared between the two weight coefficients (Lucas and Fewtrell, 1999; Cole *et al.*, 2001). In response to this criticism, Osmond reran the Helsinki data to model simultaneously birthweight and weight *gain* from birth to age 1 year (i.e. the slope change between the two points). One standard deviation higher birthweight was associated with a hazard ratio of 0.78 (0.69–0.88) for CHD, while one standard deviation in infant weight gain was associated with a hazard ratio of 0.83 (0.74–0.93) (Osmond *et al.*, 2001). The birthweight coefficient gained strength by modelling first-year weight gain in the place of year one attained weight because first-year weight gain is negatively correlated with birthweight, since catch-up growth is greatest in small newborns. In other words, both greater weight at birth, greater weight at age one, and greater weight gain between the two time-points predicted reduced CHD risk in adulthood.

In childhood, the implications of weight gain changed dramatically, and depended upon size at birth. Among boys with a higher ponderal index at birth (> 26 kg/m^3), those whose weight rank dropped in childhood appeared to have higher CHD risk. In contrast, among boys who were thin at birth, increases in weight rank increased CHD risk. The older the thin newborns were when they gained BMI in childhood, the greater was the adverse implication of the added weight. This may indicate that early increases in BMI are due to gains in muscle mass and organ size, while later increases may reflect accumulating adiposity.

How do these observations inform our understanding of the interacting implications of fetal and childhood growth for future CHD risk? Among the Helsinki findings are several useful leads:

- Weight gain in the first year of life appeared to be protective among all newborns, regardless of birthweight. This appears to refute the notion that 'catch-up growth' marks those at highest risk.
- After infancy, centile-crossing growth was associated with *increased* CHD risk among small newborns and *decreased* CHD risk among large newborns. This challenges the idea that centile crossing *per se* is a uniform risk factor for CHD, at least in childhood. However, adolescent or adult weight gain (more likely to be adipose tissue) may be similarly associated with increased CHD risk among those born small or large.
- Small infants who tracked small throughout childhood were at no, or only a modest, increased risk of future CHD. In contrast, small newborns who grew large were at considerably higher risk. This observation supports the thrifty phenotype hypothesis, as well as the possibility that consistently small people (perhaps born to genetically small parents) are not at heightened risk of CHD.

Overall, the observations from Helsinki, presaged by the earlier work from Hertfordshire and Sheffield, lend support to the notion that the child whose *in utero* growth is consistent with its postnatal growth, showing neither growth accelerations nor growth faltering, has the lowest cardiovascular risk in adulthood. This may be an indication of children whose resources were adequate enough to prevent stunting, but not so overfed as to accumulate large burdens of body fat. Studies of adult BMI, which additionally capture weight change in adolescence and adulthood, indicate that centile-crossing is harmful to all adults, but especially harmful to those born small. This lends further support to the thrifty phenotype notion, that those adapted to scarcity are ill-equipped to handle nutritional overload.

To date, only the Helsinki study has provided data to test the impact of different patterns of growth on CHD risk. Future studies may or may not replicate the Helsinki findings. Furthermore, no study has measured weights at birth, throughout childhood and adolescence, and into adulthood. Even the Helsinki study, which relied on registries to collect data about adult CHD outcomes, did not include measures of adult BMI. Other studies that have data on adult BMI and birthweight lack information on BMI through childhood. Finally, no study has yet considered the implications of longitudinal growth patterns on stroke risk.

Thus, 'the jury is still out' regarding the interpretation of the inverse association of birthweight with CVD, given that the heightened CHD risk among low birthweight babies is primarily found among those with rapid postnatal growth. Even if it is established that size at birth is an *independent* predictor of later CVD risk, we must dig deeper to understand the biological meaning behind the statistical association.

Birthweight: Sham and Straw Man

We need to maintain a healthy scepticism as we interpret the significance of birthweight. Birthweight was first seized upon for its correlation with infant mortality because it was the only reliably recorded indicator of fetal health. Where investigators might have wished for measures of maternal micronutrient intake, placental vasculopathy, umbilical artery blood flow, chorioamnionitis and levels of cytokines and glucocorticoids, they had birthweight. Birthweight is, however, not a good proxy of anything except neonatal mortality. First, birthweight is the product of many environmental and genetic factors that might, or might not, be relevant to the developing cardiovascular system. Thus, it is a non-specific marker. Secondly, as a proxy, birthweight may fail to reflect some quite potent fetal determinants of cardiovascular risk (as in several animal studies where manipulation of fetal environment affects the cardiovascular system without changing birthweight; Nwagwu *et al.*, 2000). In this sense, it is an insensitive marker. Even the widespread assumption that the observed birthweight association implicates restricted fetal growth as a programmer of future cardiovascular risk is something of a leap of faith. It could be that another factor, related only coincidentally to fetal growth and birthweight, determines future cardiovascular risk.

Thus, birthweight is both a sham and a straw man. Those who maintain that the inverse associations between birthweight and adult disease prove the role of maternal nutrition (or even fetal growth) in determining cardiovascular risk have surely promised more than birthweight can deliver. On the other hand, those who would shoot down the notion of fetal programming, by pointing out where birthweight associations are weak or inconsistent, may be committing a similar error, mistaking a weak signal from an imprecise marker as evidence against fetal programming. It seems more reasonable to consider the existence of a birthweight association only a vague pointer toward more interesting exposures. The prime suspects include genes linked to both fetal growth and cardiovascular development, maternal nutrition, placental function, infection and growth factors, all of which are likely to be interrelated. The evidence for these, more specific, risk factors, which may explain the observed birthweight associations, is reviewed elsewhere in this volume.

Future Directions

For the time being, we should continue to refine our understanding of the implications of interacting fetal, infant, childhood and adult growth on cardiovascular disease risk. In particular, it will be helpful to have data from ongoing studies that feature serial growth measures from birth to adulthood. Better yet, future studies may also include measures of fetal size obtained by ultrasound, allowing us truly to investigate 'fetal growth'. However, it will be even more useful to gather and test data with regard to the specific biological mechanisms that underlie the birthweight–cardiovascular disease association.

Other epidemiological approaches have yielded useful information in this regard. For example, the follow-up of children whose mothers were randomized to receive nutritional supplements during pregnancy (Belizan *et al.*, 1997), or preterm infants randomized to various milk regimens (Lucas, 1998; Herrmann *et al.*, 2001) give more specific information regarding prenatal or preterm nutritional exposures. Similarly, the follow-up of preterm infants whose mothers received dexamethasone injections can provide unique insights (Lucas, 1998). The tracing of adults whose mothers were pregnant during famines provides another, albeit crude, ecological look at whether restricted caloric intake programmes the fetus (Stanner *et al.*, 1997; Roseboom *et al.*, 2000). The observation of twins, whose *in utero* growth is often constrained, has provided some insights (Poulter *et al.*, 1999; Hubinette *et al.*, 2001; Johansson-Kark *et al.*, 2002). However, these studies have generally been limited by their low statistical power. While they are useful for examining cardiovascular risk factors such as blood pressure, BMI, or glucose tolerance, they have very limited ability to observe cardiovascular disease events.

Retrospective cohort studies that have stored biological samples and exposure data, such as the US National Collaborative Perinatal Project from the 1960s, will soon provide more data with regard to hormone exposures and placental characteristics. Current pregnancy cohorts, although they will not be able to observe cardiovascular events in our lifetimes, will provide much more detailed information on environmental exposures that can be used to examine cardiovascular risk factors. Genetic studies may yield insight into the question of whether the birthweight phenomenon is partly or wholly the product of genes controlling growth and cardiovascular development. Experimental data from other species may continue to generate the best data regarding specific biological mechanisms. For the foreseeable future, we will continue to 'triangulate' on the question of fetal origins of cardiovascular disease, gathering imperfect evidence from these disparate sources. Only by identifying the particular biological mechanisms underlying the apparent phenomenon of fetal programming will we be able to design appropriate public health interventions to reduce cardiovascular disease.

References

Alfredsson, L., Ahlbom, A. and Theorell, T. (1982) Incidence of myocardial infarction among male Finnish immigrants in relation to length of stay in Sweden. *International Journal of Epidemiology* 11, 225–228.

Barker, D.J.P. (1998) *Mothers, Babies and Health in Later Life*, 2nd edn. Churchill Livingstone, London.

Barker, D.J.P. and Osmond, C. (1986) Infant mortality, childhood nutrition, and ischaemic heart disease in England and Wales. *Lancet* 1, 1077–1081.

Barker, D.J.P. and Osmond, C. (1987) Death rates from stroke in England and Wales predicted from past maternal mortality. *British Medical Journal* 295, 83–86.

Barker, D.J.P., Winter, P., Osmond, C., Margetts, B.M. and Simmonds, S. (1989) Weight in infancy and death from ischaemic heart disease. *Lancet* 2, 577–580.

Bartley, M., Power, C., Davey-Smith, G. and Shipley, M. (1994) Birthweight and later socioeconomic disadvantage: evidence from the 1958 British cohort study. *British Medical Journal* 309, 1475–1478.

Belizan, J.M., Villar, J., Bergel, E., de Pino, A., Di Fulvio, S., Galliano, S.V. and Kattan, C. (1997) Long term effect of calcium supplementation during pregnancy on the blood pressure of offspring: follow up of a randomised controlled trial. *British Medical Journal* 315, 281–285.

Ben-Shlomo, Y. and Davey-Smith, G. (1991) Deprivation in infancy or in adult life: which is more important for mortality risk? *Lancet* 337, 530–535.

Cole, T.J., Fewtrell, M. and Lucas, A. (2001) Early growth and coronary disease in later life [Letter]. *British Medical Journal* 323, 572.

Dahri, S., Reusens, B., Renacle, C. and Hoet, J.J. (1995) Nutritional influences on pancreatic development and potential links with non-insulin-dependent diabetes. *Proceedings of the Nutrition Society* 54, 345–356.

Davey-Smith, G. (1997) Socioeconomic differentials. In: Kuh, D. and Ben-Shlomo, Y. (eds) *A Life Course Approach to Chronic Disease Epidemiology*. Oxford University Press, New York, pp. 242–276.

Deeming, D.C. and Ferguson, M.W.J. (1989) The mechanism of temperature dependent sex determination in crocodilians: a hypothesis. *American Zoologist* 29(973), 985.

Dodic, M., Aboutanoun, T., O'Connor, A., Wintour, E.M. and Mortiz, K.M. (2002) Programming effects of short prenatal exposure to dexamethasone in sheep. *Hypertension* 40, 729–734.

Elford, J. and Ben-Shlomo, Y. (1997) Geography and migration. In: Kuh, D. and Ben-Shlomo, Y. (eds) *A Life Course Approach to Chronic Disease Epidemiology*. Oxford University Press, New York, pp. 220–241.

Elford, J., Philips, A.N., Thompson, A.G. and Shaper, A.G. (1989) Migration and geographic variations in ischaemic heart disease in Great Britian. *Lancet* 1(343), 346.

Eriksson, J.G., Forsen, T., Tuomilehto, J., Winter, P.D., Osmond, C. and Barker, D.J.P. (1999) Catch-up growth in childhood and death from coronary heart disease: longitudinal study. *British Medical Journal* 318, 427–431.

Eriksson, J.G., Forsen, T., Tuomilehto, J., Osmond, C. and Barker, D.J.P. (2000) Early growth, adult income and risk of stroke. *Stroke* 31(4), 869–874.

Eriksson, J.G., Forsen, T., Tuomilehto, J., Osmond, C. and Barker, D.J.P. (2001) Early growth and coronary heart disease in later life: longitudinal study. *British Medical Journal* 322, 949–953.

Eriksson, M., Tibblin, G. and Cnattinguis, S. (1994) Low birthweight and ischaemic heart disease. *Lancet* 343, 731–732.

Forsdahl, A. (1977) Are poor living conditions in childhod and adolescence an important risk factor for arteriosclerotic heart disease? *British Journal of Preventive and Social Medicine* 31, 91–95.

Forsen, T., Eriksson, J.G., Tuomilehto, J., Teramo, K., Osmond, C. and Barker, D.J.P. (1997) Mother's weight in pregnancy and coronary heart disease in a cohort of Finnish men: follow up study. *British Medical Journal* 315(4112), 837–840.

Forsen, T., Eriksson, J.G., Tuomilehto, J., Osmond, C. and Barker, D.J.P. (1999) Growth *in utero* and during childhood among women who develop coronary heart disease: longitudinal study. *British Medical Journal* 314, 1403–1407.

Francis, D., Diorio, J., Liu, D. and Meaney, M.J. (1999) Nongenomic transmission across generations of maternal behavior and stress responses in the rat. *Science* 286(5442), 1155–1158.

Frankel, S., Elwood, P., Sweetnam, P., Yarnell, J. and Davey-Smith, G. (1996a) Birthweight, adult risk factors and incident coronary heart disease: the Caerphilly study. *Public Health Reports* 110, 139–143.

Frankel, S., Elwood, P., Sweetman, P., Yarnell, J. and Davey-Smith, G. (1996b) Birthweight, body-mass index in middle age and incident coronary heart disease. *Lancet* 343, 1478–1480.

Gunnarsdottir, I., Birghisdottir, B.E., Thorsdottir, I., Gudnason, V. and Benediktsson, R. (2002) Size at birth and coronary artery disese in a population with high birth weight. *American Journal of Clinical Nutrition* 76, 1290–1294.

Herrmann, T.S., Siega-Riz, A.M., Hobel, C.J., Aurora, C.J. and Dunkel-Schetter, C. (2001) Prolonged periods without food intake during pregnancy increase risk for elevated maternal cortotropin-releasing hormone concentrations. *American Journal of Obstetrics and Gynecology* 185, 403–413.

Hubinette, A., Ekbom, A., de Faire, U., Kramer, M. and Lichtenstein, P. (2001) Birthweight, early environment and genetics: a study of twins discordant for acute myocardial infarction. *Lancet* 357, 1997–2001.

Johansson-Kark, M., Rasmussen, F., de Stavola, B. and Leon, D.A. (2002) Fetal growth and systolic blood pressure in young adulthood: the Swedish Young Male Twins Study. *Paediatric and Perinatal Epidemiology* 16, 200–209.

Kind, K.L., Simonetta, G., Clifton, P.M., Robinson, J.S. and Owens, J.A. (2002) Effect of maternal food restriction on blood pressure in the adult guinea pig. *Experimental Physiology* 87, 469–477.

Koupilova, I., Leon, D.A., McKeigue, P.M. and Lithell, H.O. (1999) Is the effect of low birth weight on cardiovascular mortality mediated through high blood pressure? *Journal of Hypertension* 17, 19–25.

Kramer, M.S. and Joseph, K.S. (1996) Enigma of fetal/infant-origins hypothesis. *Lancet* 348(9037), 1254–1255.

Langley-Evans, S.C., Gardner, D.S. and Jackson, A.A. (1996) Association of disproportionate growth of fetal rats in late gestation with raised systolic blood pressure in later life. *Journal of Reproduction and Fertility* 106, 307–312.

Leon, D. and Ben-Shlomo, Y. (1997) Preadult influences on cardiovascular disease and cancer. In: Kuh, D. and Ben-Shlomo, Y. (eds) *A Life Course Approach to Chronic Disease Epidemiology*. Oxford University Press, New York, pp. 45–77.

Leon, D.A., Lithell, H.O., Vagero, D., Koupilova, I., Mohsen, R., Berglund, L., Lithell, U.B. and McKeigue, P.M. (1998) Reduced fetal growth rate and increased risk of death from ischaemic heart disease: cohort study of 1500 Swedish men and women born 1915–29. *British Medical Journal* 317(7135), 241–245.

Lucas, A. (1998) Programming by early nutrition: an experimental approach. *Journal of Nutrition* 128(suppl. 2):401S–406S.

Lucas, A. and Fewtrell, M.S. (1999) Fetal origins of adult disease – the hypothesis revisited. *British Medical Journal* 319(7204), 245–249.

Manson, J.E., Colditz, G.A., Stampfer, M.J., Willett, W., Rosner, B., Monson, R.R., Speizer, F.E. and Hennekens, C.H. (1990) A prospective study of obesity and risk of coronary heart disease in women. *New England Journal of Medicine* 322(13), 882–889.

Marmot, M.G., Syme, S.L., Kagan, A., Kato, H., Cohen, J.B. and Belsky, J. (1975) Epidemiologic studies of coronary heart disease and stroke in Japanese men living in Japan, Hawaii and California: prevalence of coronary and hypertensive heart disease and associated risk factors. *American Journal of Epidemiology* 102, 514–525.

Martyn, C.N., Barker, D.J.P. and Osmond, C. (1996) Mother's pelvic size, fetal growth, and death from stroke and coronary heart disease in men in the UK. *Lancet* 348, 1264–1268.

Nwagwu, M.O., Cook, A. and Langley-Evans, S.C. (2000) Evidence of progressive deterioration of renal function in rats exposed to a maternal low protein diet *in utero*. *British Journal of Nutrition* 83, 79–85.

Ong, K.K.L., Ahmed, M., Emmett, P.M., Preece, M.A. and Dunger, D.B. (2000) Association between postnatal catch-up and obesity in childhood: prospective cohort study. *British Medical Journal* 320, 967–971.

Osmond, C., Slattery, J.M. and Barker, D.J.P. (1990) Mortality by place of birth. In: Britton, M. (ed.) *Mortality and Geography: a Review in Mid-1980s*. The Registrar General's Decimal Supplement for England and Wales, London, pp. 96–100.

Osmond, C., Barker, D.J.P., Fall, C.H.D. and Simmonds, S.J. (1993) Early growth and death from cardiovascular disease in women. *British Medical Journal* 307, 1519–1524.

Osmond, C., Barker, D.J.P., Eriksson, J.G. and Forsen, T. (2001) Early growth and coronary heart disease in later life: author's reply (Letter). *British Medical Journal* 323, 572.

Paneth, N. and Susser, M. (1995) Early origin of coronary heart disease (the 'Barker hypothesis'). *British Medical Journal* 310(6977), 411–412.

Poulter, N., Chang, C.L., MacGregor, A.J., Sanieder, H. and Spector, T.D. (1999) Association between birth weight and adult blood pressure in twins: historical cohort study. *British Medical Journal* 319, 1330–1333.

Rich-Edwards, J.W., Stampfer, M.J., Manson, J.E., Rosner, B., Hankinson, S.E., Colditz, G.A., Willett, W.C. and Hennekens, C.H. (1997) Birthweight and the risk of cardiovascular disease in a cohort of women followed up since 1976. *British Medical Journal* 315, 396–400.

Roseboom, T.J., van der Meulen, J.H., Osmond, C., Barker, D., Ravelli, A.C.J., Schroeder-Tanka, J.M., van Montfrans, G.A., Michels, R.P. and Blecker, O.P. (2000) Coronary heart disease after prenatal exposure to the Dutch famine, 1944–45. *Heart* 84(6), 595–598.

Stanner, S.A., Bulmer, K. and Andres, C. (1997) Malnutrition *in utero* as a determinant of diabetes and coronary heart disease in adult life: the Lenigrad siege study. *British Medical Journal* 315, 1342–1349.

Stenhouse, N.S. and McCall, M.G. (1970) Differential mortality from cardiovascular disease in migrants from England and Wales, Scotland and Italy, and native-born Australians. *Journal of Chronic Disease* 23, 423–431.

Strachan, D.P., Leon, D.A. and Dodgeon, B. (1995) Mortality from cardiovascular disease among interregional migrants in England and Wales. *British Medical Journal* 310, 423–427.

Tanner, J.M. (1990) *Fetus into Man. Physical Growth from Conception to Maturity*. Harvard University Press, Cambridge, Massachusetts.

Williams, D.R., Roberts, S.J. and Davies, T.W. (1979) Deaths for ischaemic heart disease and infant mortality in England and Wales. *Journal of Epidemiology and Community Health* 33, 199–202.

5 Early-life Origins of Adult Disease: is There Really an Association Between Birthweight and Chronic Disease Risk?

RACHEL HUXLEY

Heart and Vascular Disease Programme, Institute for International Health, Sydney, NSW 2042, Australia

Introduction

Early origins of the hypothesis

The concept that events occurring in early childhood could have an impact on health in later life was originally conceived by Kermack and coworkers in the 1930s (Kermack *et al.*, 1934). It was later revived in the late 1970s by Forsdahl, who postulated that poverty in adolescence combined with later affluence contributed to coronary heart disease (CHD) mortality (Forsdahl, 1977). Within the past couple of decades the hypothesis has subsequently been revived, refined and reformulated into the fetal origins of adult disease hypothesis (Barker, 1993).

The fetal-origins hypothesis, in its initial form, postulated that maternal and fetal undernutrition, at critical time-points in pregnancy, could initiate physiological adaptations or metabolic 'programming' within the fetus that enable it to survive the less than optimal conditions of the *in utero* environment (Barker, 1993). Such adaptations, however, are suggested to result in impaired fetal growth, as reflected by a lower birthweight or a disproportionate body size at birth. Moreover, these same adaptations, that are suggested to confer a survival advantage on the fetus, are proposed to increase an individual's predisposition towards the development of CHD risk factors in adult life, including hypertension (Barker and Martyn, 1997), type 2 diabetes (Barker, 1999a) and dyslipidaemia (Barker, 1999b). By suggesting a causal role for the early-life environment in 'programming' later disease risk, the hypothesis marks a departure from more traditional theories that typically emphasize the role of adult lifestyle factors, such as cigarette smoking, high-fat diets and low levels of physical activity, in the aetiology of CHD (Magnus and Beaglehole, 2001).

The evolution of the fetal-origins hypothesis began with observations made from ecological studies, that areas of England and Wales with high rates of infant mortality in the earlier part of the 20th century were those same areas that experienced some of the highest rates of CHD mortality 60–70 years later (Barker and Osmond, 1986). As the primary cause of infant mortality at the turn of the century was low birthweight, it was hypothesized that the same mechanisms, responsible for the high rates of low birthweight and subsequent infant mortality, were also responsible for the observed high incidence of CHD mortality (Barker and Osmond, 1986). These ecological observations were subsequently followed by a series of research papers, based on findings from historical cohort studies that examined the relationship between low birthweight and CHD mortality in adults for whom birth records were available. These studies, based on birth records of men and women born in Hertfordshire, Preston and Sheffield in the 1920s and 1930s, suggested that low birthweight and a variety of other birth measurements, including increased ratio of placental weight to birthweight, small abdominal circumference, low ponderal index and reduced head circumference, were associated with elevated levels of CHD risk factors and increased CHD mortality (Barker et al., 1989a).

The innovative concept that impaired fetal and neonatal development could have a profound and sustained impact on the health of the infant in adult life has stimulated flourishing research into the possible biological mechanisms underlying fetal growth with later disease. This is of importance as, if maternal nutrition during pregnancy is indeed causally related to the subsequent health of the infant in adult life, then this could potentially provide a novel means by which to intervene in the primary prevention of CHD. Hence, determining whether the reported associations between size at birth and later disease are truly causal would have substantial implications for public health.

Over the course of the past couple of decades, the fetal-origins framework has expanded to incorporate a wide spectrum of disorders, other than cardiovascular disease, each of which has been suggested to be causally associated with impaired fetal growth (Table 5.1). In addition, much emphasis has been given to the possible influence of the early postnatal environment, in conjunction with the prenatal experience, on health outcomes (Eriksson et al., 1999). For example, some (Eriksson et al., 1999) but not all studies (Barker et al., 1989b), have reported that higher weight gain in infancy is associated with an increased likelihood of heart disease in later life. The chief aim of this chapter, however, will not be to describe the possible mechanisms that may underlie the reported associations between size at birth and later disease, but rather to investigate whether or not these associations are causal, by assessing the strength of the epidemiological evidence for some aspects of the fetal-origins hypothesis.

How do we distinguish causation from association in epidemiological studies?

In epidemiological studies, whenever a statistically significant association is reported between an exposure and an outcome, it is first necessary to consider

Table 5.1. Reported associations between impaired fetal growth with various outcomes.

Increased cardiovascular disease (CVD) mortality and possible CVD risk factors:
- Raised blood pressure (Barker and Martyn, 1997)
- Impaired glucose tolerance/type 2 diabetes/gestational diabetes (Barker, 1999a)
- Dyslipidaemia: higher cholesterol, LDL-cholesterol and triglycerides levels (Barker, 1999b)
- Obesity (Fall *et al.*, 1995)
- Higher plasma levels of fibrinogen, Factor VII and other blood-clotting factors (Martyn *et al.*, 1995)
- Renal disease/Increased mean albumin:creatinine ratio (Garrett *et al.*, 1993)
- Reduced arterial compliance (Leeson *et al.*, 1997)
- Higher plasma leptin concentrations (Lissner *et al.*, 1999)
- Increased thyroid function (Phillips *et al.*, 1993)
- Higher sympathetic nervous system activity (Phillips and Barker, 1997)
- Higher plasma cortisol levels (Phillips *et al.*, 2000)

Psychological disorders:
- Increased risk of schizophrenia (Hoek *et al.*, 1996)
- Increased risk of depression (Thompson *et al.*, 2001)
- Increased risk of suicide (Barker *et al.*, 1995a)

Respiratory disorders:
- Increased risk of asthma (Xu *et al.*, 2002)
- Increased risk of chronic obstructive pulmonary disease (Barker *et al.*, 1991)

Early menarche (dos Santos Silva *et al.*, 2002)
Early menopause (Cresswell *et al.*, 1999)
Ovarian cancer (Barker *et al.*, 1995b)
Osteoporosis (Dennison *et al.*, 2001)
Lower IQ scores (Sorensen *et al.*, 1997)
Lower rates of marriage (Phillips *et al.*, 2001)

LDL, low-density lipoprotein.

(and, where possible, discount) alternative explanations before inferring a causal relationship. Significant findings may have arisen as a result of random error (i.e. 'chance'), which is especially pertinent to small studies, or as a consequence of different forms of bias, such as selection or publication bias. Alternatively, associations may be driven by factors other than the exposure, that are related independently to both the exposure and the outcome of interest, otherwise known as confounders. This is particularly true for observational rather than experimental studies, where it is impossible to control completely for all factors that may influence the relationship in question. Only after these alternative explanations have been rejected, would there be sufficient evidence to infer reliably a causal relation between an exposure and an outcome. To do this normally requires evidence from large-scale randomized trials, or from meta-analyses of trials. However, in practice, in the absence of trial data, deducing the causal nature of relationships often rests on the findings and subsequent interpretation of data from observational epidemiological studies. As a result of the bias and confounding that are inherent within such study designs, the findings from such studies tend to be less reliable and potentially misleading (MacMahon and Collins, 2001). Therefore, although useful in generating hypotheses, in the majority of situations it would be unwise to base causal inference solely on evidence from observational studies.

Reducing error in estimates of effect size in observational epidemiology

Systematic overviews or 'meta-analyses' are becoming an increasingly common research tool in epidemiology. By systematically integrating the results of separate independent studies, the impact of random error can be reduced, and hence meta-analysis can often provide more reliable and precise estimates of an effect size than can be obtained from any individual study alone (Egger and Davey-Smith, 1997). In addition, meta-analysis is a useful process in that it can be used to identify sources of bias and important sources of heterogeneity that may give rise to differences in estimates of effect size across studies. The following section will discuss the findings from a meta-analysis of the fetal-origins literature, of the reported association between birthweight and subsequent blood pressure (Huxley et al., 2002). The possible implications that these analyses may have for the fetal-origins hypothesis of adult disease will also be discussed.

Meta-analysis of the association between birthweight and subsequent blood pressure

An inverse relationship between birthweight and later blood pressure was one of the first causal associations to be reported, and has been considered to provide the strongest evidence in support of the fetal-origins hypothesis (Leon, 1999; Robinson, 2001). An early systematic review of the literature, which included 28 studies, and information on approximately 15,000 people, suggested a 2–4 mmHg lower systolic blood pressure per kilogram higher birthweight (Law and Shiell, 1996). Furthermore, it was suggested that the effect was 'amplified' with age, that is, the association appeared to be much stronger in late adult life as compared with childhood (Law and Shiell, 1996).

An update of this review was conducted to include data from several large cohorts, including data on more that 367,000 people. It continued to suggest an inverse association between birthweight and blood pressure, with the magnitude of association being somewhere between 1 and 2 mmHg/kg, as well as continuing to support the idea that the effect is magnified with age (Huxley et al., 2000) (Fig. 5.1).

However, there were several potentially important issues that these early reviews overlooked, which may have contributed to the generation of the reported inverse association.

- Many published studies were excluded from contributing to the quantitative estimates from the earlier reviews because they did not report regression coefficients in their analyses or, in the case of longitudinal studies, they had reported the association for the same individuals at more than one age.

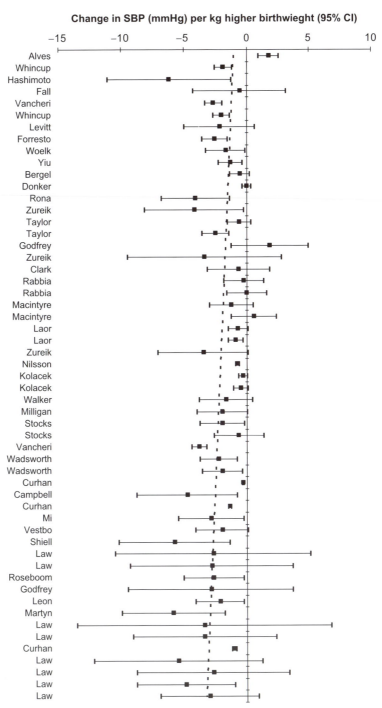

Fig. 5.1. Regression coefficients (95% confidence intervals) adjusted for current weight from studies reporting on the association between birthweight and systolic blood pressure (SBP), ordered by age.

- No allowance was made for the size of the contributing studies, which meant, in effect, that the results from the small studies (typically with only a couple of hundred of individuals) were accorded the same importance as the results from the much larger, and therefore more reliable, studies, some of which included data on several tens of thousands of people.
- The impact of potential confounders, including social class and parental blood pressure, on the size and direction of the association was not examined.
- Nearly all of the studies that had contributed to earlier estimates were adjusted for current body size. Within the individual studies, the effect of this was often to strengthen, or in some cases reverse, the direction of the association between birthweight and blood pressure.
- Twin studies were excluded from previous reviews, based on a suggestion that twins might undergo a special type of growth retardation (Vågerö and Leon, 1994). But since twins share similar pre- and postnatal environments, studies of twin pairs may help to reduce the impact of confounding, and restricting analyses to those of monozygotic twins would eliminate the potential impact of any genetic effects (Christensen et al., 2001).

To examine the impact that these issues may have had on the strength of the reported inverse association between birthweight and blood pressure, a reappraisal of the literature was conducted. The following section describes the methods used and the principal findings from this overview.

Methods

In brief, all published studies that had reported by March 2000 on the association between birthweight and subsequent blood pressure had previously been identified for two systematic reviews of the available literature. Overall, there were 55 eligible studies that had reported regression coefficients of systolic blood pressure on birthweight, and a further 48 studies that did not report regression coefficients but did indicate the direction of this association. In addition, eight studies of twins were identified and analysed separately from those of singletons. To allow comparison between the smaller and larger studies, the analyses presented here involved weighting the contribution of each study according to an estimate of its 'statistical size' (or 'information content') derived from the inverse of the variance of the regression coefficient, and combining these estimates using a 'fixed-effects' model (Shadish and Haddock, 1994; Collaborative Group on Hormonal Factors in Breast Cancer, 1997). In addition, the impact of adjustment for current body size, and for potential confounding factors, on quantitative estimates of the strength of the association was assessed by obtaining regression coefficients with, and without, such adjustments from the principal investigators of the largest, most informative, studies (i.e. those involving more than 1000 individuals).

Results

Impact of study size on the size of the association between birthweight and systolic blood pressure

One of the main arguments used in support of a causal role of birthweight on subsequent blood pressure is the apparent consistency of the reported inverse association across different study populations (Barker *et al.*, 2000). The basis for this assertion was that of the 55 regression coefficients included in the previous reviews, all but three reported an inverse association between birthweight and later blood pressure. However, when the studies are ordered by their statistical study size, what becomes apparent is that the association is much smaller in the larger studies (Huxley *et al.*, 2002) (Fig. 5.2).

In those studies that typically involved fewer than 1000 participants, the mean inverse-variance-weighted estimate was an approximately 2 mmHg lower systolic blood pressure per kilogram higher birthweight, as compared with an estimate of −0.5 mmHg/kg from those studies with more than 3000 participants. Furthermore, most of the smaller studies involved the research group that initiated the hypothesis and the weighted estimate from these studies is much larger than that for all remaining studies (Fig. 5.3).

Even after exclusion of studies from the hypothesis-generating group, there is still a significant trend towards much weaker associations in the larger studies. This finding is suggestive of the existence of publication bias, which refers to the often frequent occurrence in the scientific literature of a greater likelihood of small studies to be published if they report extreme or interesting results (Dickersin, 1997).

A frequently used method of testing for the existence of publication bias in a meta-analysis is by graphically representing the studies according to their statistical 'precision' (usually measured as the reciprocal of the standard error) and the reported size of effect. The resulting graph is known as a 'funnel plot', since, in the absence of publication bias, the distribution of studies resembles a funnel in shape (Egger *et al.*, 1997). However, if the distribution of values is heavily skewed on either side of the line of no effect, with very few studies on either side of this line, this provides some evidence for the existence of publication bias, as exemplified in Fig. 5.4.

Impact of excluded studies on the size of the association between birthweight and systolic blood pressure

In addition to the 55 studies that contributed to previous estimates for the size of an association between birthweight and blood pressure, there were a further 48 studies which were excluded from contributing because they did not report regression coefficients or had reported the association at more than one age. Of these 48 studies, only half of them had reported an inverse association (Table 5.2), with the remaining studies finding either a positive or no association between birthweight and later blood pressure. Consequently, if data from these

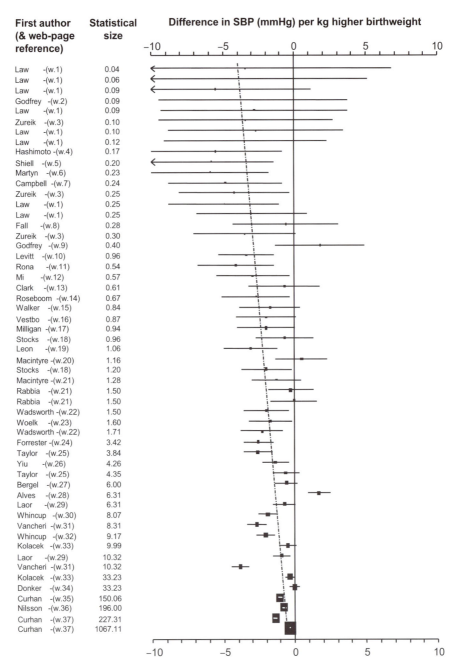

Fig. 5.2. Trend toward smaller differences in systolic blood pressure (SBP) per 1 kg difference in birthweight in larger, more informative, studies that reported regression coefficients for the association (adjusted in most cases for current weight). Statistical size of study is defined in terms of the inverse of the variance of the regression coefficient. Black squares = point estimates (with area proportional to statistical 'information', based on inverse of variance of regression coefficient, provided by each study) and horizontal line = 95% confidence interval (CI) for observed effect in each study. Dotted line = inverse-variance-weighted regression line through point estimates. The 'w' prefix refers to the web-page reference from the original study (Huxley *et al.*, 2002). (Reprinted, with permission from Elsevier, from the *Lancet* (2002) 360, 659–665.)

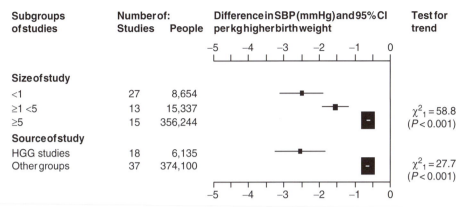

Fig. 5.3. Impact of study size and source on weighted estimates of the difference in systolic blood pressure (SBP) per 1 kg difference in birthweight (derived from studies that reported regression coefficients for the association, adjusted in most cases for current weight). Conventions are as in Fig. 5.1 for particular inverse-variance-weighted combinations of studies. Statistical size of study is defined in terms of the inverse of the variance of the regression coefficient. HGG, hypothesis-generating group of investigators. (Reprinted, with permission from Elsevier, from the *Lancet* (2002) 360, 659–665.)

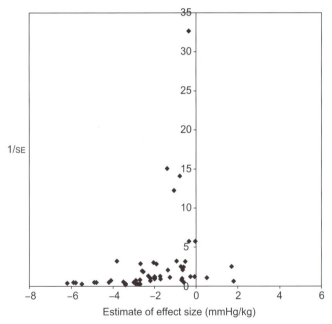

Fig. 5.4. Funnel plot of studies reporting on the size of the association between birthweight and systolic blood pressure.

excluded studies had been able to contribute to the previous quantitative estimates, then it is likely that the magnitude of the reported inverse association would have been reduced even further.

Table 5.2. Direction of association between birthweight and subsequent blood pressure in the 55 studies that contributed to previous quantitative estimates and in the 48 studies that did not.

Numbers in cohort and previous contribution	Lower SBP associated with higher birthweight	
	Yes	No
< 1000 individuals		
Contributing	35	3
Non-contributing	21	19
≥ 1000 individuals		
Contributing	17	0
Non-contributing	4	4
All studies		
Contributing	52	3
Non-contributing	25	23

SBP, systolic blood pressure.
Heterogeneity between contributing and non-contributing studies: $\chi^2_1 = 24.5$; $P < 0.0001$.

In addition to the above studies that had reported on the association between birthweight and blood pressure, one further study was identified (Said *et al.*, 1998), in which the investigators chose not to report on the association of birthweight with blood pressure, despite reporting associations with other measures of size at birth, such as ponderal index. Such selective emphasis on particular study results is likely to have introduced further bias in estimating the strength of this association, and raises the possibility that other studies may not have been reported mainly because their results were less extreme.

Impact of confounding on the size of the association between birthweight and systolic blood pressure

As discussed previously, one of the major limitations of observational studies is the difficulty in distinguishing between a causal and a chance association, as it is impossible to fully account for all known and unknown confounders of the relationship. Known confounders of an association between birthweight and blood pressure include sex and ethnicity; for example, male babies are, on average, heavier at birth and are also more likely to have higher blood pressures in later life. Other potential confounders are likely to include current and parental social class and parental blood pressure. For example, higher maternal blood pressure, both before and during pregnancy, is associated with lower birthweight and higher blood pressure in offspring (Walker *et al.*, 1998). However, besides gender, very few of the studies included in the earlier reviews had sufficient information to be able to adjust for these variables (Table 5.3).

Table 5.3. Adjustment for potential confounding factors in the 55 studies that reported regression coefficients for the association between birthweight and subsequent blood pressure.

Potential confounding factor	Number of studies adjusting for factor
Current weight	49
Sex	48
Height	13
Parental socio-economic status	7
Current socio-economic status	2
Parental blood pressure	9
Alcohol consumption	3
Race	6
Gestational age	8

Other factors adjusted for (and number of studies that adjusted for each factor): ambient temperature or exercise (four studies), sphygmomanometer cuff size (three studies), amount of TV watched, anticipated venepuncture, heart rate, maternal body mass index, parity, person who measured blood pressure, Tanner's stage of puberty or town (two studies), and Apgar score, birth rank, calcium in pregnancy, father's height, maternal age, maternal haemoglobin, maternal oedema, tar dose or time of day (one study).

Only seven studies attempted to adjust for parental social class and, similarly, only two studies included measures of current socio-economic status in their regression models, despite the impact of social class on lifestyle choices (such as smoking, physical inactivity and poor diet) that are both related to birthweight (Kramer, 1987) and independently to cardiovascular risk factors (including raised blood pressure) (Elford *et al.*, 1991; Joseph and Kramer, 1996). Moreover, indicators such as smoking and diet are only crude measures of the true differences in socio-economic status and so residual or 'left-over' confounding is likely to remain even after adjustment for these indicators is attempted. Thus, a proportion of the reported inverse association between birthweight and blood pressure may be explained by a low socio-economic status, and other known and unknown confounders, that influence both birthweight and adult lifestyle factors that are related to CHD risk (Greenland, 1980; Clarke *et al.*, 1999).

Evidence from twin studies

Previous reviews excluded studies in twin pairs due to the *post hoc* suggestion that twins may undergo a different type of intrauterine growth retardation (Vågerö and Leon, 1994). However, because twins experience similar environments before birth and in childhood and adolescence, studies within twin pairs may be less prone to the effects of confounding than studies of singletons. Furthermore, restricting analyses to studies of monozygotic twin pairs will eliminate any genetic effects on any association, which is useful as it has previously been suggested that genetic polymorphisms may explain associations between birthweight and the subsequent development of cardiovascular disease risk factors, such as insulin resistance (Frayling and Hattersley, 2001). In addition, because one twin is often born considerably lighter than the other (on average approximately 900 g), any effect of birthweight on later cardiovascular risk is probably going to be most apparent in twins. But, as with many of the studies in singletons, most studies that have been conducted in twin pairs have been relatively small, and consequently the random errors in the estimates from such studies tend to be large. As a result, the estimates from these studies differ quite markedly in terms of both the strength and the direction of association. However, when the results from all twin studies are combined, the overall mean inverse-variance-weighted estimate is very similar to that derived from the larger studies in singletons: −0.6 mmHg/kg (95% confidence interval −2.2 to 1.0) (Fig. 5.5) (Huxley et al., 2002). In addition to these twin studies, two large twin registries from Sweden and Denmark, of several thousand twin pairs, did not find twins to be at increased risk of death from cardiovascular disease or other causes, despite the significant difference in birthweight (Vågerö and Leon, 1994; Christensen et al., 1995).

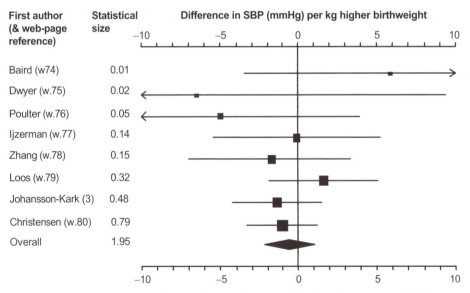

Fig. 5.5. Association between birthweight and later systolic blood pressure (SBP) in published studies of monozygotic twin pairs. Conventions as in Fig. 5.1, with a diamond indicating the inverse-variance-weighted combined point estimate and 95% CI. All of these regression coefficients were adjusted for current weight including body mass index (BMI), except for Dwyer et al., which involved adjustment for fat mass. The 'w' prefix refers to the web-page reference from the original study (Huxley et al., 2002). (Reprinted, with permission from Elsevier, from the *Lancet* (2002) 360, 659–665.)

Inappropriate adjustment for current body size

A controversial aspect in relation to studying potential associations between size at birth and later cardiovascular risk concerns the suitability of adjusting for current body weight in statistical analyses. For example, 49 of the 55 regression coefficients included in the review of the association between birthweight and blood pressure were adjusted for current body weight. Consequently, these estimates largely represent the association between birthweight and subsequent blood pressure at a given body weight. As birthweight is a positive antecedent of current body weight (Pietilainen *et al.*, 2001), and current body weight is positively associated with blood pressure (National Institute of Health, 1998), depending on the relative strength of these separate associations, adjustment for current body weight might produce a spurious inverse association between birthweight and subsequent blood pressure (Lucas *et al.*, 1999). In addition, in several studies it is often the case that an inverse association between birth size and a later disease risk factor only becomes apparent, or statistically significant, after adjustment for current weight is performed (Stocks and Davey-Smith, 1999).

Furthermore, even allowing for the existence of a small inverse association between birthweight and blood pressure at any particular current weight, this effect may well be overshadowed by the deleterious increase in blood pressure that would occur with the somewhat higher current weight associated with a higher birthweight. The net effect of removing the adjustment for current body weight in the larger studies is about a halving of the magnitude of the association, from −0.6 mmHg/kg to −0.4 mmHg/kg. If we were then to add to this the impact of residual confounding and of publication and reporting bias, it is likely that the association between birthweight and blood pressure would be further attenuated (Huxley *et al.*, 2002).

Role of measurement error on the size of the association between birthweight and systolic blood pressure

It has been argued that one possible reason for the discrepancies in the magnitude of the birthweight–blood pressure relationship between the smaller and larger studies is due to error in the measurement of either birthweight or blood pressure, or both (Hennessy, 2002). It is possible that smaller studies would have more reliable measurements of both blood pressure and birthweight, by using actual birth records, rather than self-report, to obtain information on birthweight, and by conducting more accurate assessments of blood pressure, as compared with the larger studies which may have used 'rounding' to the nearest 5 or 10 mmHg. And, indeed, errors in the assessment of birthweight would, due to 'regression dilution' bias (Clarke *et al.*, 1999), tend to produce some underestimation of the true magnitude of the association between birthweight and subsequent health outcomes. In the previous reviews (Law and Shiell, 1996; Huxley *et al.*, 2000), most of the studies obtained information on birthweight from birth records, but some – especially the much larger studies – used self-reported values or parental recall, which had been validated by comparison with birth records in smaller samples. Consequently, assessment of birthweight using these methods may involve greater errors. However, although this may explain some of the difference in the strength of the association between small and large studies, it does not seem to account for much of it. For example, the mean inverse-variance-weighted estimate for those studies which used birth records as the source of information for birthweight was –0.9 mmHg/kg, versus –0.6 mmHg/kg in those that used parental recall or self-reported birthweight. This small difference is consistent with a correlation of about 0.7 between birthweight measures obtained from birth records versus those from parental recall or self-reports (Curhan et al., 1996). Consequently, after adjusting for regression dilution, it would lead to an increase of about a third in the regression coefficient between birthweight and blood pressure. This expectation is supported by the small difference between the observed associations in studies, of more than 1000 people, that used different methods to assess blood pressure: –0.8 mmHg/kg with direct measurements versus –0.6 mmHg/kg with self-reports (Huxley et al., 2002).

In contrast, errors in the assessment of blood pressure would not be expected to produce any significant underestimation in the strength of the association, since systematic error would only add a constant to the mean blood pressure value, and random error would not change the mean value associated with any particular birthweight (Rodgers and MacMahon, 1995).

Evidence from studies of maternal nutrition in pregnancy

Evidence from animal studies has been used to provide support in favour of the fetal-origins hypothesis. For example, low-protein diets in animal studies have been linked to raised blood pressure in offspring (Langley-Evans and Jackson, 1994). However, experimental evidence in humans regarding the impact of maternal diet in pregnancy on later health outcomes in offspring is limited and often contradictory. In addition, few studies have actual information on maternal dietary intake during pregnancy, and consequently, the adequacy of fetal nutrition has had to be inferred indirectly from size at birth. At the time of writing, only a very small number of studies, which have been able to explore the impact of maternal nutrient status on offspring's blood pressure in later life, has been published. Two studies were ecological and based on populations that had been exposed to famine during the Second World War: the Dutch Famine Study (Roseboom et al., 1999) and the Leningrad Siege Study (Stanner et al., 1997). No differences in adult blood pressure were observed between individuals prenatally exposed to the Dutch famine in early, mid- or late gestation (Roseboom et al., 1999), or between those conceived before, during or after the Leningrad siege famine (Stanner et al., 1997).

The evidence from cohort studies is sparse and is not wholly consistent with the fetal-origins hypothesis. One study, comprising 626 individuals whose mothers' food intake had been recorded in pregnancy, reported that higher maternal intakes of protein were associated with raised blood pressure, but only in late gestation (Campbell *et al.*, 1996). These findings conflict with data from animal studies that have suggested that it is *low* protein intake in pregnancy that corresponds to higher blood pressure in offspring. In contrast, a follow-up study of individuals born to 400 pregnant women in Oxford, UK, during the Second World War found no associations between markers of maternal nutritional status, including protein, with blood pressure and other cardiovascular risk outcome in middle-aged offspring (Lucas and Morley, 1994). Likewise, in a randomized trial of the effects of nutrition in preterm infants, there was no difference in blood pressure in childhood between groups fed the standard or the nutritionally enhanced dietary regimens (R. Huxley, unpublished data). Of note, however, was the observation that dietary regimens producing *larger* weight gains were associated with significantly higher (rather than lower) blood pressures at follow-up in this cohort (Singhal *et al.*, 2001).

Summary

The findings from this meta-analysis suggest that previous reports of a strong, inverse association between birthweight and subsequent blood pressure are likely to have been driven by small study size, inadequate control for confounders, inappropriate adjustment for current body weight and publication bias. Although an inverse relationship between birthweight and blood pressure has been considered to provide the strongest support for the fetal-origins hypothesis, it is only one of a large number of relationships encapsulated by the hypothesis. As detailed earlier, impaired fetal growth has been suggested to be causally associated with a wide range of diseases and chronic disease risk factors. However, to determine the size and strength of each of these proposed relations necessitates similar critical overviews of the literature to be performed.

Is impaired fetal growth materially associated with cholesterol metabolism in later life?

Based on the findings from a small number of observational studies, it has been suggested that impaired fetal growth is causally associated with disturbances in cholesterol metabolism in later life (Barker *et al.*, 1993; Martyn *et al.*, 1998). In particular, findings from one small study of 219 middle-aged men and women suggested that reduced abdominal circumference (described as a proxy marker of liver size at birth) is associated with increased cholesterol concentrations (Barker *et al.*, 1993), but since abdominal circumference at birth is not routinely measured, it has not been possible to replicate these study findings. Instead, several studies have been published that have reported on the relationship between birthweight and subsequent cholesterol level. Whereas some of these studies reported inverse associations (Martyn *et al.*, 1998), others have reported positive associations (Rona *et al.*, 1996) or no apparent association (Cowin and Emmett, 2000) between birthweight and subsequent blood total cholesterol concentration. Evidence from animal studies, which has traditionally been used to provide support for the fetal-origins hypothesis, tends to suggest that maternal undernutrition and lower birthweight are associated with *lower*, not higher, cholesterol levels in offspring. For example, in animal experiments, Lucas *et al.* (1996) found that protein deficiency in pregnant rats led both to reduced birthweight and to reduced blood total cholesterol concentrations in the adult offspring. Similarly, in human populations, data from the Dutch Famine Study suggest that individuals who were exposed *in utero* to maternal undernutrition during mid- or late gestation had *lower* blood total cholesterol in adult life compared with non-exposed controls (Roseboom *et al.*, 2002). Furthermore, no association between birthweight and subsequent blood total cholesterol was found in either the Dutch Famine or the Leningrad Siege Studies (Stanner *et al.*, 1997).

A recent systematic review of 29 published studies, that had reported on the association, concluded that there was a weak inverse association between birthweight and total cholesterol that 'was of limited public-health importance when compared with the effects of childhood obesity' (Owen *et al.*, 2003). The estimated size of effect was equivalent to a 0.05 mmol/l reduction in cholesterol per kilogram higher birthweight. Since birthweight is so highly correlated with other birth measures, including abdominal circumference, there is little reason to postulate specific effects of other measures of birth size – such as abdominal circumference (which might reflect impaired hepatic growth) (Barker *et al.*, 1993) – on cholesterol metabolism in later life.

Likely significance to public health of small increases in birthweight

Over the past two decades, evidence has accumulated to suggest that poor maternal and fetal nutrition resulting in impaired fetal growth is causally associated with many adverse health outcomes, ranging from increased rates of cardiovascular disease to reduced rates of marriage (Table 5.1). Hence, from a public-health perspective it is important to examine, first, what the evidence is for the efficacy of interventions aimed at increasing birthweight, and, secondly, what impact any subsequent change in the population distribution of birthweight would have on reducing the overall burden of disease.

Most observational studies that have examined the impact of maternal diet in pregnancy on infant outcome have concluded that maternal diet has little impact on birthweight, although some studies have suggested that it is the combination of particular macronutrients that may be important (Campbell *et al.*, 1996). This finding of a null association between maternal diet and birthweight receives support from randomized trials of nutritional supplementation programmes which, overall, have shown, disappointingly, that there is little benefit to be gained in terms of increases in birthweight with the provision of dietary supplements to women (Kramer, 1993). One large trial even suggested a possible hazard of excessive protein intake in pregnancy on infants' birthweight (Rush *et al.*, 1980). The resilience of birthweight to change, following alterations in the maternal diet, can be seen in data from the Dutch famine, which showed that despite prolonged periods of severe undernourishment, women gave birth to infants whose birthweights were only reduced by, on average, 200–300 g. Currently, encouraging women to stop smoking during pregnancy remains the most effective strategy at preventing intrauterine growth retardation, with the mean difference in birthweight of offspring of women who smoked or were non-smokers in pregnancy being about 100 g (Secker-Walker and Vacek, 2003).

If we were then to allow that causal associations existed between birthweight and CHD risk factors, and that the sizes of effect are approximately those derived from meta-analysis, from a public-health perspective the expected impact of interventions that could increase birthweight would be of limited significance to overall levels of CHD mortality. If we were to assume that the size of the inverse association between birthweight and blood pressure is approximately 0.5 mmHg/kg, and that realistically, nutritional interventions and smoking cessation programmes in pregnancy can only increase birthweight by a maximum of 100 g, then the reduction in blood pressure associated with a 100 g increase in birthweight would be 0.05 mmHg, which would prevent approximately 0.2% of CHD events each year worldwide (A. Rodgers, personal communication). In contrast, modest weight loss of between 3 and 4 kg is associated with a reduction in systolic blood pressure of between 2 and 3 mmHg (De Onis *et al.*, 1998). A reduction in blood pressure of this magnitude would be expected to lower global CHD mortality by about 6% and stroke by 10% (A. Rodgers, personal communication).

A recent review of the literature of the association between birthweight and subsequent total blood cholesterol concluded that a 1 kg increase in birthweight is associated with a 0.05 mmol/l lower total blood cholesterol. If we were to assume a causal relation between these two variables of this magnitude and direction of effect, then the reduction in cholesterol associated with a 100 g increase in birthweight would be approximately 0.005 mmol/l. A meta-analysis of prospective observational studies indicated that a 0.6 mmol/l (about 10%) reduction in total blood cholesterol is associated with a 26% lower risk of CHD at ages 45–54 years (Trials of Hypertension Prevention Collaborative Research Group, 1992). From this, a reduction in cholesterol of 0.001 mmol/l would correspond to a reduction in CHD events of approximately 0.04%. In contrast, a meta-analysis of randomized dietary intervention studies in free-living populations has suggested reductions in total blood cholesterol of approximately 0.4 mmol/l (i.e. 5–6%) (Tang *et al.*, 1998), which would correspond in the long term with about a 16% lower coronary risk in the 45–54-year age group. There is also consistent evidence from randomized trials that lowering blood low-density lipoprotein (LDL) cholesterol concentrations with drugs or diet rapidly reduces the risks of vascular events and death. (Huxley *et al.*, 2004). Hence, producing material changes in blood total cholesterol that would impact on coronary risk seem likely to be more definite and easier to achieve through alterations in dietary fat intake in childhood and later life (as well as by modification of other lifestyle factors, such as increasing physical activity level) than through strategies aimed at increasing size at birth (Fig. 5.6a,b).

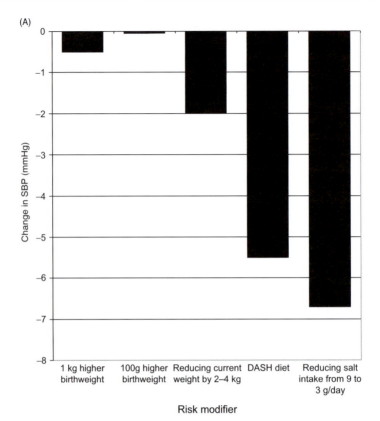

Fig. 5.6. (A) The expected reductions in systolic blood pressure (SBP) associated with modification of possible risk factors.

Further doubt regarding the relevance of birthweight to later disease comes from analyses of temporal trends of birthweight and coronary heart disease mortality. Data from the past 25 years indicate that mean birthweight has actually been increasing in both developed and developing countries, including the UK, (Power, 1994) the USA (Arbuckle and Sherman, 1989) and India (Singhal *et al.*, 1991). Recent data from Canada (Kramer *et al.*, 2002) suggest that increases in maternal anthropometry, reduced cigarette smoking and improvements in socio-economic factors are likely to be partly or wholly responsible for increases in mean birthweight, at least in westernized societies. Paralleling this rise in mean birthweight has been the dramatic increase in cardiovascular mortality (World Health Organization, 2002) over the past two decades, particularly in lower- to middle-income countries, including China and India. It is therefore difficult to attribute the huge rise in cardiovascular mortality to poor fetal growth, rather it is likely that the 'westernization' of these countries, as evidenced by the concurrent increases in smoking rates, the prevalence of obesity and the adoption of more sedentary lifestyles within these populations, is chiefly responsible for the CHD pandemic.

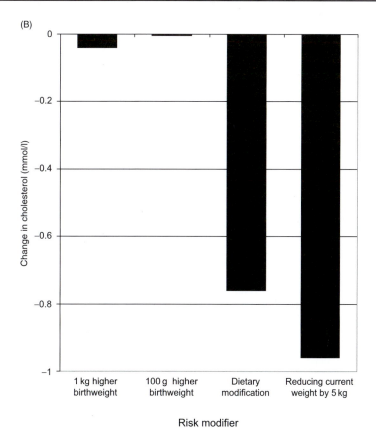

Fig. 5.6. (*Continued*) (B) The expected reductions in total cholesterol associated with modification of possible risk factors.

Conclusion

In summary, the evidence reviewed here provides little support for a significant causal role of birthweight in the determination of blood pressure and cholesterol levels in adult life, and suggests that claims of other causal associations between size at birth and disease risk factors be subject to similarly rigorous appraisals. Even allowing for a small inverse association between birthweight and risk factors, from a public-health perspective, strategies aimed at reducing the burden of chronic disease through the modification of adult lifestyle factors, such as cigarette smoking, diet and physical activity, are likely to be far more achievable and have a much greater impact than interventions aimed at reducing the burden of disease through increases in birthweight.

References

Arbuckle, T.E. and Sherman, G.J. (1989) An analysis of birth weight by gestational age in Canada. *Canadian Medical Association Journal* 140, 157–165.

Barker, D.J.P. (1993) *Fetal and Infant Origins of Adult Disease*. BMJ Books, London.

Barker, D.J. (1999a) The fetal origins of type 2 diabetes mellitus. *Annals of Internal Medicine* 130, 322–324.

Barker, D.J. (1999b) The intra-uterine origins of disturbed cholesterol homeostasis. *Acta Paediatrica* 88 483–484.

Barker, D.J. and Martyn, C.N. (1997) The fetal origins of hypertension. *Advances in Nephrology from the Necker Hospital* 26, 65–72.

Barker, D.J. and Osmond, C. (1986) Infant mortality, childhood nutrition and ischaemic heart disease in England and Wales. *Lancet* 1, 1077–1081.

Barker, D.J., Osmond, C. and Law, C.M. (1989a) The intrauterine and early postnatal origins of cardiovascular disease and chronic bronchitis. *Journal of Epidemiology and Community Health* 43, 237–240.

Barker, D.J.P., Winter, P.D., Osmond, C., Margetts, B. and Simmonds, S.J. (1989b) Weight in infancy and death from ischaemic heart disease. *Lancet* 2, 577–580.

Barker, D.J.P., Godfrey, K.M., Fall, C., Winter, P.D. and Shaheen, S.O. (1991) Relation of birth weight and childhood respiratory infection to adult lung function and death from chronic obstructive airways disease. *British Medical Journal* 303, 671–675.

Barker, D.J., Martyn, C.N., Osmond, C., Hales, C.N. and Fall, C.H. (1993) Growth *in utero* and serum cholesterol concentrations in adult life. *British Medical Journal* 307, 1524–1527.

Barker, D.J.P., Osmond, C., Rodin, I., Fall, C.H.D. and Winter, P.D. (1995a) Low weight gain in infancy and suicide in adult life. *British Medical Journal* 311, 1203.

Barker, D.J.P., Winter, P.D., Osmond, C., Phillips, D.I.W. and Sultan, H.Y. (1995b) Weight gain in infancy and cancer of the ovary. *Lancet* 345, 1087–1088.

Barker, D.J.P., Shiell, A.W., Barker, M.E. and Law, C.M. (2000) Growth *in utero* and blood pressure levels in the next generation. *Journal of Hypertension* 18, 843–846.

Campbell, D.M., Hall, M.H., Barker, D.J.P., Cross, J., Shiell, A.W. and Godfrey, K.M. (1996) Diet in pregnancy and the offspring's blood pressure 40 years later. *British Journal of Obstetrics and Gynaecology* 103, 273–280.

Christensen, K., Vaupel, J.W., Holm, N.V. and Yashin, A.I. (1995) Mortality among twins after age 6: fetal-origins hypothesis versus twin method. *British Medical Journal* 310, 432–436.

Christensen, K., Stovring, H. and McGue, M. (2001) Do genetic factors contribute to the association between birth weight and blood pressure? *Journal of Epidemiology and Community Health* 55, 583–587.

Clarke, R., Shipley, M., Lewington, S., Youngman, L., Collins, R., Marmot, M. and Peto, R. (1999) Underestimation of risk associations due to regression dilution in long-term follow-up of prospective studies. *American Journal of Epidemiology* 150, 342–353.

Collaborative Group on Hormonal Factors in Breast Cancer (1997) Breast cancer and hormone replacement therapy: collaborative reanalysis of individual data from 51 epidemiological studies including 52 705 women with breast cancer and 108 411 women without the disease. *Lancet* 350, 1047–1059.

Cowin, I. and Emmett, P. (2000) Cholesterol and triglyceride concentrations, birth weight and central obesity in pre-school children. ALSPAC Study Team. Avon Longitudinal Study of Pregnancy and Childhood. *International Journal of Obesity and Related Metabolic Disorders* 24, 330–339.

Cresswell, J.L., Egger, P., Fall, C.H., Osmond, C., Fraser, R.B. and Barker, D.J. (1999) Is the age of menopause determined in-utero? *Early Human Development* 49, 143–148.

Curhan, G.C., Chertow, G.M., Willett, W.C., Spiegelman, D., Colditz, G.A., Manson, J.E., Speizer, F.E. and Stampfer, M.J. (1996) Birth weight and adult hypertension and obesity in women. *Circulation* 94, 1310–1315.

Dennison, E.M., Arden, N.K., Keen, R.W., Syddall, H., Day, I.N., Spector, T.D. and Cooper, C. (2001) Birth weight, vitamin D receptor genotype and the programming of osteoporosis. *Paediatric and Perinatal Epidemiology* 15, 211–219.

De Onis, M., Villar, J. and Gulmezoglu, M. (1998) Nutritional interventions to prevent intrauterine growth retardation: evidence from randomized controlled trials. *European Journal of Clinical Nutrition* 52, S1, S83–93.

Dickersin, K. (1997) How important is publication bias? A synthesis of available data. *AIDS Education and Prevention* 9, 15–21.

dos Santos Silva, I., De Stavola, B.L., Mann, V., Kuh, D., Hardy, R. and Wadsworth, M.E. (2002) Prenatal factors, childhood growth trajectories and age at menarche. *International Journal of Epidemiology* 31, 405–412.

Egger, M. and Davey-Smith, G. (1997) Meta-analysis: Potential and promise. *British Medical Journal* 315, 1371–1374.

Egger, M., Davey, S.G., Schneider, M. and Minder, C. (1997) Bias in meta-analysis detected by a simple, graphical test. *British Medical Journal* 315, 629–634.

Elford, J., Whincup, P. and Shaper, A.G. (1991) Early life experience and adult cardiovascular disease: longitudinal and case-control studies. *International Journal of Epidemiology* 20, 833–844.

Eriksson, J.G., Forsen, T., Tuomilehto, J., Winter, P.D., Osmond, C. and Barker, D.J. (1999) Catch-up growth in childhood and death from coronary heart disease: longitudinal study. *British Medical Journal* 318, 427–431.

Fall, C.H.D., Osmond, C., Barker, D.J.P., Clark, P.M.S., Hales, C.N., Stirling, Y. and Meade, T.W. (1995) Fetal and infant growth and cardiovascular risk factors in women. *British Medical Journal* 310, 428–432.

Forsdahl, A. (1977) Are poor living conditions in childhood and adolescence an important risk factor for arteriosclerotic heart disease? *British Journal of Preventive and Social Medicine* 31, 91–95.

Frayling, T.M. and Hattersley, A.T. (2001) The role of genetic susceptibility in the association of low birth weight with type 2 diabetes. *British Medical Bulletin* 60, 89–101.

Garrett, P.J., Sandeman, D.D., Reza, M. and Theaker, J.M. (1993) Weight at birth and renal disease in adulthood. *Nephrology and Dialysis Transplant* 8, 920.

Greenland, S. (1980) The effect of misclassification in the presence of covariates. *American Journal of Epidemiology* 112, 564–569.

Hennessy, E. (2002) Unravelling the fetal origins hypothesis. *Lancet* 360, 2072–2073.

Hoek, H.W., Susser, E., Buck, K.A., Lumey, L.H., Lin, S.P. and Gorman, J.M. (1996) Schizoid personality disorder after prenatal exposure to famine. *American Journal of Psychiatry* 153, 1637–1639.

Huxley, R.R., Shiell, A.W. and Law, C.M. (2000) The role of size at birth and postnatal catch-up growth in determining systolic blood pressure: a systematic review of the literature. *Journal of Hypertension* 18, 815–831.

Huxley, R., Neil, A. and Collins, R. (2002) Unravelling the fetal origins hypothesis: is there really an inverse association between birth weight and subsequent blood pressure? *Lancet* 360, 659–665.

Huxley, R., Lewington, S. and Clarke, R. (2004) Cholesterol and coronary heart disease: A review of the evidence from observational studies and randomised controlled trials. *Seminars in Vascular Medicine* (in press).

Joseph, K.S. and Kramer, M.S. (1996) Review of the evidence on fetal and early child-hood antecedents of adult chronic disease. *Epidemiologic Reviews* 18, 158–173.

Kermack, W.O., McKendrick, A.G. and McKinlay, P.L. (1934) Death-rates in Great Britain and Sweden. Some general regularities and their significance. *Lancet* 1, 698–703.

Kramer, M.S. (1987) Determinants of low birth weight: methodological assessment and meta-analysis. *Bulletin of the World Health Organization* 65, 663–737.

Kramer, M.S. (1993) Effects of energy and protein intakes on pregnancy outcome: an overview of the research evidence from controlled clinical trials. *American Journal of Clinical Nutrition* 58, 627–635.

Kramer, M.S., Morin, I., Yang, H., Platt, R.W., Usher, R., McNamara, H., Joseph, K.S. and Wen, S.W. (2002) Why are babies getting bigger? Temporal trends in fetal growth and its determinants. *Journal of Paediatrics* 141, 538–542.

Langley-Evans, S.C. and Jackson, A.A. (1994) Increased systolic blood pressure in adult rats induced by fetal exposure to maternal low protein diets. *Clinical Science* 86, 217–222.

Law, C.M. and Shiell, A.W. (1996) Is blood pressure inversely related to birth weight? The strength of evidence from a systematic review of the literature. *Journal of Hypertension* 14, 935–991.

Leeson, C.P., Whincup, P.H., Cook, D.G., Donald, A.E., Papacosta, O., Lucas, A. and Deanfield, J.E. (1997) Flow-mediated dilation in 9- to 11-year-old children: the influence of intrauterine and childhood factors. *Circulation* 96, 2233–2238.

Leon, D. (1999) Twins and fetal programming of blood pressure: questioning the role of genes and maternal nutrition. *British Medical Journal* 319, 1313–1314.

Lissner, L., Karlsson, C., Lindroos, A.K., Sjostrom, L., Carlsson, B. and Bengtsson, C. (1999) Birth weight, adulthood BMI, and subsequent weight gain in relation to leptin levels in Swedish women. *Obesity Research* 7, 150–154.

Lucas, A. and Morley, R. (1994) Does early nutrition in infants born before term programme later blood pressure? *British Medical Journal* 309, 304–308.

Lucas, A., Baker, B.A., Desai, M. and Hales, C.N. (1996) Nutrition in pregnancy or lactating rats programs lipid metabolism in the offspring. *British Journal of Nutrition* 76, 605–612.

Lucas, A., Fewtrell, M.S. and Cole, T.J. (1999) Fetal-origins of adult disease – the hypothesis revisited. *British Medical Journal* 319, 245–249.

MacMahon, S. and Collins, R. (2001) Reliable assessment of the effects of treatment on mortality and major morbidity, II: observational studies. *Lancet* 357, 455–462.

Magnus, P. and Beaglehole, R. (2001) The real contribution of the major risk factors to the coronary epidemics: time to end the 'only-50%' myth. *Archives of Internal Medicine* 161, 2657–2660.

Martyn, C.N., Meade, T.W., Stirling, Y. and Barker, D.J.P. (1995) Plasma concentrations of fibrinogen and factor VII in adult life and their relation to intrauterine growth. *British Journal of Haematology* 89, 142–146.

Martyn, C.N., Gale, C.R., Jespersen, S. and Sherriff, S.B. (1998) Impaired fetal growth and atherosclerosis of carotid and peripheral arteries. *Lancet* 352, 173–178.

National Institute of Health (1998) Clinical guidelines on the identification, evaluation and treatment of overweight and obesity – the evidence report. *Obesity Research* 6, 51S–209S.

Owen, C.G., Whincup, P.H., Odoki, K., Gilg, J.A. and Cook, D.G. (2003) Birthweight and blood cholesterol level; a study in adolescents and systematic review. *Paediatrics* 111, 1081–1189.

Phillips, D.I. and Barker, D.J. (1997) Association between low birth weight and high resting pulse in adult life: is the sympathetic nervous system involved in programming the insulin resistance syndrome? *Diabetic Medicine* 14, 673–677.

Phillips, D.I., Barker, D.J. and Osmond, C. (1993) Infant feeding, fetal growth and adult thyroid function. *Acta Endocrinologia Copenhagen* 129, 134–138.

Phillips, D.I., Walker, B.R., Reynolds, R.M., Flanagan, D.E.H., Wood, P.J., Osmond, C., Barker, D.J.P. and Whorwood, C.B. (2000) Low birth weight predicts elevated plasma cortisol concentrations in adults from 3 populations. *Hypertension* 35, 1301–1306.

Phillips, D.I.W., Handelsman, D.J., Eriksson, J.G., Forsén, T., Osmond, C. and Barker, D.J.P. (2001) Prenatal growth and subsequent marital status: longitudinal study. *British Medical Journal* 322, 771.

Pietilainen, K.H., Kaprio, J., Rasanen, M., Winter, T., Rissanen, A. and Rose, R.J. (2001) Tracking of body size from birth to late adolescence. contributions of birth length, birth weight, duration of gestation, parents' body size and twinship. *American Journal of Epidemiology* 154, 21–29.

Power, C. (1994) National trends in birth weight: implications for future adult disease. *British Medical Journal* 308, 1270–1271.

Robinson, R. (2001) The fetal-origins of adult disease: no longer just a hypothesis and may be critically important in South Asia. *British Medical Journal* 322, 375–376.

Rodgers, A. and MacMahon, S. (1995) Systematic underestimation of treatment effects as a result of diagnostic test inaccuracy: implications for the interpretation and design of thromboprophylaxis trials. *Thrombosis and Haemostasis* 73(2), 167–171.

Rona, R.J., Qureshi, S. and Chinn, S. (1996) Factors related to total cholesterol and blood pressure in British 9-year-olds. *Journal of Epidemiology and Community Health* 50, 512–518.

Roseboom, T.J., van-der-Meulen, J.H., Ravelli, A.C., van-Montfrans, G.A., Osmond, C., Barker, D.J. and Bleker, O.P. (1999) Blood pressure in adults after prenatal exposure to famine. *Journal of Hypertension* 17, 325–330.

Roseboom, T.J., van der Meulen, J.H., Osmond, C., Barker, D.J., Ravelli, A.C. and Bleker, O.P. (2002) Plasma lipid profiles in adults after prenatal exposure to the Dutch famine. *American Journal of Clinical Nutrition* 72, 1101–1106.

Rush, D., Stein, Z. and Susser, M. (1980) A randomised controlled trial of prenatal nutritional supplementation in New York City. *Paediatrics* 65, 683–697.

Said, M.H., Lehingue, Y., Remontet, L. and Mamelle, N. (1998) Relations between blood pressure at 3–4 years of age and body mass at birth: a population-based study. *Revue d'Épidemiologie et de Santé Publique* 46(5), 351–360.

Secker-Walker, R.H. and Vacek, P.M. (2003) Relationships between cigarette smoking during pregnancy, gestational age, maternal weight gain, and infant birthweight. *Addictive Behaviors* 28, 55–66.

Shadish, W.R. and Haddock, C.K. (1994) Combining estimates of effect size. In: Cooper, H. and Hedges, L.V. (eds) *The Handbook of Research Synthesis*. Russel Sage Foundation, New York.

Singhal, A., Cole, T.J. and Lucas, A. (2001) Early nutrition in preterm infants and later blood pressure: two cohorts after randomised trials. *Lancet* 357, 413–419.

Singhal, P.K., Paul, V.K., Deorari, A.K., Singh, M. and Sundaram, K.R. (1991) Changing trends in intrauterine growth curves. *Indian Paediatrics* 28, 281–283.

Sorensen, H.T., Sabroe, S., Olsen, J., Rothman, K.J., Gillman, M.W. and Fischer, P. (1997) Birth weight and cognitive function in young adult life: historical cohort study. *British Medical Journal* 315, 401–403.

Stanner, S.A., Bulmer, K., Andres, C., Lantseva, O.E., Borodina, V., Poteen, V.V. and Yudkin, J.S. (1997) Does malnutrition *in utero* determine diabetes and coronary heart disease in adulthood? Results from the Leningrad siege study, a cross-sectional study. *British Medical Journal* 315, 1342–1349.

Stocks, N.P. and Davey-Smith, G. (1999) Blood pressure and birth weight in first year university students aged 18–25. *Public Health* 113, 273–277.

Tang, J.L., Armitage, J.M., Lancaster, T., Silagy, C.A., Fowler, G.H. and Neil, H.A.W. (1998) Systematic review of dietary intervention trials to lower blood total cholesterol in free-living subjects. *British Medical Journal* 316, 1213–1220.

Thompson, C., Syddall, H., Rodin, I., Osmond, C. and Barker, D.J. (2001) Birth weight and the risk of depressive disorder in late life. *British Journal of Psychiatry* 179, 450–455.

Trials of Hypertension Prevention Collaborative Research Group (1992) The effect of nonpharmacologic intervention on blood pressure of persons with high–normal level: results of the Trial of Hypertension Prevention, phase II. *Journal of the American Medical Association* 267, 1213–1220.

Vågerö, D. and Leon, D. (1994) Ischaemic heart disease and low birth weight: a test of the fetal-origins hypothesis from the Swedish Twin Registry. *Lancet* 343, 260–263.

Walker, B.R., McConnachie, A., Noon, J.P., Webb, D.J. and Watt, G.C. (1998) Contribution of parental blood pressures to association between low birth weight and adult high blood pressure: cross sectional study. *British Medical Journal* 316, 834–837.

World Health Organisation (2002) *The World Health Report: 2002. Reducing Risks, Promoting Healthy Life*. WHO, Geneva.

Xu, B., Pekkanen, J., Laitinen, J. and Jarvelin, M.R. (2002) Body build from birth to adulthood and risk of asthma. *European Journal of Public Health* 12(3), 166–170.

6 Experimental Models of Hypertension and Cardiovascular Disease

SIMON C. LANGLEY-EVANS

School of Biosciences, University of Nottingham, Sutton Bonington Campus, Loughborough LE12 5RD, UK

Introduction

As described in Chapter 4 of this volume, a number of epidemiological studies in large human cohorts have indicated that there are associations between indices of impaired fetal growth and cardiovascular disease in later life. Barker and colleagues have repeatedly reported that risk of coronary heart disease, hypertension and stroke-related mortality is increased in individuals who were of lower weight at birth or otherwise showed evidence of disproportion at birth (Barker, 2002). Although initially highly contentious, these reports of Barker and coworkers have now been widely accepted and have informed the development of health and social policy in the UK. The heavy investment of government research funds into this particular field of medical research has appeared justified on the basis of the replication of the Barker findings in other populations around the world, by independent research groups (Curhan *et al.*, 1996; Forrester *et al.*, 1996; Moore *et al.*, 1996; Leon, 1999).

Increasingly, however, questions are being raised about the validity and importance of the observed associations. Most recently Huxley *et al.* (2002) have suggested that associations between birthweight and later blood pressure are artefactual (see Chapter 5, this volume) and other critics have pointed out that the epidemiological studies may be heavily confounded by uncontrolled factors relating to social class and to genetics (Bartley *et al.*, 1994; Kramer and Joseph, 1996). Most importantly, the central tenet of the fetal origins of adult disease hypothesis is that the association between impaired fetal growth and later disease is explained by nutritionally mediated programming (Barker, 2002). This is a weak starting point for studies in humans. There is very little evidence to support the suggestion that undernutrition results in reduced birthweight or disproportionate birth, other than in populations in the developing world (Prentice *et al.*, 1987; Thame *et al.*, 1997) (see Chapter 2, this volume). In well-nourished populations, normal variations in maternal nutritional status have only a minor impact, if any, upon fetal growth (Godfrey *et al.*, 1996; Mathews *et al.*, 1999). There is evidence that exposure to undernutrition in the fetal period may associate with blood pressure in later life independently of fetal growth changes, but this is based upon small-scale studies of a somewhat serendipitous nature (Godfrey *et al.*, 1994; Campbell *et al.*, 1996). There is no information upon the long-term impact of maternal nutritional supplementation or similar interventions and, understandably, such studies are not embarked upon very readily.

Given the obvious constraints of epidemiological approaches to the study of the programming of cardiovascular disease, the development of animal models has been an essential element of research in this area. The degree of control over experimental conditions and the possibilities for invasive measurements have allowed intensive study of the pathophysiological consequences of fetal undernutrition.

Experimental Models of Programming

A broad range of experimental models has now been developed in a number of different species and it is becoming clear that quite diverse nutritional manipulations generate very similar physiological outcomes, acting through a relatively limited number of common mechanisms (Fig. 6.1). However, these studies cannot be employed as the only means of investigating cardiovascular programming. Experimental studies in humans should become the priority for the coming decade. Although studies of rodents are very informative in terms of confirming cardiovascular programming as a biological response to early undernutrition and in developing initial hypotheses regarding programming mechanisms, there are constraints on drawing parallels between animals and humans. One major drawback of the rodent studies is that these species are generally resistant to atherosclerosis and do not develop coronary heart disease. Much of the following discussion will therefore focus upon blood pressure and its regulatory mechanisms.

Dietary manipulations in rodents

Balanced dietary restriction

Modelling the human diet using animal models, although desirable, is an impossible task. In developing suitable animal models of nutritional programming, it has been argued that the approach most representative of human undernutrition is a balanced, or global, restriction of nutrient intakes (Bertram and Hanson, 2001). The suggestion is that, in human populations that are subject to chronic or episodic undernutrition, it is most likely that food intake *per se* is reduced rather than they suffer from deficiencies of specific nutrients. This is arguable, as in populations such as that of the UK, there are a number of subgroups with increased prevalence of disorders related to marginal nutrient intakes. For example, vegetarians and vegans may find it difficult to consume requirements

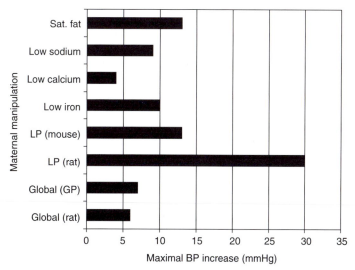

Fig. 6.1. Impact of maternal dietary manipulations in pregnant animals upon offspring blood pressure. Data shown are the maximal changes in blood pressure (BP) (systolic or mean arterial pressure) in rodent species following restriction of the diet or feeding of high-saturated fat diets. Generally, larger changes in pressure are noted following restriction of maternal intakes of specific nutrients than when global nutrient restriction is applied. Sat., saturated; LP, low protein; GP, guinea-pig. (Data were obtained from Langley-Evans *et al.*, 1994a; Crowe *et al.*, 1995; Langley-Evans, 1996; Woodall *et al.*, 1996; Dunn *et al.*, 2001; Battista *et al.*, 2002; Bergel and Belizan, 2002; Kind *et al.*, 2002.)

for protein, calcium and iron (Wagener *et al.*, 2000). Younger women may be at particular risk of micronutrient deficiencies and, given the high number of children born in the UK to mothers under the age of 18, this is of considerable relevance to the nutritional programming debate. The 2000 Diet and Nutrition Survey of British children aged 4–18 indicated that a quarter of adolescent girls had very low intakes of iron and calcium, and also highlighted magnesium intake as a cause for concern (Gregory *et al.*, 2000). Iron-deficiency anaemia is the most common nutritional disorder worldwide.

Consideration needs to be given to which human populations experimental studies should actually be modelling. At the present time, it is probably true to say that most experiments in this area are seeking to demonstrate the biological principles of programming. Some of these adopt the global restriction approach as this may be truly representative of populations exposed to periodic famine or for which food security is permanently poor. However, most of the epidemiological studies that have suggested that programming may be relevant to human disease states have focused upon populations in affluent nations, where, for the majority, food supply is assured and global nutrient restriction is unlikely.

A number of rodent models have been developed to explore the impact of global nutrient restriction upon long-term vascular functions, generally with blood pressure as the main outcome measure. One of the first studies that specifically attempted to test the fetal origins of adult disease hypothesis utilized an unusual approach to the manipulation of fetal nutrition (Persson and Jansson, 1992). The guinea-pig fetus is particularly vulnerable to the growth-retarding effects of severe maternal undernutrition (Lechner, 1984) and has often been used as a model of undernutrition in pregnancy, due to the similarities between humans and cavies in terms of their placentation (Garnica and Chan, 1996). In the guinea-pig the uterus is divided into two horns, with equal division of nutrients to the 1–3 pups that may develop in each. Persson and Jansen (1992) exploited the vulnerabilities of the guinea-pig fetus by ligating one horn of the pregnant uterus. Surgical ligation of one horn resulted in profound growth retardation of pups on that side relative to their littermates in the untreated horn. When all of the animals had their blood pressure determined in young adulthood, there was a significant relationship between the degree of growth retardation and blood pressure (Persson and Jansson, 1992). The most severely growth-retarded guinea-pigs, relative to their normal littermates, displayed the greatest increases in blood pressure relative to their normal littermates.

This study appeared to support the concept that growth retardation may be linked to later cardiovascular disease, and prompted other groups to develop nutritional models aimed primarily at limiting fetal growth in order to explore its consequences. One of the best characterized of these models was first reported by Woodall et al. (1996). In this approach, pregnant rats are provided with a greatly reduced food intake, thereby providing a balanced nutrient restriction that impacts upon all macro- and micronutrients equally. Food intake is restricted to just 30% of the ad libitum intake of pregnant rats of similar size and gestation. This has major effects upon maternal weight gain, and presumably body composition, in pregnancy.

In the rat, the first half of pregnancy is a time of anabolic metabolism, with heavy storage of both fat and protein stores (Naismith and Morgan, 1976). Weight gain is moderate (see Fig. 6.2), with approximately 25 g of stores laid down. Over the second half of pregnancy these stores are partially mobilized,

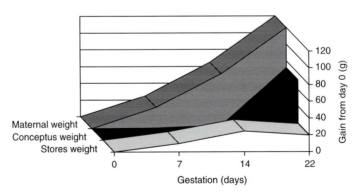

Fig. 6.2.   Gain in maternal and conceptus weight in rat pregnancy. Weight gain in pregnant rats reflects the biphasic nature of protein metabolism in this species. In early gestation anabolic processes predominate and most of the weight gain over the first half of pregnancy is attributable to the deposition of stores, and increase in fluid volume. In the second half of pregnancy stores are metabolized and a rapid increase in fetal and placental growth rate is noted from days 14 to 22.

fuelling rapid fetal growth. Remaining stores will be used for lactation. Over this period weight gain accelerates and the dams will gain approximately 70 g in weight, of which approximately 60 g will be fetal and placental material. In the global food restriction model reported by Woodall *et al.* (1996), this normal pattern of weight gain is abolished and the pregnant animals lose weight in mid-gestation, suggesting that there is only minimal, if any, deposition of the necessary stores to drive later fetal growth. The outcome is a significant reduction in weight of the offspring at birth. Blood pressure measurements indicate that in early postnatal life, the cardiovascular system is largely unaffected by the fetal growth restriction. This appears contrary to the fetal-origins hypothesis as Barker and colleagues suggest that cardiovascular changes are present even at birth and become amplified with age (Law *et al.*, 1993; Barker, 2002). However, by 30 weeks of age, the growth-retarded rat offspring exhibit a small (6 mmHg) but significant increase in blood pressure relative to the offspring of well-nourished control animals (Woodall *et al.*, 1996).

Whereas this particular global restriction model appears to support the nutritional programming hypothesis in general terms, a less severe global nutrient restriction in rat pregnancy produces less clear-cut effects. A 50% reduction of food intake in the second half of pregnancy did not increase blood pressure in the resulting offspring, despite exposure to undernutrition during the most rapid phase of fetal growth and development (Holemans *et al.*, 1999). These animals did, however, exhibit subtle changes in vascular function in the small mesenteric resistance arteries. Sensitivity to exogenous nitric oxide was increased, whereas endothelium-dependent relaxation was reduced.

This study may have been aberrant, as less severe food restriction in rat pregnancy does, in fact, impact upon blood pressure in the offspring. Rats allowed to consume 70% of *ad libitum* intake produced pups that were hypertensive relative to control animals from 13 weeks of age (Ozaki *et al.*, 2001). Blood pressure was increased by 13 mmHg in males and to a lesser extent in females. Similarly, a very mild global nutrient restriction in guinea-pig pregnancy (85% of *ad libitum* intake) also programmed later blood pressure. At around 14 weeks of age, guinea-pig pups exposed to undernutrition *in utero* had blood pressures that were 9% higher than those in control animals (Kind *et al.*, 2002).

Studies in which rodents are subject to global nutrient restriction thus appear simply to model the epidemiological studies of Barker and others. Nutrient restriction retards fetal growth, manifesting as lower birthweight. These growth-retarded animals develop high blood pressure and/or altered vascular function in later life. A common feature of all of these studies is that the cardiovascular effects of fetal undernutrition are small and are subject to some delay before their appearance in postnatal life. A rather different picture emerges with many of the studies of specific nutrient restriction.

Restriction of specific nutrients

PROTEIN. As described above, many nutrients in the human diet are likely to be limiting in terms of fetal growth and development. Much of the work with animal models that has considered the programming effects of restricting single nutrients has utilized low-protein feeding. This is of considerable relevance in the study of human health. Across the globe there is wide variation in protein intakes, with women from affluent nations consuming approximately 60–80 g/day, whereas women from poorer countries, who depend solely on plant sources, consume 40–50 g/day and may well have marginal protein intakes. Within the UK, protein intakes are lower in pregnant women from lower socio-economic classes (Table 6.1). In a 2002 study of 300 British women, we found that 6–8% had first- or third-trimester protein intakes below the UK Reference Nutrient Intake (51 g/day) and that 55% of these individuals were from the lower socio-economic groups (social classes IV and V).

Importantly, one of the few clear examples of a direct relationship between maternal nutritional status and offspring health in humans implicates protein in programming. Campbell *et al.* (1996) demonstrated that, in a cohort of men aged 43–48 years, blood pressure was inversely related to maternal animal protein intake in pregnancy, among women with high carbohydrate intakes.

Historically, low-protein diets have been widely used for inducing fetal growth retardation in rats, and numerous studies have demonstrated that severe restriction can markedly reduce fetal and placental growth. Many of these studies have compared diets containing 4–5% protein (diet by weight) with control diets containing up to 24% protein (Zeman and Stanbrough, 1969; Hastings-Roberts and Zeman, 1977; Merlet-Benichou *et al.*, 1994). These studies were not operating within physiologically likely ranges however, as the protein requirement for the rat in pregnancy is approximately 12% by weight (Clarke *et al.*, 1977). Our own studies of nutritional programming have utilized a low-protein diet based upon casein as the sole protein source. The control diet for these studies contains 18% casein, and a variety of levels of restriction have been applied, ranging from 12% to 6% by weight. Most of the work with this maternal low-protein diet (MLP) model has used a 9% casein diet (Langley-Evans, 2001). This matches the protein requirement of the non-pregnant rat and is therefore only a mild

Table 6.1. Maternal protein intakes in the first and third trimesters of pregnancy.

Socio-economic group	Trimester 1		Trimester 3	
	Protein intake (g/day)	Protein intake (% energy)	Protein intake (g/day)	Protein intake (% energy)
I	75.7 ± 13.8	14.1 ± 2.1	72.6 ± 14.3	13.8 ± 2.2
II	69.0 ± 14.0	13.8 ± 1.9	73.0 ± 14.7	15.3 ± 6.2
III M III NM	71.9 ± 14.8	14.1 ± 2.0	70.8 ± 13.2	13.5 ± 2.2
IV	68.7 ± 15.9*	13.4 ± 2.0	67.6 ± 13.8*	13.9 ± 2.3
V	64.8 ± 22.8*	13.8 ± 2.5	63.6 ± 15.6*	14.0 ± 3.1

A total of 220 and 172 women from Northampton, UK, were studied in the first and third trimesters of pregnancy, respectively. Daily protein intake was estimated using 5-day food records. Women were grouped on the basis of their partner's occupation. *Indicates significantly different to social class I ($P < 0.05$). Data are mean ± SD. Social class I represents professional occupations, class IV represents unskilled labour and V is unemployed. M represents manual, NM represents non-manual.

protein restriction. The energy content of MLP diet is matched to control diet by increasing the carbohydrate content in proportion to the protein restriction. The carbohydrate is provided as a 2:1 (w/w) mixture of starch and sucrose, and fat is provided as corn oil.

MLP diets exert effects upon fetal growth that are both quantitatively and qualitatively different to global nutrient restriction models. Feeding a 9% casein diet appears to accelerate the early growth of the fetus, such that by day 14 out of the 22 days of rat gestation, MLP-exposed fetuses are significantly larger than well-nourished controls (Fig. 6.3). This effect is amplified if the MLP feeding is targeted only to the first 7 days of gestation (Langley-Evans *et al.*, 1996a; Langley-Evans and Nwagwu 1998). More rapid fetal and placental growth continue with MLP up until day 20 gestation. In normal rat pregnancy, the fetus will double in weight over the last 2 days of gestation. MLP feeding appears to attenuate this rapid late gestation surge in growth, and fetuses that were larger than controls at day 20 were subsequently born at low to normal birthweight (Langley-Evans *et al.*, 1996a). The pattern of growth noted in MLP-exposed fetuses and their associated placentas depends to some extent upon the plane of nutrition prior to conception. Fetuses whose mothers are habituated to MLP prior to pregnancy exhibit accelerated growth for a longer period than those whose mothers begin protein restriction on the first day of pregnancy (Langley-Evans and Nwagwu, 1998). In general terms, however, MLP feeding appears to

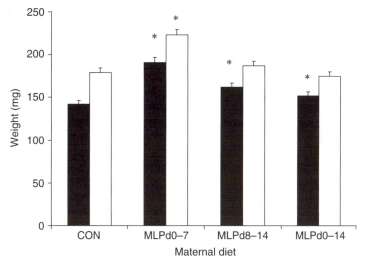

Fig. 6.3. Fetal and placental weight at day 14 gestation in rat pregnancy. Pregnant rats were fed either a control diet (CON) or maternal low-protein (MLP) diet. MLP feeding was either targeted to 7-day blocks (d0–7 or d8–14) or maintained throughout pregnancy (d0–14). Rats were killed at day 14 and fetal (shaded bars) and placental (open bars) weights determined. Data are shown as means ± SEM and * indicates a significant difference when compared with control animals (*P* < 0.05). Low-protein feeding stimulated more rapid growth of fetus and placenta. The effect was more marked when targeted to the first week of gestation only. *n* = 46–62 fetuses per group. (Data taken from Langley-Evans and Nwagwu, 1998.)

exert growth-promoting effects in early gestation and growth-retarding effects in late gestation. In the latter period of pregnancy the most vulnerable organs are those of the trunk, whereas the growth of the brain is relatively spared (Langley-Evans et al., 1996a).

The offspring of rats fed the MLP diet in pregnancy can be viewed as being undernourished only during the prenatal period. All dams, regardless of diet in pregnancy, are fed the same standard chow diet upon littering, and experiments using the MLP feeding protocol standardize litter sizes for the suckling period, to reduce the impact of fluctuations in the quality and quantity of milk by rats fed MLP in pregnancy. We have shown recently that, on postnatal day 1, the protein concentrations in milk from dams fed control and MLP diets are similar (Bellinger and Langley-Evans, unpublished observation), which supports the view that recovery from protein restriction is rapid.

The offspring of rats fed the MLP diet exhibit elevated systolic blood pressure from an early age. Among animals aged 3–4 weeks, pressures are increased by 15–30 mmHg relative to control animals (Langley-Evans et al., 1994a). This effect does not depend upon the level of protein restriction as experiments with 12, 9 or 6% casein diets suggest that they all exert a similar effect upon blood pressure (Langley and Jackson, 1994). The effect of prenatal protein restriction appears to be permanent, and blood pressures remain elevated well into adult life (Langley-Evans and Jackson, 1995). The effects of low-protein feeding on cardiovascular function are not restricted to the rat. Similar experiments have demonstrated that the feeding of MLP diet throughout mouse pregnancy also produces hypertension in the offspring. In this case, the effect is accompanied by reduced weight at birth (Dunn et al., 2001).

One of the basic elements of the programming hypothesis is that exposure to insults during critical periods of development exerts permanent physiological or metabolic effects. Rat pregnancy may be conveniently divided into three critical phases: embryogenesis, tissue differentiation and tissue maturation. Exposure to MLP during any of these phases appears to produce significant effects upon the vasculature. Kwong et al. (2000) reported that MLP feeding during the first 4 days of gestation led to significant elevation of blood pressure in the offspring at 4 weeks' postnatal age. This is remarkable, as the rat embryo at 4 days is still at the pre-implantation stage. Our own experiments show that MLP feeding from days 0–7 increased blood pressure to a similar degree as that noted when restriction was timed between days 8 and 14, a time of tissue differentiation (Langley-Evans et al., 1996b). Greater elevation of blood pressure was associated with restriction over the rapid fetal growth phase (days 15–22), but the largest programming effect of a low-protein diet was seen with restriction throughout pregnancy (Fig. 6.4).

Low-protein diets may exert some of their effects on blood pressure through structural adaptations within the vasculature and the kidney. In the kidney, reduced numbers of nephrons are present at the time of birth in the offspring rats subject to MLP feeding throughout pregnancy (Langley-Evans et al., 1996b, 2002). Mid-late gestation appears to represent a critical period of vulnerability for this organ. Nephron deficits at birth are not recovered postnatally. It is argued that to maintain renal haemodynamic functions, local blood pressure increases

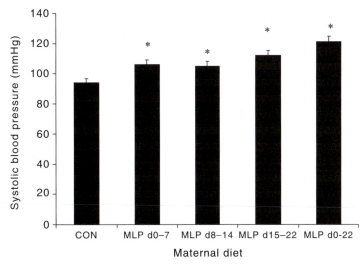

Fig. 6.4. Systolic blood pressure in rats following prenatal exposure to a maternal low-protein (MLP) diet. Pregnant rats were fed a control (CON) diet or MLP diet. MLP feeding was maintained throughout pregnancy (d0–22) or targeted to 7-day blocks (d0–7, d8–14, d15–22). Blood pressure was determined in the resulting offspring at 4 weeks of age. The data shown are mean systolic blood pressures ± SEM for 34–45 rats per group. * Indicates a significant difference when compared with the control group ($P < 0.05$). The findings indicate that protein restriction at any period in rat pregnancy may programme later hypertension, but that late gestation appears to be the most vulnerable period. (Data taken from Langley-Evans *et al.*, 1996b.)

are necessary, thereby maintaining glomerular perfusion. Rising pressures lead to loss of more nephrons and hence to still greater increases in pressure to maintain function further. Thus the animal enters a cycle of rising systemic pressure and progressive nephron loss, which eventually establishes hypertension and renal disease (Mackenzie and Brenner, 1995).

Martyn and Greenwald (2001) argue that programming of vascular structure may also contribute to hypertension. Relative deposition of elastin and collagen within the arterial wall determines stiffness and hence vascular compliance. Consistent with this hypothesis, we have demonstrated that MLP feeding in the rat produces noticeable changes within the ascending aorta from as early as 4 weeks' postnatal age. MLP-exposed rats have thinner-walled vessels, with reduced functional elasticity and significantly lower elastin content (Greenwald, Langley-Evans, Martyn and Phillips, unpublished observations).

One of the problems with rodent models of cardiovascular disease is the resistance of these species to atherosclerosis and hence coronary heart disease. In the rat low-protein diet model of nutritional programming, there has been little investigation of susceptibility to heart disease beyond studies of blood pressure and its regulation. However, it may be argued that in a atherosclerosis-prone species, some programming effect may be evident. One of the primary stages of plaque formation is oxidation of low-density lipoprotein (LDL)-cholesterol.

While some reports suggest that total cholesterol and LDL-cholesterol concentrations are lowered by prenatal protein restriction, it is clear that, overall, MLP-exposed animals have impaired antioxidant defences in adult life and are more vulnerable to oxidative processes (Langley-Evans et al., 1994b; Langley-Evans et al., 1997).

This vulnerability may also manifest as an increased rate of ageing, which is, in part, determined by oxidative processes that activate apoptosis. Aged rats exposed to MLP diet in utero exhibit abnormalities of bone mineralization (Mehta et al., 2002) and more rapid decline in renal integrity and function (Nwagwu et al., 2000) when compared to control rats of equivalent age. Moreover, life span is reduced by fetal exposure to maternal low-protein diets (Jennings et al., 1999; Sayer et al., 2001). However, in the rat it is difficult to discern the extent to which earlier death is attributable to cardiovascular programming.

Whereas many studies show that low-protein diets in pregnancy programme later hypertension in the developing fetus, this is not true of all. An extensive body of work by the late Joseph Hoet and his group in Louvain and by Hales et al. in Cambridge, has examined the nutritional programming of pancreatic function and type 2 diabetes by low-protein feeding in rat pregnancy and lactation. These studies employ a diet containing 8% protein (provided as casein), with carbohydrate provided mainly in the form of glucose and fat as soybean oil. This diet elicits structural changes within the developing pancreas, leading to glucose intolerance and insulin resistance. However, this low-protein diet does not programme blood pressure changes (Langley-Evans, 2000). This observation suggests that the overall food matrix is the critical element in nutritional programming, and that imbalances of nutrient supply act as a stressor that activates simple, probably hormonally mediated, mechanisms.

In comparing the diet used in our own studies with that of Hales and Hoet, it is clear that variation in the source of fat and/or carbohydrate may explain the discrepancies. It is therefore of considerable importance for the full composition of diets used in studies of programming to be published in papers. Other groups have also published data suggesting that a low-protein diet in utero does not programme vascular disease in rodents (Tonkiss et al., 1998). It is overly simplistic to assume that there is commonality between all rodent models utilizing low-protein diets without a greater depth of understanding of the metabolic adjustments and nutritional demands necessary to deal with suboptimal nutrition or frank malnutrition. If some nutrients are lacking in the diet and stores are depleted, others, which depend on the limiting elements for their metabolism, will effectively be present in excess. The effects of this excess may be just as important in programming as the effects of the primary nutrient deficiencies.

The finding that relatively short periods of protein restriction during fetal life can induce long-lasting elevation of blood pressure in adult life has raised interest in the role of specific amino acids. Rees et al. (1999) reported that low-protein feeding in rat pregnancy reduced the threonine concentration in fetal serum without impacting upon any other amino acid. Changes in maternal amino acid profiles suggested that threonine may be used to generate glycine, which is conditionally essential in pregnancy. Glycine is required in numerous metabolic pathways and, in both rat and human pregnancy, may be a limiting nutrient, particularly if protein intakes are low. Experiments in which MLP diet is supplemented with glycine show that this reverses the hypertensive effect of the diet upon the offspring (Jackson *et al.*, 2002). This effect was specific to glycine and was not reproduced by supplementing with an equivalent quantity of amino nitrogen in the form of urea, or a non-essential amino acid (alanine).

It has been proposed that the importance of glycine may lie in its use in the metabolism of methionine and homocysteine (Fig. 6.5) (Rees *et al.*, 1999). In the absence of an adequate supply of glycine from the diet or endogenous synthesis, first maternal and then fetal homocysteine may accumulate. This amino acid is toxic and hence likely to exert adverse effects upon fetal development. The ratio of *S*-adenosyl methionione and *S*-adenosyl homocysteine, intermediates in the methionine–homocysteine cycle, dictates that capacity for DNA methylation, which may also impact upon programming (see Chapter 14, this volume). In adults raised plasma homocysteine is a known risk factor for cardiovascular disease. It has been argued that the low-protein diet used in MLP rat experiments contains an excess of methionine, which would exacerbate fetal homocystein-aemia, and that this may explain the discrepancy between our studies and that of Hales and Hoet. However, work by McCarthy and Pickard has shown that this is not the case. Pregnant rats fed a low-protein diet that was also low in methionine produced offspring that developed hypertension equivalent to that

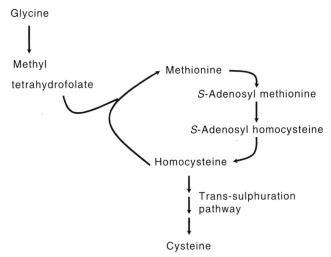

Fig. 6.5. Pathways of methionine and homocysteine metabolism. The methionine–homocysteine cycle normally permits the clearance of excess methionine through conversion to homocysteine, and then to cysteine via the trans-sulphuration pathway. When methionine supply is limited, the capacity exists to convert homocysteine to methionine through the addition of a single carbon group from methyl tetrahydrofolate, which may, in turn, be synthesized from glycine. In fetal life the trans-sulphuration pathway is not active. In situations where glycine is limiting, homocysteine formed from methionine will accumulate, as recycling back to methionine will be constrained.

induced by a standard MLP treatment (Pickard *et al.*, 1996). Similarly, we have shown that feeding an MLP diet with lower methionine content does not reverse renal defects associated with prenatal MLP exposure, and a high methionine, 18% protein diet, does not induce such defects (Langley-Evans, Makinson and McMullen, unpublished data). This indicates that the role of methionine in programming of blood pressure may be overstated by Rees *et al.* (1999).

OTHER NUTRIENTS. Feeding a low-protein diet in rodent pregnancy is not the only approach that has been used to study nutritional programming of the vasculature. Subtle shifts in the composition of the diet in pregnancy can produce potent effects. The substitution of corn oil (rich in polyunsaturated fats) with coconut oil (rich in saturated fats) in the diet of pregnant rats produces an elevation of blood pressure in their offspring (Fig. 6.6), that is the equivalent of feeding a low-protein diet (Langley-Evans, 1996). Interestingly, high-saturated fat combined with a low-protein diet does not produce any additional effect upon blood pressure.

Low intakes of micronutrients in pregnancy also appear to impact upon long-term cardiovascular health in laboratory rats. Low-iron diets, sufficient to produce anaemia in pregnant rats, reduced the early postnatal growth of the heart in the associated offspring. Initially these offspring had lower blood pressure than the offspring of iron-replete dams. However, by 6 weeks of age a

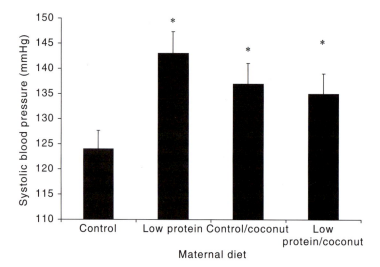

Fig. 6.6. Programming of high blood pressure in rats by feeding diets rich in saturated fatty acids. Pregnant rats were fed control or low-protein diets throughout gestation. These diets provided fat as 10% corn oil. Two further groups were fed the same diets, but providing the fat as 9% coconut oil and 1% corn oil. Blood pressure was determined in the offspring at 8 weeks of age. Data are shown as means ± SEM. * Indicates a significant difference when compared with the control group. Blood pressure was elevated in rats exposed to low-protein diets and also in rats exposed to adequate protein but supplied with coconut oil. Combining a low-protein diet with coconut oil did not reveal any additive effect of the two manipulations. (Data taken from Langley-Evans, 1996.)

significant elevation of blood pressure was observed (Crowe *et al.*, 1995). Low-sodium diets in rat pregnancy also elevated blood pressure by 7–8 mmHg in the offspring from around 6 weeks of age, through a mechanism that appears to be dependent upon renin–angiotensin system components (Battista *et al.*, 2002).

Bergel and Belizan (2002) studied the possible role of calcium in nutritional programming. Rats were fed a calcium-deficient diet, a control diet or a diet containing excess calcium for 1 month prior to mating and throughout pregnancy. Blood pressure in the offspring was measured monthly and appeared to be strongly related to maternal calcium intake. High consumption of calcium raised blood pressure slightly (4.3 mmHg at 1 year of age), whereas the offspring of calcium-deficient mothers had blood pressures 12 mmHg above the control value.

Dietary excess

One of the main discrepancies in the original fetal origins of adult disease hypothesis, as stated by Barker (2002), is the mismatch between trends in disease patterns and dietary practices. Cardiovascular disease is more prevalent in westernized countries and is associated with nutritional excess, specifically excessive intakes of fats and protein. Within the UK population, the average energy intake from fat has fallen over the past two decades, but remains in excess of the recommended 35%. Similarly, the average protein intake of British women during pregnancy (approximately 70 g/day) is well in excess of the Reference Nutrient Intake (51 g/day) and a high proportion of women may consume considerably more. In the developing world, where undernutrition is more prevalent, rates of cardiovascular disease morbidity and mortality are low. It is surprising, therefore, that there have been few attempts to model the impact of high-fat or high-protein diets in pregnancy upon later cardiovascular function and health.

Prenatal high-protein diets are generally considered to be a risk factor for low birthweight in human pregnancy (Sloan *et al.*, 2001). However, there have been no animal experiments directed at exploring the potential programming effects of excessive dietary protein. Daenzer *et al.* (2002) have demonstrated that feeding a high-protein (40% by weight) diet in rat pregnancy resulted in a greater fat mass in the offspring at 9 weeks of age. This suggests that high-protein diets may have the capacity to programme energy metabolism and may thus impact indirectly upon cardiovascular disease risk.

Similarly, there has been little evaluation of the programming effects of high-fat feeding upon cardiovascular function. Holemans *et al.* (2000) reported that feeding a high-saturated fat diet to the pregnant offspring of diabetic rats altered vascular sensitivity to acetylcholine and noradrenaline, but no assessment was made of the offspring. High-fat diets, rich in saturated or unsaturated fatty acids, fed to rats throughout pregnancy and lactation, had opposing effects on glucose metabolism, but no assessment was made of cardiovascular function markers (Siemlink *et al.*, 2002). However, our own studies of feeding a relatively low-fat diet, providing mainly saturated fatty acids, suggest that fats may play a role in programming blood pressure (Langley-Evans, 1996).

Dietary manipulations in large animal species

Large animal species arguably provide better models for human health than rodents. Rodents, with the exception of the guinea-pig, are very immature at birth. Farm animal species, such as the sheep and pig, are more mature, and their larger size allows for more detailed investigation *in utero* and in the early postnatal period.

Studies of the pig have indicated the existence of similar relationships between characteristics at birth and later cardiovascular function to those noted in humans. Poore *et al.* (2002) showed that basal mean arterial blood pressure was inversely related to birthweight and positively related to the ratio of head length to birthweight. These effects were accompanied by reduced renal angiotensin-converting enzyme activities and increased plasma noradrenaline. However, as with epidemiological studies in humans, these associations with birthweight tell us little about the mechanism of programming and are difficult to assign a cause to. In the pig there is considerable variability in birthweight, with up to threefold variation within a single litter. This variation is explained by nutrient restriction due to reduced placental size and transport. However, the nature of the nutrient restriction and prevailing endocrine milieu is not well understood.

The sheep is a much more widely studied large animal species in terms of the effects of nutrient restriction upon fetal and placental growth (Owens *et al.*, 1987). However, there is very little information upon the long-term cardiovascular impact of nutrient restriction *in utero*. The information available indicates that the endpoint of nutritional programming in this species is a reduction rather than an increase in blood pressure.

There are two main advantages associated with using the sheep as a model of programming. First, nutrient intake can be restricted very effectively through placental reduction or carunclectomy. The caruncular structure of the ovine placenta allows for the removal of a significant proportion and hence a restriction of the nutrient-transfer capability (Owens *et al.*, 1987). Secondly, with an animal of this size, it is possible to chronically instrument the developing fetus for physiological measurements. Such measurements indicate that nutrient restriction impacts upon the fetal cardiovasculature: a 15% restriction of maternal nutrient intake over the first 70 days of gestation (term 147 days) lowered basal systolic and diastolic blood pressures and reset baroreflex control mechanisms (Hawkins *et al.*, 2000).

These effects persist postnatally and, to some extent, are related to indices of fetal growth. Blood pressure is higher in sheep that were of greater weight at birth and appears related to kidney size (Gopalakrishnan *et al.*, 2002). This is directly the opposite of observations in humans. Furthermore, exposure to nutrient restriction in early pregnancy (Pearce *et al.*, 2002), resulted in lower blood pressure in lambs at 6 months of age, but, in keeping with the rat studies of Holemans *et al.* (1999), these animals demonstrated increased sensitivity to vasoconstrictors.

Hormonal manipulations and programming

It is now evident that nutritional factors are not solely responsible for the programming of the cardiovascular system. The interaction of the environment, as represented by maternal nutritional status, with the expression of key genes involved in regulation of development, is mediated by maternal hormonal status. Studies of these nutrient–hormone–gene interactions are at an early stage, but glucocorticoids and the hypothalamic–pituitary–adrenal axis have come under closest scrutiny.

Initial interest in a potential role for glucocorticoids in the fetal programming of later blood pressure arose from investigations of a rare genetic defect leading to premature death associated with early onset hypertension. The syndrome of apparent mineralocorticoid excess (AME) is characterized by the inappropriate binding of cortisol to aldosterone receptors in the kidney (New, 2002). As cortisol is secreted in concentrations in huge excess relative to aldosterone, and in response to completely different stimuli, blood pressure becomes massively and chronically elevated.

The inappropriate mineralocorticoid receptor (MR) binding that leads to the symptoms of AME is due to a lack of the enzyme 11β-hydroxysteroid dehydrogenase (11β-HSD) (New, 2002). The role of 11β-HSD is to metabolize active glucocorticoids (cortisol in humans, corticosterone in the rat) to inactive forms that do not bind the MR. Interestingly the type 2 isoform (11β-HSD-2) of this enzyme, found in kidney, is also present in placenta. Edwards *et al.* (1993) hypothesized that one of the functions of the placental enzyme is to prevent the fetal tissues from being exposed to glucocorticoids of maternal origin during early to mid-gestation. In most species the fetal adrenal becomes active in the last phase of development, and prior to this time the concentrations of active glucocorticoids present in fetal circulation are approximately one-thousandth of the concentrations seen in maternal circulation. This allows the fetal hypothalamic–pituitary–adrenal axis to develop independently of the maternal system.

Protection of the fetal tissues from maternal glucocorticoids by 11β-HSD-2 may also be critical for the normal development of other organ systems. Glucocorticoids are potent regulators of gene expression and promote tissue maturation over growth and differentiation. Exposure of the fetus at inappropriate times in development may thus retard growth and promote the development of abnormal structures and premature maturation (Liggins, 1969; Reinisch *et al.*, 1978).

At a time when the inverse association between birthweight and adult blood pressure reported by Barker and coworkers (2002) seemed secure, it was interesting to note that, in rat pregnancy, activity of 11β-HSD was inversely related to fetal weight in late gestation and positively related to placental weight (Benediktsson *et al.*, 1993). This appeared to suggest that this gatekeeper enzyme plays a key role in programming. The assertion was reinforced by the observation that treatment of pregnant rats with daily doses of dexamethasone (a synthetic glucocorticoid that is not metabolized by 11β-HSD) resulted in lower birthweights and higher blood pressure in adult life (Benediktsson *et al.*, 1993). Although the association between birthweight and blood pressure in humans may now be in some doubt (Huxley *et al.*, 2002), or might be considered something of an irrelevance, these early observations by Benediktsson *et al.* (1993) remain of major importance. It is clear from a wide range of studies of animal models that exposure to glucocorticoids has a key role in the programming of blood pressure and other aspects of health and well-being (Chapter 16, this volume).

In situations where placental 11β-HSD activity or expression is low, high blood pressure in later postnatal life appears to be the consequence (Langley-Evans *et al.*, 1996c). This is perhaps best illustrated by experiments in which the enzyme is inhibited with the liquorice derivative, carbenoxolone (CBX). Treatment of pregnant rats with CBX produces a similar physiological phenotype to that generated by nutritional manipulations, such as MLP (Lindsay *et al.*, 1996). Moreover, when CBX treatments are targeted at specific periods of rat pregnancy, the final week of gestation appears to be the critical period, during which increased glucocorticoid exposure programmes blood pressure (Langley-Evans, 1997a) (Fig. 6.7). Experiments considering the timing of nutrient restriction in rats also identify late pregnancy as a critical period (Langley-Evans *et al.*, 1996b).

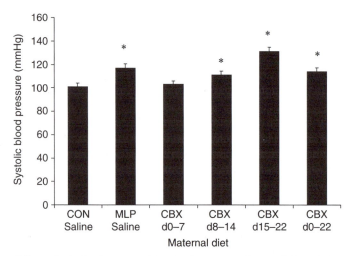

Fig. 6.7. Effect of 11β-hydroxysteroid dehydrogenase (11β-HSD) inhibition upon blood pressure. Pregnant rats were fed either a control diet (CON) or a diet low in protein (MLP). Rats fed a protein-replete diet were injected with carbenoxolone (CBX) daily, either throughout pregnancy (d0–22) or for specific 7-day periods (d0–7, d8–14, d15–22). Blood pressure was determined in the offspring at 4 weeks of age. Data are shown as mean ± SEM. * Indicates a significant difference when compared with the control group (*P* < 0.05). Blood pressure was significantly elevated in the offspring of rats subject to carbenoxolone treatment. Late-gestation treatment had the greatest programming effect upon blood pressure. (Data taken from Langley-Evans, 1997a.)

Studies of sheep are also suggestive of a role for glucocorticoids in the programming of vascular function. Moss *et al.* (2001) treated pregnant ewes with either single or repeated doses of glucocorticoids in late gestation. Repeated maternal treatments resulted in lower lamb weight at birth and reduced mean arterial blood pressure at 3 months of age. Single injections, or direct injections of the fetus with betamethasone, did not produce these effects. The lack of hypertensive effect of glucocorticoids in this species may reflect the timing of the treatment. Single dexamethasone injections between 23 and 28 days of gestation produced persistent hypertension in the resulting offspring, and this effect was associated with altered expression of angiotensin II receptors (ATR) in the brain (Dodic *et al.*, 2002).

Appropriately timed glucocorticoid treatment of pregnant animals thus produces similar physiological endpoints to those seen with nutritional manipulations. A similar pool of data for humans should be available in due course, as the same synthetic glucocorticoids are used clinically in pregnancies at risk of premature delivery. Epidemiological studies also indicate relationships between those birth characteristics that are predictive of adult cardiovascular disease and glucocorticoid status. Children who were of low weight at birth tend to excrete greater amounts of glucocorticoid metabolites (Clark *et al.*, 1996). Similarly, adults in three populations worldwide have been shown to have circulating cortisol concentrations that are inversely related to their weight at birth (Phillips *et al.*, 2000). Animal models and human observations therefore strongly indicate a common programming pathway towards high blood pressure that involves both nutritional and endocrine influences.

Common pathways to cardiovascular disease

The role of placental 11β-HSD as a gatekeeper for glucocorticoid access to the fetal tissues is pivotal in the fetal programming of hypertension. Maternal nutritional status and synthetic glucocorticoid administration appear to determine long-term cardiovascular function through a common mechanism. Undernutrition perturbs the balance of glucocorticoids between the maternal and fetal compartments by down-regulating 11β-HSD in placenta.

Feeding an MLP diet in rat pregnancy results in low activity of 11β-HSD in placenta at day 20 gestation. This is a consequence of reduced gene expression that is evident at both day 14 and day 20 (Langley-Evans *et al.*, 1996c). The ensuing increase in fetal glucocorticoid exposure has been difficult to demonstrate directly, as the small amount of fetal plasma that can be collected makes corticosterone determination difficult. However, the use of indirect measures, such as glucocorticoid-inducible enzyme activities, indicates that the fetal tissues in MLP-associated pregnancies are subject to a greater hormone exposure (Langley-Evans and Nwagwu, 1998). Importantly, the programming of blood pressure that is associated with MLP feeding in rats is a glucocorticoid-dependent phenomenon. When MLP-fed dams are treated with an inhibitor of glucocorticoid synthesis, their offspring do not develop hypertension. When these pharmacologically adrenalectomized animals are also provided with replacement doses of corticosterone, the MLP-associated hypertension is restored (Langley-Evans, 1997b) (Fig. 6.8).

The evidence thus favours the hypothesis that undernutrition acts as a glucocorticoid-mediated stressor to the fetus. The precise regulation of placental 11β-HSD is not fully understood, but it certainly appears sensitive to nutritional status in sheep, as well as in rodents (Whorwood et al., 2001). The existence of this simple hormonal signal of nutritional status may explain why such a broad range of nutritional manipulations (low protein, low calcium, global restriction, low iron) can programme physiological outcomes that are so strikingly similar (Fig. 6.9).

Glucocorticoids may also continue to act during postnatal life to mediate some of the programmed effects of fetal undernutrition. In this context, the observations of high circulating cortisol concentrations in humans of low weight at birth become of greater interest (Phillips et al., 2000). In rats exposed to the MLP diet in utero, hypertension is dependent upon postnatal glucocorticoids as well as prenatal glucocorticoid action (Fig. 6.10). Surgical adrenalectomy of young adult animals exposed to MLP in fetal life normalized their blood pressure within 14 days, without any effect upon the blood pressure of animals subjected to control diet in utero (Gardner et al., 1997). Replacement of corticosterone but not aldosterone restored the hypertensive state.

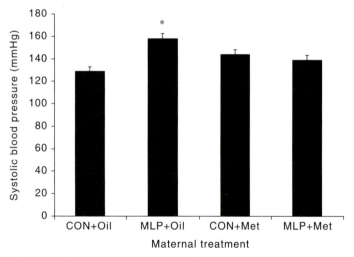

Fig. 6.8. Glucocorticoid-dependence of nutritional programming of blood pressure. Pregnant rats were fed control or maternal low-protein (MLP) diets throughout pregnancy. Rats were injected twice daily with metyrapone (Met) or arachis oil (Oil) vehicle over days 0–14 of pregnancy. Blood pressure was determined in the offspring at 7 weeks of age. Data are mean ± SEM and * indicates significantly different from all other groups (P < 0.05). Metyrapone is an inhibitor of maternal glucocorticoid synthesis. This treatment had no effect upon blood pressure in offspring of rats fed a protein-replete diet, but in offspring exposed to MLP the hypertensive effect of the diet was abolished, demonstrating the glucocorticoid-dependence of nutritional programming during the fetal period. (Data taken from Langley-Evans, 1997b.)

The postnatal effect of glucocorticoids may be mediated through a programmed hypersensitivity to the hormones. Studies of MLP-exposed rats indicate that circulating corticosterone concentrations are normal, but the activities of classical glucocorticoid-inducible enzymes in liver and brain are elevated (Langley-Evans *et al.*, 1996d). This enhancement of the effect of normal concentrations of hormone is apparently mediated through increased expression of the glucocorticoid receptor (GR) gene, and there are certainly increased numbers of receptors in key target tissues (Langley-Evans *et al.*, 1996d; Bertram *et al.*, 2001). In humans there is also evidence of increased sensitivity to exogenously administered glucocorticoids, which is consistent with the more detailed work from animal experiments (Walker *et al.*, 1998).

Increased glucocorticoid activity will promote increases in blood pressure through a range of mechanisms. Of most interest is the renin–angiotensin system, which will be dealt with in greater detail in Chapter 11 of this volume. Glucocorticoids up-regulate this system and hence promote vasoconstriction

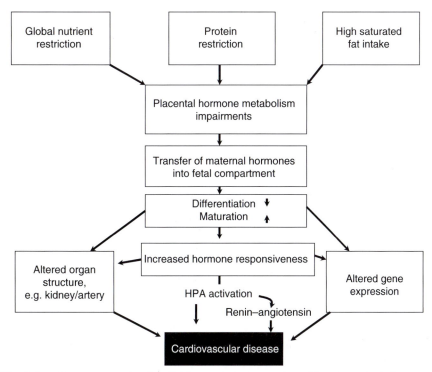

Fig. 6.9. Common mechanism linking varied maternal nutritional manipulations to later cardiovascular dysfunction. A broad range of maternal nutritional manipulations in animal species produces similar physiological endpoints. Down-regulation of key placental enzymes responsible for metabolism of hormones of maternal origin, e.g. 11β-HSD, results in increased hormone transfer into the fetal circulation. Ensuing changes to organ structure, hormone responsiveness and gene expression have all been demonstrated in animal models and are believed to contribute to the development of hypertension. HPA, hypothalamo-pituitary–adrenal.

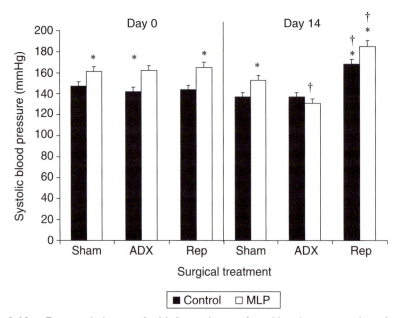

Fig. 6.10. Postnatal glucocorticoid-dependence of nutritional programming of blood pressure. Pregnant rats were fed control or low-protein (MLP) diet throughout pregnancy. At 7 weeks of age their offspring were adrenalectomized (ADX) or sham operated. ADX animals were given twice-daily injections of a replacement dose of corticosterone (Rep) or vehicle. Blood pressure was determined prior to surgery and 14 days later. Data shown are mean ± SEM for 6–8 animals per group. * Indicates a significant difference compared with sham-operated rats exposed to the control diet *in utero* (P < 0.05). † Indicates a significant difference at day 14 compared with day 0 (P < 0.05). Rats exposed to the MLP diet *in utero* had a significantly reduced blood pressure when subject to ADX, whereas the surgery had no significant effect on ADX animals exposed to the control diet. Corticosterone replacement increased blood pressure in both groups to a similar extent. (Data taken from Gardner *et al.*, 1997.)

and increases in peripheral resistance. Studies of the offspring of rats fed MLP diets in pregnancy and prenatally undernourished lambs have shown that several components of the renin–angiotensin system are up-regulated relative to controls. Angiotensin-converting enzyme, which produces the vasoactive hormone angiotensin II, is greater in the plasma and lungs of MLP-exposed rats (Langley and Jackson, 1994; Langley-Evans and Jackson, 1995). The angiotensin II receptors have also been shown to be subject to programming by under-nutrition in kidneys of both sheep and rats (Trowern *et al.*, 2000; Whorwood *et al.*, 2001) (Fig. 6.11). This may directly increase blood pressure, and we have demonstrated that MLP-exposed rats are more sensitive to the effects of low-dose intravenous angiotensin II (Gardner *et al.*, 1998). Treatment of these animals with antihypertensive drugs targeted at the renin–angiotensin system normalizes blood pressure and, if this treatment is applied during the suckling phase, the normalization is permanent (Sherman and Langley-Evans, 2000).

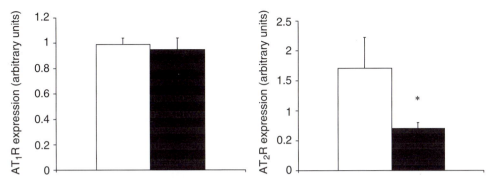

Fig. 6.11. Expression of renal angiotensin II receptors in rats exposed to low-protein diets *in utero.* Pregnant rats were fed control (open bars) or low-protein (MLP) diet (black bars) throughout gestation. Offspring were killed at 4 weeks postnatally and mRNA expression for the AT_1 and AT_2 receptors determined by reverse transcriptase-polymerase chain reaction (RT-PCR) (McMullen and Langley-Evans, unpublished data). Data are shown as mean ± SEM. * Indicates $P < 0.05$. The AT_1 receptor is classically associated with the hypertensive effects of angiotensin II, whereas AT_2 appears to be involved in attenuating this effect.

This indicates that a critical window for programming blood pressure in the rat also exists in the early postnatal period. Appropriate treatments in this period can overcome the programming effects of undernutrition in fetal life and this raises interesting prospects in terms of the future treatment of disease (Harrap, 1998).

Conclusion

An epidemiological approach to the study of cardiovascular programming has suggested that factors operating before birth are responsible for the establishment of a predisposition to hypertension and coronary heart disease in adult life. Limited evidence from human populations implicates maternal undernutrition in this process. A much larger body of experimental research utilizing animal models suggests that imbalances in maternal nutrition may programme raised blood pressure in a variety of species. The detailed mechanism linking fetal exposure to undernutrition and later cardiovascular dysfunction is unclear, but there is strong evidence to suggest that glucocorticoid transfer from mother to fetus is of major importance.

References

Barker, D.J.P. (2002) Fetal programming of coronary heart disease. *Trends in Endocrinology and Metabolism* 13, 364–368.

Bartley, M., Power, C., Davey-Smith, G. and Shipley, M. (1994) Birthweight and later socioeconomic disadvantage: evidence from the 1958 British cohort study. *British Medical Journal* 309, 1475–1478.

Battista, M.-C., Oligny, L.L., St-Louis, J. and Brochu, M. (2002) Intrauterine growth restriction in rats is associated with hypertension and renal dysfunction in adulthood. *American Journal of Physiology* 283, E124–E131.

Benediktsson, R., Lindsay, R.S., Noble, J., Seckl, J.R. and Edwards, C.R.W. (1993) Glucocorticoid exposure *in utero*: new model for adult hypertension. *Lancet* 341, 339–341.

Bergel, E. and Belizan, J.M. (2002) A deficient maternal calcium intake during pregnancy increases blood pressure of the offspring in adult rats. *British Journal of Obstetrics and Gynaecology* 109, 540–545.

Bertram, C.E. and Hanson, M.A. (2001) Animal models and programming of the metabolic syndrome. *British Medical Bulletin* 60, 103–121.

Bertram, C., Trowern, A.R., Copin, N., Jackson, A.A. and Whorwood, C.B. (2001) The maternal diet during pregnancy programs altered expression of the glucocorticoid receptor and type 2 11 beta-hydroxysteroid dehydrogenase: potential molecular mechanisms underlying the programming of hypertension *in utero*. *Endocrinology* 142, 2841–2853.

Campbell, D.M., Hall, M.H., Barker, D.J.P., Cross, J., Shiell, A.W. and Godfrey, K.M. (1996) Diet in pregnancy and the offspring's blood pressure 40 years later. *British Journal of Obstetrics and Gynaecology* 103, 273–280.

Clark, P.M., Hindmarsh, P.C., Shiell, A.W., Law, C.M., Honour, J.W. and Barker, D.J.P. (1996) Size at birth and adrenocortical function in childhood. *Clinical Endocrinology* 45, 721–726.

Clarke, H.E., Coates, M.E., Eva, J.K., Ford, D.J., Milner, C.K., O'Donoghue, P.N., Scott, P.P. and Ward, R.J. (1977) Dietary standards for laboratory animals: report of the Laboratory Animals Centre Diets Advisory Committee. *Laboratory Animals* 11, 1–28.

Crowe, C., Dandekar, P., Fox, M., Dhingra, K., Bennet, L. and Hanson, M.A. (1995) The effects of anaemia on heart, placenta and body weight, and blood pressure in fetal and neonatal rats. *Journal of Physiology* 488, 515–519.

Curhan, G.C., Chertow, G.M., Willett, W.C., Spiegelman, D., Colditz, G.A., Manson, J.E., Speizer, F.E. and Stampfer, M.J. (1996) Birth weight and adult hypertension and obesity in women. *Circulation* 94, 1310–1315

Daenzer, M., Ortmann, S., Klaus, S. and Metges, C.C. (2002) Prenatal high protein exposure decreases energy expenditure and increases adiposity in young rats. *Journal of Nutrition* 132, 142–144.

Dodic, M., Aboutanoun, T., O'Connor, A., Wintour, E.M. and Moritz, K.M. (2002) Programming effects of short prenatal exposure to dexamethasone in sheep. *Hypertension* 40, 729–734.

Dunn, R.L., Langley-Evans, S.C., Jackson, A.A. and Whorwood, C.B. (2001) Hypertension in the mouse following intrauterine exposure to a low protein diet. *Proceedings of the Nutrition Society* 60, 51A.

Edwards, C.R.W., Benediktsson, R., Lindsay, R.S. and Seckl, J.R. (1993) Dysfunction of placental glucocorticoid barrier: link between fetal environment and adult hypertension. *Lancet* 341, 355–357.

Forrester, T.E., Wilks, R.J., Bennett, F.I., Simeon, D., Osmond, C., Allen, M., Chung, A.P. and Scott, P. (1996) Fetal growth and cardiovascular risk factors in Jamaican schoolchildren. *British Medical Journal* 312, 156–160.

Gardner, D.S., Jackson, A.A. and Langley-Evans, S.C. (1997) Maintenance of maternal diet-induced hypertension in the rat is dependent upon glucocorticoids. *Hypertension* 30, 1525–1530.

Gardner, D.S., Jackson, A.A. and Langley-Evans, S.C. (1998) Prenatal under-nutrition alters postnatal sensitivity to angiotensin II. *Clinical Science* 94 (suppl. 38), M7.

Garnica, A.D. and Chan, W.Y. (1996) The role of the placenta in fetal nutrition and growth. *Journal of the American College of Nutrition* 16, 206–222.

Godfrey, K.M., Forrester, T., Barker, D.J.P., Jackson, A.A., Landman, J.P., Hall, J.St.E., Cox, V. and Osmond, C. (1994) The relation of maternal nutritional status during pregnancy to blood pressure in childhood. *British Journal of Obstetrics and Gynaecology* 101, 398–403.

Godfrey, K.M., Robinson, S., Barker, D.J.P., Osmond, C. and Cox, V. (1996) Maternal nutrition in early and late pregnancy in relation to placental and fetal growth. *British Medical Journal* 312, 410–414.

Gopalakrishnan, G., Pearce, S., Dandrea, J., Mostyn, A., Walker, R.M., Ramsay, M.M., Symonds, M.E. and Stephenson, T. (2002) Influence of maternal nutrition during early to mid-gestation on blood pressure control of offspring of juvenile offspring in sheep. *Journal of Physiology* 539, 121–122.

Gregory, J., Lowe, S., Bates, C.J. and Walker, A. (2000) National diet and nutrition survey: young people aged 4 to 18 years. HMSO, London.

Harrap, S.B. (1998) Preventing adult disease: windows of opportunity. *Clinical Science* 94, 337–338.

Hastings-Roberts, M.M. and Zeman, F.J. (1977) Effects of protein deficiency, pair-feeding, or diet supplementation on maternal, fetal and placental growth in rats. *Journal of Nutrition* 107, 973–982.

Hawkins, P., Steyn, C., Ozaki, T., Saito, T., Noakes, D.E. and Hanson, M.A. (2000) Effect of maternal undernutrition in early gestation on ovine fetal blood pressure and cardiovascular reflexes. *American Journal of Physiology* 279, R340–R348.

Holemans, K., Gerber, R., Meurrens, K., De Clerck, F., Poston, L. and Van Assche, F.A. (1999) Maternal food restriction in the second half of pregnancy affects vascular function but not blood pressure of rat female offspring. *British Journal of Nutrition* 81, 73–79.

Holemans, K., Gerber, R., O'Brien-Coker, I., Mallet, A., Van Bree, R., Van Assche, F.A. and Poston, L. (2000) Raised saturated-fat intake worsens vascular function in virgin and pregnant offspring of streptozocin-diabetic rats. *British Journal of Nutrition* 84, 285–296.

Huxley, R., Neil, A. and Collins, R. (2002) Unravelling the fetal origins hypothesis: is there really an inverse association between birth weight and subsequent blood pressure? *Lancet* 360, 659–665.

Jackson, A.A., Dunn, R.L., Marchand, M.C. and Langley-Evans, S.C. (2002) Increased systolic blood pressure in rats induced by maternal low protein diet is reversed by dietary supplementation with glycine. *Clinical Science* 103, 633–639.

Jennings, B.J., Ozanne, S.E., Dorling, M.W. and Hales, C.N. (1999) Early growth determines longevity in male rats and may be related to telomere shortening in the kidney. *FEBS Letters* 448, 4–8.

Kind, K.L., Simonetta, G., Clifton, P.M., Robinson, J.S. and Owens, J.A. (2002) Effect of maternal feed restriction on blood pressure in the adult guinea pig. *Experimental Physiology* 87, 469–477.

Kramer, M.S. and Joseph, K.S. (1996) Enigma of fetal/infant-origins hypothesis. *Lancet* 348, 1254–1255.

Kwong, W.Y., Wild, A.E., Roberts, P., Willis, A.C. and Fleming, T.P. (2000) Maternal undernutrition during the preimplantation period of rat development causes blastocyst abnormalities and programming of postnatal hypertension. *Development* 127, 4195–4202.

Langley, S.C. and Jackson, A.A. (1994) Increased systolic blood pressure in adult rats induced by fetal exposure to maternal low protein diet. *Clinical Science* 86, 217–222.

Langley-Evans, S.C. (1996) Intrauterine programming of hypertension in the rat: nutrient interactions. *Comparative Biochemistry and Physiology* 114A, 327–333.

Langley-Evans, S.C. (1997a) Maternal carbenoxolone treatment lowers birthweight and induces hypertension in the offspring of rats fed a low protein diet. *Clinical Science* 93, 423–429.

Langley-Evans, S.C. (1997b) Hypertension induced by fetal exposure to a maternal low protein diet, in the rat, is prevented by pharmacological blockade of glucocorticoid synthesis. *Journal of Hypertension* 15, 537–544.

Langley-Evans, S.C. (2000) Critical differences between two low protein diet protocols in the programming of hypertension in the rat. *International Journal of Food Science and Nutrition* 51, 11–17.

Langley-Evans, S.C. (2001) Fetal programming of cardiovascular function through exposure to maternal undernutrition. *Proceedings of the Nutrition Society* 60, 505–513.

Langley-Evans, S.C. and Jackson, A.A. (1995) Captopril normalises systolic blood pressure in rats with hypertension induced by fetal exposure to maternal low protein diets. *Comparative Biochemistry and Physiology* 110A, 223–228

Langley-Evans, S.C. and Nwagwu, M. (1998) Impaired growth and increased activities of glucocorticoid sensitive enzyme activities in tissues of rat fetuses exposed to maternal low protein diets. *Life Science* 63, 605–615.

Langley-Evans, S.C., Phillips, G.J. and Jackson, A.A. (1994a) *In utero* exposure to maternal low protein diets induces hypertension in weanling rats, independently of maternal blood pressure changes. *Clinical Nutrition* 13, 319–324.

Langley-Evans, S.C., Wood, S. and Jackson, A.A. (1994b) Enzymes of the gamma-glutamyl cycle are progammed *in utero* by maternal nutrition. *Annals of Nutrition and Metabolism* 39, 28–35.

Langley-Evans, S.C., Gardner, D.S. and Jackson, A.A. (1996a) Association of disproportionate growth of fetal rats in late gestation with raised systolic blood pressure in later life. *Journal of Reproduction and Fertility* 106, 307–312.

Langley-Evans, S.C., Welham, S.J.M., Sherman, R.C. and Jackson, A.A. (1996b) Weanling rats exposed to maternal low protein diets during discrete periods of gestation exhibit differing severity of hypertension. *Clinical Science* 91, 607–615.

Langley-Evans, S.C., Phillips, G.J., Benediktsson, R., Gardner, D.S., Edwards, C.R.W., Jackson, A.A. and Seckl, J.R. (1996c) Protein intake in pregnancy, placental glucocorticoid metabolism and the programming of hypertension in the rat. *Placenta* 17, 169–172.

Langley-Evans, S.C., Gardner, D.S. and Jackson, A.A. (1996d) Evidence of programming of the hypothalamic–pituitary–adrenal axis by maternal protein restriction during pregnancy. *Journal of Nutrition* 126, 1578–1585.

Langley-Evans, S.C., Phillips, G.J. and Jackson, A.A. (1997) Fetal exposure to a maternal low protein diet alters the susceptibility of the young adult rat to sulphur dioxide-induced lung injury. *Journal of Nutrition* 127, 202–209.

Langley-Evans, S.C., Langley-Evans, A.J. and Marchand, M.C. (2002) Nutritional programming of blood pressure and renal morphology. *Archives of Physiology and Biochemistry* 111, 8–16.

Law, C.M., de Swiet, M., Osmond, C., Fayers, P.M., Barker, D.J.P., Cruddas, A.M. and Fall, C.H.D. (1993) Initiation of hypertension *in utero* and its amplification throughout life. *British Medical Journal* 306, 24–27.

Lechner, A.J. (1984) Growth retardation and mortality in guinea pigs following prenatal starvation. *Nutrition Report International* 30, 1435–1447.

Leon, D.A. (1999) Fetal growth and later disease: epidemiological evidence from Swedish cohorts. In: O'Brien, P.M.S., Wheeler, T. and Barker, D.J.P. (eds) *Fetal Programming: Influences on Development and Disease in Later Life*. RCOG Press, London, pp. 12–29.

Liggins, G.C. (1969) Premature delivery of foetal lambs infused with glucocorticoids. *Journal of Endocrinology* 45, 515–523.

Lindsay, R.S., Lindsay, R.M., Edwards, C.R.W. and Seckl, J.R. (1996) Inhibition of 11β-hydroxysteroid dehydrogenase in pregnant rats and the programming of blood pressure in the offspring. *Hypertension* 27, 1200–1204.

Mackenzie, H.S. and Brenner, B.M. (1995) Fewer nephrons at birth: a missing link in the etiology of essential hypertension? *American Journal of Kidney Disease* 26, 91–98.

Martyn, C.N. and Greenwald, S.E. (2001) A hypothesis about a mechanism for the programming of blood pressure and vascular disease in early life. *Clinical and Experimental Pharmacology and Physiology* 28, 948–951.

Mathews, F., Yudkin, P. and Neil, A. (1999) Influence of maternal nutrition on outcome of pregnancy: prospective cohort study. *British Medical Journal* 319, 339–343.

Mehta, G., Roach, H.I., Langley-Evans, S.C., Reading, I., Oreffo, R.O.C., Aihie-Sayer, A., Clarke, A.M.P. and Cooper, C. (2002) Intrauterine exposure to a maternal low protein diet reduces adult bone mass and alters growth plate morphology. *Calcified Tissue International* 79, 493–498.

Merlet-Benichou, C., Gilbert, T., Muffat-Joly, M., Lelievre-Pegorier, M. and Leroy, B. (1994) Intrauterine growth retardation leads to a permanent nephron deficit in the rat. *Pediatric Nephrology* 8, 175–180.

Moore, V.M., Miller, A.G., Boulton, T.J.C., Cockington, R.A., Hamilton Craig, I., Magarey, A.M. and Robinson, J.S. (1996) Placental weight, birth measurements and blood pressure at age 8 years. *Archives of Disease in Childhood* 74, 538–541.

Moss, T.J.M., Sloboda, D.M., Gurrin, L.C., Harding, R., Challis, J.R.G. and Newnham, J.P. (2001) Programming effects in sheep of prenatal growth restriction and glucocorticoid exposure. *American Journal of Physiology* 281, R960–R970.

Naismith, D.J. and Morgan, B.L.G. (1976) The biphasic nature of protein metabolism during pregnancy in the rat. *British Journal of Nutrition* 36, 563–566.

New, M.I. (2002) Hypertension in congenital adrenal hyperplasia and apparent mineralocorticoid excess. *Annals of the New York Academy of Science* 970, 145–154.

Nwagwu, M.O., Cook, A. and Langley-Evans, S.C. (2000) Evidence of progressive deterioration of renal function in rats exposed to a maternal low protein diet *in utero*. *British Journal of Nutrition* 83, 79–85.

Owens, J.A., Falconer, J. and Robinson, J.S. (1987) Effect of restriction of placental growth on fetal and uteroplacental metabolism. *Journal of Developmental Physiology* 9, 225–238.

Ozaki, T., Nishina, H., Hanson, M.A. and Poston, L. (2001) Dietary restriction in pregnant rats causes gender-related hypertension and vascular dysfunction in offspring. *Journal of Physiology* 530, 141–152.

Pearce, S., Walker, R.M., Stephenson, T., Symonds, M.E. and Ramsay, M.M. (2002) Relationship between blood pressure and fetal weight in the late gestation ovine fetus. *Journal of Physiology* 539, 128P.

Persson, E. and Jansson, T. (1992) Low birth weight is associated with elevated adult blood pressure in the chronically catheterized guinea-pig. *Acta Physiologica Scandinavica* 115, 195–196.

Phillips, D.I.W., Walker, B.R., Reynolds, R.M., Flanagan, D.E.H., Wood, P.J., Osmond, C., Barker, D.J.P. and Whorwood, C.B. (2000) Low birth weight predicts elevated plasma cortisol concentrations in adults from 3 populations. *Hypertension* 35, 1301–1306.

Pickard, C.L., Devoto, M.K. and McCarthy, H.D. (1996) Post-weaning dietary manipulation reduces blood pressure in rats with hypertension of fetal origin. *Proceedings of the Nutrition Society* 55, 103A.

Poore, K.R., Forhead, A.J., Gardner, D.S., Giussani, D.A. and Fowden, A.L. (2002) The effects of birth weight on basal cardiovascular function in pigs at 3 months of age. *Journal of Physiology* 539, 969–978.

Prentice, A.M., Cole, T.J., Foord, F.A., Lamb, W.H. and Whitehead, R.G. (1987) Increased birthweight after prenatal dietary supplementation of rural African women. *American Journal of Clinical Nutrition* 46, 912–925.

Rees, W.D., Hay, S.M., Buchan, V., Antipatis, C. and Palmer, R.M. (1999) The effects of maternal protein restriction on the growth of the rat fetus and its amino acid supply. *British Journal of Nutrition* 81, 243–250.

Reinisch, J.M., Simon, N.G. and Karwo, W.G. (1978) Prenatal exposure to prednisone in humans and animals retards intra-uterine growth. *Science* 202, 436–438.

Sayer, A.A., Dunn, R.L., Langley-Evans, S.C. and Cooper, C. (2001) Intrauterine exposure to a maternal low protein diet shortens lifespan in rats. *Gerontology* 47, 9–14.

Sherman, R.C. and Langley-Evans, S.C. (2000) Antihypertensive treatment in early postnatal life modulates prenatal dietary influences upon blood pressure, in the rat. *Clinical Science* 98, 269–275.

Siemlink, M., Verhoef, A., Dormans, J.A.M.A., Span, P.N. and Piersma, A.H. (2002) Dietary fatty acid composition during pregnancy and lactation in the rat programs growth and glucose metabolism in the offspring. *Diabetologia* 45, 1397–1403.

Sloan, N.L., Lederman, S.A., Leighton, J., Himes, J.H. and Rush, D.A. (2001) The effect of prenatal dietary protein intake on birth weight. *Nutrition Research* 21, 129–139.

Thame, M., Wilks, R.J., McFarlane-Anderson, N., Bennett, F.I. and Forrester, T.E. (1997) Relationship between maternal nutritional status and infants' weight and body proportions at birth. *European Journal of Clinical Nutrition* 51, 134–138.

Tonkiss, J., Trzcinska, M., Galler, J.R., Ruiz-Opazo, N. and Herrera, V.L.M. (1998) Prenatal malnutrition-induced changes in blood pressure – dissociation of stress and nonstress responses using radiotelemetry. *Hypertension* 32, 108–114.

Trowern, A., Sherman, R., Bertram, C., Dunn, R., Gardner, D., Langley-Evans, S.C. and Whorwood, C.B. (2000) The intra-uterine environment programs angiotenin II receptor-mediated hypertension in later life. *Third International Symposium on Angiotensin II Antagonism*, QE2 Conference Centre, London.

Wagener, I.E., Bergmann, R.L., Kamtsiuris, P., Eisenreich, B., Andres, B., Eckert, C., Dudenhausen, J.W. and Bergmann, K.E. (2000) Prevalence and risk factors of iron deficiency among young mothers. *Gesundheitswesen* 62, 176–178.

Walker, B.R., Phillips, D.I.W., Noon, J.P., Panarelli, M., Andrew, R., Edwards, H.V., Holton, D.W., Seckl, J.R., Webb, D.J. and Watt, G.C.M. (1998) Increased glucocorticoid activity in men with cardiovascular risk factors. *Hypertension* 31, 891–895.

Whorwood, C.B., Firth, K.M., Budge, H. and Symonds, M.E. (2001) Maternal undernutrition during early to mid-gestation programs tissue-specific alterations in the expression of the glucocorticoid receptor, 11 beta-hydroxysteroid dehydrogenase isoforms, and type 1 angiotensin II receptor in neonatal sheep. *Endocrinology* 142, 2854–2864.

Woodall, S.M., Johnston, B.M., Breier, B.H. and Gluckman, P.D. (1996) Chronic maternal undernutrition in the rat leads to delayed postnatal growth and elevated blood pressure of offspring. *Pediatric Research* 40, 438–443.

Zeman, F.J. and Stanbrough, E.C. (1969) Effect of maternal protein deficiency on cellular development in the fetal rat. *Journal of Nutrition* 99, 274–282.

7 Associations between Fetal and Infant Growth and Non-insulin-dependent Diabetes

Simon C. Langley-Evans

School of Biosciences, University of Nottingham, Sutton Bonington Campus, Loughborough LE12 5RD, UK

Introduction

Earlier chapters in this volume have set out the case for long-term programming effects of the early environment upon health and disease. These arguments, based upon both epidemiological and experimental data, have led to the suggestion that exposure to less than optimal nutrition during fetal life may programme increased risk of hypertension and coronary heart disease. As shown in Chapter 4, most of the epidemiology relating to the programming of cardiovascular disease has been focused upon exploring relationships between markers of poor fetal growth, principally birthweight, and later disease. Whereas these associations have come under close critical scrutiny and may be considerably weaker than originally reported (Huxley *et al.*, 2002), associations between infant anthropometric indices at birth and over the first year of life may provide more robust indicators of risk of developing glucose intolerance, insulin resistance and type 2 diabetes.

Evidence of Programming

There is a wealth of data relating to the aetiology of type 2 (non-insulin-dependent) diabetes in human populations. This condition is a disorder of insulin and glucose metabolism, which is characterized by glucose intolerance and insulin resistance, and is an independent risk factor for coronary heart disease (Stolar and Chilton, 2003). As insulin plays an important role in determining fetal growth (Fowden, 1989), and because there is a known familial predisposition to the condition (Gloyn, 2003), type 2 diabetes was an early target for investigations of possible links between early life events and disease processes.

The Hertfordshire and Preston cohorts

The first large-scale evaluation of the relationship between early life and adult diabetes was reported by Hales and coworkers (Hales, 1991), who studied a cohort of men aged 64 years who had been born in Hertfordshire, an area of England where unique birth records had been obtained and preserved. Glucose tolerance tests were performed on these men and it was noted that the proportion of men with impaired glucose tolerance (2-hour plasma glucose between 7.8 and 11.0 mM) or with frank diabetes (2-hour plasma glucose in excess of 11.0 mM) increased with decreasing birthweight (Hales, 1991). The relationship between birthweight and 2-hour glucose concentration was continuous across all birthweight categories and, most strikingly, the men who had been smallest at birth were 6.6 times more likely to have impaired glucose tolerance or type 2 diabetes than were those who had been heaviest at birth (Fig. 7.1), even after correction for adult body mass index.

Normal glucose metabolism is dependent upon the function of the endocrine pancreas. In humans the development of the pancreas continues into postnatal life, with approximately half of the adult β-cell mass being attained by the age of 1 year (Van Assche and Aerts, 1979). Within the Hertfordshire cohort it was apparent that growth between birth and the age of 1 year was also related to the risk of developing glucose intolerance, or type 2, diabetes (Hales, 1991). Glucose concentrations 30 min and 2 h after a 75 g glucose load were significantly greater in men who were smaller at the age of 1 year, and these individuals also tended to have lower plasma insulin concentrations after 2 h.

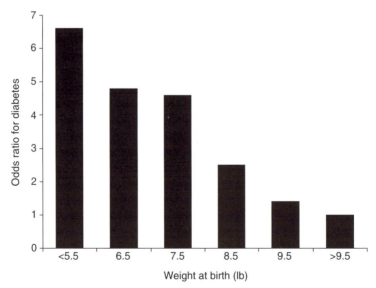

Fig. 7.1.   Odds ratios for type 2 diabetes among 64-year-old men from the Hertfordshire cohort. Decreasing weight at birth increased risk of diabetes in later life. Odds ratios were corrected for current body mass index. (Data redrawn from Hales, 1991.)

This relationship between infant weight and glucose clearance was modulated by adult body mass index, such that the highest plasma glucose concentrations following loading were noted in men who had been of low birthweight, low weight at 1 year and with highest body mass index at age 64 (Hales, 1991). This suggests that factors in early life combine with an adult lifestyle that favours obesity, to increase susceptibility to glucose intolerance and diabetes.

The metabolic syndrome, or 'syndrome X', is characterized by glucose intolerance, hypertension and raised serum triglycerides and is most commonly noted in obese individuals. The Hertfordshire cohort defined the metabolic syndrome on the basis of fasting plasma triglycerides over 1.4 mM, 2-hour glucose concentrations over 7.8 mM and systolic blood pressure over 160 mmHg (Barker *et al.*, 1993). Using this definition, a striking relationship between the prevalence of the syndrome and birthweight was noted, with an odds ratio, comparing the men who had been smallest at birth with those who were largest at birth (Fig. 7.2), of 18.0 (Barker *et al.*, 1993). In considering the metabolic syndrome, only small shifts in weight at birth appeared to greatly increase later risk.

Information available for the Hertfordshire cohort was limited to weight at birth and at the age of 1 year. A further cohort of men and women studied in Preston, in northern England, provided the opportunity to study individuals for whom more detailed birth anthropometry was available, including placental weights, length at birth and head circumference (Phipps *et al.*, 1993). Glucose tolerance testing of 266 of these individuals showed, as with the Hertfordshire data, that glucose intolerance was more common among those of lower weight

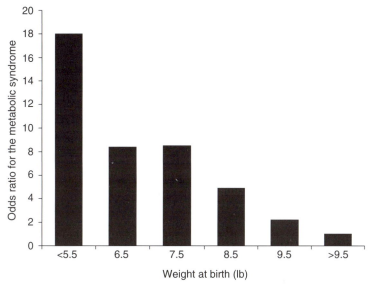

Fig. 7.2. Odds ratios for the metabolic syndrome among 64-year-old men from the Hertfordshire cohort. Decreasing weight at birth increased risk of the metabolic syndrome in later life. Odds ratios were corrected for current body mass index. (Data redrawn from Barker *et al.*, 1993.)

at birth, but, more importantly, revealed that relative thinness or shortness at birth was predictive of impaired glucose handling (Phipps *et al.*, 1993).

The Hertfordshire and Preston cohorts have also been used to explore the possible mechanistic basis of the relationship between events in fetal life and later diabetes. Studies with animals have suggested that exposure to adverse conditions *in utero* has a negative impact upon the developing pancreas, such that the β-cell mass is reduced (Snoeck *et al.*, 1990). The likely consequence of this is that the ability of the pancreas to secrete insulin will be reduced. There is some evidence that, in humans, fetal growth retardation reduces the number of pancreatic β-cells and also that patients with non-insulin-dependent diabetes have a reduced β-cell mass relative to weight-matched healthy controls (Kloppel *et al.*, 1985; Hellerström *et al.*, 1988). Determination of plasma 32–33-split pro-insulin in samples from the men in the Hertfordshire cohort revealed a significant inverse association with weight at 1 year (Hales, 1991). The finding of elevated concentrations in men who had been small in infancy, particularly in those who had a higher body mass index as adults, suggested that a poor early environment could programme β-cell dysfunction, and that the programming of type 2 diabetes is a consequence of impaired pancreatic development. However, this assertion was not supported by data from the Preston cohort, which found no association between insulin secretion following a glucose challenge and any anthropometric measures at birth (Phillips *et al.*, 1994).

In contrast to the lack of strong evidence to link fetal development to insulin deficiency, there is a reasonable body of data to support the assertion that insulin resistance may be programmed *in utero*. In addition to data from Preston and Hertfordshire, studies of Mexican–American and non-Hispanic white people in San Antonio, Texas, have shown that there is a higher prevalence of insulin resistance syndrome among those of lower birthweight, although this finding was heavily dependent upon current body mass index (Valdez *et al.*, 1994).

Insulin resistance and the associated hyperinsulinaemia have been argued to be the main basis of the other features of the metabolic syndrome (Reaven, 1988). Hypertension, abnormalities of fat metabolism and cholesterol transport may all lie downstream of insulin resistance, and, as such, the programming of the insulin axis *in utero* may be a critical step in determining disease risk (Reaven, 1988). It is therefore of considerable importance to understand how insulin resistance may develop. One possibility is that growth-retarding influences in early life may have a negative impact on the development of muscle mass.

It is well known from studies of farm animals that undernutrition in pregnancy leads to the production of offspring that have reduced muscle mass, with lower numbers of muscle fibres and a redistribution of the type of fibres present (Hegarty and Allen, 1978; Handel and Stickland, 1987; Dwyer *et al.*, 1994). The numbers of muscle fibres within a specific muscle are set at around the time of birth in most mammals, with the exception of rodents (Brameld *et al.*, 2003). Postnatal growth of muscle involves increases in fibre size rather than increases in the numbers of fibres. Hence the processes of myogenesis take place predominantly *in utero* and are followed by postnatal hypertrophy.

The formation of muscle fibres takes place in two phases, with primary fibres forming first and secondary fibres developing around the primaries (Maltin *et al.*,

2001; Picard *et al.*, 2002; Wigmore and Evans, 2002). There are specific myoblast precursors for the different populations of fibres. In humans and large animal species, the embryonic myoblasts form primary muscle fibres in early to mid-gestation, and fetal myoblasts form secondary muscle fibres in mid- to late gestation. In general, the primary fibres tend to become slow, oxidative (type I) muscle fibres, while the secondary fibres tend to become faster fibre types (types IIA, IIB) (Brameld *et al.*, 2003). However, there is plasticity in postnatal life such that primary fibres have the potential to become fast fibres in 'fast' muscles, and secondary fibres to become slow fibres in 'slow' muscles (Maltin *et al.*, 2001; Picard *et al.*, 2002). Rodent muscle appears vulnerable to undernutrition, including *in utero* manipulations of the maternal diet that are known to programme glucose intolerance in the resulting offspring (Vickers *et al.*, 2001; Bayol *et al.*, 2003). Muscle from animals subjected to global undernutrition in fetal life contains a reduced density of fibres, although the types of fibres present are generally unchanged (Bayol *et al.*, 2003). However, we have shown recently that a low-protein diet *in utero* altered the ratio of type I to type II fibres in rat muscle (Hurley, Brameld and Langley-Evans, unpublished observation).

Insulin resistance in humans is associated with a lesser proportion of type I muscle fibres and an increase in the proportion of IIB (Lillioja *et al.*, 1987). Muscle is the major insulin-sensitive tissue, and it has been suggested that a reduction in overall muscle mass, and hence a change in the substrate utilization and metabolism of skeletal muscle, may provide a link between early life events, later insulin resistance and associated sequelae. This possibility has been investigated in small numbers of individuals recruited from the Preston cohort. In both men and women, muscle mass, estimated by urinary creatinine excretion, was related to weight at birth, but not to thinness at birth (Phillips, 1995). However, reduced muscle mass was not related to glucose intolerance or insulin resistance in this group. Similarly, biopsies taken from a further subset of this cohort revealed no association between activity of glycogen synthase and markers of intrauterine growth (Phillips *et al.*, 1996). Glycogen synthase is a rate-limiting step for insulin action within muscle. Together, these data suggest that programmed changes in muscle do not underpin associations between early life events and human diabetes, and further investigations are, instead, focusing heavily upon the possible programming of adiposity as a mediator of insulin resistance.

Studies of children and young adults

Studies such as those of the cohorts in Preston and Hertfordshire are likely to be confounded by a number of important factors. Relationships between characteristics at birth and risk of glucose intolerance and insulin resistance 50–70 years later are complicated by the interaction with adult lifestyle, socio-economic status and adiposity, in a manner that cannot be wholly controlled for statistically. The epidemiological link between events in fetal life and infancy is thus greatly strengthened by observations that show similar trends among children and younger adults.

Two studies have demonstrated that even in very young children, variation in glucose tolerance can be related to characteristics at birth. In the UK, a group of 7-year-olds from Salisbury were subjected to a standard oral glucose tolerance test (Law et al., 1995). Remarkably, there was a significant inverse relationship between plasma glucose concentrations at 30 min post-loading and ponderal index at birth. For both girls and boys, the clearance of the glucose challenge was impaired in those who had been thinnest at birth. Similarly, a study of 4-year-old children in Pune, India, showed that 30-min glucose concentrations were inversely related to birthweight, in a manner analogous to the Hertfordshire study of adult men (Yajnik et al., 1995). This study also indicated that insulin concentrations were inversely related to birthweight, suggesting that these young children were already firmly on the path to insulin resistance and type 2 diabetes.

Studies of young adults also suggest that insulin resistance may be programmed in utero. Flanagan et al. (2000) reported a study of 163 20-year-olds from Adelaide, Australia, in which low birthweight and relative shortness at birth were related to low insulin sensitivity and increased insulin secretion, independently of current body mass index or fat distribution (Flanagan et al., 2000). However, these effects tended to be gender-specific and were not observed in young women.

The observations of children are of major importance, as they largely remove the confounding factors associated with postnatal growth, adolescence and the attainment of adult body mass and adiposity. The close temporal association of impaired glucose metabolism and insulin resistance with birth and fetal events permits a stronger argument that the two are linked, particularly in the light of animal experiments in this area (see Chapter 8, this volume). It is apparent that the prenatal and postnatal environments interact to a high degree in the determination of type 2 diabetes risk. Bavdekar et al. (1999) studied 477 8-year-old children in India, and found that lower weight at birth was associated with impaired glucose tolerance, raised plasma insulin and insulin resistance, as estimated using the Homeostasis Model Assessment (HOMA) scale. The highest levels of insulin resistance were noted in those children who were smallest at birth and with highest fat mass at age 8. These data indicate that, in India, as in westernized countries, the greatest concern is the increasing level of obesity among children (Bundred et al., 2001; Wright et al., 2001), which may superimpose an independent risk of metabolic syndrome over and above that determined by prenatal programming factors. Given the suggestion that obesity itself may be subject to prenatal programming influences (Jackson et al., 1996; Martorell et al., 2001) (see Chapters 9 and 10, this volume) it is interesting to speculate that risk of type 2 diabetes may be determined in utero via multiple routes.

The Mechanism of Programming

The fetal insulin hypothesis

In seeking an explanation for the association between fetal growth impairments and later disease, it is attractive to seek a simple mechanism that explains both factors. In the area of diabetes there has been considerable interest and invest-ment in the exploration of genetic basis for insulin resistance syndromes (Gloyn, 2003). In the context of fetal programming of type 2 diabetes, Hattersley and Tooke (1999) have proposed that the underlying reason for the association between impaired fetal growth and later disease is that there are genes that cause both low birthweight and type 2 diabetes, and this proposal has been termed the 'fetal insulin hypothesis'. Insulin is known to be an important growth factor in fetal life (Fowden, 1989) and genetic defects of insulin secretion or action could limit fetal growth, the accrual of muscle mass and determine insulin resistance later in life. This view is supported by the finding that mutations in the gene encoding glucokinase have been identified as contributors to both low birthweight and maturity-onset diabetes (Hattersley *et al.*, 1998).

One of the weaknesses of the fetal insulin hypothesis is that mutations such as that of glucokinase are extremely rare, whereas type 2 diabetes is increasingly common. Extensive searches for other gene candidates have, as yet, failed to yield promising results. Given the manner of inheritance of insulin-related genes, the fetal insulin hypothesis would suggest that a child's birthweight and insulin-mediated growth pattern would be inversely related to paternal insulin resistance (Yajnik *et al.*, 2001). Among Pima Indians this is the case, and the children of diabetic fathers tend to be of low weight, after appropriate adjustment for mater-nal gestational diabetes (Lindsay *et al.*, 2000). Detailed studies of the contribu-tion of maternal and paternal genes to fetal growth patterns in India suggest that paternal body size, and specifically body mass index, predicts infant size at birth, whereas paternal metabolic indices (including insulin resistance) were only weakly related (Yajnik *et al.*, 2001). These studies therefore, do not appear to support the fetal insulin hypothesis.

At the present time there are no clear genetic markers for insulin resistance. Direct testing of the fetal insulin hypothesis through appropriately sensitive molecular genetic analyses is therefore currently impossible. In contrast, the thrifty phenotype hypothesis, described below, presents a framework of ideas that is testable through the currently available models, human cohorts and technologies.

Thrifty phenotype hypothesis

The 'thrifty phenotype hypothesis' was proposed by Hales and Barker in 1992, in order to account for the epidemiological observations arising from the Hertfordshire cohort. The thrifty phenotype hypothesis postulates that type 2 diabetes and the metabolic syndrome have a predominantly environmental basis. Variations in fetal growth, such as low birthweight or disproportion, pro-vide a useful and easily measured marker for disease risk, as opposed to retarded growth and metabolic disorders having a common genetic cause (Hales and Barker, 1992).

The basis of the hypothesis is the occurrence of fetal malnutrition. If a grow-ing fetus is malnourished, it is likely to adopt a number of adaptive strategies in order to maximize its chances of postnatal survival. Fetal malnutrition may arise from several diverse causes, including maternal malnutrition and placental dysfunction, but will elicit a relatively small number of adaptive responses. Primarily, it is believed that the fetus has the capacity to selectively redistribute nutrients to preserve the function of key organs (Rudolph, 1984). This has the effect of altering relative growth rates of different organs, such that some are compromised while others maintain normal development. Brain growth is most likely to be preserved at the expense of other organs, such as liver, pancreas and muscle, and this phenomenon is termed brain sparing (Rudolph, 1984).

There do not seem to be any significant and convincing data to demonstrate the existence of brain sparing in humans, and the phenomenon is largely inferred from the co-occurrence of disproportionate head size at birth and disease processes or physiological effects. The example generally cited in this context is the relationship between increased head circumference at birth and later atopy (Langley-Evans, 1997). This is felt to show the consequences of selective nutrient diversion away from the immune system in order to spare brain growth. However, studies of thymic development suggest that there is no mismatch between the growth of this tissue and that of the head in atopic individuals (Benn et al., 2001). The lack of clear evidence is primarily because accurate measurements of body proportions at birth have rarely, if ever, been combined with sequential ultrasonography to identify fetuses whose growth has been constrained in utero. However, animal studies have shown that where specific nutritional insults are applied during fetal development, growth of the truncal organs is affected more severely than that of the brain (Langley-Evans et al., 1996).

The consequence of such a redistribution of nutrients will be a reduction of functional capacity in metabolically active organs and, as a result, metabolic programming will occur. In order to preserve basic functions in the face of reduced functional capacity, cells and tissues must harness the available resources more effectively. Such adaptations will therefore favour thrift, or in other words, a capacity to metabolize and store energy substrates more efficiently. Metabolic changes in the offspring increase its chances of surviving conditions of poor postnatal nutrition, but these adaptations are detrimental to health in the long term if the individual experiences overnutrition and/or becomes obese postnatally (Fig. 7.3).

The thrifty phenotype hypothesis is something that can be readily assessed in the context of available epidemiological data. Ecological data from several populations are highly suggestive that type 2 diabetes may be a consequence of an adaptation to conditions where metabolic thrift would be a survival advantage (Zimmet et al., 1984; Cohen et al., 1988). In rural populations in Africa (McLarty et al., 1989) and other areas, such as the highlands of Papua New Guinea, rates of type 2 diabetes are frequently below 1%. Within such communities, scarcity of food for pregnant women, at least in comparison to developed nations, is commonplace and remains the norm for their offspring. The thrifty phenotype that these offspring may acquire in utero is therefore not challenged.

The westernization of populations that were previously underdeveloped and where undernutrition was rife, is frequently associated with an explosion of obesity and type 2 diabetes. The best-studied examples of this phenomenon are populations in the Pacific region, such as the Nauruan islanders. Nauru was an

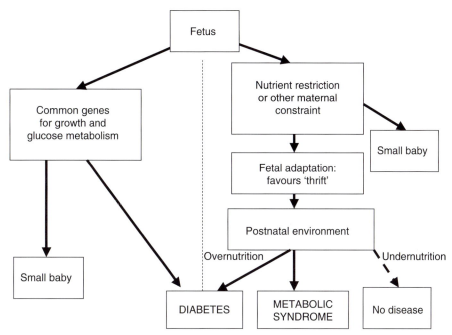

Fig. 7.3. The fetal origins of diabetes. Routes to diabetes from fetal life may be the consequence of the expression of genes that encode for both fetal growth factors and controllers of glucose metabolism (fetal insulin hypothesis: left side of figure), or may result from the acquisition of a thrifty phenotype (right side of figure).

impoverished community reliant on a subsistence lifestyle prior to the 1950s, when it became wealthy on the back of phosphate mining. The transition to affluence brought with it an epidemic of non-insulin-dependent diabetes (Zimmet *et al.*, 1984).

Studies of twins are also generally supportive of a thrifty phenotype as the basis for type 2 diabetes, as opposed to a largely genetic origin. A study of Italian twins, aged 32 years, suggested that the intrauterine environment had a more powerful influence on glucose metabolism than their genetic background (Bo *et al.*, 2000). Consideration of monozygotic and dizygotic twins pairs, that were discordant for diabetes or glucose intolerance, showed that the members of each pair showing hyperinsulinaemia and hyperglycaemia following an oral glucose tolerance test, had lower birthweights than their siblings with normal glucose tolerance and insulin responses. In other words, insulin resistance was more prevalent in the twins of lower birthweight, whose growth *in utero* may be considered to have been constrained. The smaller twins also had higher levels of triglycerides, insulin, total cholesterol and C-peptide, suggesting that they may have gone on to develop the full metabolic syndrome (Bo *et al.*, 2000).

Similar findings were reported from a Danish study of middle-aged monozygotic and dizygotic twins who also were discordant for type 2 diabetes (Poulsen *et al.*, 1997). As with the Italian study, the diabetic twins in each pair tended to be of lower birthweight. In this particular study, a greater period of time had elapsed between birth and development of disease, and the postnatal environment was poorly defined, allowing some doubt as to the strength of the influence of the intrauterine environment. However, in the Italian study the postnatal environmental conditions were known and were similar in the insulin-resistant and unaffected twins, thereby indicating that intrauterine environmental conditions do have a major influence on susceptibility to metabolic abnormalities in adult life (Poulsen et al., 1997; Bo et al., 2000).

Evidence from the studies of individuals born during the Dutch famine of 1945 also provides general support for the thrifty phenotype hypothesis. This relatively short period of moderate undernutrition at the end of the Second World War is described in more detail in Chapter 9 of this book. The occurrence of a famine situation in a well-developed European nation presents a unique opportunity for follow-up and evaluation of possible programming effects on the population who were exposed in utero. Oral glucose tolerance tests of men and women who had been in utero during the period of the famine showed that these individuals had high plasma glucose concentrations at 2 h, with the greatest impact being on the offspring whose mothers were caught by the famine in the last trimester of pregnancy (Roseboom et al., 2001). Within this Dutch population, as with other cohorts, the strongest predictor of glucose intolerance was low weight at birth and obesity in adult life, suggesting an interaction of pre-natal and postnatal factors. In this population however, there is clear and unequivocal evidence that the poor intrauterine growth was, at least in part, the product of nutrient restriction. As such, the pre–postnatal interaction is consistent with the concept of programming thrift in utero, that is inappropriate for the excess nutrition of adult life in an affluent environment that is profoundly different from that which prevailed in the fetal period.

The late 20th and early 21st centuries have seen a rapidly escalating epidemic of insulin resistance and obesity in India (Yajnik, 2001). This, too, seems consistent with the acquisition of a thrifty phenotype in early life. Small size at birth, deprivation and relatively poor maternal nutrition have been predominant features in this population for many generations, but modern Indians appear to be particularly prone to adiposity in later life. This is especially apparent in Indian populations who have migrated to the UK, where they are the population group most at risk of obesity and its associated disease sequelae (Bhopal et al., 1999). However, it is difficult to dissociate what may be indicators of the programming of a thrifty phenotype from possible genetic effects. A study of trends in birthweights across first and second generations of Asian migrants to the UK showed no trend for an increase, and second-generation babies remained significantly smaller at birth than the national average (Margetts et al., 2002). It is not possible to distinguish a genetic influence from poor socio-economic indicators as risk factors for insulin resistance in such a population.

Future Perspectives

The association between early growth and the later development of type 2 diabetes is well established and appears more robust than equivalent studies of cardiovascular disease. Low weight at birth, or thinness at birth, are good markers of later risk for insulin resistance, particularly if coupled to a rapid increase in adiposity during childhood. As they go through a transition in diet and lifestyle, populations in China and the Indian subcontinent may be at particular risk of an epidemic of insulin resistance and associated disease in the early decades of the 21st century, possibly due to effects of programming that promote metabolic thrift. Developing an understanding of the mechanisms, whether genetic or epigenetic, through which risk of type 2 diabetes or the metabolic syndrome may be transmitted between generations is therefore of prime importance for the development of global disease-prevention strategies. The development of appropriate animal models for intrauterine programming of insulin resistance will provide the main vehicle for elucidating the molecular basis of these processes.

References

Barker, D.J.P., Clark, P.M.S., Cox, L.J., Fall, C., Osmond, C. and Winter, P.D. (1993) Type 2 (non-insulin-dependent) diabetes mellitus, hypertension and hyperlipidaemia (syndrome x): relation to reduced fetal growth. *Diabetologia* 36, 62–67.

Bavdekar, A., Yajnik, C.S., Fall, C.H.D., Bapat, S., Pandit, A.N., Deshpande, V., Bhave, S., Kellingray, S.D. and Joglekar, C. (1999) Insulin resistance syndrome in 8-year-old Indian children – small at birth, big at 8 years, or both? *Diabetes* 48, 2422–2429.

Bayol, S., Jones, D., Goldspink, G. and Stickland, N. (2003) Influence of maternal nutrition on postnatal skeletal muscle growth. *Archives of Animal Breeding* 46, 158.

Benn, C.S., Jeppesen, D.L., Hasselbalch, H., Olesen, A.B., Nielsen, J., Bjorksten, B., Lisse, I. and Aaby, P. (2001) Thymus size and head circumference at birth and the development of allergic diseases. *Clinical and Experimental Allergy* 31, 1862–1866.

Bhopal, R., Unwin, N., White, M., Yallop, J., Walker, L., Alberti, K.G.M.M., Harland, J., Patel, S., Ahmad, N., Turner, C., Watson, B., Kaur, D., Kulkarni, A., Laker, M. and Tavridou, A. (1999) Heterogeneity of coronary heart disease risk factors in Indian, Pakistani, Bangladeshi, and European origin populations: cross sectional study. *British Medical Journal* 319, 215–220.

Bo, S., Cavallo-Perin, P., Scaglione, L., Ciccone, G. and Pagano, G. (2000) Low birthweight and metabolic abnormalities in twins with increased susceptibility to type 2 diabetes. *Diabetic Medicine* 17, 365–370.

Brameld, J.M., Fahey, A.J., Langley-Evans, S.C. and Buttery, P.J. (2003) Nutritional and hormonal control of muscle growth and fat deposition. *Archives of Animal Breeding* 46, 143–156.

Bundred, P., Kitchiner, D. and Buchan, I. (2001) Prevalence of overweight and obese children between 1989 and 1998. *British Medical Journal* 322, 326.

Cohen, M.P., Stern, E., Rusecki, Y. and Ziedler, A. (1988) The high prevalence of diabetes in young Ethiopian migrants to Israel. *Diabetes* 37, 824–828.

Dwyer, C.M., Stickland, N.C. and Fletcher, J.M. (1994) The influence of maternal nutrition on muscle fiber number development in the porcine fetus and on subsequent postnatal growth. *Journal of Animal Science* 72, 911–917.

Flanagan, D.E., Moore, V.M., Godsland, I.F., Cockington, R.A., Robinson, J.S. and Phillips, D.I.W. (2000) Fetal growth and the physiological control of glucose tolerance in adults: a minimal model analysis. *American Journal of Physiology* 278, E700–E706.

Fowden, A.L. (1989) The role of insulin in prenatal growth. *Journal of Developmental Physiology* 12, 173–182.

Gloyn, A.L. (2003) The search for type 2 diabetes genes *Ageing Research Reviews* 2, 111–127.

Hales, C.N. (1991) Fetal and infant growth and impaired glucose tolerance at age 64 years. *British Medical Journal* 303, 1019–1022.

Hales, C.N. and Barker, D.J.P. (1992) Type 2 (non-insulin-dependent) diabetes mellitus: the thrifty phenotype hypothesis. *Diabetologia* 35, 595–601

Handel, S.E. and Stickland, N.C. (1987) Muscle cellularity and birth weight. *Animal Production* 44, 311–317.

Hattersley, A.T. and Tooke, J.E. (1999) The fetal insulin hypothesis: an alternative explanation of the association of low birthweight with diabetes and vascular disease. *Lancet* 353, 1789–1792.

Hattersley, A.T., Beards, F., Appleton, M., Harvey, R. and Ellard, S. (1998) Mutations in the glucokinase gene of the fetus result in reduced birthweight. *Nature Genetics* 19, 268–270.

Hegarty, P.V.J. and Allen, C.E. (1978) Effect of pre-natal runting on post-natal development of skeletal muscles in swine and rats. *Journal of Animal Science* 46, 1634–1640.

Hellerström, C., Swenne, I. and Andersson, A. (1988) Islet cell replication and diabetes. In: Lefebvre, P.J. and Pipellers, D.G. (eds) *The Pathology of the Endocrine Pancreas in Diabetes*. Springer Verlag, Heidelberg, Germany, pp. 141–170.

Huxley, R., Neil, A. and Collins, R. (2002) Unravelling the fetal origins hypothesis: is there really an inverse association between birth weight and subsequent blood pressure? *Lancet* 360, 659–665.

Jackson, A.A., Langley-Evans, S.C. and McCarthy, H.D. (1996) Nutritional influences in early life upon obesity and body proportions. In: Chadwick, D.J. and Cardew, G. (eds) *Origins and Consequences of Obesity*, Ciba Foundation Symposium 201. John Wiley & Sons, Chichester, UK, pp. 118–129.

Kloppel, G., Lohr, M., Habich, K., Oberholzer, M. and Heitz, P.U. (1985) Islet pathology and pathogenesis of type 1 and type 2 diabetes mellitus revisited. *Survey and Synthesis of Pathology Research* 4, 110–125.

Langley-Evans, S.C. (1997) Fetal programming of immune function and respiratory disease. *Clinical and Experimental Allergy* 27, 1377–1379.

Langley-Evans, S.C., Gardner, D.S. and Jackson, A.A. (1996) Association of disproportionate growth of fetal rats in late gestation with raised systolic blood pressure in later life. *Journal of Reproduction and Fertility* 106, 307–312.

Law, C.M., Gordon, G.S., Shiell, A.Q., Barker, D.J.P. and Hales, C.N. (1995) Thinness at birth and glucose tolerance in seven year old children. *Diabetic Medicine* 12, 24–29.

Lillioja, S., Young, A.A., Cutler, S.L., Ivy, J.L., Abbott, W.G.H., Zawadzki, J.K., Ykijarvinen, H., Christin, L., Secomb, T.W. and Bogardens, C. (1987) Skeletal muscle capillary density and fibre type are possible determinants of *in vivo* insulin resistance in man. *Journal of Clinical Investigation* 80, 415–424.

Lindsay, R.S., Dabelea, D., Roumain, J., Hanson, R.L., Bennet, P.H. and Knowlwer, W.C. (2000) Type 2 diabetes and low birth weight. The role of paternal inheritance in the association of low birth weight and diabetes. *Diabetes* 49, 445–449.

Maltin, C.A., Delday, M.I., Sinclair, K.D., Steven, J. and Sneddon, A.A. (2001) Impact of manipulations of myogenesis *in utero* on the performance of adult skeletal muscle. *Reproduction* 122, 359–374.

Margetts, B.M., Yusof, S.M., Al Dallal, Z. and Jackson, A.A. (2002) Persistence of lower birth weight in second generation South Asian babies born in the United Kingdom. *Journal of Epidemiology and Community Health* 56, 684–687.

Martorell, R., Stein, A.D. and Schroeder, D.G. (2001) Early nutrition and later adiposity. *Journal of Nutrition* 131, 874S–880S.

McLarty, D.G., Kintange, H.M., Mtinangi, B.L., Mahem, W.J., Swai, A.B.M., Masuki, G., Kilima, P.M., Chuwa, L.M. and Alberti, K.G.M.M. (1989) Prevalence of diabetes and impaired glucose tolerance in rural Tanzania. *Lancet* 1, 871–874.

Phillips, D.I.W. (1995) Relation of fetal growth to adult muscle mass and glucose tolerance. *Diabetic Medicine* 12, 686–690.

Phillips, D.I.W., Hirst, S., Clark, P.M.S., Hales, C.N. and Osmond, C. (1994) Fetal growth and insulin secretion in adult life. *Diabetologia* 37, 592–596.

Phillips, D.I.W., Borthwick, A.C., Stein, C. and Taylor, R. (1996) Fetal growth and insulin resistance in adult life: relationship between glycogen synthase activity in adult skeletal muscle and birthweight. *Diabetic Medicine* 13, 325–329.

Phipps, K., Barker, D.J.P., Hales, C.N., Fall, C.H.D., Osmond, C. and Clark, P.M.S. (1993) Fetal growth and impaired glucose tolerance in men and women. *Diabetologia* 36, 225–228.

Picard, B., Lefaucheur, L., Berri, C. and Duclos, M.J. (2002) Muscle fibre ontogenesis in farm animal species. *Reproduction, Nutrition, Development* 42, 415–431.

Poulsen, P., Vaag, A., Kyvik, K.O., Jensen, D.M. and Beck-Nielsen, H. (1997) Low birth weight is associated with NIDDM in discordant monozygotic and dizygotic twin pairs. *Diabetologia* 40, 439–446.

Reaven, G.M. (1988) Role of insulin resistance in human disease. *Diabetes* 37, 1595–1607.

Roseboom, T.J., van der Meulen, J.H.P., Ravelli, A.C.J., Osmond, C., Barker, D.J.P. and Bleker, O.P. (2001) Effects of prenatal exposure to the Dutch famine on adult disease in later life: an overview. *Molecular and Cellular Endocrinology* 185, 93–98.

Rudolph, A.M. (1984) The fetal circulation and its response to stress. *Journal of Developmental Physiology* 6, 11–19.

Snoeck, A., Remacle, C., Reusens, B. and Hoet, J.J. (1990) Effect of a low protein diet during pregnancy on the rat fetal endocrine pancreas. *Biology of the Neonate* 5, 107–118.

Stolar, M.W. and Chilton, R.J. (2003) Type 2 diabetes, cardiovascular risk, and the link to insulin resistance. *Clinical Therapeutics* 25 (suppl. B), B4–B31.

Valdez, R., Athens, M.A., Thompson, G.H., Bradshaw, B.S. and Stern, M.P. (1994) Birthweight and adult health outcomes in a biethnic population in the USA. *Diabetologia* 37, 624–631.

Van Assche, F.A. and Aerts, L. (1979) The fetal endocrine pancreas. *Contributions to Gynecology and Obstetrics* 5, 44–57.

Vickers, M.H., Reddy, S., Ikenasio, B.A. and Breier, B.H. (2001) Dysregulation of the adipoinsular axis – a mechanism for the pathogenesis of hyperleptinemia and adipogenic diabetes induced by fetal programming. *Journal of Endocrinology* 170, 323–332.

Wigmore, P.M. and Evans, D.J.R. (2002) Molecular and cellular mechanisms involved in the generation of fiber diversity during myogenesis. *International Review of Cytology* 216, 175–232.

Wright, C.M., Parker, L., Lamont, D. and Craft, A.W. (2001) Implications of childhood obesity for adult health: findings from the thousand families cohort study. *British Medical Journal* 323, 1280–1284.

Yajnik, C.S. (2001) The insulin resistance epidemic in India: fetal origins, later lifestyle or both? *Nutrition Reviews* 59, 1–9.

Yajnik, C.S., Fall, C.H.D., Vaidya, U., Pandit, A.N., Bavdekar, A., Bhat, D.S., Osmond, C., Hales, C.N. and Barker, D.J.P. (1995) Fetal growth and glucose and insulin metabolism in 4-year-old Indian children. *Diabetic Medicine* 12, 330–336.

Yajnik, C.S., Coyaji, K.J., Joglekar, C.V., Kellingray, S. and Fall, C. (2001) Paternal insulin resistance and fetal growth: problem for the 'fetal insulin' and the 'fetal origins' hypotheses. *Diabetologia* 44, 1197–1201.

Zimmet, P., King, H., Taylor, R., Raper, L.R., Balkau, B., Borger, J., Heriot, W. and Thoma, K. (1984) The high prevalence of diabetes mellitus, impaired glucose tolerance and diabetic retinopathy in Nauru: the 1982 survey. *Diabetes Research* 1, 13–18.

8 Programming of Diabetes: Experimental Models

BRIGITTE REUSENS, LUISE KALBE AND CLAUDE REMACLE

Laboratoire de Biologie Cellulaire, Université Catholique de Louvain, Place Croix du Sud 5, B-1348, Louvain-la-Neuve, Belgium

Introduction

The mechanism by which fetal malnutrition increases the risk for glucose intolerance and type 2 diabetes is not well understood. Besides the insulin resistance that has been postulated to develop as a consequence of the lack of nutrient availability during early life, a primary insult in β-cell development has also been observed. Fetal malnutrition would lead to inappropriate β-cell ontogeny, resulting in a population of β-cells that does not cope adequately with metabolic or oxidative stress later in life. Since, obviously, this hypothesis can not be verified in humans, various animal models have been established.

The time course of development is different from one species to another. For instance, humans and guinea-pigs are born more mature than rats or mice. The same is true at the level of the endocrine pancreas. In humans, the initial formation of the endocrine cells in the pancreas occurs at 10 weeks' gestation (Bouwens *et al.*, 1997). In the guinea-pig, islet formation and remodelling also begin at an early stage of gestation and continue for a longer time after birth. In rodents, the islets develop relatively late in gestation and undergo a remodelling 2 weeks after birth. This means that the critical window for islet development is narrower in rodents than in other species. This could be an advantage for the identification of mechanisms involved when the consequences of nutritional or other experimental manipulations are analysed. However, results from such studies should be viewed with caution until confirmed in other species, before extrapolating them to humans.

Development of the Endocrine Pancreas in the Rat

Endocrine cells of the pancreas are organized in highly vascularized and innervated microorgans distributed throughout the exocrine tissue. These microorgans, called 'islets of Langerhans', contain four endocrine cell types and represent only 1% of the pancreatic tissue at adulthood: α-cells produce glucagon, β-cells produce insulin, δ-cells produce somatostatin and PP-cells produce pancreatic polypeptide. The most abundant cell is the β-cell, which represents 60–80% of the islet cell population. The development of the pancreas is a fascinating event, starting from a pool of common progenitor cells (multipotent endodermal progenitors) which will be committed into the endocrine or exocrine cell lineage or duct cell. Then, within the endocrine compartment, the cells will have to differentiate further into α-, β-, δ- or PP-cells. This is regulated by the expression of distinct genes, under the control of a hierarchy of various and specific networks of transcription factors. It is thus obvious that any disturbance in the environment of the future endocrine cell, for instance by intrauterine malnutrition or other injuries, will alter the relative participation of factors involved in this network, and may drive the β-cell mass into the corner, contributing to β-cell failure and diabetes later in life.

Figure 8.1 illustrates the different steps of pancreas development The pancreas develops from two anlagen of the primitive gut, which fuse to form both the exocrine and endocrine pancreas. In the mouse and rat, the dorsal pancreatic bud appears at embryonic day (E) 9.5 closely followed by the ventral bud. The buds fuse together at E16.5. A branched structure is distinguishable at E14.5 and the endocrine cells can be identified by E15.5. The endocrine tissue is derived from epithelial duct cells by rotation of the polarity of the mitotic axis. These cells will divide to form small clusters budding out from the pancreatic ducts. These immature endocrine cell clusters become vascularized and coexpress several pancreatic hormones and neuropeptides, eventually becoming 'islets of Langerhans' (Reusens *et al.*, 2000).

One of the important components of the early specification of the pancreatic programme within the region of the gut endoderm involves the exclusion of the expression of the hedgehog gene family (*Shh* and *Ihh*). The *hh* signalling molecules are expressed throughout the primitive gut endoderm except in the regions destined to become the pancreas (endocrine and exocrine). In other words, the *hh* molecules promote the intestinal differentiation but impair pancreatic development. The classical way of specifying a particular cell fate within the field of initially equivalent cells is the lateral specification mediated by the Notch pathway. Notch signalling involves the cell expressing high quantities of ligands (Delta or Serrate) that signal to activate Notch receptors on the neighbouring cells in which the activated intracellular Notch receptors (IC) suppress the primitive cell fate (Edlund, 2001). In the Notch-signalling pathway, IC interacts with the DNA-binding protein RBP-Jx to activate expression of repressor genes such as *hes* genes that, in turn, repress expression of other genes that otherwise will promote the primary fate. Notch signalling controls the choice between differentiated endocrine and progenitor cell fate in the developing pancreas. Blocking the activation of Notch receptor results in high neurogenin-3 gene (*ngn3*) expression, and promotes the endocrine fate. Neurogenin-3 downstream of the endoderm factors will specify which cells in the pancreatic epithelium will differentiate into endocrine cells and will initiate the differentiation programme. In contrast, cells with active Notch signalling adopt the exocrine fate and/or

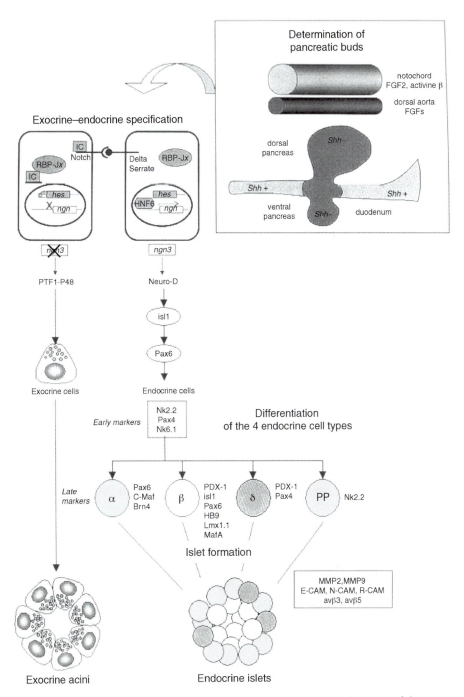

Fig. 8.1. Schematic representation of the different steps in the development of the pancreas (adapted from Grapin-Botton *et al.*, 2001; Wilson *et al.*, 2003). See text for explanation.

remain as undifferentiated progenitor cells (Edlund, 2001). As stated before, the endocrine cells delaminate from the epithelium upon differentiation and migrate into the mesenchyme where they cluster. This migration is likely to result in a decrease in the Notch signal among the progenitor cells and will allow the formation of the islets.

The final fate of the individual endocrine cells is determined by the expression of a series of transcription factors specific for each type of endocrine cell. Some of them are early markers, such as Pax4, Nk2.2 and Nk6.1, co-expressed with neurogenin-3, whereas others are late markers, such as Pax6, isl1, HB9 and PDX-1. The transcription factor network is highly complex and several factors involved are expressed more than once during the differentiation process and play more than one role. One of the key players is the homeodomain transcription factor PDX-1, which is not only important in the regulation of insulin gene expression, but is also required for the differentiation of the mature pancreas. At embryonic day 8.5 in the mouse (1 day before the appearance of the dorsal pancreatic bud), cells of the endoderm are already committed to the pancreatic fate (Reusens *et al.*, 2000) and will give rise to all pancreatic tissues. These cells already express *Pdx-1*, also known as *Sft-1*, *Idx-1* or *Ipf-1* (Sandler and German, 1997), and *hb9* (Wilson *et al.*, 2003) under the control of signals coming from the surrounding tissues. Cells expressing *Pdx-1* between E9.5 and E11.5 give rise to pancreatic duct, endocrine islets and exocrine acinar cells. Cells expressing *Pdx-1* at E8.5, or after E11.5, only give rise to exocrine acini or endocrine islets. Stated otherwise, the duct progenitors express detectable PDX-1 only around E10.5, while the endocrine and exocrine progenitors express PDX-1 throughout embryogenesis. The lineage for pancreatic duct and the rest of the pancreas must thus separate before E12.5 (Gu *et al.*, 2003). Expression of *Pdx-1* in undifferentiated ductal epithelium is associated with the glucose transporter GLUT 2. By day 15 in the rat, both remain in the developing β-cell but are lost in the acinar cell.

Early morphogenetic signalling in the formation of the pancreas may depend on the interplay between peptide growth factors and tissue transcription factors, an interaction which is apparent throughout islet formation. Indeed, it was found in chick and mouse embryo that activin-βB (a member of the transforming growth factor family (TGFβ)) and fibroblast growth factor-2 are notochord factors that can repress endodermal *Shh*, permitting expression of pancreas genes, including *Pdx-1* and *insulin* (Hebrok *et al.*, 1998). Other growth factors, such as platelet-derived growth factor (PDGF), vascular endothelial growth factor (VEGF) and fibroblast growth factor (FGF)-7, which are expressed within the pancreatic stroma adjacent to the ductal epithelium, may also intervene. The ongoing proliferation and developmental differentiation of β-cells, once formed, is highly dependent on the expression of the insulin-like growth factors (IGFs) within the islets, as we will see below.

β-Cell Function and Insulin Action

In adults, β-cells store insulin and C-peptide within their granules. After stimulation by glucose uptake via the low-affinity glucose transporter GLUT 2, glucose enters the cell, is phosphorylated by glucokinase, and metabolized, leading to a rise in the ATP/ADP ratio. This increase induces a blockage of the K^+ ATP-dependent channels, which in turn will lead to membrane depolarization and, subsequently, to the activation of the voltage-dependent Ca^{2+} channels. Ca^{2+} will enter into the β-cell and stimulate the release of insulin by exocytosis. In addition to glucose, amino acids have been shown to stimulate insulin release in the absence of glucose, the most potent secretagogues being leucine, arginine and lysine (Fajans and Floyd, 1972). In the fetus, insulin secretion is more sensitive to amino acids than to glucose (de Gasparo *et al.*, 1978), its full response to glucose beginning after birth. Fetal pancreas is capable of insulin synthesis and release in response to agents that increase cyclic AMP, activate protein kinase-C or raise calcium levels. In humans, as well as in rats, fetal β-cells show an immature or poor response to nutrients, especially to glucose. In contrast to the adult pancreas, fetal β-cells never display a biphasic pattern (Hughes, 1994).

Insulin promotes the storage of glucose as glycogen in the liver and muscle, the incorporation of amino acids into the muscle proteins and the accumulation of triglycerides in adipose tissues. In muscle and adipose tissue, the action of insulin on glucose uptake is mediated through the translocation of the glucose transporter GLUT4 from the intracellular site to the plasma membrane. To achieve this action, insulin binds to the α and β receptors (type α predominates during development, while type β predominates in adulthood). These receptors are composed of an extracellular ligand-binding domain that controls the activity of an intracellular tyrosine kinase. Insulin fixation on the α-subunit of the receptor activates the β-subunit kinase activity and induces tyrosine phosphorylation of the insulin receptor substrate (IRS) family (IRS1, 2, 3 and/or 4). IRS-1 and IRS-2 function as scaffold proteins to coordinate separate branches of the insulin cascades (and IGFs). IRS proteins couple insulin to the phosphatidylinositol (PI) 3-kinase and extracellular signal-regulated kinase (ERK) cascades. The phosphorylation of IRS proteins recruits the phosphatidylinositol 3-kinase (PI3K) by its association with the regulatory subunit p85a. PI3K is central in the action of insulin, including the stimulation of glucose uptake and inhibition of lipolysis (Shepherd *et al.*, 1998). It is a heterodimereric enzyme, comprising a regulatory subunit (p85) and a catalytic subunit (p110). PI3K activation is an absolute requirement for the insulin-induced translocation of GLUT4, from both the endosomal and GLUT4 storage vesicules, to the plasma membrane. However, subsequent steps are vague, as various serine kinases have been involved, including PKB, PKC-λ and PKC-ξ (White and Myers, 2001).

Early Malnutrition Programmes: the Endocrine Pancreas and its β-cells

In the rat fetus, the β-cell mass increases rapidly at the end of gestation, due to both replication and recruitment of undifferentiated β-cell precursors in the pancreatic duct. Following birth, the growth rate of each islet cell population, including β-cells, declines within 3–4 days. A wave of apoptosis occurs in the neonatal rat islets between 2 and 3 weeks of age (Scaglia *et al.*, 1997). Since the total number of β-cells is not substantially modified during this period of time, this suggests that replication and neogenesis compensate for the loss. It is obvious that the development of the β-cell mass contributes to the accumulation of the islet mass in adulthood. Therefore, any deficiency occurring *in utero* or soon after birth is unlikely to be completely compensated for later in life. Alteration of the β-cell mass by maternal malnutrition in humans had already been demonstrated more than 25 years ago (Winick and Noble, 1966; Weinkove *et al.*, 1974), but the mechanisms involved in this alteration were only deciphered when animal models were developed.

The cellular area staining immunopositively for insulin increases twofold over the 2 days before birth in normal rats (Kaung, 1994). A maternal low-protein diet (LP, 8% of protein instead of 20% in the control diet) modifies this process of β-cell expansion. The islet area was reduced by 30–50% between 19.5 and 21.5 days of gestation in fetal offspring from protein-restricted dams (Snoeck *et al.*, 1990; Petrik *et al.*, 1999; Boujendar *et al.*, 2002). This is due partially to a relative deficiency in α-, β- and somatostatin-secreting cells, although the β-cell population was the most severely affected (Petrik *et al.*, 1999). As a consequence, the total islet and β-cell mass were depleted at birth. When the protein restriction was maintained until weaning, the deficiency was even more pronounced. Cells traversing the S phase of the replication cycle were investigated after tritiated thymidine or bromodeoxyuridine (BrdU) incorporation in these LP fetal and neonatal islet cells. The replication rate of islet cells was reduced by almost 50% in the malnourished offspring, and preferentially in the β-cell, which is consistent with the reduction in the endocrine cell mass. Further analysis has revealed that the cell cycle was lengthened in the LP islets because more β-cells from LP pups contained cyclin D1 (a marker of G_1 phase) but fewer islet cells contained NIMA-related kinase 2 (NEK2; an indicator of cells in G_2 and mitosis) (Petrik *et al.*, 1999).

A modulation of the β-cell area by the maternal diet might also involve β-cell death. After a low rate of apoptosis in fetal islets, a dramatic increase in apoptosis occurs after birth, with a return to a minimal level by weaning. This was also observed in the malnourished pups. Although the timing of the neonatal wave was not affected by the maternal diet, the rate of islet cell apoptosis was increased in LP-exposed offspring at *every* age analysed. This suggests that the event is quantitatively dependent upon, but qualitatively independent of, the diet. This is further supported by the fact that the presence of inducible nitric oxide synthase (iNOS), which precedes the peak of apoptosis in normal islets by 2 days (Petrik *et al.*, 1998), was not changed in LP islets (Petrik *et al.*, 1999).

The timing of the neonatal wave of apoptosis coincides not only with an increase of iNOS but also with the disappearance of the expression of insulin-like growth factor-II (IGF-II) in the endocrine pancreas. IGF-II can act functionally as a growth factor, but also as a survival factor to prevent apoptosis in β-cells (Petrik *et al.*, 1998) and in other cell types (Geier *et al.*, 1992; Jung *et al.*, 1996). We have demonstrated reduced expression of IGF-II mRNA, and a lower number of islet cells positive for the protein in the pancreas of LP pups. This suggests that the increased apoptosis and the reduced β-cell proliferation seen in islets of LP rats may be linked functionally to this reduction of IGF-II expression (Petrik *et al.*, 1999).

The development of fetal islet cells is dependent on the availability of glucose. However, at 17–18 days of gestation in the rat, amino acids appear to be more important than glucose in stimulating β-cell differentiation and proliferation (de Gasparo *et al.*, 1978). In protein-restricted animals, plasma glucose levels were normal but the amino acid profile was perturbed in the feto-maternal unit (Reusens *et al.*, 1995). Maternal and fetal total amino acid levels were not perturbed by the maternal diet but several amino acids were significantly decreased. Essential amino acids levels were reduced by 10% in the fetal plasma on the last day of gestation. Taurine, which does not participate in protein synthesis, but which is very important for several tissues during development (Sturman, 1993), was the most affected, being reduced by 30% in the fetal and maternal plasma by protein deficiency. It was shown that amino acids, but not glucose, potentiate the release of immunoreactive IGF-II from isolated fetal rat islets (Hogg *et al.*, 1993). Interestingly, as mentioned above, less IGF-II was observed in the pancreas of fetuses that grew in an intrauterine milieu where amino acids were limiting. Supplementation of the drinking water of the LP-fed pregnant rat by 25 g/l of taurine prevented the reduction of the β-cell mass by enhancing β-cell proliferation and decreasing islet cell apoptosis. We demonstrated that this could be achieved partially by the normalization of the number of islet cells expressing IGF-II (Boujendar *et al.*, 2002) (Figs 8.2–8.4).

The endocrine pancreas is a richly vascularized tissue. In adult islets, irrigation represents 10% of the total blood flow, while the endocrine mass represents only 1% of the total mass of the pancreas. Pancreatic cell–endothelial cell

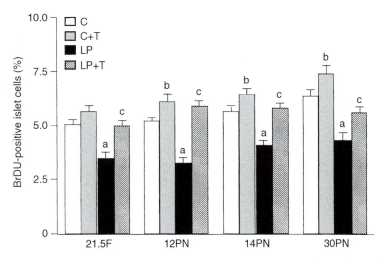

Fig. 8.2. Effect of a maternal low-protein (LP) diet during gestation and lactation on islet cell proliferation of the progeny, and its prevention by taurine (T). F, Fetus; PN, postnatal; BrDU, bromodeoxyuridine. a, $P < 0.05$, LP versus control (C); b, $P < 0.05$, C + T versus C; c, $P < 0.05$, LP + T versus LP. (Reproduced from Boujendar *et al.*, Figure 5 in *Diabetologia* (2002) 45, p. 861, Springer-Verlag.)

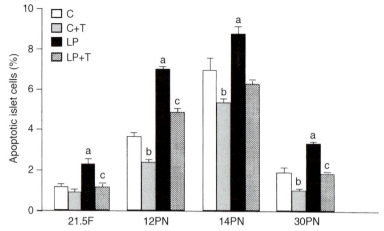

Fig. 8.3. Effect of a maternal low protein (LP) diet during gestation and lactation on the islet cell apoptotic rate of the progeny, and its prevention by taurine (T). F, Fetus; PN, postnatal. a, $P < 0.05$, LP versus control (C); b, $P < 0.05$, C + T versus C; c, $P < 0.05$, LP + T versus LP. (Reproduced from Boujendar *et al.*, Figure 7 in *Diabetologia* (2002) 45, p. 863, Springer-Verlag.)

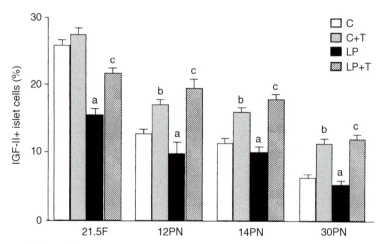

Fig. 8.4. Effect of a maternal low protein (LP) diet during gestation and lactation on the percentage of islet cells positive for insulin-like growth factor-II (IGF-II) in the progeny, and its prevention by taurine (T). F, Fetus; PN, postnatal. a, $P < 0.05$, LP versus control (C); b, $P < 0.05$, C + T versus C; c, $P < 0.05$, LP + T versus LP. (Reproduced from Boujendar *et al.*, Figure 10 in *Diabetologia* (2002) 45, p. 863, Springer-Verlag.)

interactions begin long before islets are functionally mature, and are maintained throughout islet formation. Recently, blood vessels have been shown not only to provide metabolic sustenance, but also inductive signals for the development of endocrine pancreas. Vascular endothelial growth factor (VEGF) is a major factor in these endothelium–endocrine cell interactions (Lammert *et al.*, 2001). At

E8.5–E9.5 of mouse development, pancreatic buds develop precisely where endoderm previously contacted the endothelium of the dorsal aorta and two vitelline veins (Lammert *et al.*, 2001, 2003). Thus pancreatic and vascular development cooperate during embryogenesis.

Islet blood vessel development has been shown to be very sensitive to the lack of protein availability *in utero,* as the volume occupied by blood vessels was lower in islets from LP-exposed fetuses, and this was associated with a reduction in the blood vessel number (Snoeck *et al.*, 1990; Boujendar *et al.*, 2003). The proportion of VEGF-positive cells was reduced in fetal islets from LP rats compared to controls, suggesting that the impaired vascularization could be a consequence of the reduction of VEGF production by the surrounding β-cells, since VEGF stimulates the growth of the endothelial cells. VEGF could play a role in β-cell differentiation from duct precursor cells because its receptor, Flk-1, is found on these cells and VEGF is able to stimulate their proliferation (Oberg *et al.*, 1994; Oberg-Welsh *et al.*, 1997). In parallel, we investigated the VEGF receptor, Flk-1, in the pancreas of the LP offspring. We found that the percentage of cells immunopositive for Flk-1 was decreased in the islets, while it was increased in the duct cells. Maternal protein deprivation thus induces an up-regulation of the Flk-1 expression in duct cells as a reaction to the decreased endocrine cell mass. However, such an up-regulation seemed inefficient to maintain a normal β-cell mass, probably because the level of VEGF was too low (Boujendar *et al.*, 2003).

Islet vascularization is also sensitive to the depletion of taurine that occurs in the LP fetus, since addition of this amino acid to the LP diet of the dam was sufficient to restore a well-vascularized endocrine pancreas in the progeny. Taurine supplementation of the LP dams led to a normalization of the number of the blood vessels, and the proportion of cells positive for VEGF and its receptor in islets. However, it is again unclear whether the prevention of the alteration of the vascular system by taurine in the LP islets is the cause, or the consequence, of the restoration of the β-cell mass by this specific amino acid (Boujendar *et al.*, 2003).

As mentioned previously, the transcription factor, pancreatic and duodenal homeobox 1 (PDX-1), is important for the development and the maintenance of β-cells. The expression of this factor was also modulated in the offspring when the dam was a fed another low-protein diet (Arantes *et al.*, 2002) containing 6% of protein during pregnancy and lactation. At birth and after 28 days of life, islet volume and PDX-1 protein expression were reduced in pups fed this diet during gestation and lactation. In contrast, *Pdx-1* mRNA levels in the islets from 28-day-old low-protein rats were no different from those of controls. If the low-protein diet was present only during fetal life, PDX-1 protein expression in pancreatic islets, the volume of islets and insulin secretion were restored in recovered rats, whereas PDX-1 mRNA levels were higher than in normal rats. These results suggest links between diminished PDX-1 protein expression, reduction in islet volume and impaired insulin secretion in pups exposed to a low-protein diet.

The deleterious effect of fetal malnutrition on the development of the β-cell mass is also apparent in other animal models of fetal malnutrition. Fetuses whose mothers were caloric restricted by 50% during the last week of gestation were growth retarded. Such animals were also born with important alterations in the development of their endocrine pancreas, including a lower β-cell mass, brought about by different mechanisms than those observed in the case of protein deprivation (Garofano et al., 1997). In this model, the reduction in β-cell mass appears to be due to reduced neogenesis expressed through a smaller number of islets rather than a lower rate of islet cell proliferation and increased apoptosis, as occurred with protein deprivation. Interestingly, the islet blood vascularization was not affected (Kalbe et al., 2003). In a study comparing the effect of maternal low-protein but isocaloric, low calorie and low-protein–calorie-restricted diets, Bertin et al. (2002) demonstrated that, although the three approaches to inducing fetal malnutrition all induced 50% reduction of the fetal β-cell mass, plasma taurine was only depleted in the fetuses that were protein deprived. Taurine can thus not be involved in the reduction of β-cell mass observed in caloric-restricted fetuses, and other factors have been suggested. During development, a negative role of glucocorticoids on the fetal β-cell has been demonstrated (Blondeau et al., 2001). Maternal food restriction increased maternal and fetal corticosterone levels (Lesage et al., 2001). A normalization of the glucocorticoid levels in the intrauterine growth retardation (IUGR) calorie-restricted fetus restored a normal β-cell mass that was associated with the correction of the decreased β-cell neogenesis (Blondeau et al., 2001).

To better address the key issue of the fetal programming of the endocrine pancreas, two approaches were used. In a first step, we highlighted the short-term programming by culturing fetal β-cells, which were thus withdrawn from the influence of a disturbed metabolic maternal environment. In a second step, by feeding the offspring with a normal diet after birth or after weaning and analysing the adult progeny, long-term consequences were revealed. This will be addressed in the next part of this chapter.

Pancreatic cells cultured for 7 days proliferate and differentiate into pseudo-islets rich in β-cells (Hellerström, 1979). Although they were cultured in the same medium as the control islets and were free of the poor maternal milieu, low-protein islet cells retained the lower proliferation rate (Cherif et al., 2001) and the higher apoptotic rate (Merezak et al., 2001) that were observed in vivo. In addition, insulin secretion in response to glucose and various amino acids was dramatically altered in islets of the LP fetus, depending on the secretagogues used. The lowering of insulin release was more pronounced when the islets were challenged with amino acids than with glucose (Cherif et al., 1998, 2001). Although a reduction of cAMP concentration was detected in these islets, and might explain, in part, the reduced insulin release, we demonstrated that the main defect in insulin secretion was at the level of exocytosis (Cherif et al., 2001). The persisting reduction of the insulin secretion and replication, as well as the increased apoptotic rate of fetal β-cells in LP offspring, even when they had been withdrawn from the maternal environment and cultured for 1 week, demonstrates that protein restriction during pregnancy induced lasting impairments. The secretory and proliferative actions of the fetal β-cells are stimulated by amino acids (Fajans and Floyd, 1972; Swenne et al., 1980). Since a decrease in essential, branched amino acids and taurine was reported in the LP feto-maternal unit (Reusens et al., 1995), lower sensitivity to several amino acids might have been due to their low availability during development. However, a low level of taurine was also involved, since taurine supplementation of the LP diet of the pregnant rat restored a completely normal insulin secretion from these fetal islets.

Early Malnutrition Programmes, Glucose Metabolism and Insulin Action: Type 2 Diabetes

Type 2 diabetes is characterized by hyperglycaemia, resulting from insulin resistance, β-cell dysfunction or both. β-Cell dysfunction occurs because of an inability to synthesize and secrete active insulin in sufficient amounts to meet the increased demand for insulin (Kahn, 1998). In addition, type 2 diabetic patients often show a reduced β-cell number compared to weight-matched non-diabetic patients. This suggests that these patients had fewer cells prior to the onset of diabetes, or that they failed to enhance their β-cell mass in response to the demand (Clark *et al.*, 1988). Individuals with type 2 diabetes are not at increased risk for autoimmune diseases, but do have higher prevalence of metabolic abnormalities, including obesity, hypertension and dyslipidaemia. It should be mentioned, however, that a recent study showed that one-third of patients aged 15–34 with clinical type 2 diabetes had objectively type 1 diabetes on the basis of the evolution of their anti-islets antibodies; namely, islet cell antibody (ICA), glutamic acid decarboxylase (GAD) and insulin antibody (IA) (Borg *et al.*, 2003).

The underdevelopment of the endocrine pancreas as a response to malnutrition may be a survival advantage in early life, but may be a risk factor for the appearance of diabetes later on. The long-term effect of the early malnutrition depends on the critical time windows at which the poor diet was applied. If protein restriction in rat pregnancy was reversed at birth, the imbalance between β- and α-cell populations observed at birth was restored by 3 months of age (Dahri *et al.*, 1991), but females had a lower insulin secretion in response to an oral glucose tolerance test. If the low-protein diet was maintained until weaning, the adult offspring retained a reduced number of pancreatic β-cells and an increased α-cell number (Berney *et al.*, 1997) and both males and females exhibited a blunted insulin secretion in response to the oral glucose challenge (Reusens and Remacle, 2001a). This suggests that the LP diet causes fundamental changes in the programming of the β-cell phenotype, with critical periods both in fetal and neonatal life. Changes in such programming of the β-cells were also observed following fetal and postnatal calorie restriction. The β-cell mass, which was depressed by 66% at weaning, remained reduced by 35% at 3 months despite adequate calorie intake after weaning. However, an increased proliferation rate was observed in the tail of the pancreas, which was not sufficient to fully restore a β-cell mass since the latter remained significantly reduced (Garofano *et al.*, 1998).

Despite lower insulin secretion in the young offspring protein-malnourished early in life, such animals present better glucose tolerance (Shepherd *et al.*, 1997). In contrast, young offspring from mothers that received only 50% of calories during the last week of gestation featured the same pattern for insulin, but with a normal glucose tolerance (Garofano *et al.*, 1999). To understand this apparent discrepancy between lower insulin secretion and better glucose tolerance, several authors have further investigated the insulin-sensitive tissues in the case of maternal protein restriction. Lower plasma insulin concentration and the increased glucose infusion rates needed to maintain euglycaemia in hyper-insulinaemic clamps suggest an increased sensitivity of peripheral tissues to insulin in the young low-protein-exposed offspring (Holness, 1996). This focuses attention on the three key organs involved in glucose homeostasis: the muscle, the liver and the adipose tissue.

At the level of the muscle and the adipocytes, protein-restricted offspring have an enhanced basal glucose uptake. The number of insulin receptors expressed in these tissues was very considerably increased, as was the number of glucose transporters (GLUT 4) in the plasma membrane (Ozanne *et al.*, 1996). Such alterations are likely to have made a significant contribution to the improvement in glucose tolerance observed in the animals' young adult life.

Despite having increased expression of insulin receptors, adipocytes from protein-restricted offspring have revealed a selective insulin resistance in studies of lipolysis (Ozanne *et al.*, 1999, 2000). The mechanism of this resistance is unknown, but an alteration in the expression and activities of various components of the insulin-signalling pathway seems to be involved (Ozanne *et al.*, 1997; Shepherd *et al.*, 1997). Indeed, increased basal and stimulated levels of insulin-receptor-substrate-1-associated phosphatidylinositol 3-kinase (PI3K) activities and increased Akt/protein kinase B activities have been reported. In addition, adipocytes from low-protein-exposed offspring have a relatively low level of the p110-β catalytic subunit of the PI3K.

Resistance of the liver to the effect of glucagon on stimulation of glucose output has also been described in early protein-restricted offspring, and has been associated with a decreased hepatic glucagon receptor number (Ozanne *et al.*, 1996). These animals also exhibited an increased insulin receptor number. In addition, the livers of the low-protein-exposed offspring had larger, but fewer hepatic lobules than those of the controls (Burns *et al.*, 1997). This was associated with functional differences such as changes in enzyme activity. Increased phosphoenol-pyruvate carboxykinase (PEPCK) and decreased hepatic gluco-kinase (GK) activity were observed at weaning and at 3 months. Interestingly, it was demonstrated that the gluconeogenic enzyme PEPCK is an important target gene under potent glucocorticoid regulation (Friedman *et al.*, 1993) and its expression is inhibited by insulin (Girard *et al.*, 1991).

So, early protein restriction induces a number of different effects on glucose metabolism and insulin action, including alteration in the regulation of the hepatic and muscle glucose and disturbance in the suppression of the adipose-tissue lipolysis. The limited capacity of the β-cells to regenerate following poor development of the endocrine pancreas after early malnutrition leaves the offspring with a suboptimal complement of functional units in the pancreas. This will not be a real handicap as long as the individual is young, thin and does not face ageing, overfeeding and pregnancy. Should such events occur, the offspring would develop insulin resistance which would evolve to glucose intolerance and diabetes.

Indeed, whereas glucose tolerance in young adults appeared unaffected, or even enhanced, by the protein deprivation, it deteriorated more rapidly with age than that of controls. Sugden and Holness (2002) showed that exposure to protein restriction during early life alone led to a relative insulin resistance and hyperinsulinaemia associated with a normal glucose tolerance at 5 months of age, but only in males. The animals became glucose intolerant at 15 months (Hales *et al.*, 1996) and suffered from frank diabetes at 17 months (Petry *et al.*, 2001). The response seemed also to be sex-dependent. The hyperglycaemia was associated with relative hyperinsulinaemia in male low-protein-exposed offspring and with relative hypoinsulinaemia in female offspring.

The fetal adaptation to malnutrition takes place to favour survival with poor or cyclic availability of food. The 'thrifty phenotype' hypothesis proposed that following such an adaptation, excessive food availability later in life may be detrimental for health (Hales and Barker, 1992). This part of the hypothesis has been tested in models of malnourished rats receiving several enriched diets in later life. The offspring of dams fed 5% protein during gestation and lactation and fed a high-sucrose or a high-fat diet at adulthood had an impaired glucose tolerance. Feeding a standard lab chow in adult life resulted in normal glucose tolerance in animals subject to protein restriction earlier in life. Glucose-stimulated insulin release was reduced in islets of previously malnourished rats fed sucrose or fat (Wilson and Hughes, 1997). Here again, poor fetal and neonatal nutrition led to impaired pancreatic β-cell function persisting into adulthood. In another study, 8 weeks of feeding a high saturated-fat diet to low-protein-exposed offspring was necessary to provoke an impaired glucose tolerance associated with reduced insulin-stimulated glucose uptake (Holness and Sugden, 1999). Anti-lipolytic effects of insulin were impaired in these animals.

Long-term consequences of the early malnutrition were also apparent in offspring of mothers receiving 50% of the calories needed during the last week of gestation and during lactation (Garofano *et al.*, 1998, 1999). At 3 months, male offspring had fewer β-cells, the reduction being greater when the caloric restriction was maintained until weaning. In fact, the β-cell mass, which normally increases between 3 and 12 months, failed to do so, partially because the apoptotic rate was higher and increased further with ageing (Garofano *et al.*, 1999). Insulin secretion in response to an oral glucose injection was depressed at 3 months but, as in low-protein-exposed offspring, no glucose intolerance was observed. At 12 months, the offspring featured increased fasting glycaemia and a dramatically impaired glucose tolerance associated with a profound insulin-openia (Garofano *et al.*, 1999). When the calorie restriction was more severe (30% of the *ad libitum* available food) and was applied from the first day of gestation until birth, 4-month-old male offspring developed obesity, hyper-insulinaemia and hyperlipidaemia, which was amplified by hypercaloric nutrition postnatally (Vickers *et al.*, 2000). However, such offspring did not exhibit an abnormal fasting plasma glucose level, but the hyperglycaemia induced by the hypercaloric diet after weaning was aggravated by the early malnutrition (Vickers *et al.*, 2001). The authors proposed that fetal programming may lead to β-cell dysfunction which, in this case, is induced by hyperlipidaemia. The fact that leptin suppresses insulin production from β-cells (Poitout *et al.*, 1998) and that leptin receptors are present on pancreatic β- and δ-cells (Leclercq-Meyer *et al.*, 1996; Emilsson *et al.*, 1997) suggests a functional relationship between circulating leptin and insulin secretion. Leptin receptors are evenly distributed throughout the pancreatic islets. In adult offspring from calorie-deprived mothers, however, a higher number of leptin-positive cells were identified as δ-cells and this was amplified by a post-weaning high calorie diet (Vickers *et al.*, 2001).

Fetal malnutrition as a consequence of utero-placental insufficiency also programmes the development of the endocrine pancreas and glucose metabolism later in life. Bilateral uterine artery ligation performed on day 19 of gestation in rats leads to intrauterine growth retardation. In this model, IUGR offspring remained growth retarded until 7 weeks after birth, after which they began to recover a normal body weight. They developed marked fasting hyperglycaemia and hyperinsulinaemia at 10 weeks, which deteriorated into glucose intolerance and insulin resistance at 15 weeks. By 26 weeks of age, the IUGR rats were obese (Boloker *et al.*, 2002). Interestingly, the IUGR rats presented a lower insulin secretion in response to an intraperitoneal glucose challenge at 1 week, and a blunted insulin secretion at 26 weeks, whereas at 15 weeks they were clearly insulin resistant and glucose intolerant. In this specific experimental condition, the nutrient deprivation was present during a short time window at the end of the development of the β-cell, which corresponded to an expansion phase of the β-cell mass. No measurement of the β-cell mass was performed at birth but, although no difference was detected at 1 and 7 weeks postnatally, a reduction by 50% at 15 weeks and by 70% at 26 weeks was reported (Simmons *et al.*, 2001). At 14 days postnatally, intrauterine growth-retardation pups exhibited a reduced β-cell proliferation, but a normal apoptotic rate. The expression of *Pdx-1*, the critical regulator of the pancreatic development and β-cell development, was dramatically reduced at 14 days and remained affected at 3 months (Stoffers *et al.*, 2003). Injections of Exendin-4, a long-acting glucagon-like peptide 1 (GLP-1) analogue which promotes expansion of pancreatic β-cell mass, just after birth prevented the defects in the development of the β-cell mass observed postnatally. As a consequence, the glucose intolerance and diabetes observed in the adult were also prevented (Stoffers *et al.*, 2003). Here again, long-lasting consequences of early fetal malnutrition at the level of the endocrine pancreas may be prevented by specific intervention during development.

In conclusion, fetal malnutrition due to maternal protein restriction, caloric restriction or limited availability of nutrients to the fetus jeopardizes the development of the β-cell mass, with consequences for insulin secretion and glucose metabolism later in life.

Transgenerational Programming of the Endocrine Pancreas

The lasting consequences of fetal malnutrition are not limited to the first generation, and seem to persist in a second generation. The vulnerability of the β-cell mass acquired early in life may only be frankly revealed in a situation of increased insulin demand, such as obesity, pregnancy or ageing. The exhaustion of the β-cell mass and the deterioration of the glucose tolerance with obesity and ageing have already been discussed above. Pregnancy is a particular situation during which the endocrine pancreas has to adapt in response to the high demand of insulin coming from the fetus for its anabolism. This specific adaptation can be achieved by several mechanisms. A lowering of the threshold at which glucose stimulates insulin secretion occurs in early pregnancy and, as a consequence, increased insulin synthesis and secretion take place. This is achieved by an up-regulation of β-cell proliferation (Parsons *et al.*, 1992; Sorenson and Brelje, 1997). β-Cell mass doubles by the end of gestation in rats (Bone and Taylor, 1976; Aerts *et al.*, 1997) and this increase is controlled by placental lactogens I and II (Brelje *et al.*, 1993). Altered β-cell mass resulting from protein and calorie deprivation in early life, or placental insufficiency, is a limiting factor for this adaptation.

When 3-month-old offspring from dams fed a low-protein diet during gestation became pregnant, they exhibited a very low insulin secretion after an oral glucose challenge performed at 18.5 days of gestation, and became glucose intolerant (Dahri *et al.*, 1995). Adaptation of the endocrine pancreas was not fully achieved, as evidenced by the fact that the pancreatic insulin content in mothers fed a low-protein diet during fetal life was significantly lower than in the control mothers (Reusens and Remacle, 2001b). This abnormal intrauterine milieu impacted upon the next generation. Just before birth, the pups whose grandmothers were protein restricted during pregnancy also clearly exhibited lower plasma insulin levels, probably as a consequence of the reduced development of their own endocrine pancreas. These rats therefore had a tendency to be hyperglycaemic (Bone and Taylor, 1976). Indeed, fetal pancreatic insulin content and volume density of the β-cell mass were significantly reduced. An intergenerational effect of the abnormal metabolic intrauterine milieu was thus apparent.

Adaptation to pregnancy was also compromised in the calorie-restricted rat model. Although a normal adaptation was seen at 4 months in mothers that were previously malnourished during development, at 8 months they were no longer able to increase their β-cell mass (Blondeau *et al.*, 1999). A study was undertaken to characterize the cellular mechanism responsible for the absence of adaptation. In normally fed pregnant rats, Avril *et al.* (2002) reported a preferential increase in β-cell proliferation in the head of the pancreas at day 12 of gestation. Such an enhanced proliferation rate leads to an important increase in the β-cell fraction on the last day of gestation. Perinatal malnutrition impaired this subsequent adaptation to pregnancy by decreasing the β-cell proliferation in the head of the pancreas at the critical time, i.e. day 12 of pregnancy. In addition, the lack of adaptation in the mother was associated with abnormal α- and β-cell development in the second generation at the fetal stage (Blondeau *et al.*, 2002). The β-cell mass and pancreatic insulin content were reduced. A decreased number of cells expressing PDX-1, which are likely to be precursors for endocrine cells, has been reported in these pancreases at 17 day of gestation. This may partially explain the lower β- and α-cell fraction.

In the model of placental insufficiency, the female progeny are also less able to cope with pregnancy. In fact, pregnancy prematurely precipitated the development of diabetes in IUGR offspring that was only clearly apparent by month 6 in non-pregnant rats (Boloker *et al.*, 2002). Pregnant rats exhibited a clear insulin resistance and glucose intolerance. The consequences of the disturbed metabolic intrauterine milieu were apparent when the second generation was analysed. Pups were born slightly heavier and remained heavier throughout life. They were insulin resistant very early in life and they featured progressive glucose intolerance. At 1 week of age, β-cell mass was slightly increased, but because β-cell proliferation declined progressively compared to control offspring, the β-cell mass was dramatically reduced at 26 weeks (Boloker *et al.*, 2002).

Early Malnutrition and Susceptibility to Type 1 Diabetes

Clinical and animal studies have shown that type 1 diabetes is an autoimmune disease in which both genetic and environmental factors, such as nutrition, participate in the pathogenesis and development of the disease. In type 1 diabetes, β-cells are rapidly and selectively destroyed by apoptosis because of the invasion of islets by immune cells releasing free radicals and cytokines, and also because they have poor defence mechanisms. Type 1 diabetes is not, as is generally believed, a disorder limited to young people. Recent studies support a model in which the disease can occur at any age and that some patients diagnosed with type 2 diabetes actually have type 1 diabetes (Turner *et al.*, 1997). The traditional view of type 1 diabetes postulates that an environmental agent triggers the onset of disease in genetically susceptible individuals. However, more recent observations from humans and in animals support a more complex model, wherein the penetration and expression of heritable aberrations, in combination with inherent target organ defects, are part of the life-long influence of multiple environmental factors (Atkinson and Eisenbarth, 2001).

In contrast to type 2 diabetes, there is little epidemiological evidence to suggest a relation between poor nutrition in early life and the occurrence of type 1 diabetes later in life. Only viral infections, such as coxsackie B4, might support the idea of early programming of type 1 diabetes in humans (Hyöty and Taylor, 2002). In spontaneously diabetic animals, the hypothesis of early programming of type 1 diabetes was also proposed, with an exaggerated wave of postnatal apoptosis suggested to be at the origin of insulitis later in life (Trudeau *et al.*, 2000).

In view of the defects in the endocrine pancreas, particularly the increased apoptotic rate that we have highlighted in offspring from mother fed a low-protein diet, we asked the question about the possibly increased susceptibility of the β-cells to the effects of agents known to be involved in type 1 diabetes. When β-cells from the fetus of a protein-deprived mother were challenged in culture with a nitric oxide (NO) donor or interleukin-1β (IL-1β), they exhibited a higher apoptotic rate than the control fetal β-cells (Merezak *et al.*, 2001). Moreover, the increased susceptibility was maintained throughout life, despite adequate feeding after weaning, since adult islets were also more vulnerable in the presence of cytokines (Merezak *et al.*, 2002). The lack of protein during development has thus generated a β-cell population that is more sensitive to cytokines, perhaps because of a low level of IGF-II (Petrik *et al.*, 1999) and a low level of taurine present during development. Indeed, taurine, which is a sulphur amino acid, has antioxidant properties (Huxtable, 1992). When added to the culture medium, it prevented the destruction of β-cells by NO and IL-1β in fetal and in adult islets. The protective role of taurine against NO- and cytokine-induced apoptosis was attributed to the sulphydryl group. Indeed, methionine, which also possesses this sulphydryl group, was also able to prevent apoptosis; however, the effect was less marked than with taurine. β-Alanine, an analogue of taurine lacking the sulphydryl moiety, was unable to provide any protection (Merezak *et al.*, 2001). Moreover, supplementation of the low-protein diet with taurine, which restored a normal β-cell mass with adequate numbers of cells positive for IGF-II, a normal vascularization and a normal insulin secretion at birth, prevented the hyper-sensitivity of the fetal and adult islets to cytokines (Merezak *et al.*, 2001, 2002). An adequate level of taurine during fetal and early life thus seems a critical parameter to achieving normal development and function of the endocrine pancreas. Should that not be present, vulnerability, at the level of proliferation, defence and secretion, would ensue.

Conclusions

Epidemiological studies have revealed strong relationships between poor fetal growth and subsequent development of metabolic syndrome, glucose intoler-ance and type 2 diabetes (Hales *et al.*, 1996; Merezak *et al.*, 2002). Persisting effects of early malnutrition become translated into pathology and thereby determine chronic disease risk (Barker *et al.*, 1993). These epidemiological observations identify the phenomena of fetal programming without explaining the underlying mechanisms that establish their causal link. Animal models have been established and studies have demonstrated that reduction in the availability of nutrients during fetal development programmes the endocrine pancreas and the insulin-sensitive tissues. Independently of the type of fetal malnutrition

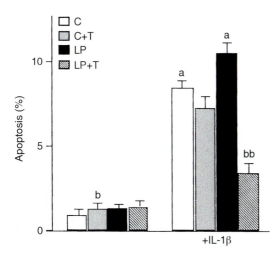

Fig. 8.5. Effect of taurine (T) supplementation on the sensitivity to cytokines of fetal islet cells from control (C) and low-protein-exposed (LP) offspring. a, $P < 0.001$ versus without cytokines; b, $P < 0.05$ versus without taurine; bb, $P < 0.05$ versus without taurine.

(whether there are not enough calories or protein in food or after placental deficiency), malnourished pups are born with a defect in their β-cell mass that will never completely recover, and insulin-sensitive tissues will be definitively altered. Despite the similar defects arising from different approaches to induction of fetal malnutrition, different mechanisms seem to operate and be responsible for the observed endpoints of glucose intolerance and insulin insensitivity. A lack of taurine in the case of protein restriction, and high levels of glucocorticoids in the case of the calorie-restriction model have been the focus of much interest. Interestingly, addition of taurine to the maternal low-protein diet, or the normalization of the maternal plasma glucocorticoid level in the calorie-restricted mother, prevents the alterations of the endocrine pancreas observed without these interventions.

References

Aerts, L., Vercruysse, L. and Van Assche, F.A. (1997) The endocrine pancreas in virgin and pregnant offspring of diabetic pregnant rats. *Diabetes Research and Clinical Practice* 38, 9–19.

Arantes, V.C., Teixeira, V.P., Reis, M.A., Latorraca, M.Q., Leite, A.R., Carneiro, E.M., Yamada, A.T. and Boschero, A.C. (2002) Expression of PDX1 is reduced in pancreatic islets from pups of rat dams fed a low protein diet during gestation and lactation. *Journal of Nutrition* 132, 3030–3035.

Atkinson, M.A. and Eisenbarth, G.S. (2001) Type 1 diabetes: new perspectives on disease pathogenesis and treatment. *Lancet* 358, 221–229.

Avril, I., Blondeau, B., Duchene, B., Czernichow, P. and Bréant, B. (2002) Decreased β-cell proliferation impairs the adaptation to pregnancy in rats malnourished during perinatal life. *Journal of Endocrinology* 174, 215–223.

Barker, D.J.P., Hales, C.N., Fall, C.H., Osmond, C., Philips, K. and Clark, P.M. (1993) Type 2 (non-insulin-dependent) diabetes mellitus, hypertension and hyperlipidemia (syndrome X): relation to reduced fetal growth. *Diabetologia* 36, 62–67.

Berney, D.M., Desai, M., Palmer, D.J., Greenwald, S., Brown, A., Hales, C.N. and Berry, C.L. (1997) The effects of maternal protein deprivation on the fetal rat pancreas: major structural changes and their recuperation. *Journal of Pathology* 183, 109–115.

Bertin, E., Gangnerau, M.N., Bellon, G., Bailbe, D., Arbelot de Vacqueur, A. and Portha, B. (2002) Development of β-cell mass in fetuses of rats deprived of protein and/or energy in last trimester of pregnancy. *American Journal of Physiology* 283, R623–R630.

Blondeau, B., Garofano, A., Czernichow, P. and Bréant, B. (1999) Age-dependant inability of the endocrine pancreas to adapt to pregnancy: a long term consequence of perinatal malnutrition in the rat. *Endocrinology* 40, 4208–4213.

Blondeau, B., Lesage, J., Czernichow, P., Dupouy, J.P. and Bréant, B. (2001) Glucocorticoids impair fetal β cell development in rat. *American Journal of Physiology* 281, E592–E599.

Blondeau, B., Avril, I., Duchene, B. and Bréant, B. (2002) Endocrine pancreas development is altered in foetuses from rats previously showing intra-uterine growth retardation in response to malnutrition. *Diabetologia* 45, 394–401.

Boloker, J., Shira, J.G. and Simmons, R. (2002) Gestational diabetes leads to the development of diabetes in adulthood in the rat. *Diabetes* 51, 1499–1506.

Bone, A. and Taylor, K. (1976) Metabolic adaptation to pregnancy shown by increased biosynthesis of insulin islets of Langerhans isolated from pregnant rats. *Nature* 262, 501–502.

Borg, H., Arnqvit, H.J., Bjork, E., Bolinder, J., Eriksson, J.W., Nystrom, L., Jeppsson, J.O. and Sundkvist, G. (2003) Evaluation of the new ADA and WHO criteria for classification of diabetes mellitus in young adult people (15–34 yrs) in the Diabetes Incidence Study in Sweden (DISS). *Diabetologia* 46, 173–181.

Boujendar, S., Reusens, B., Merezak, S., Ahn, M.T., Arany, E., Hill, D. and Remacle, C. (2002) Taurine supplementation to a low protein diet during fetal and early postnatal life restores a normal proliferation and apoptosis of rat pancreatic islets. *Diabetologia* 45, 856–866.

Boujendar, S., Arany, E., Hill, D., Remacle, C. and Reusens, B. (2003) Taurine supplementation of a low protein diet fed to rat dams normalized the vascularization of the fetal endocrine pancreas. *Journal of Nutrition* 133, 2820–2825.

Bouwens, L., Lu, W.G. and De Krijger, R.R. (1997) Proliferation and differentiation in the human fetal endocrine pancreas. *Diabetologia* 40, 398–404.

Brelje, T.C., Scharp, D.W., Lacy, P.E., Ogren, L., Talamantes, F., Robertson, M., Friesen, H.G. and Sorenson, R.L. (1993) Effect of homologous placental lactogens, prolactins and growth hormones on islet β-cell division and insulin secretion in rat, mouse and human islets: implication for placental lactogen regulation of islet function during pregnancy. *Endocrinology* 132, 879–887.

Burns, S.P., Desai, M., Cohen, R.D., Hales, C.N., Iles, R.A., Germain, J.P., Going, T.C. and Bailey, R.A. (1997) Gluconeogenesis, glucose handling and structural changes in livers of the adult offspring of rats partially deprived of protein during pregnancy and lactation. *Journal of Clinical Investigation* 100, 1768–1774.

Cherif, H., Reusens, B., Ahn, M.T., Hoet, J.J. and Remacle, C. (1998) Effect of taurine on the insulin secretion of islets of fetuses from dams fed a low protein diet. *Endocrinology* 159, 341–348.

Cherif, H., Reusens, B., Dahri, S. and Remacle, C. (2001) A protein-restricted diet during pregnancy alters *in vitro* insulin secretion from islets of fetal Wistar rat. *Journal of Nutrition* 131, 1555–1559.

Clark, A., Wells, C.A., Buley, I.D., Cruickshank, J.K., Vanhegan, R.I., Matthews, D.R., Cooper, G.J., Holman, R.R. and Turner, R.C. (1988) Islet amyloid, increased A-cells, reduced B-cell and exocrine fibrosis: quantitative changes in the pancreas in type 2 diabetes. *Diabetes Research* 9, 151–159

Dahri, S., Snoeck, A., Reusens, B., Remacle, C. and Hoet, J.J. (1991) Islet function in offspring of mothers on low protein diet during gestation. *Diabetes* 40, 115–120.

Dahri, S., Reusens, B., Remacle, C. and Hoet, J.J. (1995) Nutritional influences on pancreatic development and potential links with non-insulin dependent diabetes. *Proceedings of the Nutrition Society* 54, 345–356.

de Gasparo, M., Milner, G.R., Norris, P.D. and Milner, R.D.G. (1978) Effect of glucose and amino acids on fœtal rat pancreatic growth and insulin secretion *in vitro*. *Journal of Endocrinology* 77, 241–248.

Edlund, H. (2001) Factors controlling pancreatic cell differentiation and function. *Diabetologia* 44, 1071–1079.

Emilsson, V., Liu, Y.L., Cawthorne, M.A., Morton, N.M. and Davenport, M. (1997) Expression of the functional leptin receptor mRNA in pancreatic islets and direct inhibitory action of leptin on insulin secretion. *Diabetes* 46, 313–316.

Fajans, S.S. and Floyd, J.C. (1972) Stimulation of islet cell secretion by nutrients and by gastro-intestinal hormone release during gestation. In: Steiner, D.F. and Freinkel, N.

(eds) *Handbook of Physiology.* American Physiology Society, Washington, DC, p. 473.

Friedman, J.E., Yun, J.S., Patel, Y.M., McGrane, M.M. and Hanson, R.W. (1993) Glucocorticoids regulate the induction of phosphoenolpyruvate carboxykinase (GTP) gene transcription during diabetes. *Journal of Biological Chemistry* 268, 12952–12957.

Garofano, A., Czernichow, P. and Bréant, B. (1997) In utero undernutrition impairs rat β-cell development. *Diabetologia* 40, 1231–1234.

Garofano, A., Czernichow, P. and Bréant, B. (1998) Beta-cell mass and proliferation following late fetal and early postnatal malnutrition in the rat. *Diabetologia* 34, 373–384.

Garofano, A., Czernichow, P. and Bréant, B. (1999) Effect of ageing on beta-cell mass and function in rats malnourished during the perinatal periods. *Diabetologia* 42, 711–718.

Geier, A., Haimshon, M., Beery, R. and Lunenfeld, B. (1992) Insulin like growth factor 1 inhibits cell death induced by cycloheximide in MCF-7 cells – a model system for analyzing control of cell death. *In Vitro Cellular and Developmental Biology. Animal* 28A, 725–729.

Girard, J., Perdereau, D., Narkewicz, M., Coupe, C., Ferre, P., Decaux, J.F. and Bossard, P. (1991) Hormonal regulation of liver phosphoenolpyruvate carboxykinase and glucokinase gene expression at weaning in the rat. *Biochimie* 73, 71–76

Grapin-Botton, A., Majithia, A.R. and Melton, D.A. (2001) Key events of pancreas formation are triggered in gut endoderm by ectopic expression of pancreatic regulatory genes. *Genes and Development* 15, 44–54.

Gu, G., Brown, J.R. and Melton, D.A. (2003) Direct lineage tracing reveals the ontogeny of pancreatic cell fates during mouse embryogenesis. *Mechanisms of Development* 120, 35–43.

Hales, C.N. and Barker, D.J.P. (1992) Type 2 non-insulin-dependent diabetes mellitus: the thrifty phenotype hypothesis. *Diabetologia* 35, 595–601.

Hales, C.N., Desai, M., Ozanne, S.E. and Crowther, N.J. (1996) Fishing in the stream of diabetes: from measuring insulin to the control of fetal organogenesis. *Biochemical Society Transactions* 24, 341–350.

Hebrok, M., Kim, S.G. and Douglas, A.M. (1998) Notochord repression of endodermal Sonic hedgehog permits pancreas development. *Genes and Development* 12, 1705–1713.

Hellerström, C. (1979) Methods for large scale isolation of pancreatic islets by tissue culture of fetal rat pancreas. *Diabetes* 28, 769–776.

Hogg, J., Han, V.K.M., Clemmons, D. and Hill, D.J. (1993) Interactions of glucose, insulin like growth factors (IGFs) and IGF binding proteins in the regulation of DNA synthesis by isolated fetal rat islets of Langerhans. *Journal of Endocrinology* 138, 401–412.

Holness, M.J. (1996) Impact of early growth retardation on glucoregulatory control and insulin action in mature rats. *American Journal of Physiology* 270, E946–E954.

Holness, M.J. and Sugden, M.C. (1999) Antecedent protein restriction during early development of impaired insulin action after high-fat feeding. *American Journal of Physiology* 276, E85–E93.

Hughes, S.J. (1994) The role of reduced glucose transporter content and glucose metabolism in the immature secretory responses of fetal rat pancreatic islets. *Diabetologia* 37, 134–140.

Huxtable, R.J. (1992) Physiological actions of taurine. *Physiological Reviews* 72, 101–163.

Hyöty, H. and Taylor, K.W. (2002) The role of viruses in human diabetes. *Diabetologia* 45, 1353–1361.

Jung, Y., Miura, M. and Yuan, J. (1996) Suppression of Il-1β converting enzyme mediated cell death by insulin like growth factor. *Journal of Biological Chemistry* 271, 5112–5117.

Kahn, B.B. (1998) Type 2 diabetes: when insulin secretion fails to compensate for insulin resistance. *Cell* 92, 593–596.

Kalbe, L., Gesina, E., Dumontier, D., Merezak, S., Reusens, B. and Remade, C. (2003) The lower fetal beta-cell mass is differently programmed by maternal protein restriction and general food restriction in the rat. *Diabetologia* 46, A171.

Kaung, H.L. (1994) Growth dynamic of pancreatic islet cell population during fetal and neonatal development of the rat. *Developmental Dynamics* 200, 163–175.

Lammert, E., Cleaver, O. and Melton, D. (2001) Induction of pancreatic differentiation by signals from blood vessels. *Science* 294, 564–567.

Lammert, E., Cleaver, O. and Melton, D. (2003) Role of endothelial cells in early pancreas and liver development. *Mechanisms of Development* 120, 59–64.

Leclercq-Meyer, V., Considine, R.V., Sener, A. and Malaisse, W.J. (1996) Do leptin receptors play a functional role in the endocrine pancreas? *Biochemical and Biophysical Research Communications* 224, 522–527.

Lesage, J., Blondeau, B., Grino, M., Bréant, B. and Dupouy, J.P. (2001) Maternal undernutrition during gestation induces fetal overexpression to glucocorticoids and intrauterine growth retardation, and disturbs the hypothalamo-pituitary adrenal axis in the newborn rat. *Endocrinology* 142, 1692–1702.

Merezak, S., Hardikar, A., Yajnick, C.S., Remacle, C. and Reusens, B. (2001) Intraurerine low protein diet increases fetal β cell sensitivity to NO and IL-1-β: the protective role of taurine. *Journal of Endocrinology* 171, 299–308.

Merezak, S., Reusens, B., Ahn, M.T. and Remacle, C. (2002) Effect of low protein diet and taurine in early life on the sensitivity of adult islet to cytokines. *Diabetologia* 45, A 450.

Oberg, C., Waltenberger, J., Claesson-Welsh, C. and Welsh, M. (1994) Expression of protein kinase in islet cells: possible role of the Flk-1 receptor for β cell maturation from duct cells. *Growth Factors* 10(2), 115–126.

Oberg-Welsh, C., Sandler, S., Andersson, A. and Welsh, M. (1997) Effect of vascular endothelial growth factor on pancreatic duct cell replication and the insulin production of fetal islet-like clusters *in vitro*. *Molecular and Cellular Endocrinology* 126, 125–132.

Ozanne, S.E., Wang, C.L., Coleman, N. and Smith, G.D. (1996) Altered muscle insulin sensitivity in the male offspring of protein-malnourished rats. *American Journal of Physiology* 271, E1128–1134.

Ozanne, S.E., Nave, B.T., Wang, C.L., Shepherd, P.R., Prins, J. and Smith, G.D. (1997) Poor fetal nutrition causes long term changes in expression of insulin signaling components in adipocytes. *American Journal of Physiology* 273, E46–E51.

Ozanne, S.E., Wang, C.L., Dorling, M.W. and Petry, C.J. (1999) Dissection of the metabolic actions of insulin I in adipocytes from early growth retarded male rats. *Journal of Endocrinology* 162, 313–319.

Ozanne, S.E., Dorling, M.W., Wang, C.L. and Petry, C.J. (2000) Depot specific effects of early growth retardation on adipocyte insulin action. *Hormone and Metabolic Research* 32, 71–75.

Parsons, J.A., Brelje, T.C. and Sorenson, R.L. (1992) Adaptation of islets of Langerhans to pregnancy: increased islet cell proliferation and insulin secretion correlates with the onset of placental lactogen secretion. *Endocrinology* 130, 1459–1466.

Petrik, J., Arany, E., McDonald, T.J. and Hill, D.J. (1998) Apoptosis in the pancreatic islet cells of the neonatal is associated with a reduced expression of insulin-like growth factor II that may act as a survival factor. *Endocrinology* 139, 2994–3004.

Petrik, J., Reusens, B., Arany, E., Remacle, C., Coelho, C., Hoet, J.J. and Hill, D. (1999) A low protein diet alters the balance of islet cell replication and apoptosis in the fetal and neonatal rat and is associated with a reduced pancreatic expression of insulin-like growth factor II. *Endocrinology* 140, 4861–4873.

Petry, C.J., Ozanne, S.E. and Hales, C.N. (2001) Programming of intermediary metabolism. *Molecular and Cellular Endocrinology* 185, 81–91.

Poitout, V., Rouault, C., Guerre-Millo, M., Briaud, I. and Reach, G. (1998) Inhibition of insulin secretion by leptin in normal rodent islets of Langerhans. *Endocrinology* 139, 822–826.

Reusens, B. and Remacle, C. (2001a) Intergenerational effects of adverse intrauterine environment on perturbation of glucose metabolism. *Twin Research* 4, 406–411.

Reusens, B. and Remacle, C. (2001b) Effects of maternal nutrition and metabolism on the developing endocrine pancreas. In: Barker, D. (ed.) *Fetal Origins of Cardiovascular and Lung Disease*. Marcel Dekker, New York, pp. 339–358.

Reusens, B., Dahri, S., Snoeck, A., Bennis-Taleb, N., Remacle, C. and Hoet, J.J. (1995) Long-term consequences of diabetes and its complications may have a fetal origin: experimental evidence. In: Cowett, R.M. (ed.) *Diabetes*. Raven Press, New York, pp. 187–198.

Reusens, B., Hoet, J.J. and Remacle, C. (2000) Anatomy, developmental biology and pathology of the pancreatic islets. In: De Groot, L.J., Besser, M., Burger, H.G., Jameson, L.J., Loriaux, L.J., Marshall, J.C., Odell, W.D., Potts, J.T. and Rubenstein, A.H. (eds) *Endocrinology*. Saunders, Philadelphia, Pennsylvania, pp. 5024–5035.

Sandler, M. and German, S. (1997) The β cell transcriptor factors and the development of the pancreas. *Journal of Molecular Medicine* 75, 327–340.

Scaglia, L., Cahill, C.J., Finegood, D.T. and Bonner-Weir, S. (1997) Apoptosis participates in the remodelling of the endocrine pancreas in the neonatal rat. *Endocrinology* 138, 1736–1741.

Shepherd, P.R., Crowther, N.J., Desai, M. and Hales, C.N. (1997) Altered adipocyte properties in the offspring of protein malnourished rats. *British Journal of Nutrition* 78, 121–129.

Shepherd, P.R., Withers, D.J. and Siddle, K. (1998) Phosphoinositide 3-kinase: the key switch mechanism in insulin signalling. *Biochemical Journal* 333, 471–490.

Simmons, R.A., Templeton, L.J. and Gertz, S.J. (2001) Intrauterine growth retardation leads to the development of type 2 diabetes in rat. *Diabetes* 50, 2279–2286.

Snoeck, A., Remacle, C., Reusens, B. and Hoet, J.J. (1990) Effect of low protein diet during pregnancy on the fetal rat endocrine pancreas. *Biology of the Neonate* 57, 107–118.

Sorenson, R.L. and Brelje, T.C. (1997) Adaptation of islets of Langerhans to pregnancy: beta-cell growth enhanced insulin secretion and the role of lactogenic hormones. *Hormone and Metabolic Research* 29, 301–307.

Stoffers, D.A., Desai, B.M., DeLeon, D.D. and Simmons, R. (2003) Neonatal Exendin-4 prevents the development of diabetes in the intrauterine growth-retarded rat. *Diabetes* 52, 734–740.

Sturman, G.A. (1993) Taurine in development. *Physiological Reviews* 73, 119–147.

Sugden, M.C. and Holness, M.J. (2002) Gender-specific programming of insulin secretion and action. *Journal of Endocrinology* 175, 757–767.

Swenne, I., Bone, A.J., Howell, S.L. and Hellerström, C. (1980) Effects of glucose and amino acids on the biosynthesis of DNA and insulin in fetal rat islets maintained in tissue culture. *Diabetes* 29, 686–692.

Trudeau, J., Dutz, J.P., Arany, E., Hill, D., Fieldus, W. and Finegood, D. (2000) Perspectives in diabetes. Neonatal β cell apoptosis. A trigger for auto-immune diabetes. *Diabetes* 49, 1–7.

Turner, R., Stratton, I., Horton, V., Manley, S., Zimmet, P., Mackay, I.R., Shattock, M., Bottazzo, G.F. and Holman, R. (1997) UKPDS 25: autoantibodies to islet cell cytoplasm and glutamic acid decarboxylase for prediction of insulin requirement in type 2 diabetes. *Lancet* 350, 1288–1293.

Vickers, M.H., Breier, B.H., Cutfield, W.S., Hofman, P.L. and Gluckman, P.D. (2000) Fetal origin of hyperphagia, obesity and hypertension and its postnatal amplification by hypercaloric nutrition. *American Journal of Physiology* 279, 231–242.

Vickers, M.H., Reddy, S., Ikenasio, B.A. and Breier, B.H. (2001) Dysregulation of the adipoinsular axis – a mechanism for the pathogenesis of hyperleptinemia and adipogenic diabetes induced by fetal pogramming. *Journal of Endocrinology* 170, 323–332.

Weinkove, C., Weinkove, E.A. and Pimstone, B.L. (1974) Microassays for glucose and insulin. *South African Medical Journal* 48, 365–368.

White, M.S. and Myers, M.G. (2001) The molecular basis of insulin action. In: De Groot, L.J., Besser, M., Burger, H.G., Jameson, L.J., Loriaux, L.J., Marshall, J.C., Odell, W.D., Potts, J.T. and Rubenstein, A.H. (eds) *Endocrinology*. Saunders, Philadelphia, Pennsylvania, pp. 712–727.

Wilson, M.E., Scheel, D. and German, M.S. (2003) Gene expression cascades in pancreas development. *Mechanisms of Development* 120, 65–80.

Wilson, M.R. and Hughes, S.J. (1997) The effect of maternal protein deficiency during pregnancy and lactation on glucose tolerance and pancreatic islets function in adult rat offspring. *Journal of Endocrinology* 154, 177–185.

Winick, M. and Noble, A. (1966) Cellular response in rats during malnutrition at various ages. *Journal of Nutrition* 89, 300–306.

9 Birthweight and the Development of Overweight and Obesity

Department of International Health, Emory University, Rollins School of Public Health, Atlanta, GA 30322, USA

Introduction

This chapter will discuss the relation between size at birth, the most widely used marker of the outcome of growth during the 9 months of gestation, and size later in life, among humans. The starting point for this discussion is that the predominance of evidence (as described elsewhere in this book) suggests that birthweight, and perhaps specific exposures prior to birth, are consistently related to the development of a range of diseases. Lower birthweight is generally associated with increased risk, but is simply a marker of nutritional status around the time of birth and is not a critical causal factor. It is also abundantly clear that overweight and obesity are positively associated with the risk of these same diseases. This chapter will provide examples of the research we and others have conducted in this area, and relate the findings to the overall discussion of the importance in humans of early life experience to the development of adult disease. A separate chapter of this book (Chapter 10) reviews some of the animal evidence on this topic.

Overweight and Obesity

Obesity is an excess of body fat. The determination of the exact quantity and distribution of body fat in living persons is not feasible, and close approximations involve technology-intensive assessment methods (such as underwater weighing or its newer cousin, air-displacement plethysmography (the Bod-Pod®), dual-energy X-ray absorptiometry (DEXA) and others) that are not suitable for large-scale field-based studies. Typically, simple anthropometric methods are employed. Measurements are obtained of weight, height and selected skinfolds and circumferences, and these are converted by the use of calibration equations to derive indicators of adiposity. Of these, the most common are the body mass index (BMI, weight (in kg) divided by the square of height (in m)), and the ratio of the circumferences (in cm) at the waist and the hip (waist–hip ratio, WHR).

The BMI provides an overall indicator of excess body mass. In some individuals, particularly bodybuilders and professional athletes, a high value can reflect increased musculature, but, in general, higher BMI is highly correlated with excess adiposity measured against alternative approaches, and is only weakly correlated with height. This is true across global regions and ethnic groups, and for men and women. The World Health Organization has adopted a classification of nutritional status according to BMI (Table 9.1) (World Health Organization Consultation of Obesity, 1997).

The waist–hip ratio (WHR) provides an indicator of the distribution of body fat. Typically, men have a higher value than women. Within each gender, a higher ratio value indicates greater deposition of adipose tissue centrally, while a lower value suggests that any adipose tissue is deposited peripherally. It is generally accepted that central adipose tissue is more closely related to the aetiology of the metabolic diseases associated with insulin resistance (diabetes, hypertension, cardiovascular disease) than is excess peripheral adipose tissue (National Heart Lung and Blood Institute, 1998). Taken together, these two simple indicators (BMI and WHR) obtained from four anthropometric measurements, that may be readily obtained in both research and clinical settings, provide reproducible and standardized measures for epidemiological study and for clinical prediction and monitoring (National Heart Lung and Blood Institute, 1998).

Global Prevalence of Obesity and Underweight in Adulthood

Obesity is fast becoming a global epidemic (Popkin and Doak, 1998). In the USA, the prevalence of obesity exceeds 25%, and reaches 50% among African-American women (Flegal *et al.*, 2002). The prevalence of overweight and obesity has doubled since the early 1970s (Flegal *et al.*, 2002), and has increased by 61% since 1991 (Mokdad *et al.*, 2002). The longitudinal data available worldwide, with all the limitations inherent in these studies, suggest increases in the prevalence of overweight and obesity in all parts of the globe, among developed and developing countries alike (Martorell and Stein, 2001; Popkin, 2001). The rapidity of these changes strongly implicates adult factors, specifically sedentary lifestyles and excess caloric consumption, in this epidemic.

Table 9.1. WHO classification of nutritional status based on body mass index (World Health Organization Consultation of Obesity, 1997).

Undernourished	< 18.5 kg/m^2
Normal	≥ 18.5 kg/m^2 and < 25.0 kg/m^2
Overweight	≥ 25.0 kg.m^2 and < 30.0 kg/m^2
Grade 1 Obesity	≥ 30.0 kg/m^2 and < 35.0 kg/m^2
Grade 2 Obesity	≥ 35.0 kg/m^2 and < 40.0 kg/m^2
Grade 3 Obesity	≥ 40.0 kg/m^2

The obesity epidemic notwithstanding, adult chronic undernutrition continues to coexist with overweight and obesity, and continues to be prevalent in some South-East Asian countries and some regions of sub-Saharan Africa, such as Ethiopia (World Health Organization Consultation of Obesity, 1997).

Birthweight and Adult Overweight and Obesity

Observational data

The vast majority of studies that have related birthweight to measures of adiposity in later life (almost always BMI, but occasionally other measures) have reported a positive association. This literature has been reviewed elsewhere (Martorell *et al.*, 2001; Rogers, 2003). The correlations are modest, but are consistent across studies and populations. There is also a positive correlation between birthweight and adult height (Paz *et al.*, 1993), and an inverse correlation between birthweight and the WHR has been observed in several studies (e.g. Kuh *et al.*, 2002).

Much of the literature on size at birth and later outcomes, including overweight and obesity, is limited in the quality of the source measurements of size at birth. Birthweight is the most consistently available and reported measure. However, birthweight is a composite measure, as it reflects both length and ponderosity. These two components may be confidently predicted to differ in their associations with size later in life, and the inability to differentiate between them in some studies is likely to account for many inconsistencies in the literature.

What happens in twins?

Twins represent a special case of observational research where differences in size at birth can be particularly informative, as they share exposures that affect the mother's external environment. Monozygotic twins share complete genetic information, and hence any difference in size reflects variation in maternal nutritional supply to the two developing fetuses. Dizygotic twins are no more genetically alike than any other siblings, of course, and hence differences in size at birth reflect both nutrition and genetic potential. They do provide complete control for period effects in the life of the mother and age-related effects in the lives of the twins themselves.

In general, the results from the twin studies are supportive of data from studies of singletons. Overall, there is a positive association between birthweight and later BMI when twins are considered as individuals (Pietilainen *et al.*, 2001; Whitfield *et al.*, 2001). Loos *et al.* (2001a, 2002) observed that the twin heavier at birth will be taller and have a lower WHR than the lighter twin, with no additional effect of zygosity and chorionicity (Loos *et al.*, 2001b). However, a Swedish study found only a weak positive association between the within-pair difference in birthweight and later BMI, and then only in monozygotic twins (Johansson and Rasmussen, 2001).

Experimental data

The observational literature is limited in its ability to differentiate between the effects of nutrition and other causes of variation in birthweight on adult BMI and other markers of obesity. Animal experiments (such as those reviewed elsewhere in this book) are informative, but species specificity is always a concern, as are questions as to the relevance of the dose and the timing of any experimental manipulation to the human experience. Experimental studies in humans are, of course, the gold standard, but in this field are plagued with logistical and ethical constraints. Two sets of research data, one quasi-experimental and one truly experimental, address, at least in part, some of the constraints of the observational research. One approach is to study the consequences of naturally occurring severe food restriction, in the context of famine, while the other is to follow individuals who participated (either themselves, or by proxy due to their mother's participation while pregnant or lactating) in supplementation trials.

Famine

Famines provide a severe, indeed 'critical' (Susser, 1973) test of the hypothesis that maternal nutrition is the causal factor in the development of any long-term effect of birthweight on adult health status. Limitations of the study of famines include: (i) famines are unpredictable, so baseline data cannot readily be collected; (ii) most famines in recent times have been associated with major societal upheavals (war, revolution) and hence there are multiple exposures that cannot be completely disentangled; and (iii) most famines have occurred in societies where individuals cannot be traced through population registers or other approaches. The ability to trace cohorts exposed to two famines that occurred during the Second World War facilitated research that has addressed at least some of these limitations.

THE SIEGE OF LENINGRAD.   Between 1940 and 1942 the German army laid siege to the city of Leningrad (now St Petersburg). Tens of thousands of people died of starvation and of disease exacerbated by nutrient deficiencies. While the birth rate dropped precipitously, some pregnancies did occur and the mean birthweight dropped by 500 g.

Survivors of the siege were traced and studied in the mid-1990s, at which time they were in their mid-50s (Stanner et al., 1997). Three groups were studied. Group 1 were born prior to the onset of the siege, and hence were not exposed in utero but were exposed in early postnatal life. Group 2 were born during the siege, and Group 3 consisted of a control group of individuals born during the same period, but in areas under German control and hence not subject to famine. Groups 1 and 2 were recruited through survivor organizations, while Group 3 was recruited through general practitioners and work sites. Approximately 31% (361 of 1157) of those identified as being born before or during the siege or were studied successfully. Response rates for the 'place controls' were not provided. A comprehensive clinical examination of prevalence of cardiovascular disease and its risk factors was conducted. Few differences between the groups emerged. Of particular interest for this chapter is the comparison of various measures of body fat distribution. There was no difference in the distribution of BMI or of WHR across the three study groups (Table 9.2). There was a tendency for the ratio of the subscapular to triceps skinfolds to be lower in men born during the siege than in men born at the same time but outside Leningrad, while in women the reverse was true. There was no difference in height among the three groups.

THE DUTCH FAMINE. The Netherlands were invaded by Germany in the first years of the Second World War, and a stable civil administration was established and continued to function throughout the occupation period. Towards the end of the war, after the landing of Allied forces in Normandy in June 1944 and their advance northwards through France and Belgium, the Dutch readied themselves for liberation. In support of the Allied advance, the Dutch government in exile called for a rail strike. In retaliation, the Germans imposed a blockade on food transports. However, the Allied advance stalled at the Rhine, and the Allied troops continued their advance directly eastward, bypassing The Netherlands. However, even after the Germans lifted the food embargo, distribution did not return to normal, The winter of 1944/45 was particularly severe, and the Dutch canals froze in November. The food situation in the major urban areas of western Holland deteriorated rapidly. While a ration system had been functioning adequately for most of the war period, the reduced supplies meant that the *per capita* ration was progressively reduced, such that by October 1944 it went below 1000 kcal/day, and at times reached as low as 500 kcal/day, until the blockade was lifted with liberation on 8 May, 1945 and massive airdrops of food aid began. While additional rations were always provided for pregnant women and young children, the extent of redistribution within the household is not generally known.

The short duration of the famine (5–7 months, depending on one's definition) permits examination of potentially differing consequences of exposure to famine late in gestation and at or around conception. Exposure to famine in late gestation was strongly related to birthweight, which was not reduced by exposure in other trimesters (Smith, 1947). At the height of the famine, birthweights were reduced by up to 300 g. Indeed, there is some suggestion that birthweights

Table 9.2. Exposure to famine during the Siege of Leningrad and markers of adiposity at age 50 (from Stanner *et al.*, 1997).

		Born during famine (*n* = 169)	Born prior to famine (*n* = 192)	Born outside famine area (*n* = 188)
BMI	Men	24.6 (23.6–25.6)	25.4 (24.2–26.6)	25.2 (24.1–26.3)
(mean, 95% CI)	Women	26.9 (26.1–27.7)	27.0 (26.2–27.8)	26.7 (25.9–27.5)
Waist–hip ratio	Men	0.86 (0.84–0.88)	0.88 (0.84–0.92)	0.87 (0.85–0.89)
(mean, 95% CI)	Women	0.79 (0.77–0.81)	0.78 (0.76–0.80)	0.79 (0.75–0.83)
Subscapular:triceps	Men	1.26 (1.11–1.41)	1.32 (1.20–1.44)	1.41 (1.31–1.51)
skinfolds ratio	Women	1.01 (0.93–1.09)	0.93 (0.87–0.99)	0.88 (0.82–0.94)

BMI, body mass index; CI, confidence interval.

were elevated among those conceived during the famine, who were not subject to food restriction in late gestation.

The specific circumstances of the Dutch famine have lent themselves to several investigations of the long-term impact. The first team to do so related data collected at military conscription at age 18 (Ravelli *et al.*, 1976). While restricted by design to males (women in The Netherlands are not subject to conscription), this study benefited from national coverage, full compliance, and standardized and systematic assessment. Among these men, the prevalence of overweight (using 120% of the Metropolitan Life Insurance Company relative weight for height as the threshold) was elevated, from 1.5% to 3%, among conscripts who had had at least some exposure in the middle trimester (Fig. 9.1). The authors interpreted this as due to an effect of the famine on perturbation of hypothalamic function.

Two studies have followed famine-exposed cohorts through to later life. For a study with a primary focus on reproductive outcomes, Lumey *et al.* (1993) traced a cohort of women who had all been born at the Wilhelmina Gasthuis, the maternity hospital of the University of Amsterdam, in the period before, during and after the famine. These women were interviewed in their homes, and reported their own heights and weights, as well as their weight at age 18. Height was unrelated to famine exposure, while weight at both age 18 and at interview (at mean age 43 years) was increased among women exposed to famine in their first trimester of gestation (Ravelli *et al.*, 1992).

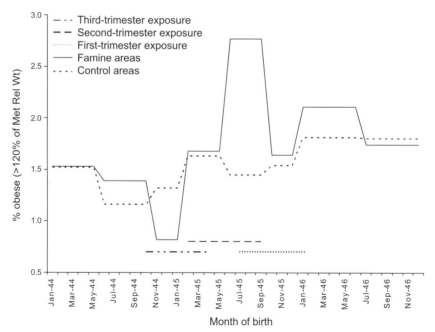

Fig. 9.1.   Exposure to famine *in utero* and obesity at age 18. Met Rel Wt, Metropolitan Life Insurance Company relative weight for height. (Drawn from data in Ravelli *et al.*, 1976.)

Subsequently, this study population was enriched with a comparable cohort of men born in the same hospital, and the men and women were invited to attend a clinical examination (Ravelli *et al.*, 1999). A total of 741 men and women participated, of whom approximately 68–120 were exposed in each trimester. Exposure to famine in the first trimester was associated with increased weight, and hence BMI, in women, but not in men, and there was no effect of famine exposure in other trimesters (Table 9.3). After adjustment for covariates, including BMI, there was a slight tendency for WHR to be elevated among both men and women exposed in early gestation.

Taken together, these studies suggest that exposure to famine early in gestation does indeed increase the risk for obesity later in life. This finding is most robust among the conscripts, primarily due to the large sample size. The two other studies provided estimates somewhat in conflict with the data from the conscripts with respect to the timing of the effect, and the Ravelli paper did not find any effect in men, but small sample sizes in each exposure cohort resulted in imprecise estimates of effect.

All of these studies are subject to one potentially fatal flaw. As noted by Stein *et al.* (1975), conception rates declined in the famine period, more dramatically among the manual labouring classes. To the extent that the outcome of interest is related to social class of the parents rather than to nutrition *per se*, confounding might result. An example of this is clearly seen in the data on mental performance among the recruits (Stein *et al.*, 1972). A substantial improvement in the scores on Raven's Progressive Matrices, a test of pattern recognition that is widely used as a formal test of intelligence, was observed among recruits conceived during the famine. This could be completely explained by the father's occupation. Presumably, wealthier families retained adequate resources to maintain levels of nutrition compatible with fecundity even at the height of the famine, to a greater extent than did the families where the main breadwinner was a labourer.

Nutritional supplementation

Clearly, caloric restriction prior to or during pregnancy cannot be contemplated in experimental research in humans. However, the reverse, of supplementing

Table 9.3. Exposure to the Dutch Famine of 1944/45 among births at the Wilhelmina Gasthuis, Amsterdam, and adult body size (from Ravelli *et al.*, 1999).

	Exposure to famine				
	Born before ($n = 210$)	Late gestation ($n = 120$)	Mid-gestation ($n = 110$)	Early gestation ($n = 68$)	Conceived after ($n = 233$)
Weight (kg)	79.0	79.0	76.8	84.2	80.6
Height (cm)	171.0	170.9	168.6	171.0	170.9
BMI (kg/m^2)	26.7	26.7	26.6	28.1	27.2
Overweight (%)	65	63	64.6	75	67
WHR	0.87	0.88	0.87	0.88	0.88

BMI, body mass index; WHR, waist–hip ratio.

undernourished women with food or specific nutrients, is relatively standard practice. While the focus of most supplementation research has been on the short-term outcomes of birthweight and child development, a few studies have now been followed for long enough to enable study of the effects into adulthood. Our research group, for example, has been following the participants of the INCAP Longitudinal Study, a community-randomized controlled trial of nutritional supplementation in Guatemala conducted between 1969 and 1977 (Martorell *et al.*, 1995). The original focus of the study was to test the hypothesis that improved protein–energy nutrition, during pregnancy and the first 7 years of life, would result in improved mental performance. Secondary hypotheses related to the effect of this nutritional supplementation on growth and physical development.

In the study, four villages, stratified by size (two large and two small), were randomized to receive either Atole or Fresco supplement. Atole was a high-energy, high-protein supplement, which contained 91 kcal of energy and 6.4 g protein per 100 ml, whereas Fresco contained 33 kcal of energy per 100 ml and no protein. Both Atole and Fresco were fortified with vitamins and minerals. Supplement type was assigned at random, with village as the unit of randomization. The target population of the intervention was pregnant or lactating women and children up to age 7 years. Both supplements were available year-round, and consumption was *ad libitum*. Supplements were distributed and consumed twice daily in a centrally located feeding hall in each village. Supplement intake to the nearest 10 ml was recorded for all pregnant and lactating women and their offspring up to age 7 years. Heights and weights of the mothers and children were recorded at select intervals, including birth.

We have conducted several rounds of follow-up among this cohort. In 1988, when many were still adolescents, we showed that growth was improved among those who received Atole in the first 3 years of childhood (Schroeder *et al.*, 1995; Schroeder and Martorell, 1999). Within the randomized design of the study there was no effect of supplementation type on birthweight, but a within-treatment analysis, in which the (self-selected) quantity of supplement was related to birth size, suggested an effect of energy intake, with no added effect of the protein in the Atole supplement. There was an increase in fat-free mass in adolescence among those receiving Atole (Rivera *et al.*, 1995), although the analysis was complicated by the need to take into account the age range of the cohort.

By 1996, when the next wave of data collection commenced, all the cohort members had reached adulthood and adult stature. We measured adult anthropometry in the context of a study of pregnancy, reproductive outcomes, and child development conducted among women resident in the four study villages between 1996 and 1999, and a survey of cardiovascular disease risk factors conducted among male and female cohort members living in the study villages or in Guatemala City. At a simplistic level, we observed a crude association between birthweight and BMI (Stein *et al.*, 2002).

We recently assessed the role of growth in stature in three phases (prenatal life, the first 2 years, and the period from age 2 to adulthood), in influencing adult body composition in 267 members of the original cohort (Li *et al.*, 2003).

As the three growth periods are correlated, we used a multiple-stage least squares regression approach to ensure independence of effects. Briefly, a model was developed in which period 1 growth was regressed on period 2 growth, and the residual retained. This residual became the independent effect of period 2. This process was repeated for period 3, resulting in three variables that were orthogonal to each other. We considered measures of length, weight and ponderosity at birth, and a wide array of measures of adiposity, including fat-free mass and fat mass, derived from prediction equations developed for this population using hydrostatic weighting.

We found that birth size (weight or length) and length at age 2 were independently related to attained height, weight and fat-free mass in both men and women (Table 9.4). Ponderal index at birth was not associated with any anthropometric measure in adulthood, suggesting that the main determinant of adult anthropometry was prenatal growth in length rather than weight per se. Neither size at birth nor size at 2 years was associated with the WHR. In general, measures of growth from birth to age 2 were more strongly associated with adult anthropometry than were birth measures.

Tracking of Overweight/Obesity throughout Childhood

A vast literature has documented that measures of overweight and obesity 'track' (i.e. maintain relative rank order) from early childhood through to adulthood (Charney et al., 1976; Guo et al., 1994; Whitaker et al., 1997; Qing and Karlberg, 1999). This phenomenon is usually interpreted as evidence of the need to intervene early in life to prevent the development of intractable obesity later in life (National Heart Lung and Blood Institute, 1998). The degree of tracking (usually measured in terms of the correlation between measures at two points in time) increases with increasing age at the younger of the two time points. Infant obesity is only modestly predictive of overweight later in life, unless one or both parents are obese, but as children reach adolescence, obesity appears to become established, and in the absence of treatment and modification, continues to track.

Table 9.4. Effects of prenatal and postnatal growth on adult anthropometry (effect sizes per 1 SD in each determinant, 95% confidence intervals) among 267 men and women followed prospectively in Guatemala (from Li et al., 2003).

Adult	Men (n = 136)		Women (n = 131)	
	Length at birth (1 SD = 2.3 cm)	Growth from birth to 2 years (1 SD = 1.9 cm)	Length at birth (1 SD = 3.5 cm)	Growth from birth to 2 years (1 SD = 2.8 cm)
Height (cm)	2.8 (1.9–3.6)	2.7 (1.9–3.6)	1.5 (0.8–2.1)	2.2 (1.4–3.1)
Weight (kg)	1.5 (0.5–2.6)	3.1 (1.4–4.4)	2.6 (0.7–4.4)	3.5 (1.7–5.4)
Fat-free mass (kg)	1.7 (1.0–2.4)	2.0 (1.1–3.0)	0.9 (0.1–1.7)	1.7 (1.0–2.4)
Fat mass (kg)	−0.05 (−0.6–0.5)	1.1 (0.4–1.8)	1.6 (0.4–2.8)	1.9 (0.6–2.4)
% Body fat	−0.4 (−1.1–0.4)	1.0 (0.1–2.0)	1.3 (0.2–2.3)	1.2 (0.1–2.2)

Horse racing

The literature on the association between birthweight and later BMI is consistent with a phenomenon characterized as 'horse-racing' (Peto, 1981). Birth is but one point along the continuum of growth and development. If one considers growth to start at conception, and to occur at different rates for different people (determined, presumably, by the interaction between genetic potential, maternal body size and nutrition, prenatal factors such as placentation and exposure to toxins, and postnatal factors such as nutrition and burden of infection), then it is clear that rank order in size (the representation at a single point in time of the cumulative process of growth until that time) will correlate across any two time periods, including birth and adulthood (Fig. 9.2).

This model also explains why the tracking correlation coefficients increase as the study cohort ages – there is simply more variance at older ages, and hence less likelihood that measurement and other sources of error will outweigh the true signal. If, however, we consider tracking to be normal, what is, in fact, of interest is perturbation of tracking. In other words, if tracking is to be expected, then a positive association between size at birth and size later in life is not of clinical or epidemiological significance (Hofman and Valkenburg, 1983; Shea *et al.*, 1998). Indeed, the research team following the Helsinki birth cohort, who has available multiple measures of height and weight in childhood, has shown that specific aberrant patterns of growth are associated with the later development of adult disease (Eriksson *et al.*, 1999). These analyses do not, in themselves, address the question of the causal role of birth size on adult obesity, but do strongly suggest that postnatal growth and birth size need to be considered in models more complex than first-order linear regressions.

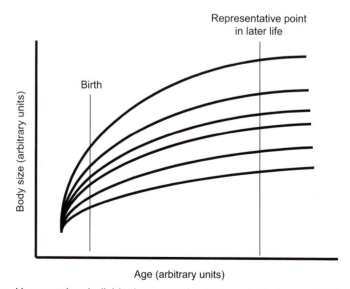

Fig. 9.2. Horse-racing: individuals start at the same point but grow at different rates, thus differences become established early in life and track thereafter.

Modifiability of Association – the Role of Breastfeeding

A growing body of evidence is suggesting that breastfeeding is associated with lower risk of overweight and obesity in later life (Kramer, 1981; Gillman *et al.*, 2001; Liese *et al.*, 2001; Martorell *et al.*, 2001; Armstrong and Reilly, 2002). Martin *et al.* (2002) have observed that breastfeeding is also associated with increased stature as adults, although they note that both breastfeeding and stature are strongly related to social class, and thus confounding by unmeasured factors also associated with social class is possible. This is despite the fact that in the first few months of life breastfed infants are typically heavier than bottle-fed infants (Cole *et al.*, 2002), and the finding also appears to be independent of birthweight. Prolonged breastfeeding, which is not the norm in the USA or Great Britain, may be required to reap the full benefit (Elliott *et al.*, 1997). The mechanism for the benefit is as yet unclear. It has been suggested that breastfed infants are better able to regulate intakes and recognize signs of satiety (Dewey, 2003).

Birthweight, Adult BMI and Research into the Early Origins of Disease

Much of the literature relating birthweight to the development of hypertension, type 2 diabetes mellitus or cardiovascular disease has noted that the inverse association commonly observed is only apparent, or is stronger, when current measures of adiposity (usually BMI) are 'controlled for' in multiple regression models. Examples include the data from the US Nurses' Health Study (Curhan *et al.*, 1996), among many others. There has long been debate as to the implications of such 'adjusted birthweights' for both future explanatory research and for public health.

From a purely statistical argument, adding an additional variable, assuming other conditions of the model hold, implies that this parameter is 'held constant' when evaluating the impact of the first variable. Thus, the interpretation of the birthweight coefficient in a model with birthweight, adult BMI and adult blood pressure levels would be the change in blood pressure conditional upon a unit change in birthweight (typically 1 kg), among people of the same adult BMI. However, as individuals of low birthweight and high birthweight have travelled along different trajectories to get to be the same BMI in adulthood, the interpretation of the coefficients is not straightforward, and is critically dependent on several factors. These are the true overall effect of birthweight on the outcome of interest, the true association between birth size and adult adiposity, the true association between adult adiposity and the outcome of interest and, finally, the extent of measurement error in each of these variables.

Several investigators have attempted to specify the statistical and physiological interpretation of a regression model including both birthweight and a measure of adiposity later in life. Lucas *et al.* (1999) in an often-cited paper, develop an argument that what is needed is an interaction term between the early life measure and the later measure. They suggest that this interaction term can be interpreted as the effect of the change in status over time, and that, if serial measures of body size are available, one can assess when the effect of body size on the endpoint of interest 'flips' from being inverse to being positive. Recently, this approach has been applied to the British 1958 Birth Cohort Study (Hypponen *et al.*, 2003).

Catch-up growth and percentile rank change

One issue that needs to be mentioned here is that of 'catch-up' growth. This term, originally invoked to include only the short-term recovery from short-term faltering of an individual's growth line following acute illness (Mata *et al.*, 1972), has more recently been used to denote any upward changing of percentile ranking (Eriksson *et al.*, 1999; Adair and Cole, 2003). As the ideal growth pattern of children has not been determined (growth curves in current use portray percentiles based on statistical norms rather than prescriptive values), use of 'catch-up growth' as a category implies that the growth in the earlier period was inadequate and that the child has now resumed 'normal growth'. However, merely considering change in rank order rather than inclusion of a baseline would imply that a child born at the 50th percentile who has grown to reach the 80th percentile would also be considered to have experienced catch-up growth. This distinction also highlights the need to consider relations between birth size, adult size and adult health outcome separately for countries or populations with a high prevalence of low birthweight and postnatal growth failure. In these (typically developing country) settings, catch-up growth is a requirement for short-term survival (Victora *et al.*, 2001), and there has not yet been widespread development of childhood obesity (Martorell *et al.*, 2000).

Implications for Public Health Policies and Programmes

The global epidemic of obesity is clearly multifactorial in origin. While there is substantial evidence that birthweight and later overweight and obesity are statistically associated, the causal role of birthweight (as distinct from its role as a marker of growth *in utero*) is unclear. It is hard to imagine a scenario in which public health advocates would work for a reduction in birthweight in order to combat adult-onset obesity. A shift of the birthweight distribution to the left would be associated with vastly increased short-term risks to the larger numbers of infants who would be born at low birthweight.

Much of the evidence to date stresses that it is infants who fail to grow along their established rank percentile who are at particular risk. Those who drop percentile rankings are at increased short-term risk of illness and death. Those whose growth curves suggest an increase in percentile rank are at particular risk for the development of early-onset obesity, diabetes and hypertension. Taken together, these findings reinforce the need for children in developing and in developed countries to continue to have their growth monitored at regular intervals and for changes in growth rank to be detected and the reasons identified.

The best evidence to date suggests that breastfeeding is associated with lower rates of obesity in childhood and adolescence (Dewey, 2003). Exclusive breastfeeding to at least 4 months, and continued breastfeeding to 12 or even 24 months, have multiple benefits to the child and to the mother, and should be encouraged regardless of the long-term effects on obesity. To the extent that there is a causal role for breastfeeding in the prevention of obesity, this is merely another reason among many, that may be of particular salience to upper- and middle-class women in developed and developing countries, who may be particularly responsive to health messages concerning the long-term risks associated with obesity in their children.

References

Adair, L.S. and Cole, T.J. (2003) Rapid child growth raises blood pressure in adolescent boys who were thin at birth. *Hypertension* 41, 451–456.

Armstrong, J. and Reilly, J.J. (2002) Breastfeeding and lowering the risk of childhood obesity. *Lancet* 359, 2003–2004.

Charney, E., Goodman, H.C., McBride, M., Lyon, B. and Pratt, R. (1976) Childhood antecedents of adult obesity: do chubby infants become obese adults? *New England Journal of Medicine* 295, 6–9.

Cole, T.J., Paul, A.A. and Whitehead, R.G. (2002) Weight reference charts for British long-term breastfed infants. *Acta Paediatrica* 91, 1296–1300.

Curhan, G.C., Chertow, G.M., Willett, W.C., Spiegelman, D., Colditz, G.A., Manson, J.E., Speizer, F.E. and Stampfer, M.J. (1996) Birth weight and adult hypertension and obesity in women. *Circulation* 94, 1310–1315.

Dewey, K.G. (2003) Is breastfeeding protective against child obesity? *Journal of Human Lactation* 19, 9–18.

Elliott, K.G., Kjolhede, C.L., Gournis, E. and Rasmussen, K.M. (1997) Duration of breastfeeding associated with obesity during adolescence. *Obesity Research* 5, 538–541.

Eriksson, J.G., Forsen, T., Tuomilehto, J., Winter, P.D., Osmond, C. and Barker, D.J.P. (1999) Catch-up growth in childhood and death from coronary heart disease: longitudinal study. *British Medical Journal* 318, 427–431.

Flegal, K.M., Carroll, M.D., Ogden, C.L. and Johnson, C.L. (2002) Prevalence and trends in obesity among US adults, 1999–2000. *Journal of the American Medical Association* 288, 1723–1727.

Gillman, M.W., Rifas-Shiman, S.L., Camargo, C.A. Jr, Berkey, C.S., Frazier, A.L., Rockett, H.R., Field, A.E. and Colditz, G.A. (2001) Risk of overweight among adolescents who were breastfed as infants. *Journal of the American Medical Association* 285, 2461–2467.

Guo, S.S., Roche, A.F., Chumlea, W.C., Gardner, J.D. and Siervogel, R.M. (1994) The predictive value of childhood body mass index values for overweight at age 35 y. *American Journal of Clinical Nutrition* 59, 810–819.

Hofman, A. and Valkenburg, H.A. (1983) Determinants of change in blood pressure during childhood. *American Journal of Epidemiology* 117, 735–743.

Hypponen, E., Power, C. and Davey-Smith, G. (2003) Prenatal growth, BMI, and risk of type 2 diabetes by early midlife. *Diabetes Care* 26, 2512–2517.

Johansson, M. and Rasmussen, F. (2001) Birthweight and body mass index in young adulthood: the Swedish young male twins study. *Twin Research* 4, 400–405.

Kramer, M.S. (1981) Do breast-feeding and delayed introduction of solid foods protect against subsequent obesity? *Journal of Pediatrics* 98, 883–887.

Kuh, D., Hardy, R., Chaturvedi, N. and Wadsworth, M.E.J. (2002) Birth weight, childhood growth and abdominal obesity in adult life. *International Journal of Obesity* 26, 40–47.

Li, H., Stein, A.D., Barnhart, H.X., Torun, B., Ramakrishnan, U. and Martorell, R. (2003) Prenatal and postnatal growth retardation and adult body size and composition. *American Journal of Clinical Nutrition* 77, 1498–1505.

Liese, A.D., Hirsch, T., von Mutius, E., Keil, U., Leupold, W. and Weiland, S.K. (2001) Inverse association of overweight and breast feeding in 9- to 10-y-old children in Germany. *International Journal of Obesity and Related Metabolic Disorders* 25, 1644–1650.

Loos, R.J., Beunen, G., Fagard, R., Derom, C. and Vlietinck, R. (2001a) Birth weight and body composition in young adult men – a prospective twin study. *International Journal of Obesity and Related Metabolic Disorders* 25, 1537–1545.

Loos, R.J., Beunen, G., Fagard, R., Derom, C. and Vlietinck, R. (2001b) The influence of zygosity and chorion type on fat distribution in young adult twins: consequences for twin studies. *Twin Research* 4, 356–364.

Loos, R.J., Beunen, G., Fagard, R., Derom, C. and Vlietinck, R. (2002) Birth weight and body composition in young women: a prospective twin study. *American Journal of Clinical Nutrition* 75, 676–682.

Lucas, A., Fewtrell, M.S. and Cole, T.J. (1999) Fetal origins of adult disease – the hypothesis revisited. *British Medical Journal* 319, 245–249.

Lumey, L.H., Ravelli, A.C., Wiessing, L.G., Koppe, J.G., Treffers, P.E. and Stein, Z.A. (1993) The Dutch famine birth cohort study: design, validation of exposure, and selected characteristics of subjects after 43 years follow-up. *Paediatric Perinatology and Epidemiology* 7, 354–367.

Martin, R.M., Davey-Smith, G., Mangtani, P., Fankel, S. and Gunnell, D. (2002) Association between breast feeding and growth: the Boyd–Orr cohort study. *Archives of Disease in Childhood Fetal and Neonatal Edition* 87, F193–F201.

Martorell, R. and Stein, A.D. (2001) The emergence of diet-related chronic diseases in developing countries. In: Bowman, B. and Russell, R. (eds) *Present Knowledge in Nutrition*, 8th edn. International Life Sciences Institute, Washington, DC.

Martorell, R., Habicht, J.P. and Rivera, J.A. (1995) History and design of the INCAP longitudinal study (1969–77) and its follow-up (1988–89). *Journal of Nutrition* 125 (suppl.), 1027S–1041S.

Martorell, R., Kettel Khan, L., Hughes, M.L. and Grummer-Strawn, L.M. (2000) Overweight and obesity in preschool children from developing countries. *International Journal of Obesity and Related Metabolic Disorders* 24, 959–967.

Martorell, R., Stein, A.D. and Schroeder, D.G. (2001) Early nutrition and later adiposity. *Journal of Nutrition* 131, 874S–880S.

Mata, L.J., Urrutia, J.J., Albertazzi, C., Pellecer, O. and Arellano, E. (1972) Influence of recurrent infections on nutrition and growth of children in Guatemala. *American Journal of Clinical Nutrition* 25, 1267–1275.

Mokdad, A.L., Ford, E.S., Bowman, B.A., Dietz, W.H., Vinicor, F., Bales, V.S. and Marks, J.S. (2002) Prevalence of obesity, diabetes, and obesity-related health risk factors, 2003. *Journal of the American Medical Association* 289, 76–79.

National Heart Lung and Blood Institute (1998) *Clinical Guidelines on the Identification, Evaluation, and Treatment of Overweight and Obesity in Adults*. NIH Publication No. 98–4083. National Heart, Lung, and Blood Institute, Washington, DC.

Paz, I., Seidman, D., Danon, Y.L., Laor, A., Stevenson, D.K. and Gale, R. (1993) Are children born small for gestational age at increased risk of short stature? *American Journal of Diseases in Childhood* 147, 337–339.

Peto, R. (1981) The horse-racing effect. *Lancet* 2, 467–468.

Pietilainen, K.H., Kaprio, J., Rasanen, M., Winter, T., Rissanen, A. and Rose, R.J. (2001) Tracking of body size from birth to late adolescence: contributions of birth length, birth weight, duration of gestation, parents' body size, and twinship. *American Journal of Epidemiology* 154, 21–29.

Popkin, B.M. (2001) The nutrition transition and obesity in the developing world. *Journal of Nutrition* 131, 871S–873S.

Popkin, B.M. and Doak, C.M. (1998) The obesity epidemic is a worldwide phenomenon. *Nutrition Reviews* 56, 106–114.

Qing, H. and Karlberg, J. (1999) Prediction of adult overweight during the pediatric years. *Pediatric Research* 46, 697.

Ravelli, A.C.J., Stam, G.A., Stein, Z.A. and Lumey, L.H. (1992) Birthweight, adult weight and offspring birthweight after in-utero exposure to the Dutch famine of 1944–1945. *Journal of Perinatal Medicine* 20(suppl. 1), 205.

Ravelli, A.C., van Der Meulen, J.H., Osmond, C., Barker, D.J. and Bleker, O.P. (1999) Obesity at the age of 50 y in men and women exposed to famine prenatally. *American Journal of Clinical Nutrition* 70, 811–816.

Ravelli, G.P., Stein, Z.A. and Susser, M.W. (1976) Obesity in young men after famine exposure in utero and early infancy. *New England Journal of Medicine* 295, 349–353.

Rivera, J.A., Martorell, R., Ruel, M.T., Habicht, J.P. and Haas, J.D. (1995) Nutritional supplementation during the preschool years influences body size and composition of Guatemalan adolescents. *Journal of Nutrition* 125 (suppl.), 1068S–1077S.

Rogers, I. (2003) The influence of birthweight and intrauterine environment on adiposity and at distribution in later life. *International Journal of Obesity and Related Metabolic Disorders* 27, 755–777.

Schroeder, D.G. and Martorell, R. (1999) Fatness and body mass index from birth to young adulthood in a rural Guatemalan population. *American Journal of Clinical Nutrition* 70, 137S–144S.

Schroeder, D.G., Martorell, R., Rivera, J.A., Ruel, M.T. and Habicht, J.P. (1995) Age differences in the impact of nutritional supplementation on growth. *Journal of Nutrition* 125(suppl.), 1051S–1059S.

Shea, S., Rabinowitz, D., Stein, A.D. and Basch, C.E. (1998) Components of variability in the systolic blood pressures of preschool children. *American Journal of Epidemiology* 147, 240–249.

Smith, C.A. (1947) Effects of wartime starvation in Holland on pregnancy and its products. *American Journal of Obstetrics and Gynecology* 53, 599–608.

Stanner, S.A., Bulmer, K., Andres, C., Lantseva, O.E., Borodina, V., Pteen, V.V. and Yudkin, J.S. (1997) Does malnutrition in utero determine diabetes and coronary heart disease in adulthood? Results from the Leningrad siege study, a cross sectional study. *British Medical Journal* 315, 1342–1349.

Stein, A.D., Conlisk, A.J., Torun, B., Schroeder, D.G., Grajeda, R. and Martorell, R. (2002) Cardiovascular disease risk factors are related to adult adiposity but not birth weight in young Guatemalan adults. *Journal of Nutrition* 132, 2208–2214.

Stein, Z., Susser, M., Saenger, G. and Marolla, F. (1972) Nutrition and mental performance. *Science* 178, 708–713.

Stein, Z., Susser, M., Saenger, G. and Marolla, F. (1975) *Famine and Human Development*. Oxford University Press, New York.

Susser, M. (1973) *Causal Thinking in the Health Sciences: Concepts and Strategies in Epidemiology.* Oxford University Press, New York.

Victora, C.G., Barros, F.C., Horta, B.L. and Martorell, R. (2001) Short-term benefits of catch-up growth for small-for-gestational-age infants. *International Journal of Epidemiology* 30, 1325–1330.

Whitaker, R.C., Wright, J.A., Pepe, M.S., Seidel, K.D. and Dietz, W.H. (1997) Predicting obesity in young adulthood from childhood and parental obesity. *New England Journal of Medicine* 337, 869–873.

Whitfield, J.B., Treloar, S.A., Zhu, G. and Martin, N.G. (2001) Genetic and non-genetic factors affecting birth-weight and adult body mass index. *Twin Research* 4, 365–370.

World Health Organization Consultation of Obesity (1997) *Preventing and Managing the Global Epidemic of Obesity.* Report of the World Health Organization Consultation of Obesity. WHO, Geneva.

10 Maternal Nutrition in Pregnancy and Adiposity in Offspring

BERNHARD H. BREIER, STEFAN O. KRECHOWEC AND MARK H. VICKERS

Liggins Institute for Medical Research, Faculty of Medical and Health Sciences, University of Auckland, Private Bag 92019, Grafton, Auckland, New Zealand

Introduction

There is increasing evidence that metabolic and cardiovascular diseases which commonly manifest in adult life have their roots before birth. The 'fetal origins of adult disease' (FOAD) or 'fetal programming' paradigm is based on the observation that environmental changes can reset the developmental path during intrauterine development, leading to obesity and cardiovascular and metabolic disorders later in life. This pathogenesis is not based on genetic defects but on altered genetic expression, seen as a result of fetal adaptation to adverse intrauterine influences. After initial controversy when these relationships were first suggested, both prospective clinical and experimental studies have clearly shown that the propensity to develop abnormalities of cardiovascular, endocrine and metabolic homeostasis in adulthood are increased when fetal development has been adversely affected (Barker, 2000; Godfrey and Barker, 2000).

The mechanisms underlying fetal programming and the relative role of genetic versus environmental factors remain speculative. One general thesis is that in response to an adverse intrauterine environment the fetus adapts its physiological development to maximize its immediate chances for survival. These adaptations may include resetting of metabolic homeostasis and endocrine systems and the down-regulation of growth, commonly reflected in altered birth phenotype. This prenatal plasticity of the fetus may allow environmental factors to alter the physiological function of the conceptus in preparation for suboptimal environmental conditions after birth. It is thought that while these changes in fetal physiology may be beneficial for short-term survival *in utero*, they may be maladaptive in postnatal life, contributing to poor health outcomes when offspring are exposed to catch-up growth, diet-induced obesity and other factors (Gluckman, 2001).

Experimental Evidence for Fetal Programming of Obesity

Animal models have been used extensively to investigate the basic physiological principles of the FOAD hypothesis. The variety of models that have been developed is essential to the search for the mechanistic links between prenatal and postnatal influences and the pathophysiological complications in later life. Although epidemiological data suggest that fetal programming occurs within the normal range of birth size (Barker, 1998), most experimental work has tended to focus on significant restriction of fetal growth, in the assumption that the nature of the insults that impair fetal growth are likely to be those that trigger fetal programming. Alterations in maternal nutrition are commonly used experimentally to induce intrauterine growth retardation (IUGR), as it is an experimentally practical and reproducible way to induce nutrient limitation to the fetus and thus change its developmental trajectory. In this context, IUGR is not essential to fetal programming, but is merely a surrogate for evidence that fetal development may have been affected.

Several animal models of early growth restriction have been developed in an attempt to elucidate its relationship with adult-onset disease and provide a framework for investigating the underlying mechanisms. In rats hypertension, insulin resistance and obesity have been induced in offspring by maternal undernutrition (Woodall *et al.*, 1996a,b; Vickers *et al.*, 2000), a low-protein diet (Langley-Evans *et al.*, 1996), maternal uterine artery ligation (Rajakumar *et al.*, 1998), maternal dexamethasone (DEX) treatment (Nyirenda *et al.*, 1998) or prenatal exposure to the cytokines interleukin (IL)-6 and tumour necrosis factor (TNF)-α (Dahlgren *et al.*, 2001). Studies in rats fed a low-protein diet during pregnancy indicate that increased levels of insulin receptors in adipocytes or enhanced insulin sensitivity of adipocytes can be observed in programmed offspring (Ozanne *et al.*, 1997). As discussed below, we have shown, in the rat, that feeding offspring of undernourished mothers a hypercaloric diet amplifies prenatal influences on hypertension, hyperinsulinaemia and obesity (Vickers *et al.*, 2000, 2001a,b).

There are also increasing experimental data in other species. In guinea-pigs, IUGR caused by uterine artery ligation or maternal undernutrition results in reduced glucose tolerance, increased sensitivity to cholesterol loading (Kind *et al.*, 1999) and elevated blood pressure in offspring (Persson and Jansson, 1992). DEX treatment of pregnant ewes in early gestation results in elevated blood pressure (Dodic *et al.*, 1999) and altered regulation of lipolysis (Gatford *et al.*, 2000) in the adult offspring. Recent work by Bispham *et al.* (2003) has shown that, irrespective of maternal nutrition in late gestation, fetuses sampled from ewes with nutrient restriction in early gestation possessed more adipose tissue, whereas when ewes were fed to appetite throughout gestation, fetal adipose tissue deposition and leptin mRNA abundance were both reduced. These changes suggested that offspring of nutrient-restricted mothers were at increased risk of developing obesity in later life. This study also suggested that the increased incidence of obesity in adults born to mothers exposed to the Dutch famine during early pregnancy (Roseboom *et al.*, 2000) may be a direct consequence of adaptations in the endocrine sensitivity of fetal adipose tissue (Bispham *et al.*, 2003).

The exact nature of the maternal factors that change prenatal development and determine postnatal pathophysiology remains uncertain. In particular, the extent to which fetal adipose tissue can be re-programmed as a consequence of altered maternal nutrition has not been elucidated (Bispham *et al.*, 2003). Most experimental studies have focused on either altered maternal nutrition or increased glucocorticoid exposure. It has been argued that maternal nutrition is not a limiting factor for human fetal growth except under extreme conditions (Ravelli *et al.*, 1999). However, recent epidemiological studies have found relationships between nutritional status during pregnancy in non-famine conditions, adverse outcomes at birth and later disease risk (Campbell *et al.*, 1996; Godfrey *et al.*, 1996). These observations have raised the possibility that subtle changes in the materno-placental supply of nutrients may alter fetal metabolism and endocrine status with postnatal health consequences compatible with the FOAD hypotheses (Rich-Edwards *et al.*, 1997; Eriksson *et al.*, 2001).

Recent studies have suggested that the timing for the programming of postnatal function by an adverse prenatal environment might differ between different regulatory systems. For example, maternal nutrient restriction during the Dutch famine did not affect basal blood pressure but it impaired glucose tolerance in adult offspring (Ravelli *et al.*, 1976). Famine exposure in late gestation led to a greater impairment of glucose tolerance than during early or mid-gestation. The rate of obesity was higher in men exposed in the first half of gestation and lower in men exposed in the last trimester of gestation as compared to non-exposed men (Inagaki *et al.*, 1986). Thus, while fetal exposure to a substrate-limited environment at most stages of development appears to lead to adult dysregulation of metabolism, the precise mechanisms responsible may vary with the timing of exposure.

Another way in which an adverse maternal environment can influence fetal development is through the action of maternal glucocorticoids. Similar to that seen in the human, animal studies indicate that fetal undernutrition leads to lifelong changes in the fetal hypothalamic–pituitary–adrenal (HPA) axis which, in turn, reset homeostatic mechanisms controlling blood pressure (Edwards *et al.*, 1993; Seckl, 1994). The fetus is partly protected from exposure to maternal glucocorticoids by the placental enzyme 11β-hydroxysteroid dehydrogenase type 2 (11β-HSD-2), which converts maternal glucocorticoids to inactive 11-keto products (Seckl *et al.*, 1995). In pregnant rats, administration of 11β-HSD-2 inhibitors that block placental inactivation of endogenous glucocorticoids, reduced birthweight and resulted in hypertension and impaired glucose tolerance in the adult offspring (Lindsay *et al.*, 1996). Treatment of pregnant rats with DEX, a synthetic glucocorticoid that can cross the placenta, also reduced birthweight and caused hypertension, hyperglycaemia and hyperinsulinaemia in adult offspring, which were amplified by obesity (Seckl *et al.*, 2000).

There is some evidence that the role of undernutrition and glucocortiocoids as triggers may be interdependent. DEX-injected pregnant rats eat less and gain less weight than controls. Conversely, acute protein restriction or undernutrition during the last week of pregnancy in the rat elevates maternal corticosterone levels. Offspring are small at birth and show disturbed development of the HPA axis during postnatal life (Lesage *et al.*, 2001). Furthermore, protein restriction during pregnancy reduces placental 11β-HSD-2 activity and thus increases fetal exposure to maternal glucocorticoids (Seckl *et al.*, 1995). Recent data suggest that hyperglycaemia in 6-month-old rats exposed to DEX *in utero* is not due to attenuated peripheral glucose disposal. However, increased glucocorticoid receptors (GRs) and attenuated fatty acid uptake, specifically in visceral adipose, are consistent with insulin resistance in this crucial metabolic depot and could contribute indirectly to increased hepatic glucose output (Cleasby *et al.*, 2003).

Nutritional Programming

Fetal undernutrition has been highlighted as the primary factor involved in the early life origins of adult disease. Within the laboratory, fetal undernutrition can most commonly be achieved through maternal dietary restriction during pregnancy. Manipulation of maternal nutrition during pregnancy has been known to alter fetal growth and development for some time (Dobbing, 1981). At present, rodent models investigating the mechanistic links between maternal undernutrition and adult disease generally utilize one of two dietary protocols: global undernutrition or isocaloric low-protein diets. The maternal low-protein (MLP) diet during pregnancy and lactation is one of the most extensively utilized models of nutritional programming (Snoeck *et al.*, 1990; Langley and Jackson, 1994; Desai *et al.*, 1996; Ozanne *et al.*, 1996a; Petry *et al.*, 2001). This model involves *ad libitum* feeding to pregnant rats of a low-protein diet, containing 5–8% (w/w) protein (casein), generally a little under half the protein content but equivalent in energy content to a control diet containing 18–20% (w/w) protein (Snoeck *et al.*, 1990; Langley-Evans, 2000). Offspring from protein-restricted mothers are around 15–20% lighter at birth (Desai *et al.*, 1996). Maintenance of a MLP diet during lactation enhances this weight difference and permanently restricts later growth. If restricted offspring are cross-fostered to mothers fed a control diet, offspring exhibit rapid catch-up growth (Desai *et al.*, 1996). This catch-up growth appears to have a detrimental effect on life span, resulting in premature death, which is associated with accelerated loss of kidney telomeric DNA (Jennings *et al.*, 1999).

Restricted-protein-exposed offspring exhibit significantly elevated blood pressure at an early age, in comparison to controls (Langley and Jackson, 1994). However, the precise composition of the low-protein diet is critical in determining the cardiovascular outcome for the offspring, with methionine, folic acid, fatty acids and carbohydrate sources all implicated as modifiers of the low-protein effect (Langley-Evans, 2000). This highlights the importance that the balance of micronutrients plays in determining the long-term health effects of maternal nutrition during pregnancy. Investigations into fetal programming of hypertension in offspring consistently reveal a reduction in renal mass, increased apoptosis without a balancing increase in cell proliferation and reductions in glomeruli number (Langley-Evans *et al.*, 1999a). Changes in kidney structure and development are also associated with enhanced activity of the renin–angiotensin system (RAS) (Langley-Evans *et al.*, 1999b). Increased expression of glucocorticoid receptors (GRs) in the kidney and lung, accompanied by reduced expression of 11β-HSD-2 in the kidney and adrenals, is associated with an enhancement of glucocorticoid-mediated increases in blood pressure (Bertram *et al.*, 2001). These molecular responses are compatible with the idea that alterations in the function of the HPA axis may be central to the pathological mechanism involved in generating the phenotype of the MLP model.

Carbohydrate metabolism in offspring is also altered by a MLP diet during pregnancy. Fasting plasma insulin and glucose levels are lower in MLP offspring and are associated with improved insulin sensitivity in early adulthood. However, programmed offspring exhibit a greater age-dependent loss of glucose tolerance (Hales *et al.*, 1996). By 15 months of age, in rats, glucose tolerance in restricted offspring is significantly diminished compared to that of controls, and is associated with hyperinsulinaemia in males and hypoinsulinaemia in females (Hales *et al.*, 1996). The mechanisms behind these phenotypic observations include altered development of the pancreas and an enhancement of insulin signalling. The MLP diet programmes pancreatic function in restricted offspring through a reduction in β-cell proliferation, islet size and vascularity, coupled with an enhancement of β-cell apoptosis (Snoeck *et al.*, 1990). Functionally restricted islets demonstrate depressed insulin secretion and secretory responses *in vitro* (Snoeck *et al.*, 1990). Peripheral insulin sensitivity in low-protein-exposed offspring is enhanced through increased insulin receptor expression in the liver, skeletal muscle and adipose, which is accompanied by an increase in insulin-stimulated glucose uptake through increased GLUT 4 translocation (Ozanne *et al.*, 1996b). Subsequently, it has been shown that a defect in glucose-mediated insulin secretion from islets of adult low-protein-exposed offspring only manifests when an additional dietary insult, such as high-fat feeding, is introduced postnatally (Ozanne, 2001).

Insulin sensitivity of adipocytes in MLP offspring has been studied in much greater detail. The findings of these studies show that enhanced activation of insulin receptor substrate-1 (IRS-1)-associated phosphoinositol 3-kinase (PI3K) activity may be the key to improvements in insulin sensitivity (Ozanne *et al.*, 2001). However, alterations in PI3K subunit expression indicate that the adipocytes of restricted offspring may be resistant to insulin's antilipolytic effects (Ozanne *et al.*, 2001). A MLP diet during gestation has been shown to augment the sensitivity of fetal islet cells to nitric oxide (NO) and to IL-1β (Merezak *et al.*, 2001). Interestingly, taurine supplementation to a MLP diet during fetal and early postnatal life restores a normal proliferation and apoptosis of rat pancreatic islets (Boujendar *et al.*, 2002). The mechanisms by which taurine acts on DNA synthesis and apoptosis rate of endocrine cells appears to involve insulin-like growth factor (IGF)-II, Fas regulation but not inducible nitric oxide synthase (iNOS).

Hepatic development is also altered in protein-restricted offspring, with apparent changes in the expression and function of a range of liver enzymes (Burns *et al.*, 1997). Functionally, hepatic glucose output is altered, with a relative resistance to glucagon stimulation being observed (Burns *et al.*, 1997).

Experimental observations in the MLP diet model of fetal programming highlight many potential mechanisms that may be involved in the pathogenesis of hypertension and diabetes. These mechanisms include both physical and functional changes to various organ and endocrine systems.

Global undernutrition at various times during pregnancy is another widely used approach to induce nutritional programming. Various different models have been developed, with different levels of undernutrition during different periods of pregnancy. A mild nutritional restriction, to 70% of normal intake in the first 18 days of pregnancy in the rat, results in offspring with significant growth retardation at birth that catch up to controls at postnatal day 20 (Ozaki et al., 2001). Restricted offspring exhibit elevated blood pressure in adult life, with an increased vasoconstriction response to potassium and thromboxane A_2 mimetics. These abnormalities increase with age and are most pronounced in male offspring (Ozaki et al., 2001). Another model using a nutritional restriction to 50% of normal ad libitum intake in the second half of gestation had no effect on blood pressure, with only subtle alterations in vasoconstrictive ability being observed (Holemans et al., 1999). In another study a 50% restriction of a normal diet from day 15 of pregnancy showed that 21-day-old rat fetuses had significantly decreased pancreatic insulin content (Blondeau et al., 2001).

We have developed a rodent model of fetal programming using maternal undernutrition throughout pregnancy. At birth, offspring of undernourished mothers (UN offspring) had fetal and placental weights that were 25–30% lower than offspring of ad libitum-fed mothers (AD offspring). A lack of catch-up growth despite a standard postnatal diet (Woodall et al., 1996a) was accompanied by a transient reduction in circulating IGF-I and hepatic IGF-I mRNA expression, which normalized at weaning. Consistent with this observation, we also showed that UN offspring had a reduced responsiveness to growth hormone (GH) during the neonatal period, possibly reflecting delayed maturation of the somatotrophic axis, which was fully restored before puberty (Woodall et al., 1996a, 1998). In addition, UN offspring developed elevated blood pressure in adult life (Weder and Schork, 1994; Woodall et al., 1999).

Postnatal Nutrition

We can distinguish two conceptually different types of interactions between prenatal and postnatal nutrition in the pathogenesis of metabolic disorders and obesity. Diet-induced obesity during postnatal life can amplify the prenatal induction of disease susceptibility (Vickers et al., 2000). Alternatively, prenatal influences can facilitate the disease process that is induced by postnatal nutrition, such as the development of obesity and insulin resistance in individuals who are exposed to a high-fat diet during postnatal life. The direction of the interactions between prenatal and postnatal influences is most probably dependent on timing and severity of each factor.

In historically undernourished, recently urbanized populations, such as those of India, where individuals of low birthweight are exposed to a high-fat Western diet, the incidence of obesity and type 2 diabetes is reaching epidemic proportions (Yajnik, 2000). Work by Yajnik and colleagues has shown that although Indian babies are born of low birthweight, they exhibit relatively increased visceral adiposity and hyperinsulinaemia at birth (Yajnik *et al.*, 2002). Such observations have been explained by the 'thrifty-phenotype' hypothesis proposed by Hales and Barker (1992) and may illustrate the long-term disadvantage of postnatal 'catch-up' growth. Although there is considerable debate whether catch-up growth in early postnatal life is beneficial or not, most studies suggested that postnatal 'catch-up' growth is associated with adverse outcomes in later life (Bonora *et al.*, 1994; Eriksson *et al.*, 1999; Ong *et al.*, 2001; Soto *et al.*, 2003).

Epidemiological studies have shown that the greatest insulin resistance is observed in people of low birthweight who develop obesity as adults (Phillips, 1998). Hofman *et al.* (1997) have shown that short pre-pubertal IUGR children have impaired insulin sensitivity. In rats, the combinations of prenatal undernutrition with retarded fetal growth, and of good postnatal nutrition with accelerated growth, lead to a striking reduction in life span (Hales *et al.*, 1996; Jennings *et al.*, 1999). The well-established notion that diets high in saturated fats play a key role in the development of insulin resistance and obesity has recently been extended to the frequency of food intake. Zammit *et al.* (2001) suggested that the pathogenesis of insulin resistance may be related to a pattern of frequent snacking, which results in a continuous post-prandial state for most of the day. This prevents the attainment of low basal interprandial insulin levels, even in normal individuals. Prolonged exposure of the liver to high basal insulin, through its stimulatory effect on hepatic triglycerides and very-low-density lipoprotein (VLDL) secretion, may contribute to the initial induction of muscle insulin resistance (Zammit *et al.*, 2001).

In our studies, we introduced offspring of undernourished rats (UN) to a hypercaloric (high fat/high protein) diet after weaning to investigate whether enhanced nutritional supply would facilitate postnatal catch-up growth. This led to development of obesity during adult life (Fig. 10.1) (Vickers *et al.*, 2000, 2001b). UN offspring also developed hypertension, hyperinsulinaemia, hyperleptinaemia and hyperphagia, independent of postnatal diet (Fig. 10.2). Postnatal hypercaloric nutrition amplified the existing cardiovascular, metabolic and endocrine abnormalities of UN offspring (Vickers *et al.*, 2000). Interestingly, hyperphagia was established before puberty, independent of caloric content of the diet, and increased with advancing age (Vickers *et al.*, 2000). The increased plasma insulin and leptin concentrations were paralleled by markedly enhanced immunolabelling for leptin in the peripheral cells of the pancreatic islets (Vickers *et al.*, 2001a). Hyperleptinaemia has been proposed to reflect an endocrine endeavour to reduce insulin secretion through direct action on pancreatic β-cells (Seufert *et al.*, 1999). Since leptin inhibits glucose-stimulated insulin secretion *in vitro* (Pallett *et al.*, 1997), we hypothesized that the local increase of immunoreactive leptin in pancreatic δ-cells may be a paracrine mechanism to reduce hypersecretion of insulin (Vickers *et al.*, 2001a). The hyperleptinaemia and hyperinsulinaemia seen in UN offspring may be a mechanism induced by a nutrient-deprived fetal environment to store large quantities of triglycerides when food is plentiful, thus representing a competitive advantage ('thrifty phenotype')

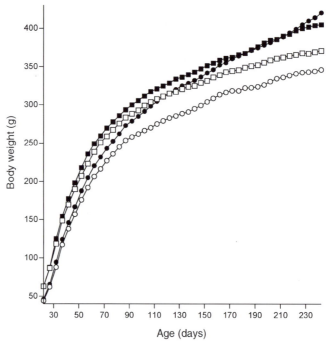

Fig. 10.1. Body weight gain in the offspring of *ad libitum*-fed (AD) and under-nourished (UN) mothers, fed either a control or high-fat diet postnatally. Note the marked weight gain in UN animals fed a high-fat diet. AD control (□), AD high-fat (■), UN control (○), UN high-fat (●).

in preparation for a nutrient-deprived postnatal environment (Hales and Barker, 1992). However, when hypercaloric nutrition persists for long periods of time, adipogenic diabetes may develop. Our work to date cannot resolve whether the primary defect in this cascade is in appetite regulation, fat accumulation, altered leptin or insulin action. We have shown that therapy with IGF-I or GH can ameliorate obesity, hyperphagia and hypertension induced by fetal programming and high-fat nutrition, but the precise mechanisms underlying these effects are yet to be resolved (Vickers *et al.*, 2001b, 2002).

In a recent study, we reduced the food intake of UN offspring after weaning to 70% of *ad libitum* intake (hypocaloric diet) to investigate whether reduced postnatal nutrition could prevent the development of the metabolic disorders induced by prenatal maternal undernutrition (M.H. Vickers and B.H. Breier, unpublished observations). As expected, body weight and fat pad mass decreased in UN offspring on the hypocaloric diet. However, we were surprised to see that these animals still developed hyperinsulinaemia, increased leptin/fat pad ratio and elevated blood pressure as adults. This is the first evidence to suggest that the prenatal influences of maternal undernutrition on metabolic pathogenesis may persist into adult life, even if postnatal growth is limited. The public health implications of these preliminary observations are enormous,

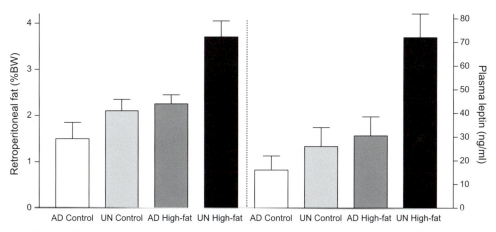

Fig. 10.2. Retroperitoneal fat pad mass and plasma leptin concentrations in offspring from undernourished (UN) or *ad libitum*-fed mothers (AD) at 120 days of age, fed either a control or high-fat diet during postnatal life. BW, body weight.

since they suggest that the balance of postnatal nutrition is critical and that either under- or overnutrition in the face of adverse prenatal influences may be detrimental to long-term health.

Early Origins of the Metabolic Syndrome

Maternal malnutrition in animals manifests as insulin resistance, hyper-leptinaemia, obesity, hypertension and appetite disorders in offspring. Thus, animal models of fetal programming display a phenotype in offspring that closely mimics the clinical symptoms of the metabolic syndrome seen in humans born with low birthweight (Reaven, 1993; Smith *et al.*, 1999). The metabolic syndrome is the term used by the World Health Organization (WHO) to describe the clustering of clinical cardiovascular risk factors that occur in individuals with impaired insulin sensitivity (Alberti and Zimmet, 1998). These risk factors include obesity, dyslipidaemia, hypertension and microalbuminuria (Groop and Orho-Melander, 2001). The prevalence of the metabolic syndrome, its associated disorders and their impact on national health and well being is now increasing in epidemic proportions worldwide. The WHO has estimated that by 2025 there will be 300 million people worldwide suffering from health problems associated with the metabolic syndrome (Seidell, 2000). This trend is most pronounced in countries undergoing a rapid economic transition to a Western-style market economy and is associated with a move to a westernized lifestyle and diet (Seidell, 2000; Zimmet *et al.*, 2001). The changes accompanying westernization include a sedentary lifestyle, significantly improved nutrition and, in some cases, a switch to foods of greater energy density containing high levels of saturated fats and simple sugars (Riccardi and Rivellese, 2000). These factors that are associated with westernization are believed to be the key environmental influences driving the staggering increases in obesity, type 2 diabetes and metabolic syndrome seen in the developing nations of the world (Zimmet *et al.*, 2001).

The associations between westernization and the incidence of obesity, diabetes, metabolic syndrome and coronary heart disease (CHD) have led these disorders to be termed 'the diseases of affluence' (Barker, 1994). When the socio-economic dimensions of these disorders are investigated, interesting links begin to emerge between economic status and disease risk. In both affluent countries and in those counties undergoing economic transition, obesity and type 2 diabetes are highest in those with low socio-economic status (Zimmet *et al.*, 2001). Those with a high socio-economic status appear to be less suscepti-ble to these diseases (Zimmet *et al.*, 2001). Rather than being associated with affluence, these observations indicate a relation between poor socio-economic status and increased susceptibility to chronic cardiovascular and metabolic disease.

The fundamental origins of the metabolic syndrome and its complex multi-factorial pathogenesis have yet to be determined. Current opinion has favoured the role of a genetic susceptibility, a thrifty genotype, particularly apparent in some ethnic groups (Neel, 1999; Groop and Orho-Melander, 2001). This hypothesis proposes that a number of thrifty gene variants act together to alter glucose and fat metabolism, generating systemic metabolic thrift. Thrifty changes may include alterations in the metabolic function of critical organs, such as the pancreas, adipose tissue, liver or skeletal muscle. Overall, this genotype is char-acterized by an energy-conserving metabolism providing an enhanced capacity to store and retain surplus energy as fat (Neel, 1999; Groop and Orho-Melander, 2001). When this thrifty genotype is exposed to the abundance of calories typical of a Western pattern of nutrition, obesity soon develops, leading to diabetes and the metabolic syndrome (Groop and Orho-Melander, 2001). The thrifty genotype hypothesis promotes the idea that the primary origins of the metabolic syndrome lie in a gene–environment interaction. The list of candidate thrifty genes believed to play a role in this process is quite extensive and includes those for leptin and its receptor, pro-opiomelanocortin (POMC) and the melanocortin receptor (MC4), β-adrenergic receptors, TNF-α, peroxisomal proliferator activated receptor γ (PPAR-γ), IRS-1 and many more (Groop, 2000). To date, monogenetic mutations and polymorphisms in candidate genes have been linked with the metabolic syndrome in only a few rare cases. Current genetic approaches to understanding the pathophysiology of the metabolic syndrome focus on the interplay of multiple candidate gene loci that act together to increase an individual's susceptibility to environmental triggers.

Hales and Barker (1992) proposed an alternative hypothesis for the origins of the metabolic syndrome, the thrifty phenotype hypothesis. This hypothesis is similar to that of the thrifty genotype, in that the metabolic syndrome is seen as the result of a critical interaction between an inherent susceptibility and environ-mental trigger. However, as opposed to a genetic susceptibility, Hales and Barker (1992) propose a developmental susceptibility, a metabolically thrifty phenotype programmed *in utero* by fetal undernutrition. The programming of fetal metabolism with a thrifty phenotype, characterized by a reduced metabolic capacity, is seen as an adaptive response to suboptimal intrauterine nutrition, and is believed to be aimed at conserving metabolic energy for critical organ growth and development, aiding in the ultimate survival of the fetus (Hales and Barker, 1992). If poor nutrition is maintained after birth, a thrifty phenotype is believed to offer a metabolic advantage in a nutrient-poor environment (Hales and Barker, 1992).

However, exposure of the thrifty phenotype to a postnatal environment consisting of an excessive nutritional plane overloads the reduced metabolic capacity of the thrifty individual, resulting in the preferential storage of surplus energy as fat (Hales and Barker, 1992). Low socio-economic status contributing to poor maternal nutrition and fetal undernutrition, in combination with the subsequent improvement of nutrition that accompanies economic development, can now be identified as another potential mechanism driving the staggering increases in the incidence of the metabolic syndrome seen in developing nations (Hales and Barker, 1992). In the light of the current understanding of time trends, geographic and socio-economic association, the thrifty phenotype hypothesis provides important insight into the potential origins of a worldwide epidemic.

The 'couch potato' syndrome

We have recently reported experimental evidence suggesting that maternal undernutrition can induce sedentary behaviour, hyperphagia and concomitant obesity in offspring, independent of postnatal dietary influences (Vickers *et al.*, 2003). We had shown previously that maternal undernutrition throughout pregnancy in the rat results in hypertension, hyperinsulinaemia and hyperleptinaemia in the offspring when they reach adulthood (Vickers *et al.*, 2000). Obesity was not present until after puberty and was associated with hyperphagia. In the course of these studies we noted that the onset of the abnormal eating behaviours occurred prior to puberty, thus preceding the development of obesity. This led us to speculate that the prenatal maternal environment might also affect other components of behaviour associated with the metabolic syndrome.

Voluntary locomotor activity was assessed in rat prenatally undernourished offspring at various ages from the peri-pubertal period to adulthood. This was done following three habituation trials using Optimax behavioural testing apparatus. The animals were fed either a standard diet or a hypercaloric diet throughout postnatal life. Offspring of undernourished mothers were significantly more sedentary in postnatal life than those born of *ad libitum*-fed mothers, for all parameters measured, and this was independent of postnatal diet. Analysis of food intake revealed hyperphagia in mature offspring that had been exposed to maternal undernutrition. This was independent of postnatal diet, although it was exacerbated by hypercaloric nutrition (Fig. 10.3). Importantly, in the animals tested at a peri-pubertal age, diminished locomotor activity was already present prior to the development of maturity-onset obesity and was significantly reduced in males compared to females (Fig. 10.4).

These results suggest that maternal undernutrition can lead to the development of both overeating and diminished exercise, behaviour concomitant with

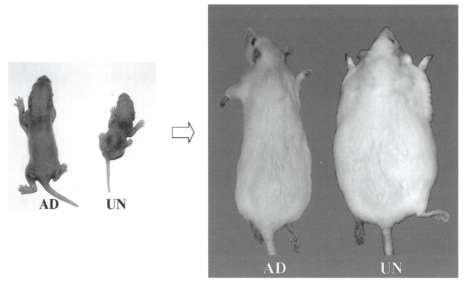

Fig. 10.3. Offspring of undernourished (UN) mothers are significantly lighter and shorter at birth than those born from *ad libitum* (AD)-fed mothers. UN offspring develop increased fat deposition concomitant with hyperleptinaemia and hyperphagia in adult life.

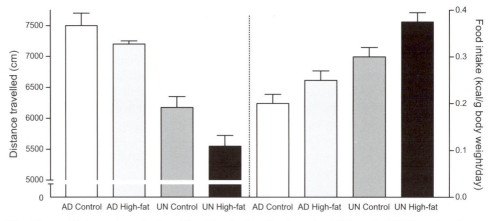

Fig. 10.4. Distance travelled and food intake in offspring of *ad libitum*-fed (AD) and under-nourished (UN) mothers, at 135 days of age, fed either a control or high-fat diet postnatally. UN offspring are hyperphagic and significantly less active than AD offspring, and the effect is amplified by exposure to a high-fat diet.

the physiological features of the metabolic syndrome. The former observation raises the intriguing possibility that some behaviours and lifestyle choices that exacerbate the metabolic syndrome in humans may not be voluntary but may be an inherent part of the syndrome, and may have a prenatal origin. Our recent studies suggest that the 'couch potato' syndrome may have its origins during prenatal development. This has major implications for public health policy. Health-care funding may be better spent on improving pregnancy care rather than waiting until metabolic and cardiovascular disorders manifest in offspring years or decades later.

Endocrine and Metabolic Mechanisms

The precise mechanisms underlying the programming of adult disease by maternal nutrient restriction remain a matter of debate. Maternal undernutrition or low-protein diet during the last trimester in the pregnant rat leads to reduction of fetal pancreatic β-cell mass (Petrik *et al.*, 1999) and increased apoptosis of immature β-cells (Cherif *et al.*, 1998). While insulin-stimulated glucose uptake in adipocytes is increased during early postnatal life due to increased insulin receptor number (Ozanne *et al.*, 1997), there is greater age-dependent loss of glucose tolerance and later insulin resistance (Hales *et al.*, 1996; Ozanne *et al.*, 2001). The reduced insulin action is associated with reduced phosphatidyl-inositol 3-kinase (PI3K) and protein kinase B (PKB) activation and altered fatty acid metabolism (Ozanne *et al.*, 1998).

Another important target of prenatal events is the liver, where glucocorticoids regulate several metabolic processes, including hepatic enzymes regulating carbohydrate and fat metabolism. Rats exposed to DEX in the last trimester of pregnancy show increased phosphoenolpyruvate carboxykinase (PEPCK) gene transcription and increased activity of this rate-limiting enzyme of gluconeogenesis in the liver (Nyirenda *et al.*, 1998). These animals have adult hyperglycaemia and increased hepatic glucocorticoid receptor expression. Similarly, structural changes in the liver and altered expression patterns of gluconeogenic enzymes and glucose handling have been reported after a maternal low-protein diet (Burns *et al.*, 1997).

Neuroendocrine regulatory systems are also vulnerable to disturbances in early life, which can lead to permanent structural changes, including reduced cerebral vascularity (Bennis-Taleb *et al.*, 1999) and dysfunction of central nervous system regulation. Maternal low-protein nutrition results in structural changes in the mediobasal hypothalamic nuclei in weanling offspring, and fewer neurons immunopositive for neuropeptide Y in the arcuate hypothalamic nucleus (Plagemann *et al.*, 2000). These neuroendocrine changes are accompanied by the development of obesity and diabetogenic disturbances later in life. The HPA axis is particularly susceptible to prenatal influences. For example, neonatal disturbance of mother–pup interactions permanently alters plasma adrenocorticotrophic hormone (ACTH) and corticosterone concentrations and glucocorticoid receptor (GR) levels in hippocampus, paraventricular nucleus (PVN) and pituitary (Meaney, 2001). Similar GR abnormalities have been described following either nutritional manipulation or glucocorticoid administration to the mother. Maternal glucocorticoids alter the utilization of alternative exon 1 sequences coding for promotor regions on the GR gene in offspring (McCormick *et al.*, 2000). This is strong evidence that programming can cause permanent alterations in gene expression and could explain the increase in basal plasma corticosterone levels in adulthood that may contribute directly to hypertension and hyperglycaemia (Seckl *et al.*, 1999).

It is well established that prenatal stress can influence the development of neural systems that control endocrine responses to stress and regulate behavioural traits (Ladd *et al.*, 2000; Meaney, 2001). Maternal glucocorticoid administration or prenatal stress in rats leads to development of decreased locomotor activity and increased defaecation and avoidance behaviour in an 'open field' test (Welberg and Seckl, 2001; Welberg *et al.*, 2001). An animal model of fetal programming by maternal tumour necrosis factor (TNF)-α administration showed reduced locomotor activity of offspring (Dahlgren *et al.*, 2001). While recent studies in the rat have focused on maternal behaviour during the neonatal period, which influences the HPA axis activity and anxiety behaviour (Meaney, 2001), there is little published experimental information on the effects of maternal nutrition on offspring behaviour. One group reported that maternal low-protein nutrition during pregnancy in the rat led to changes in exploratory behaviour, social interactions and avoidance behaviour in offspring (Almeida *et al.*, 1996a,b). Since it is well established that diet-induced obesity in animals leads to a reduction in locomotor activity (Remke *et al.*, 1988), these studies are in general agreement with our observation of increased eating behaviour in offspring of undernourished mothers and our observation of their decreased locomotor activity, as discussed above.

Programming of the Adipoinsular Axis and Altered Adipogenesis

It is important to note that very few animal studies have addressed interactions between pre- and postnatal nutrition. However, other studies that have investigated diet-induced obesity point to a link between peripheral leptin resistance and insulin resistance in the development of obesity. The physiological role of hyperleptinaemia associated with caloric excess has been proposed to relate to the protection of non-adipocytes from lipid oversupply that would lead to steatosis and lipotoxicity (Unger and Orci, 2001). Elevated leptin production as a result of short-term caloric excess prevents the up-regulation of lipogenesis and increases fatty acid oxidation, thus reducing lipid supply to peripheral tissue during caloric excess (Unger and Orci, 2001). In diet-induced obesity, peripheral leptin function is, at first, normal. However, prolonged caloric excess results in dysregulation of post-receptor leptin signalling. This causes accumulation of triglycerides and lipid metabolites, providing fatty acid substrate for the damaging effects of non-oxidative metabolism, leading to functional impairment of non-adipose tissue and a progression to type 2 diabetes and cardiovascular disease (Unger, 2001).

A range of genetic components of obesity has been identified (Flatt and Bailey, 1981; Kawano *et al.*, 1992; Akiyama *et al.*, 1996), and research on alterations in biochemical pathways caused by single gene mutations in animal models has contributed significantly towards knowledge of physiological mechanisms of obesity (Campfield *et al.*, 1998). It is well established that leptin acts at the level of the hypothalamus to regulate appetite and energy homeostasis (Ahima and Flier, 2000). The long-form, or signalling form, of the leptin receptor

(OB-Rb) is expressed in high levels in several cell groups of the hypothalamus and in various tissues throughout the body (Baskin *et al.*, 1999a,b; Vickers *et al.*, 2001a). Under normal physiological conditions, increased leptin signalling in the medial hypothalamus is associated with reduced neuropeptide Y (NPY) and agouti-related (AgRP) protein production (Hahn *et al.*, 1998) but increased cocaine- and amphetamine-regulated transcript (CART) and pro-opiomelanocortin (POMC) production (Schwartz *et al.*, 1997; Thornton *et al.*, 1997; Wang *et al.*, 1999). These leptin-induced changes in neuropeptides lead to decreased food intake and increased energy expenditure.

In obese individuals, elevated plasma leptin is proposed to uncouple leptin action on its receptors in the hypothalamus, thereby disrupting signal trans-duction pathways that exert effects on satiety and energy expenditure (Ahima and Flier, 2000). Direct leptin signalling in peripheral tissues has only recently been demonstrated. For example, increased leptin signalling in muscle tissue has been shown to blunt lipogenesis and stimulate lipid oxidation (Muoio *et al.*, 1997). There is also growing evidence for a feedback system between leptin and insulin which links the brain and the endocrine pancreas with other peripheral insulin- and leptin-sensitive tissues in the control of feeding behaviour, metabolic regulation and body energy balance (Kieffer and Habener, 2000). This endo-crine system has been termed the adipoinsular axis (Kieffer and Habener, 2000). When adipose stores decrease, falling leptin concentrations permit increased insulin production, resulting in the deposition of additional fat. Conversely, the suppressive effects of leptin on insulin production are mediated by the autonomic nervous system and by direct actions via leptin receptor on β-cells (Kieffer and Habener, 2000). Our data suggest that fetal programming by maternal under-nutrition throughout gestation may lead to dysregulation of the adipoinsular feedback system. Relative leptin resistance by pancreatic β–cells may contribute to hyperinsulinism, which further exacerbates adipogenesis. The hypeinsulinism and hyperleptinaemia may also trigger the pathogenesis of hyperphagia.

Increasing evidence points to two main peripheral metabolic pathways in the pathogenesis of diabetic complications in diet-induced obesity, namely insulin signalling through its tyrosine kinase receptor (IR) and leptin signalling through OB-Rb. Cross-talk between the two pathways has been discovered recently, which suggests potential avenues for homeostatic modulation of their individual functions (Szanto and Kahn, 2000). However, the extent of the inter-dependence between the two systems in physiological and pathophysiological settings remains poorly characterized and not all of the interactions between the two pathways may exist at any one time in an individual tissue.

Binding of leptin to OB-Rb results in the activation of Janus kinase (JAK)-2 which, in turn, tyrosine phosphorylates the intracellular domain of the receptor at two sites, each of which mediate distinct signalling pathways, namely the MAP kinase (MAPK) pathway and the signal transducers and activators of transcrip-tion (STAT)-3/suppressor of cytokine signalling (SOCS)-3 pathway (Wang *et al.*, 2000). The latter is a leptin-regulated inhibitor of leptin signalling *in vivo* and therefore its overproduction is a potential mechanism for leptin resistance (Bjorbaek *et al.*, 1997, 1999; Li and Friedman, 1999; Banks *et al.*, 2000).

However, in muscle, insulin induces SOCS-2 and SOCS-3 through STAT-5 activation, by a mechanism that is independent of its major signalling mechanisms (PI3K and MAPK pathways), thereby creating a complex interplay of signals with potential to blunt the leptin response (Sadowski *et al.*, 2001).

Another focus for interplay between these two pathways is at the level of the insulin receptor substrates (IRS-1 and IRS-2). Leptin has been shown to interact with IRS-1, IRS-2, PI3K and MAPK (Kim *et al.*, 2000; Szanto and Kahn, 2000). Exposure to leptin modifies the IRS response to insulin, causing increased binding of PI3K to IRS-1, while simultaneously inhibiting phosphorylation and PI3K binding to IRS-2. Moreover, leptin alone can activate PKB/Akt and glycogen synthase 3 by a pathway that appears to be different from that of insulin. A picture therefore emerges of divergent leptin and insulin action on IRSs and their downstream kinases, leading to a complex of overlapping, but distinct, interactions between the two signalling systems.

Summary and Conclusions

Numerous epidemiological studies have described a relationship between adverse prenatal factors and the development of metabolic disease and obesity in later life. Both prospective clinical studies and experimental research have clearly shown that the propensity to develop abnormalities of cardiovascular, endocrine and metabolic homeostasis in adulthood is increased when fetal development has been adversely affected. The pathogenesis is not based on genetic defects but on altered genetic expression as a consequence of an adaptation to environmental changes during fetal development.

Studies of the interaction between maternal undernutrition throughout pregnancy followed by postnatal hypercaloric nutrition in the rat have shown that offspring from undernourished mothers are growth retarded at birth and develop obesity, hypertension, hyperleptinaemia, hyperinsulinaemia and hyperphagia during postnatal life. Recent evidence also suggests an alteration in locomotor activity and eating behaviour. Close associations between a major rise in circulating insulin and leptin concentrations, and a large increase in appetite and fat mass, provide evidence for disturbed endocrine communication between the hypothalamus, adipose tissue and the endocrine pancreas in the pathogenesis of programming-induced obesity. Hypercaloric nutrition during postnatal life greatly amplifies prenatal effects on metabolic abnormalities, obesity, overeating and diminished exercise behaviour.

Fetal programming research offers a novel approach to investigating the mechanistic basis of metabolic disorders, hyperphagia and diminished exercise behaviour which, in human populations, predominantly arise from environmental factors and lifestyle choices. The use of animal models can establish model conditions that will reliably provide high contrasts of phenotypes. Such studies offer an exciting potential for new advances in our understanding of critical determinants and mechanisms for human obesity and metabolic disorders.

References

Ahima, R.S. and Flier, J.S. (2000) Leptin. *Annual Review of Physiology* 62, 413–437.

Akiyama, T., Tachibana, I., Shirohara, H., Watanabe, N. and Otsuki, M. (1996) High-fat hypercaloric diet induces obesity, glucose intolerance and hyperlipidemia in normal adult male Wistar rat. *Diabetes Research and Clinical Practice* 31, 27–35.

Alberti, K.G. and Zimmet, P.Z. (1998) Definition, diagnosis and classification of diabetes mellitus and its complications. Part 1: diagnosis and classification of diabetes mellitus provisional report of a WHO consultation. *Diabetic Medicine* 15(7), 539–553.

Almeida, S.S., Tonkiss, J. and Galler, J.R. (1996a) Prenatal protein malnutrition affects exploratory behavior of female rats in the elevated plus-maze test. *Physiology and Behavior* 60, 675–680.

Almeida, S.S., Tonkiss, J. and Galler, J.R. (1996b) Prenatal protein malnutrition affects avoidance but not escape behavior in the elevated T-maze test. *Physiology and Behavior* 60, 191–195.

Banks, A.S., Davis, S.M., Bates, S.H. and Myers, M.G.J. (2000) Activation of downstream signals by the long form of the leptin receptor. *Journal of Biological Chemistry* 275, 14563–14572.

Barker, D.J. (1994) Outcome of low birthweight. *Hormone Research* 42, 223–230.

Barker, D.J.P. (1998) *Mothers, Babies and Health in Later Life*. Churchill Livingstone, Edinburgh, UK.

Barker, D.J. (2000) *In utero* programming of cardiovascular disease. *Theriogenology* 53, 555–574.

Baskin, D.G., Hahn, T.M. and Schwartz, M.W. (1999a) Leptin sensitive neurons in the hypothalamus. *Hormone and Metabolic Research* 31, 345–350.

Baskin, D.G., Breininger, J.F. and Schwartz, M.W. (1999b) Leptin receptor mRNA identifies a subpopulation of neuropeptide Y neurons activated by fasting in rat hypothalamus. *Diabetes* 48, 828–833.

Bennis-Taleb, N., Remacle, C., Hoet, J.J. and Reusens, B. (1999) A low-protein isocaloric diet during gestation affects brain development and alters permanently cerebral cortex blood vessels in rat offspring. *Journal of Nutrition* 129, 1613–1619.

Bertram, C., Trowern, A.R., Copin, N., Jackson, A.A. and Whorwood, C.B. (2001) The maternal diet during pregnancy programs altered expression of the glucocorticoid receptor and type 2 11beta-hydroxysteroid dehydrogenase: potential molecular mechanisms underlying the programming of hypertension *in utero*. *Endocrinology* 142(7), 2841–2853.

Bispham, J., Gopalakrishnan, G.S., Dandrea, J., Wilson, V., Budge, H., Keisler, D.H., Broughton Pipkin, F., Stephenson, T. and Symonds, M.E. (2003) Maternal endocrine adaptation throughout pregnancy to nutritional manipulation: consequences for maternal plasma leptin and cortisol and the programming of fetal adipose tissue development. *Endocrinology* 144(8), 3575–3585.

Bjorbaek, C., Uotani, S., da Silva, B. and Flier, J.S. (1997) Divergent signaling capacities of the long and short isoforms of the leptin receptor. *Journal of Biological Chemistry* 272, 32686–32695.

Bjorbaek, C., El-Haschimi, K., Frantz, J.D. and Flier, J.S. (1999) The role of SOCS-3 in leptin signaling and leptin resistance. *Journal of Biological Chemistry* 274, 30059–30065.

Blondeau, B., Lesage, J., Czernichow, P., Dupouy, J.P. and Breant, B. (2001) Glucocorticoids impair fetal beta-cell development in rats. *American Journal of Physiology* 281, E592–E599.

Bonora, M., Boule, M. and Gautier, H. (1994) Ventilatory strategy in hypoxic or hypercapnic newborns. *Biology of the Neonate* 65, 198–204.

Boujendar, S., Reusens, B., Merezak, S., Ahn, M.T., Arany, E., Hill, D. and Remacle, C. (2002) Taurine supplementation to a low protein diet during foetal and early postnatal life restores a normal proliferation and apoptosis of rat pancreatic islets. *Diabetologia* 45(6), 856–866.

Burns, S.P., Desai, M., Cohen, R.D., Hales, C.N., Iles, R.A., Going, T.C. and Bailey, R.A. (1997) Gluconeogenesis, glucose handling, and structural changes in livers of the adult offspring of rats partially deprived of protein during pregnancy and lactation. *Journal of Clinical Investigation* 100, 1768–1774.

Campbell, D.M., Hall, M.H., Barker, D.J., Cross, J., Shiell, A.W. and Godfrey, K.M. (1996) Diet in pregnancy and the offspring's blood pressure 40 years later. *British Journal of Obstetrics and Gynaecology* 103, 273–280.

Campfield, L.A., Smith, F.J. and Burn, B. (1998) Stategies and potential molecular targets for obesity treatment. *Science* 280, 1383–1387.

Cherif, H., Reusens, B., Ahn, M.T., Hoet, J.J. and Remacle, C. (1998) Effects of taurine on the insulin secretion of rat fetal islets from dams fed a low-protein diet. *Journal of Endocrinology* 159, 341–348.

Cleasby, M.E., Kelly, P.A., Walker, B.R. and Seckl, J.R. (2003) Programming of rat muscle and fat metabolism by *in utero* overexposure to glucocorticoids. *Endocrinology* 144(3), 999–1007.

Dahlgren, J., Nilsson, C., Jennische, E., Ho, H.P., Eriksson, E., Niklasson, A., Bjorntorp, P., Albertsson Wikland, K. and Holmang, A. (2001) Prenatal cytokine exposure results in obesity and gender-specific programming. *American Journal of Physiology* 281, E326–E334.

Desai, M., Crowther, N.J., Lucas, A. and Hales, C.N. (1996) Organ-selective growth in the offspring of protein-restricted mothers. *British Journal of Nutrition* 76, 591–603.

Dobbing, J. (1981) Maternal nutrition in pregnancy – eating for two? *Early Human Development* 5(2), 113–115.

Dodic, M., Wintour, E.M., Whitworth, J.A. and Coghlan, J.P. (1999) Effect of steroid hormones on blood pressure. *Clinical and Experimental Pharmacology and Physiology* 26, 550–552.

Edwards, C.R., Benediktsson, R., Lindsay, R.S. and Seckl, J.R. (1993) Dysfunction of placental glucocorticoid barrier: link between fetal environment and adult hypertension? *Lancet* 341, 355–357.

Eriksson, J.G., Forsen, T., Tuomilehto, J., Winter, P.D. and Barker, D.J. (1999) Catch-up growth in childhood and death from coronary heart disease: longitudinal study. *British Medical Journal* 318, 427–431.

Eriksson, J.G., Forsen, T., Tuomilehto, J., Osmond, C. and Barker, D.J. (2001) Early growth and coronary heart disease in later life: longitudinal study. *British Medical Journal* 322, 949–953.

Flatt, P.R. and Bailey, C.J. (1981) Development of glucose intolerance and impaired plasma insulin response to glucose in obese hyperglycaemic (ob/ob) mice. *Hormone and Metabolic Research* 13, 556–560.

Gatford, K.L., Wintour, E.M., De Blasio, M.J., Owens, J.A. and Dodic, M. (2000) Differential timing for programming of glucose homoeostasis, sensitivity to insulin and blood pressure by *in utero* exposure to dexamethasone in sheep. *Clinical Science* 98, 553–560.

Gluckman, P.D. (2001) Editorial: nutrition, glucocorticoids, birth size, and adult disease. *Endocrinology* 142, 1689–1691.

Godfrey, K.M. and Barker, D.J.P. (2000) Fetal nutrition and adult disease. *American Journal of Clinical Nutrition* 71, 1344s–1352s.

Godfrey, K., Robinson, S., Barker, D.J., Osmond, C. and Cox, V. (1996) Maternal nutrition in early and late pregnancy in relation to placental and fetal growth. *British Medical Journal* 312, 410–414.

Groop, L. (2000) Pathogenesis of type 2 diabetes: the relative contribution of insulin resistance and impaired insulin secretion. *International Journal of Clinical Practice* 113, 3–13.

Groop, L. and Orho-Melander, M. (2001) The dysmetabolic syndrome. *Journal of Internal Medicine* 250(2), 105–120.

Hahn, T.M., Breininger, J.F., Baskin, D.G. and Schwartz, M.W. (1998) Coexpression of Agrp and NPY in fasting-activated hypothalamic neurons. *Nature Neuroscience* 1, 271–272.

Hales, C.N. and Barker, D.J. (1992) Type 2 (non-insulin-dependent) diabetes mellitus: the thrifty phenotype hypothesis. *Diabetologia* 35, 595–601.

Hales, C.N., Desai, M., Ozanne, S.E. and Crowther, N.J. (1996) Fishing in the stream of diabetes: from measuring insulin to the control of fetal organogenesis. *Biochemical Society Transactions* 24, 341–350.

Hofman, P.L., Cutfield, W.S., Robinson, E.M., Bergman, R.N., Menon, R.K., Sperling, M.A. and Gluckman, P.D. (1997) Insulin resistance in short children with intrauterine growth retardation. *Journal of Clinical Endocrinology and Metabolism* 82, 402–406.

Holemans, K., Gerber, R., Meurrens, K., De Clerck, F., Poston, L. and Van Assche, F.A. (1999) Maternal food restriction in the second half of pregnancy affects vascular function but not blood pressure of rat female offspring. *British Journal of Nutrition* 81(1), 73–79.

Inagaki, S., Kito, S., Kubota, Y., Girgis, S., Hillyard, C.J. and MacIntyre, I. (1986) Autoradiographic localization of calcitonin gene-related peptide binding sites in human and rat brains. *Brain Research* 374, 287–298.

Jennings, B.J., Ozanne, S.E., Dorling, M.W. and Hales, C.N. (1999) Early growth determines longevity in male rats and may be related to telomere shortening in the kidney. *FEBS Letters* 448, 4–8.

Kawano, K., Hirashima, T., Mori, S., Saitoh, Y., Kurosumi, M. and Natori, T. (1992) Spontaneous long-term hyperglycemic rat with diabetic complications; Otsuka Long–Evans Tokushima Fatty (OLETF) strain. *Diabetes* 41, 1422–1428.

Kieffer, T.J. and Habener, J.F. (2000) The adipoinsular axis: effects of leptin on pancreatic beta-cells. *American Journal of Physiology* 278, E1–E14.

Kim, Y.-B., Uotani, S., Pierroz, D.D., Flier, J.S. and Kahn, B.B. (2000) *In vivo* administration of leptin activates signal transduction directly in insulin sensitive tissues: overlapping but distinct pathways from insulin. *Endocrinology* 141, 2328–2339.

Kind, K.L., Clifton, P.M., Katsman, A.I., Tsiounis, M. and Owens, J.A. (1999) Restricted fetal growth and the response to dietary cholesterol in the guinea pig. *American Journal of Physiology* 277, R1675–R1682.

Ladd, C.O., Huot, R.L., Thrivikraman, K.V., Nemeroff, C.B., Meaney, M.J. and Plotsky, P.M. (2000) Long-term behavioral and neuroendocrine adaptations to adverse early experience. *Progress in Brain Research* 122, 81–103.

Langley, S.C. and Jackson, A.A. (1994) Increased systolic blood pressure in adult rats induced by fetal exposure to maternal low protein diets. *Clinical Science* 86, 217–222.

Langley-Evans, S.C. (2000) Critical differences between two low protein diet protocols in the programming of hypertension in the rat. *International Journal of Food Science and Nutrition* 51, 11–17.

Langley-Evans, S.C., Gardner, D.S. and Jackson, A.A. (1996) Association of disproportionate growth of fetal rats in late gestation with raised systolic blood pressure in later
life. *Journal of Reproduction and Fertility* 106, 307–312.

Langley-Evans, S.C., Welham, S.J. and Jackson, A. (1999a) Fetal exposure to a maternal
low protein diet impairs nephrogenesis and promotes hypertension in the rat. *Life
Science* 64, 965–974.

Langley-Evans, S.C., Sherman, R.C., Welham, S.J., Nwagwu, M.O., Gardner, D.S. and
Jackson, A.A. (1999b) Intrauterine programming of hypertension: the role of the
renin–angiotensin system. *Biochemical Society Transactions* 27, 88–93.

Lesage, J., Blondeau, M., Grino, B., Breant, B. and Dupouy, J.P. (2001) Maternal
undernutrition during late gestation induces fetal overexposure to glucocorticoids
and intrauterine growth retardation, and disturbs the hypothalamo-pituitary adrenal
axis in the newborn rat. *Endocrinology* 142, 1692–1702.

Li, C. and Friedman, J.M. (1999) Leptin receptor activation of SH2 domain containing protein tyrosine phosphatase 2 modulates Ob receptor signal transduction.
Proceedings of the National Academy of Sciences USA 96, 9677–9682.

Lindsay, R.S., Lindsay, R.M., Edwards, C.R.W. and Seckl, J.R. (1996) Inhibition of
11beta-hydroxysteroid dehydrogenase in pregnant rats and the programming of
blood pressure in the offspring. *Hypertension* 27, 1200–1204.

McCormick, J.A., Lyons, V., Jacobson, M.D., Noble, J., Diorio, J., Nyirenda, M.,
Weaver, S., Ester, W., Yau, J.L., Meaney, M.J., Seckl, J.R. and Chapman, K.E.
(2000) 5'-Heterogeneity of glucocorticoid receptor messenger RNA is tissue
specific: differential regulation of variant transcripts by early-life events. *Molecular
Endocrinology* 14, 506–517.

Meaney, M.J. (2001) Maternal care, gene expression, and the transmission of individual
differences in stress reactivity across generations. *Annual Review of Neuroscience*
24, 1161–1192.

Merezak, S., Hardikar, A.A., Yajnik, C.S., Remacle, C. and Reusens, B. (2001) Intrauterine low protein diet increases fetal beta-cell sensitivity to NO and IL-1 beta: the
protective role of taurine. *Journal of Endocrinology* 171(2), 299–308.

Muoio, D.M., Dohm, G.L., Fiedorek, F.T.J., Tapscott, E.B., Coleman, R.A. and Dohn,
G.L. (1997) Leptin directly alters lipid partitioning in skeletal muscle. *Diabetes* 46,
1360–1363.

Neel, J.V. (1999) Diabetes mellitus: a 'thrifty' genotype rendered detrimental by
'progress'? *Bulletin of the World Health Organization* 77(8), 694–703.

Nyirenda, M.J., Lindsay, R.S., Kenyon, C.J., Burchell, A. and Seckl, J.R. (1998) Glucocorticoid exposure in late gestation permanently programs rat hepatic phosphoenol-
pyruvate carboxykinase and glucocorticoid receptor expression and causes glucose
intolerance in adult offspring. *Journal of Clinical Investigation* 101, 2174–2181.

Ong, K.K., Ahmed, M.L., Emmett, P.M., Preece, M.A. and Dunger, D.B. (2001)
Association between postnatal catch-up growth and obesity in childhood:
prospective cohort study. *British Medical Journal* 320, 967–971.

Ozaki, T., Nishina, H., Hanson, M.A. and Poston, L. (2001) Dietary restriction in pregnant
rats causes gender-related hypertension and vascular dysfunction in offspring.
Journal of Physiology 530(1), 141–152.

Ozanne, S. (2001) Metabolic programming in animals. *British Medical Bulletin* 60,
143–152.

Ozanne, S.E., Smith, G.D., Tikerpae, J. and Hales, C.N. (1996a) Altered regulation of
hepatic glucose output in the male offspring of protein-malnourished rat dams.
American Journal of Physiology 270, E559–E564.

Ozanne, S.E., Wang, C.L., Coleman, N. and Smith, G.D. (1996b) Altered muscle insulin sensitivity in the male offspring of protein-malnourished rats. *American Journal of Physiology* 271(6), E1128–E1134.

Ozanne, S.E., Nave, B.T., Wang, C.L., Shepherd, P.R., Prins, J. and Smith, G.D. (1997) Poor fetal nutrition causes long-term changes in expression of insulin signaling components in adipocytes. *American Journal of Physiology* 273, E46–E51.

Ozanne, S.E., Martensz, N.D., Petry, C.J., Loizou, C.L. and Hales, C.N. (1998) Maternal low protein diet in rats programmes fatty acid desaturase activities in the offspring. *Diabetologia* 41, 1337–1342.

Ozanne, S.E., Dorling, M.W., Wang, C.L. and Nave, B.T. (2001) Impaired PI 3-kinase activation in adipocytes from early growth-restricted male rats. *American Journal of Physiology* 280, E534–E539.

Pallett, A.L., Morton, N.M., Cawthorne, M.A. and Emilsson, V. (1997) Leptin inhibits insulin secretion and reduces insulin mRNA levels in rat isolated pancreatic islets. *Biochemical and Biophysical Research Communications* 238, 267–270.

Persson, E. and Jansson, T. (1992) Low birth weight is associated with elevated adult blood pressure in the chronically catheterised guinea pig. *Acta Physiologica Scandinavica* 145, 195–196.

Petrik, J., Reusens, B., Arany, E., Remacle, C., Coelho, C. and Hoet, J.J. (1999) A low protein diet alters the balance of islet cell replication and apoptosis in the fetal and neonatal rat and is associated with a reduced pancreatic expression of insulin-like growth factor-II. *Endocrinology* 140, 4861–4873.

Petry, C.J., Dorling, M.W., Pawlak, D.B., Ozanne, S.E. and Hales, C.N. (2001) Diabetes in old male offspring of rat dams fed a reduced protein diet. *International Journal of Experimental Diabetes Research* 2(2), 139–143.

Phillips, D.I. (1998) Birth weight and the future development of diabetes. A review of the evidence. *Diabetes Care* 21(suppl. 2), B150–B155.

Plagemann, A., Harder, T., Rake, A., Melchior, K., Rohde, W. and Dorner, G. (2000) Hypothalamic nuclei are malformed in weanling offspring of low protein malnourished rat dams. *Journal of Nutrition* 130, 2582–2589.

Rajakumar, P.A., He, J., Simmons, R.A. and Devaskar, S.U. (1998) Effect of utero-placental insufficiency upon brain neuropeptide Y and corticotropin-releasing factor gene expression and concentrations. *Pediatric Research* 44, 168–174.

Ravelli, A.C., van der Meulen, J.H., Osmond, C., Barker, D.J. and Bleker, O.P. (1999) Obesity at the age of 50 y in men and women exposed to famine prenatally. *American Journal of Clinical Nutrition* 70, 811–816.

Ravelli, G.P., Stein, Z.A. and Susser, M.W. (1976) Obesity in young men after famine exposure *in utero* and in early infancy. *New England Journal of Medicine* 295, 349–353.

Reaven, G.M. (1993) Role of insulin resistance in human disease (syndrome X): an expanded definition. *Annual Review of Medicine* 44, 121–131.

Remke, H., Wilsdorf, A. and Muller, F. (1988) Development of hypothalamic obesity in growing rats. *Experimental Pathology* 33, 223–232.

Riccardi, G. and Rivellese, A.A. (2000) Dietary treatment of the metabolic syndrome – the optimal diet. *British Journal of Nutrition* 83(suppl 1), S143–S148.

Rich-Edwards, J.W., Stampfer, M.J., Manson, J.E., Rosner, B., Hankinson, S.E., Colditz, G.A., Willett, W.C. and Hennekens, C.H. (1997) Birth weight and risk of cardiovascular disease in a cohort of women followed up since 1976. *British Medical Journal* 315, 396–400.

Roseboom, T.J., van der Meulen, J.H., Osmond, C., Barker, D.J.P., Ravelli, A.C. and Bleker, O.P. (2000) Plasma lipid profiles in adults after prenatal exposure to the Dutch famine. *American Journal of Clinical Nutrition* 72, 1101–1106.

Sadowski, C.L., Choi, T.S., Le, M., Wheeler, T.T., Wang, L.H. and Sadowski, H.B. (2001) Insulin induction of SOCS-2 and SOCS-3 mRNA expression in C2C12 skeletal muscle cells is mediated by Stat5. *Journal of Biological Chemistry* 276, 20703–20710.

Schwartz, M.W., Seeley, R.J., Woods, S.C., Weigle, D.S., Campfield, L.A., Burn, P. and Baskin, D.G. (1997) Leptin increases hypothalamic pro-opiomelanocortin mRNA expression in the rostral arcuate nucleus. *Diabetes* 46, 2119–2123.

Seckl, J.R. (1994) Glucocorticoids and small babies. *Quarterly Journal of Medicine* 87, 259–262.

Seckl, J.R., Benediktsson, R., Lindsay, R.S. and Brown, R.W. (1995) Placental 11 beta-hydroxysteroid dehydrogenase and the programming of hypertension. *Journal of Steroid Biochemistry and Molecular Biology* 155, 447–455.

Seckl, J.R., Nyirenda, M.J., Walker, B.R. and Chapman, K.E. (1999) Glucocorticoids and fetal programming. *Biochemical Society Transactions* 27, 74–78.

Seckl, J.R., Cleasby, M. and Nyirenda, M.J. (2000) Glucocorticoids, 11beta-hydroxysteroid dehydrogenase, and fetal programming. *Kidney International* 57, 1412–1417.

Seidell, J.C. (2000) Obesity, insulin resistance and diabetes – a worldwide epidemic. *British Journal of Nutrition* 83(suppl. 1), S5–S8.

Seufert, J., Kieffer, T.J. and Habener, J.F. (1999) Leptin inhibits insulin gene transcription and reverses hyperinsulinemia in leptin-deficient ob/ob mice. *Proceedings of the National Academy of Sciences USA* 96, 674–679.

Smith, U., Axelsen, M., Carvalho, E., Eliasson, B., Jansson, P.A. and Wesslau, C. (1999) Insulin signaling and action in fat cells: associations with insulin resistance and type 2 diabetes. *Annals of the New York Academy of Sciences* 892, 119–126.

Snoeck, A., Remacle, C., Reusens, B. and Hoet, J.J. (1990) Effect of a low protein diet during pregnancy on the fetal rat endocrine pancreas. *Biology of the Neonate* 57, 107–118.

Soto, N., Bazaes, R.A., Pena, V., Salazar, T., Avila, A., Iniguez, G., Ong, K.K., Dunger, D.B. and Mericq, M.V. (2003) Insulin sensitivity and secretion are related to catch-up growth in small-for-gestational-age infants at age 1 year: results from a prospective cohort. *Journal of Clinical Endocrinology and Metabolism* 88(8), 3645–3650.

Szanto, I. and Kahn, C.R. (2000) Selective interaction between leptin and insulin signaling pathways in a hepatic cell line. *Proceedings of the National Academy of Sciences USA* 97, 2355–2360.

Thornton, J.E., Cheung, C.C., Clifton, D.K. and Steiner, R.A. (1997) Regulation of hypothalamic proopiomelanocortin mRNA by leptin in ob/ob mice. *Endocrinology* 138, 5063–5066.

Unger, R.H. (2001) Lipotoxicity in the pathogenesis of obesity-dependent NIDDM. Genetic and clinical implications. *Diabetes* 44, 863–870.

Unger, R.H. and Orci, L. (2001) Lipotoxic diseases of nonadipose tissues in obesity. *International Journal of Obesity and Related Metabolic Disorders* 24, S28–S32.

Vickers, M.H., Breier, B.H., Cutfield, W.S., Hofman, P.L. and Gluckman, P.D. (2000) Fetal origins of hyperphagia, obesity and hypertension and its postnatal amplification by hypercaloric nutrition. *American Journal of Physiology* 279, E83–E87.

Vickers, M.H., Reddy, S., Ikenasio, B.A. and Breier, B.H. (2001a) Dysregulation of the adipoinsular axis – a mechanism for the pathogenesis of hyperleptinemia and adipogenic diabetes induced by fetal programming. *Journal of Endocrinology* 170, 323–332.

Vickers, M.H., Ikenasio, B.A. and Breier, B.H. (2001b) IGF-1 treatment reduces hyperphagia, obesity, and hypertension in metabolic disorders induced by fetal programming. *Endocrinology* 142, 3964–3973.

Vickers, M.H., Ikenasio, B.A. and Breier, B.H. (2002) Adult growth hormone treatment reduces hypertension and obesity induced by an adverse prenatal environment. *Journal of Endocrinology* 175, 615–623.

Vickers, M., Breier, B., McCarthy, D. and Gluckman, P. (2003) Sedentary behavior during postnatal life is determined by the prenatal environment and exacerbated by postnatal hypercaloric nutrition. *American Journal of Physiology* 285, R271–R273.

Wang, Z.W., Zhou, Y.T., Kakuma, T., Lee, Y., Higa, M., Kalra, S.P., Dube, M.G., Kalra, P.S. and Unger, R.H. (1999) Comparing the hypothalamic and extrahypothalamic actions of endogenous hyperleptinemia. *Proceedings of the National Academy of Sciences USA* 96, 10373–10378.

Wang, Z., Zhou, Y.T., Kakuma, T., Lee, Y., Kalra, S.P., Kalra, P.S., Pan, W. and Unger, R.H. (2000) Leptin resistance of adipocytes in obesity: role of suppressors of cytokine signaling. *Biochemical and Biophysical Research Communications* 277, 20–26.

Weder, A.B. and Schork, N.J. (1994) Adaptation, allometry and hypertension. *Hypertension* 24, 145–156.

Welberg, L.A. and Seckl, J.R. (2001) Prenatal stress, glucocorticoids and the programming of the brain. *Journal of Neuroendocrinology* 13, 113–128.

Welberg, L.A., Seckl, J.R. and Holmes, M.C. (2001) Prenatal glucocorticoid programming of brain corticosteroid receptors and corticotrophin-releasing hormone: possible implications for behaviour. *Neuroscience* 104, 71–79.

Woodall, S.M., Breier, B.H., Johnston, B.M. and Gluckman, P.D. (1996a) A model of intrauterine growth retardation caused by chronic maternal undernutrition in the rat: effects on the somatotropic axis and postnatal growth. *Journal of Endocrinology* 150, 231–242.

Woodall, S.M., Johnston, B.M., Breier, B.H. and Gluckman, P.D. (1996b) Chronic maternal undernutrition in the rat leads to delayed postnatal growth and elevated blood pressure of offspring. *Pediatric Research* 40, 438–443.

Woodall, S.M., Bassett, N.S., Gluckman, P.D. and Breier, B.H. (1998) Consequences of maternal undernutrition for fetal and postnatal hepatic insulin-like growth factor-I, growth hormone receptor and growth hormone binding protein gene regulation in the rat. *Journal of Molecular Endocrinology* 20, 313–326.

Woodall, S.M., Breier, B.H., Johnston, B.M., Bassett, N.S., Barnard, R. and Gluckman, P.D. (1999) Administration of growth hormone or IGF-I to pregnant rats on a reduced diet throughout pregnancy does not prevent fetal intrauterine growth retardation and elevated blood pressure in adult offspring. *Journal of Endocrinology* 163, 69–77.

Yajnik, C. (2000) Interactions of perturbations in intrauterine growth and growth during childhood on the risk of adult-onset disease. *Proceedings of the Nutrition Society* 59, 257–265.

Yajnik, C.S., Lubree, H.G., Rege, S.S., Naik, S.S., Deshpande, J.A., Deshpande, S.S., Joglekar, C.V. and Yudkin, J.S. (2002) Adiposity and hyperinsulinemia in Indians are present at birth. *Journal of Clinical Endocrinology and Metabolism* 87, 5575–5580.

Zammit, V.A., Waterman, I.J., Topping, D. and McKay, G. (2001) Insulin stimulation of hepatic triacylglycerol secretion and the etiology of insulin resistance. *Journal of Nutrition* 131, 2074–2077.

Zimmet, P., Alberti, K.G. and Shaw, J. (2001) Global and societal implications of the diabetes epidemic. *Nature* 414(6865), 782–787.

11 Renal Disease and Fetal Undernutrition

LORI L. WOODS

Division of Nephrology and Hypertension, L463 Oregon Health and Science University, Portland, OR 97239-3098, USA

Introduction

Although it has now been about a decade and a half since Barker and colleagues first reported the inverse relationship between early growth patterns and the incidence of adult heart disease (Barker et al., 1989), the long-term implications of prenatal undernutrition for kidney disease in adulthood are still not well known. However, the little information that is available suggests that intrauterine growth retardation (IUGR) or low birthweight in humans is associated with a reduced number of nephrons (Hinchliffe et al., 1992; Manalich et al., 2000), an increased rate of proteinuria (Hoy et al., 1998, 1999) and renal failure (Lackland et al., 2000) later in life. This chapter will first examine what is known about the effects of early undernutrition on renal development, morphology and physiology. It will then consider some possible mechanisms involved in this programming. Finally, the chapter will explore how the known abnormalities associated with prenatal undernutrition may lead to renal disease.

Models of Fetal Undernutrition

To provide some points of reference with which to examine the existing data, it is useful to consider the various experimental models that have been used to study the long-term effects of fetal undernutrition on the offspring. Fetal undernutrition can be induced either by maternal undernutrition, by interference with utero-placental blood flow, or by nutrient transfer at the maternal–fetal interface in an otherwise well-nourished mother. Animal models of maternal undernutrition have generally involved either global food restriction, at anywhere from 30 to 70% of ad libitum intakes, in the rat or sheep, or restriction of protein intake by adjustment of the protein content of the diet, with the food itself being given ad libitum. Restriction of protein intake has been most often used in the rat, and the protein level chosen has ranged from about 5% (6% casein) to 12%, with what has been considered the 'normal' level usually set at about 19% (21% casein), but sometimes reaching 30%. Recently a model of maternal protein restriction in the pig has been used, with maternal protein intake reduced from 14% to 0.5–1% (Bagby et al., 2004). Restriction of maternal food or protein intake has been employed for all or part of gestation, sometimes with a clear intent to isolate a specific window or critical period of development, and at other times without a clear reason for the protocol chosen. At any rate, with such a large variation in the protocols used, it is unsurprising that there are inconsistencies in the results have been reported. In considering the findings of different studies, it will thus be crucial to give attention to the specifics of the dietary protocols employed in each case.

A possible role for maternal dietary fat intake in fetal programming has also been considered (Khan et al., 2003), and further work in this area is likely to be forthcoming. Variations in maternal Na⁺ intake can also programme for offspring hypertension, and we have begun to explore potential mechanisms involved in this (Woods and Weeks, 2004). Finally, some attention has been given to possible roles for micronutrients or vitamins in programming the offspring; in particular a role for vitamin A has been postulated (Lelievre-Pegorier et al., 1998).

In addition to maternal undernutrition, several other methods have also been used to induce fetal undernutrition. These include surgical removal of most of the uterine caruncles (the implantation sites for the placenta) prior to pregnancy or placental embolization in the sheep (Robinson et al., 1979; Louey et al., 2003), and ligation of one uterine artery in the rat (Merlet-Benichou et al., 1994). Some of these methods of interfering with placental function affect the entire pregnancy, whereas others affect only the later portion of gestation. Although the focus of this chapter is on fetal programming by maternal diet, findings in these other models will be referred to if they contribute to our understanding of the effects seen with maternal dietary restriction.

Effects of Fetal Undernutrition on Renal Structure and Function

It has long been recognized that fetal undernutrition, in the rat, leads to abnormalities in renal structure and function after birth. In 1968, Zeman first reported that rat offspring of mothers that were severely protein-restricted (6% casein diet) throughout pregnancy had kidneys that contained fewer glomeruli than offspring of mothers on a normal diet (24% casein). This investigator acknowledged the difficulty of quantifying morphologic components using the techniques available. However, it was estimated that in kidneys of newborn protein-restricted pups, the total number of glomeruli per section was reduced by 18%, and that the percentage accounted for by immature glomeruli was increased from 31% to 46% of the total. The nephrogenic zone also appeared to occupy a larger proportion of the total width of the cortex, indicating that the kidneys were less mature in offspring of protein-deprived mothers. The finding of a decreased number of cross-sections of proximal tubules was taken as an indication that the proximal tubules were fewer in number or shorter in the protein-deprived newborn offspring, providing further evidence of renal immaturity. Staining for acid and alkaline phosphatases was reduced or absent, also thought to indicate immaturity (Zeman, 1968). Figure 11.1 shows photomicrographs from near-term fetal rats in our laboratory, also illustrating the relative immaturity of the kidneys in offspring of protein-restricted mothers.

In more recent years, several laboratories have also reported a reduced number of nephrons in offspring of protein-restricted mothers, using a variety of methods. Merlet-Benichou et al. (1994) caused intrauterine growth retardation (IUGR) in rats either by ligation of one uterine artery or by feeding the mother a severely protein-restricted diet (5% protein versus a 22% protein control diet) from day 8 of gestation onward. Fetuses in the uterine horn with the ligated artery were 29% smaller and had 37% fewer glomeruli than those in the intact horn. By 2 weeks of age, pups from the ligated horns were still 23% smaller and had 30% fewer glomeruli. Glomerular volume was reported to be increased. Likewise, offspring of protein-deprived mothers were 28% smaller at birth and had 22% fewer glomeruli; by 2 weeks of age they were still 18% smaller and had 18% fewer glomeruli than offspring of mothers fed the normal diet. In this study, glomeruli were counted using an acid digestion method (Merlet-Benichou et al., 1994). Glomerular filtration rate (GFR) was reduced by about 50% in the 2-week-old pups from the ligated uterine horns, but renal function was not measured in the offspring of protein-deprived mothers. In another study, Vehaskari et al. (2001) fed a severely protein-restricted diet (6% protein) to pregnant rats for the last half of gestation. Using the maceration method, they estimated that the total number of glomeruli was decreased by nearly 30% in both male and female offspring at 8 weeks of age. Measurements of GFR were not done, but these investigators reported that plasma creatinine levels were similar in all groups.

Although methods using acid maceration or dissociation are relatively simple and may allow qualitative comparisons between groups, they are subject to considerable bias. The 'gold standard' techniques for determination of glomerular number and volume employ stereological methods, and the importance of using such unbiased techniques has recently come to the forefront (Madsen, 1999). Using these methods, we have recently confirmed that the relatively severe degree of maternal protein restriction used in the above studies, when fed throughout or during the last half of pregnancy, indeed causes a reduction of 30–45% in the number of nephrons in the offspring (Woods et al., 2004a). Although this effect is present in both males and females, it tends to be greater in males. We also found that absolute GFR is reduced in both male and female offspring of severely protein-restricted mothers. GFR normalized to body weight was significantly reduced in male offspring subjected to prenatal undernutrition, and tended to be reduced in females.

Although it seems clear from the above studies that severe maternal protein restriction during pregnancy leads to a reduced number of nephrons in the offspring, the effects of a more modest protein restriction are less easily delineated. Langley-Evans et al. (1999) counted glomeruli in 3–5 sections from fixed kidneys and reported that nephron number was significantly reduced by 16% in

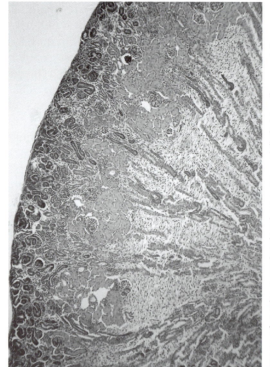
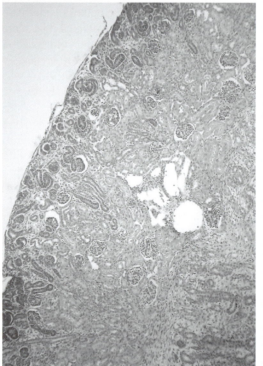

Fig. 11.1. Representative photomicrographs of kidneys of 23-day rat fetuses of mothers maintained on a normal (left panel) or protein-restricted (right panel) diet throughout pregnancy. The renal cortex is not only thinner in the fetus of the protein-restricted mother, but the nephrogenic zone, the compact outer layer of immature tubules and glomeruli, comprises a greater proportion of the cortex, indicating a less-mature kidney. (Courtesy of Drs Douglas Weeks and Hua Guo.)

mature offspring of mothers that had received 9% casein throughout pregnancy. Data for males and females were combined, so gender differences were either not present or not assessed. However, the average number of glomeruli in control kidneys in that study was considerably lower than that reported by other investigators, casting some doubt on the reliability of the method. However, these findings have been confirmed using both an acid digestion method and an unbiased stereological technique (Zimanyi *et al.*, 2000; Woods *et al.*, 2004b). GFR was measured only in females, at 19 weeks of age, and no differences were found between the offspring of control and protein-restricted mothers.

A study of Sprague–Dawley rats from our laboratory showed general agreement with the results of this study of Langley-Evans *et al.* Using stereological methods, we found that an 8.5% protein (9% casein) maternal diet caused a 13% reduction in birthweight and a 25% reduction in nephron number in male offspring (Woods *et al.*, 2001a). The average individual volume of the glomeruli was increased, so that the total volume of all glomeruli was not different from that in normal animals. Glomerular hypertrophy and hyperfiltration are well-known responses to a reduction in nephron number (Hostetter *et al.*, 1981). In contrast, female offspring of these modestly protein-restricted mothers had a normal number of glomeruli, which were of normal size (Woods *et al.*, 2004b). Thus, use of stereological techniques and a modest protein restriction revealed a gender difference in programming, which will be discussed further later in this chapter. We also found that although GFR was not different between female offspring of normal and protein-restricted mothers, it was reduced by about 10% in male offspring of protein-restricted mothers compared to controls. Although this did not reach statistical significance, this difference is at the limits of detection of these techniques. A decrease of this magnitude would be physiologically significant, as a decrease of only 10% in whole-kidney GFR coupled with a decrease of 25% in nephron number implies that GFR of the individual nephrons was increased in these animals compared to controls. This increased single-nephron GFR may have important implications for the progression of renal disease, as discussed later in this chapter.

Zimanyi *et al.* (2000) also used stereological techniques to determine glomerular number in offspring of modestly protein-restricted Wistar–Kyoto rats. In this case, the mothers were fed the diet from before breeding throughout pregnancy, and for the first 2 weeks of lactation. As this dietary restriction protocol encompassed the entire period of nephrogenesis (from approximately mid-gestation to about 7–10 days after birth) in the rat, it would, if anything, be expected to have a greater impact on nephron number than protein restriction during pregnancy alone (Moritz and Wintour, 1999). Abnormally large or small pups were culled, which may have reduced variability, and only male offspring were studied. Despite the small number of animals studied, these investigators also found that nephron number was significantly reduced by about 30% in offspring of protein-restricted mothers (Zimanyi *et al.*, 2000).

In summary, it seems clear that severe maternal protein restriction during pregnancy causes a reduced number of nephrons in both male and female offspring. Renal function is also reduced. In contrast, a modest maternal protein restriction appears to reduce nephron number and renal function only in male offspring, whereas females appear to be relatively protected from this maternal insult.

What are the Key Nutrients in Programming of Altered Renal Structure, Renal Disease and Hypertension?

Although it has been clearly established that the protein content of the maternal diet can have a major impact on renal development and ultimate renal structure, not all investigators agree that protein intake is the only, or even the major, player in programming for adult disease. Maintaining a test diet isocaloric to the control diet while reducing protein content requires an increase in other nutrients, usually carbohydrate. Thus, some have suggested that factors other than the protein content in the maternal diet are critical in programming the fetus. Langley-Evans (2000) compared the effects of two low-protein diets that were equal in terms of protein (casein) content but differed in terms of fat, carbohydrate and methionine content. He found that the low-protein diet that contained more fat and starch programmed the offspring for increased systolic blood pressure compared to its own control diet, whereas the one containing more sugar did not cause increased blood pressure compared to its own control (normal protein) diet. This suggests that the balance of nutrients in the diet may be critical in determining the long-term effects of maternal undernutrition on the offspring. On the other hand, we and others have found that global maternal food restriction (limiting total food intake rather than altering the composition of the food) leads to similar effects on the offspring blood pressure as protein restriction (Woodall *et al.*, 1996; Woods and Weeks, 2004b). This suggests that the amount of protein consumed by the pregnant mother is critical to the outcome of her offspring, although there may also be factors in some dietary formulations that can ameliorate some of the detrimental effects of a low maternal protein intake.

It should be noted that Tonkiss *et al.* (1998) measured blood pressure using radiotelemetry in male rat offspring of mothers that had been severely protein-restricted (6% casein) before and throughout pregnancy. They found no significant differences in blood pressure between the protein-restricted offspring and controls during the light phase of the day (a time of sleep in these nocturnal animals), but diastolic pressure was significantly higher in protein-restricted offspring than controls during the dark (active) phase of the day. Also, the protein-restricted animals had higher systolic and diastolic pressures in response to a stressor. The authors suggested that the more dramatic differences in blood pressure found by other investigators using the tail-cuff method may be due, in large part, to stress. However, in our studies the animals are chronically instrumented, and although loosely restrained, they have been trained and acclimatized to these conditions. Thus, stress is reduced, although probably not entirely prevented. Moreover, as, in humans, a substantial portion of the day is generally spent awake and often experiencing the routine stresses of daily life, it seems reasonable that the blood pressures of the rats during mild stress may be quite applicable to the human condition.

A high maternal Na^+ intake can also programme the offspring for hypertension (Woods and Weeks, 2004a). Although the mechanisms are unknown, it does not appear to involve a reduced nephron endowment, as glomerular number is normal in these offspring (Woods and Weeks, 2004a). The other nutrient that has received some attention for its possible role in programming the fetal kidney is vitamin A. Lelievre-Pegorier *et al.* (1998) fed a vitamin A-deficient diet to female rats before mating and throughout pregnancy. Glomeruli were counted using the acid maceration technique in pups at 14 days of age. These investigators reported that the number of nephrons was reduced in vitamin A-deficient offspring compared to controls. Interestingly, in pups of normal mothers injected with retinoic acid on day 11 of gestation, nephron number was actually reported to be increased compared to pups of normal mothers which were not treated with retinoic acid. Thus, maternal intake of specific vitamins or other micronutrients may play a role in programming renal structure and function in the offspring.

Prenatal Undernutrition and Adult Hypertension

The changes in the kidney that occur in response to prenatal protein restriction are likely to have important implications for hypertension later in life. The kidney is widely recognized as the major long-term controller of arterial blood pressure (Guyton *et al.*, 1972). Although most textbooks state that the average number of nephrons in a human kidney is about 1 million, the range within the population is actually quite large: between 300,000 and 1,200,000 (Brenner *et al.*, 1988; Nyengaard and Bendtsen, 1992; Brenner and Chertow, 1994). Brenner *et al.* (1988) have postulated that the reduced 'endowment' of nephrons at birth in certain individuals may account, at least in part, for the tendency to develop essential hypertension later in life. The mechanisms by which this could occur are illustrated in Fig. 11.2. A reduced number of nephrons due to fetal undernutrition or other causes would provide a decreased total filtration surface area, which would cause renal sodium retention. Blood pressure would increase until the forces for ultrafiltration were sufficient to overcome the reduced surface area, and the individual was again in sodium and water balance. Thus, normal excretion of salt and water would be maintained only at the expense of a higher blood pressure. Systemic hypertension itself promotes glomerular hypertension and glomerulosclerosis, which further reduces the functioning surface area, thus perpetuating a vicious cycle of increasing arterial pressure and progressive glomerular damage. Thus, by reducing the nephron endowment, fetal undernutrition could programme for hypertension as well as increased risk for renal disease later in life.

Renal Mechanisms of Programming for Hypertension

We first became interested in the effects of maternal undernutrition on the developing kidney because of our interest in the mechanisms of hypertension. It had

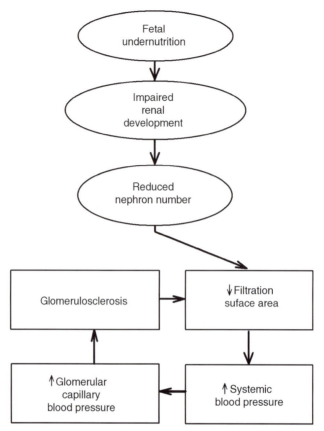

Fig. 11.2. Flow chart illustrating how a reduced number of nephrons caused by fetal undernutrition could lead to hypertension and progressive renal disease. (Adapted from Brenner *et al.*, 1988; Brenner and Chertow, 1994.)

been shown that modest maternal dietary protein restriction in pregnancy caused systolic hypertension in the offspring (Langley and Jackson, 1994), but the mechanisms were unknown. In light of the overwhelming evidence that the kidney is the major long-term controller of arterial blood pressure (Guyton *et al.*, 1972), the kidney was the logical place to begin our investigation into mechanisms of prenatally programmed hypertension. Additionally, Brenner *et al.* (1988) had recently put forth the postulate that hypertension in humans may be related to a reduced endowment of nephrons from birth, described above.

Combining what had been reported about maternal protein deprivation causing fewer glomeruli (Zeman, 1968) with the report that offspring of protein-restricted mothers develop hypertension (Langley and Jackson, 1994), and the idea that a reduced nephron endowment may be associated with hypertension (Brenner *et al.*, 1988), we formulated the following hypothesis (illustrated in Fig. 11.3). We postulated that a reduced maternal protein intake in pregnancy is somehow translated to the fetus, presumably by some signalling molecule, across the placenta. This signal could be something as simple as a change in

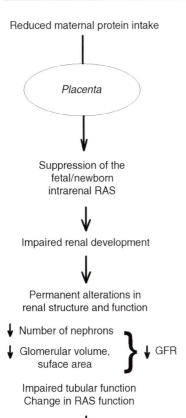

Reduced maternal protein intake

Placenta

Suppression of the
fetal/newborn
intrarenal RAS

Impaired renal development

Permanent alterations in
renal structure and function

↓ Number of nephrons

↓ Glomerular volume,
   suface area
} ↓ GFR

Impaired tubular function
Change in RAS function

Hypertension

Fig. 11.3. Hypothesis illustrating the mechanisms by which fetal undernutrition could lead to adult hypertension. RAS, renin–angiotensin system; GFR, glomerular filtration rate. (Adapted from Woods *et al.*, 2001a.)

amino acid transport, although other investigators have postulated a role for increased exposure of the fetus to maternal cortisol or corticosterone (in the rat) (Benediktsson *et al.*, 1993). Whatever the signal, we postulated that the renin–angiotensin system (RAS) of the fetus is suppressed when maternal protein intake is reduced. Either the circulating RAS or the intrarenal RAS could be altered, but as it is the intrarenal RAS that is generally thought to be important in long-term regulation of arterial pressure, by causing structural changes, it seemed likely that this would be the system that would be involved here. Several laboratories had shown that angiotensin II (AngII) was critical for normal renal development (Fogo *et al.*, 1990; Friberg *et al.*, 1994; Tufro-McReddie *et al.*, 1994, 1995; Nishimura *et al.*, 1999), so it was logical to propose that suppression of the intrarenal RAS during the developmental period would lead to impaired renal development. It is appropriate to point out here that nephrogenesis is completed before birth in the sheep and human, so that no new nephrons are formed postnatally in these species (Moritz and Wintour, 1999). In contrast, in the rat, nephrogenesis takes place from about mid-gestation until some 7–10 days after birth. Thus, maternal dietary restriction may continue to influence renal development in this species during the first half of the lactation period. Impaired development would, in turn, result in permanent changes in renal structure and, consequently, in renal function. This could take several forms, including a reduced number of nephrons, a reduced glomerular volume or capillary surface area, impaired tubular function and altered RAS function. Not all of these changes might be expected to be present, but any one of them could lead, in turn, to chronic hypertension. Early reports of apparent reductions in numbers of glomeruli in offspring of protein-deprived rat mothers, as well as the hypothesis of Brenner *et al.* (1988) that a smaller nephron endowment at birth might account for adult hypertension, suggested that nephron number should be the primary focus for study.

Studies in our laboratory have used a model of modest maternal protein restriction (8.5% protein) throughout pregnancy in the Sprague–Dawley rat (Woods *et al.*, 2001a). Kidneys were harvested from newborn animals for assessment of the intrarenal RAS, and mean arterial pressure and renal function were measured in chronically instrumented adult offspring. In this particular study, only male offspring were used. Our findings are shown in Fig. 11.4. Renal renin, renin mRNA and AngII levels were reduced in the newborn offspring of protein-restricted mothers, compared to offspring of mothers fed the normal diet, in keeping with our initial hypothesis. In adult male offspring of modestly pro-tein-restricted mothers, the total number of glomeruli, measured using unbiased stereological methods, was reduced by about 25%, and conscious, resting mean arterial blood pressure was elevated by about 10 mmHg. We also found a 10% reduction in glomerular filtration rate (GFR) in the low-protein-exposed offspring. Again, the fact that nephron number was reduced by a greater percentage than the GFR indicates that the individual nephrons were hyper-filtering. Although this is a well-recognized response to nephron loss, it may con-tribute to progressive renal disease (Hostetter *et al.*, 1981). Importantly, using gold-standard techniques, we thereby confirmed reports by other investigators, using the tail-cuff method, of elevations in systolic blood pressure (Langley and Jackson, 1994), and of reductions in glomerular (nephron) number counted in sections of kidney (Langley-Evans *et al.*, 1999) in offspring of modestly protein-restricted mothers, and we showed for the first time that all of the key elements in our hypothesis were present in the same animal model.

Our next task in testing the hypothesis was to establish a cause-and-effect relationship among the various elements. Our first approach, to show that sup-pression of the RAS during the window of nephrogenesis leads to a reduced nephron number and hypertension, was to pharmacologically block this system during development using the AngII receptor antagonist, losartan. We found that in normal male and female offspring treated with losartan for the first 12 days of postnatal life, the total number of nephrons in adulthood (22 weeks) was reduced by 42%, GFR was reduced by 27%, and mean arterial pressure was elevated by 14 mmHg (Woods and Rasch, 1998). Thus, suppression of the RAS within the window of nephrogenesis caused a reduced number of nephrons, impaired renal function and hypertension.

To determine whether a reduction in the number of nephrons, from birth, leads to adult hypertension, in our next series of experiments we surgically reduced the nephron number by 50% by performing a uninephrectomy in normal rat pups on the first day of postnatal life (Woods, 1999; Woods *et al.*, 2001b). These animals developed a salt-sensitive hypertension as early as 8 weeks of age, and this hypertension preceded the onset of renal disease, which did eventually occur, at least in males. In females and young males, total GFR was reduced by only about 25–30%, whereas in older males it was reduced by

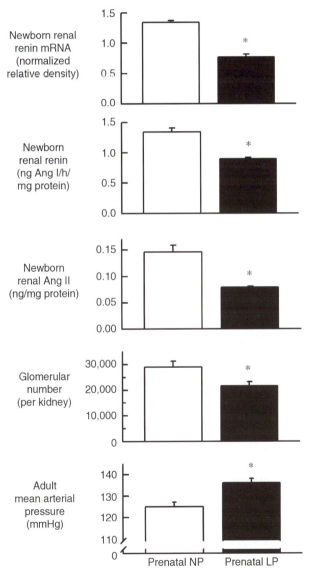

Fig. 11.4. Newborn intrarenal renin–angiotensin system components and adult glomerular number and blood pressure in male offspring of modestly protein-restricted (LP, 8.5% protein) rat dams. *$P < 0.05$ compared to male offspring of mothers fed the normal diet (NP). (Adapted from Woods *et al.*, 2001a.)

about 50%. Thus, although reports regarding a possible hypertensive effect of uninephrectomy in adulthood are mixed (Vincenti *et al.*, 1983; Hakim *et al.*, 1984; Smith *et al.*, 1985; Williams *et al.*, 1986), removal of 50% of the nephron mass, when done at birth, leads unequivocally to adult hypertension in the rat. A recent study in the sheep has confirmed this finding. Uninephrectomy during the period of nephrogenesis in the ovine fetus leads to increased mean arterial pressures at 6 and 12 months of age (Moritz *et al.*, 2002). Thus, a cause-and-effect relationship among the key elements of our hypothesis was established.

There are two principles that are fundamental to the concept of fetal (or perinatal) programming. First, an insult occurs during a critical window of development and such windows differ for different organ systems. Secondly, such an insult causes permanent changes in the structure and function of specific organs. Work with the low-protein-exposed rat models in our laboratory and that of Langley-Evans has shown that maternal protein restriction does indeed cause permanent changes in structure and function of the offspring kidneys. That the insult must occur during a critical period has been implied in the above discussion, but the issue has not yet been addressed directly. To look specifically at this issue, we designed experiments in which rat fetuses were exposed to a more severe maternal protein restriction that either specifically targeted or specifically avoided the window of nephrogenesis (Woods *et al.*, 2004a). We postulated that if impaired renal development and a reduced nephron number are central in the aetiology of the hypertension induced by fetal undernutrition, then the future blood pressure set point of an animal should be sensitive to maternal protein intake only during the window of nephrogenesis. Thus, pregnant rats were fed a low-protein diet either throughout pregnancy, only during the first half of gestation (before nephrogenesis), or only during the last half of gestation (during nephrogenesis). Arterial pressure, renal function and nephron number in the adult offspring were compared to those in offspring of mothers receiving the normal protein diet throughout pregnancy (Woods *et al.*, 2004a). Figure 11.5 shows that arterial pressure was increased and nephron number and GFR were reduced in male offspring that were exposed to maternal protein restriction during the last half of, or throughout, gestation, whereas they were normal in offspring that were exposed only during the first half of gestation. Thus, in our study, the window of sensitivity of future adult blood pressure to maternal protein restriction coincided with nephrogenesis. These findings further support the importance of impaired renal development and permanent reductions in nephron number in programming for hypertension by maternal diet.

Interestingly, Langley-Evans *et al.* (1996) did a similar study in which they fed a 9% casein diet to pregnant rats during either the first, second or third week of gestation. This showed that exposure to protein restriction during any of the three trimesters caused systolic hypertension in male offspring, although the largest effect was seen in offspring exposed throughout pregnancy. The reasons for the discrepancies between this study and ours are not clear, although there were a number of technical differences. Perhaps the most important difference is that their animals were studied at 4 weeks of age, whereas our animals were 22 weeks old. Thus, the differences they noted may have been transient, whereas our data may represent more long-term, steady-state responses to maternal

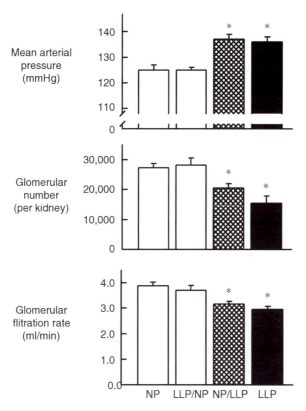

Fig. 11.5. Blood pressure, glomerular number and renal function in adult male offspring of rat dams fed a protein-restricted diet (6% protein) during the first half of pregnancy (LLP/NP), the second half of pregnancy (NP/LLP) or throughout pregnancy (LLP), compared to offspring of mothers fed a normal diet (NP, 19% protein). *$P < 0.05$ compared to NP. (Adapted from Woods *et al.*, 2004a.)

protein deprivation. In another study, Kwong *et al.* (2000) reported that feeding a 9% casein diet to pregnant rats for only the first 4.25 days of pregnancy was sufficient to programme the male, but not the female, offspring for increased systolic blood pressure. The technical aspects of this study were similar to those in the study of Langley-Evans *et al.* (1996) and, again, the animals were studied at a younger age than in our study. It is puzzling that the control females in that study had considerably higher blood pressures than the control males. Interestingly, fetal undernutrition induced by uteroplacental embolization in sheep does not appear to cause adult hypertension (Louey *et al.*, 2003). This may be related to the fact that such embolization experiments have been performed near the end of gestation, and thus there was not a great deal of overlap with the period of nephrogenesis.

There is strong evidence that modest maternal protein restriction programmes the offspring for hypertension by suppression of the intrarenal RAS during development, leading to impaired renal development, a reduced endowment of nephrons, and consequent hypertension in adulthood. However, the possibility that other mechanisms may also come into play cannot be excluded, and more work is needed to resolve the apparent differences in results among the studies that have been done to date.

Little is known to date about possible changes in renal tubular function that may be induced by fetal undernutrition. Manning et al. (2002) have examined a potential role for abnormal up-regulation of sodium transporters in offspring of rats undergoing a severe protein restriction for the last half of pregnancy. These studies have reported that both mRNA and protein levels of the bumetanide-sensitive $Na^+-K^+-2Cl^-$ cotransporter (BSC1) and the thiazide-sensitive Na^+-Cl^- cotransporter (TSC) – the apical Na^+ transporters of the thick ascending limb and the distal convoluted tubule, respectively – were up-regulated in offspring of protein-restricted mothers (Manning et al., 2002). Importantly, increased levels of these proteins and their mRNAs were increased at 4 weeks of age, before any difference in arterial pressures could be detected, suggesting that the changes were not a response to hypertension. Presumably, such increases in sodium transporters could promote sodium retention and consequent hypertension. In contrast, abundances of the type III sodium–hydrogen exchanger (NHE3) and the α-, β- and γ-subunits of the amiloride-sensitive epithelial Na^+ channel (ENaC) were not significantly different between groups. Thus, changes in post-natal gene expression within the kidney programmed by prenatal undernutrition could contribute to the increased blood pressure in offspring later in life. However, more work is needed to clarify the precise role of altered tubular function in causing the hypertension programmed by fetal exposure to maternal dietary restriction.

The Role of Maternal Glucocorticoids in Programming the Offspring for Hypertension and Renal Abnormalities

Several investigators have postulated an important role for fetal exposure to excess maternal glucocorticoids in the mechanism(s) through which maternal undernutrition programmes for offspring hypertension (Benediktsson et al., 1993; C. Bertram et al., 2001). Although the role of maternal glucocorticoids in programming is addressed in detail elsewhere in this volume (Chapter 16), it warrants a few words here as well, in particular because some of our own recent data may refute the importance of this proposed mechanism. Briefly, it is generally thought that maternal glucocorticoids are normally largely inactivated by the placental enzyme 11β-hydroxysteroid dehydrogenase (11β-HSD) before they reach the fetus. However, under conditions in which maternal glucocorticoid levels are markedly elevated and/or placental 11β-HSD activity is reduced, the fetus may be exposed to excess maternal glucocorticoids, which could, in turn, programme for hypertension. Indeed, it has long been recognized that human infants exposed to prednisone in utero have reduced birthweights and a higher incidence of being 'small for dates' (Reinisch et al., 1978). Additionally, placental 11β-HSD activity has been shown to be reduced in human pregnancies that are complicated by IUGR (Shams et al., 1998), although this is not universally reported (Stewart et al., 1995; Rogerson et al., 1997; McCalla et al., 1998).

Administration of dexamethasone (a synthetic glucocorticoid not inactivated by the placental enzyme) to pregnant rats on normal diets throughout or during the last part of pregnancy leads to offspring of lower birthweight than normal, who are hypertensive later in life (Benediktsson et al., 1993; Levitt et al., 1996). Dexamethasone also causes a reduced number of nephrons in the offspring (Celsi et al., 1998). Additionally, administration of the 11β-HSD inhibitor, carbenoxolone, to normal pregnant rats, either throughout gestation or during the last part of pregnancy, produces offspring that are hypertensive, although it apparently does not do so if carbenoxolone is only given during early pregnancy (Lindsay et al., 1996; Langley-Evans, 1997). These and other findings have led some investigators to conclude that fetal exposure to maternal glucocorticoids plays an important role in programming for offspring hypertension. However, the relatively high doses of these drugs that were used in the studies mentioned are of concern. At these doses, these drugs impair maternal food intake and weight gain, and the mothers are often in poor health. In a very recent study, we injected dexamethasone at 100 µg/kg/day (the dose most commonly used in the above studies) into pregnant rats either during the first or last part of gestation (Woods and Weeks, 2004b). Food intake was reduced, and animals always lost weight or failed to gain the normal amount of weight during the period of injection. Administration of dexamethasone early in gestation did not programme the offspring for hypertension, but administration later in pregnancy did. Pair-feeding of another group of pregnant animals to the late pregnancy dexamethasone-treated group, showed that adult offspring of these mothers had hypertension that was equivalent to that in the offspring of dexamethasone-treated mothers. Thus, the reduction in food intake in these animals appeared to be able to account for the hypertensive programming effects on the offspring, suggesting that maternal glucocorticoids may not play a major role in programming by maternal diet. At the very least, these data suggest that maternal glucocorticoids and dietary protein restriction act through the same mechanisms to programme the offspring for hypertension.

Do Experimental Manipulations Mimic Naturally Occurring Phenomena?

Aside from the epidemiological studies in humans indicating an inverse relationship between early growth, on the one hand, and adult hypertension and renal disease on the other, very little information is available regarding naturally occurring IUGR and these adult outcomes. A recent study in the pig suggested an inverse relationship between mean arterial pressure at 3 months of age and birthweight, although the lack of robustness of the data was disappointing (Poore et al., 2002). In the rat, animals whose birthweight was less than 90% of the mean for their litters have blood pressures that are higher than gender-matched littermate controls of normal birthweight. This is true in litters from untreated mothers and in offspring resulting from a variety of maternal treatments, such as protein restriction, dexamethasone administration and sodium loading (Woods and Weeks, 2004c). One study in the rat has suggested that birthweight is not related to glomerular number and volume (Jones *et al.*, 2001). However, although these investigators used stereological methods, the design of the study was such that there was not a large difference in mean size between the 'low birthweight' and 'normal birthweight' groups, and many animals in the 'low birthweight' group were actually larger than many animals in the 'normal birthweight' group. Thus, a real effect of birthweight on nephron number may have been obscured. In human subjects, it has recently been shown, using stereological techniques, that patients diagnosed with hypertension have significantly fewer nephrons than do normotensive controls (Keller *et al.*, 2003). Although this finding does not prove cause and effect, it is reassuring to find that a reduced nephron number and hypertension again occur in parallel.

Does Fetal Undernutrition Programme for Renal Disease?

Given that fetal undernutrition has been shown to cause a reduced nephron endowment and hypertension, it seems likely that it would also lead to an increased risk for some types of renal disease. Although very little is presently known about the implications of fetal undernutrition for renal disease, emerging evidence supports the idea that maternal dietary restriction indeed programmes the offspring for increased renal risk as well.

In the rat, Lucas *et al.* (2001) found that male offspring of mothers that underwent a 50% food restriction throughout pregnancy had a reduced GFR per body weight compared to controls at 3 and 18 months of age. In ageing animals (18 months), the percentage of glomeruli showing focal or global glomerulosclerosis was greater in the offspring of restricted mothers. Nwagwu *et al.* (2000) found that offspring of modestly protein-restricted mothers had increased blood urea nitrogen levels and urine albumin excretion by 20 weeks of age, suggesting progressive deterioration of renal function in these animals. As shown in Fig. 11.6, we have also found that offspring of mothers that were severely protein restricted during the last part of, or throughout, pregnancy had significantly more tubular dilatation, tubular atrophy, interstitial fibrosis and scarring than did offspring of normal mothers (Woods *et al.*, 2004a). This injury was more prominent in males, and appeared to worsen with age.

Only a very few studies to date have examined the possibility of prenatal programming for subsequent renal disease in humans. Using histomorphometric methods, Manalich *et al.* (2000) studied the kidneys of low birthweight and normal birthweight newborn infants. They found a significant positive relationship between birthweight and number of glomeruli in the subcapsular cortex and a negative correlation between birthweight and glomerular volume. Although the method did not allow calculation of the total number of glomeruli in the kidney, in the sections examined, babies weighing less than 2500 g at birth had 12% fewer glomeruli than those weighing more than 2500 g. Greater percentages of the mothers of the low birthweight infants smoked, and/or had essential or gestational hypertension, all of which might contribute to low birthweight, than mothers of normal birthweight infants. Thus, cause-and-effect relationships in this study were not clear. It also was not clear whether genetic or environmental

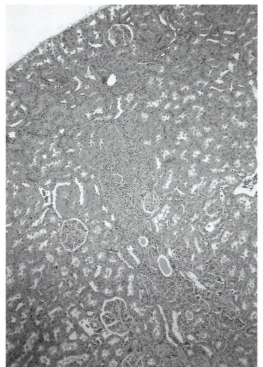

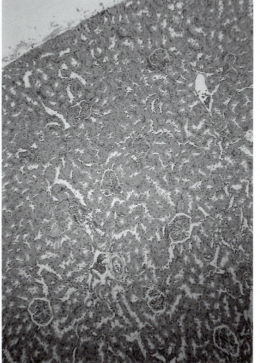

Fig. 11.6. Representative photomicrographs of kidneys of adult male rat offspring of mothers maintained on a normal (left panel) or protein-restricted (right panel) diet throughout pregnancy. The kidney of the protein-restricted offspring has significantly more tubular dilatation, tubular atrophy, interstitial fibrosis and scarring. (Courtesy of Drs Douglas Weeks and Hua Guo.)

mechanisms (or both) were responsible for the relationships found. However, these data were at least consistent with the idea that low birthweight is associated with a reduced nephron endowment. Hinchliffe et al. (1992) used stereological methods to study renal development in IUGR. Although the number of subjects was small, the number of nephrons was significantly reduced by an average of about 35% in babies that were intrauterine growth-retarded, compared to babies of normal weight (Hinchliffe et al., 1992). Thus, it does appear that there is also an inverse relationship between fetal growth and nephron number in humans.

The incidence of chronic renal failure is known to be particularly high in several populations, including Aborigines of Australia's Northern Territory and residents of the south-eastern United States. These populations have provided some insight into possible relationships between low birthweight and suscepti-bility to renal disease in humans. Hoy et al. (1999) studied a community of Aborigines for which birthweights were available. In this population, birthweights ranged from 1.5 to 4.1 kg, with the mean being approximately 2.7 kg. About one-third of the study participants were classified as 'low birthweight' (less than 2.5 kg). Urine albumin to creatinine ratio, an index of renal disease, tended to be higher in the low birthweight group, and this relationship was significant after accounting for age, sex, body mass index and blood pressures. In a matched-pair analysis (low versus normal birthweight pairs matched for age and sex), the rate of overt albuminuria ($\geq$ 300 mg albumin per g creatinine) was over twice as high in the low birthweight individuals (Hoy et al., 1999). Preliminary studies have not shown a difference in nephron number among Australian Aborigine, African American and white populations (J.F. Bertram et al., 2001), but larger sample sizes may eventually reveal such differences.

Lackland et al. (2000) studied patients in South Carolina who were diag-nosed with renal failure and undergoing dialysis, and compared their birth-weights with those of controls that did not have end-stage renal disease (ESRD), who were matched for age, sex and race. The odds ratio for renal failure was highest in subjects who weighed less than 2500 g at birth, and decreased with increasing birthweight. There was, however, evidence of a U-shaped trend, with an elevated odds ratio in the group with the largest birthweights ($\geq$ 4000 g). This was particularly evident in the subjects in whom diabetes was the primary cause of the renal failure. The percentage of the ESRD subjects who were African-American was disproportionately high. Approximately 30% of the population in South Carolina are African-Americans, whereas 70% of the ESRD subjects were. However, this is consistent with the relatively high incidence of ESRD in African-Americans in the USA overall.

Low birthweight may also pose an added risk for renal disease in subjects with diabetes, in whom the renal risk is already elevated. Rossing et al. (1995) reported an increase in the risk for renal disease in women with type 1 diabetes whose birthweights were below the 10th percentile, compared to those with larger birthweights. In Pima Indians with type 2 diabetes, birthweight and elevated urinary albumin excretion showed a U-shaped relationship (Nelson et al., 1998). The high urinary albumin excretion rate associated with low birthweight was suggested to reflect intrauterine programming, whereas that associated with high birthweight was thought to reflect intrauterine exposure to maternal diabetes.

Zidar *et al.* (1998) have shown that among children with IgA nephropathy, those with a birthweight below the 10th percentile have an increased risk for developing hypertension and glomerulosclerosis, suggesting that low birthweight introduces factors that contribute to the progression of another form of renal disease. Thus, although relative fetal undernutrition and other factors that limit fetal growth may not always lead directly to renal disease, it appears that they may predispose to more serious disease in patients who develop renal disease from other causes.

Gender Differences in Programming for Renal Disease and Hypertension by Fetal Undernutrition

As alluded to earlier, emerging evidence indicates that there are gender differences in nutritional programming for renal disease and hypertension. In humans and animals, males generally have somewhat higher blood pressures than females of the same age, and considerable evidence suggests that the sex hormones play a role in regulation of blood pressure. Thus it is not surprising that sex differences appear to exist within the phenomenon of fetal programming. For example, our studies in the rat have shown that a modest maternal protein restriction in pregnancy programmes the male but not the female offspring for a reduced nephron number and hypertension in adulthood (Woods *et al.*, 2001a, 2004b). In contrast, a more severe protein restriction programmes both male and female offspring for fewer nephrons and hypertension in adulthood (Woods *et al.*, 2004a). Thus, females may be relatively protected from the long-term effects of *in utero* exposure to maternal dietary protein restriction. Recent evidence suggests that this gender difference is due to differences in the intrarenal renin–angiotensin system during development in males and females. In males this system is suppressed by maternal dietary protein restriction, whereas in females renal renin mRNA, renin and angiotensin II remain at normal levels (Woods *et al.*, 2004b). It seems likely that this programming is related to the number of nephrons with which the offspring are endowed (males with a reduced number and females with a normal number), because we have also shown that surgical reduction in the number of nephrons from birth leads to salt-sensitive hypertension in both male and female animals (Woods, 1999; Woods *et al.*, 2001b). However, the blood pressure elevation is greater in males, and they also develop proteinuria and histological evidence of renal damage by 20 weeks of age, whereas the females do not (Woods, 1999; Woods *et al.*, 2001b). There are also gender differences in programming by maternal salt intake in pregnancy. A moderately high maternal Na^+ intake during pregnancy and lactation leads to hypertension in male but not in female offspring (unpublished observations). On the other hand, a very high maternal Na^+ intake programmes both male and female offspring for increased blood pressure (Woods and Weeks, 2004a).

Other investigators have also reported gender differences in programming for hypertension by maternal diet. In offspring of rats that were modestly food-restricted (70% of the normal intake for the first 18 days of pregnancy), males became hypertensive at a younger age than did their female littermates (Ozaki *et al.*, 2001). Interestingly, in offspring of rats fed a lard-rich diet, the females became hypertensive whereas the males did not (Khan *et al.*, 2003). The precise mechanisms responsible for gender differences in fetal programming are not known, although the sex hormones oestrogen and testosterone are likely to play a role. This will be an important area for future study.

In summary, low birthweight in humans is associated with an increased risk for hypertension and renal disease in adulthood. Based largely on animal studies of maternal dietary restriction, the following scenario seems likely. Programming of offspring for these diseases occurs through suppression of the intrarenal renin–angiotensin system during a critical window of development, resulting in impaired renal development and a reduced nephron endowment, which, in turn increases the risk for hypertension and renal disease in later life. In general, females may be less susceptible than males, requiring a stronger or longer insult to cause discernible programming. More work is needed to further delineate the molecular mechanisms involved, and to investigate possible therapeutic interventions that could potentially prevent or reverse these abnormalities.

References

Bagby, S.P., LeBard, L.S., Luo, Z., Woods, L.L., McPherson, E., Corless, C. and Ogden, B.E. (2004) Maternal protein restriction in a microswine model: early asymmetric growth restriction and adult hypertension. *Pediatric Research* (submitted).

Barker, D.J.P., Winter, P.D., Osmond, C., Margetts, B. and Simmonds, S.J. (1989) Weight in infancy and death from ischaemic heart disease. *Lancet* 2, 577–580.

Benediktsson, R., Lindsay, R.S., Noble, J., Seckl, J.R. and Edwards, C.R.W. (1993) Glucocorticoid exposure *in utero*: new model for adult hypertension. *Lancet* 341, 339–341.

Bertram, C., Trowern, A.R., Copin, N., Jackson, A.A. and Whorwood, C.B. (2001) The maternal diet during pregnancy programs altered expression of the glucocorticoid receptor and type 2 11β-hydroxysteroid dehydrogenase: potential molecular mechanisms underlying the programming of hypertension *in utero*. *Endocrinology* 142, 2841–2853.

Bertram, J.F., Johnson, K., Hughson, M.D. and Hoy, W.E. (2001) Renal glomerular number and size in Australian Aborigines, African Americans and white populations from the same locations: a preliminary report. *Image Analysis and Stereology* 20, 153–156.

Brenner, B.M. and Chertow, G.M. (1994) Congenital oligonephropathy and the etiology of adult hypertension and progressive renal injury. *American Journal of Kidney Disease* 23, 171–175.

Brenner, B.M., Garcia, D.L. and Anderson, S. (1988) Glomeruli and blood pressure: less of one, more the other? *American Journal of Hypertension* 1, 335–347.

Celsi, G., Kistner, A., Aizman, R., Eklof, A.-C., Ceccatelli, S., De Santiago, A. and Jacobson, S.H. (1998) Prenatal dexamethasone causes oligonephronia, sodium retention, and higher blood pressure in the offspring. *Pediatric Research* 44, 317–322.

Fogo, A., Yoshida, Y., Yared, A. and Ichikawa, I. (1990) Importance of angiogenic action of angiotensin II in the glomerular growth of maturing kidneys. *Kidney International* 38, 1068–1074.

Friberg, P., Sundelin, B., Bohman, S.-O., Bobik, A., Nilsson, H., Wickman, A., Gustafsson, H., Petersen, J. and Adams, M.A. (1994) Renin–angiotensin system in neonatal rats: induction of a renal abnormality in response to ACE inhibition or angiotensin II antagonism. *Kidney International* 45, 484–492.

Guyton, A.C., Coleman, T.G., Cowley, A.W. Jr, Scheel, K.W., Manning, R.D. Jr and Normal, R.A. Jr (1972) Arterial pressure regulation. Overriding dominance of the kidneys in long-term regulation and in hypertension. *American Journal of Medicine* 52, 584–594.

Hakim, R.M., Goldszer, R.C. and Brenner, B.M. (1984) Hypertension and proteinuria: long-term sequelae of uninephrectomy in humans. *Kidney International* 25, 930–936.

Hinchliffe, S.A., Lynch, M.R.J., Sargent, P.H., Howard, C.V. and Van Velzen, D. (1992) The effect of intrauterine growth retardation on the development of renal nephrons. *British Journal of Obstetrics and Gynaecology* 99, 296–301.

Hostetter, T.H., Olson, J.L., Rennke, H.G. and Venkatachalam, M.A. (1981) Hyper-filtration in remnant nephrons: a potentially adverse response to renal ablation. *American Journal of Physiology* 241, F85–F93.

Hoy, W.E., Rees, M., Kile, E., Mathews, J.D., McCredie, D.A., Pugsley, D.J. and Wang, Z. (1998) Low birthweight and renal disease in Austalian aborigines. *Lancet* 352, 1826–1827.

Hoy, W.E., Rees, M., Kile, E., Mathews, J.D. and Wang, Z. (1999) A new dimension to the Barker hypothesis: low birthweight and susceptibility to renal disease. *Kidney International* 56, 1072–1077.

Jones, S.E., Nyengaard, J.R., Flyvbjerg, A., Bilous, R.W. and Marshall, S.M. (2001) Birth weight has no influence on glomerular number and volume. *Pediatric Nephrology* 16, 340–345.

Keller, G., Zimmer, G., Mall, G., Ritz, E. and Amann, K. (2003) Nephron number in patients with primary hypertension. *New England Journal of Medicine* 348, 101–108.

Khan, I.Y., Taylor, P.D., Dekou, V., Seed, P.T., Lakasing, L., Graham, D., Dominiczak, A.F., Hanson, M.A. and Poston, L. (2003) Gender-linked hypertension in offspring of lard-fed pregnant rats. *Hypertension* 41, 168–175.

Kwong, W.Y., Wild, A.E., Roberts, P., Willis, A.C. and Fleming, T.P. (2000) Maternal undernutrition during the preimplantation period of rat development causes blastocyst abnormalities and programming of postnatal hypertension. *Development* 127, 4195–4202.

Lackland, D.T., Bendall, H.E., Osmond, C., Egan, B.M. and Barker, D.J.P. (2000) Low birth weights contribute to the high rates of early-onset chronic renal failure in the Southeastern United States. *Archives of Internal Medicine* 160, 1472–1476.

Langley, S.C. and Jackson, A.A. (1994) Increased systolic blood pressure in adult rats induced by fetal exposure to maternal low protein diet. *Clinical Science* 86, 217–222.

Langley-Evans, S.C. (1997) Maternal carbenoxolone treatment lowers birthweight and induces hypertension in the offspring of rats fed a protein-replete diet. *Clinical Science* 93, 423–429.

Langley-Evans, S.C. (2000) Critical differences between two low protein diet protocols in the programming of hypertension in the rat. *International Journal of Food Science and Nutrition* 51, 11–17.

Langley-Evans, S.C., Welham, S.J.M., Sherman, R.C. and Jackson, A.A. (1996) Weanling rats exposed to maternal low-protein diets during discrete periods of gestation exhibit differing severity of hypertension. *Clinical Science* 91, 607–615.

Langley-Evans, S.C., Welham, S.J.M. and Jackson, A.A. (1999) Fetal exposure to a maternal low protein diet impairs nephrogenesis and promotes hypertension in the rat. *Life Science* 64, 965–974.

Lelievre-Pegorier, M., Vilar, J., Ferrier, M.-L., Moreau, E., Freund, N., Gilbert, T. and Merlet-Benichou, C. (1998) Mild vitamin A deficiency leads to inborn nephron deficit in the rat. *Kidney International* 54, 1455–1462.

Levitt, N.S., Lindsay, R.S., Holmes, M. and Seckl, J.R. (1996) Dexamethasone in the last week of pregnancy attenuates hippocampal glucocorticoid receptor gene expression and elevates blood pressure in the adult offspring in the rat. *Neuroendocrinology* 64, 412–418.

Lindsay, R.S., Lindsay, R.M., Edwards, C.R.W. and Seckl, J.R. (1996) Inhibition of 11β-hydroxysteroid dehydrogenase in pregnant rats and the programming of blood pressure in the offspring. *Hypertension* 27, 1200–1204.

Louey, S., Cock, M.L. and Harding, R. (2003) Postnatal development of arterial pressure: Influence of the intrauterine environment. *Archives of Physiology and Biochemistry* 111, 53–60.

Lucas, S.R.R., Miraglia, S.M., Zaladek Gil, F. and Coimbra, T.M. (2001) Intrauterine food restriction as a determinant of nephrosclerosis. *American Journal of Kidney Disease* 37, 467–476.

Madsen, K.M. (1999) The art of counting. *Journal of the American Society of Nephrology* 10, 1124–1125.

Manalich, R., Reyes, L., Herrera, M., Melendi, C. and Fundora, I. (2000) Relationship between weight at birth and the number and size of renal glomeruli in humans: a histomorphometric study. *Kidney International* 58, 770–773.

Manning, J., Beutler, K., Knepper, M.A. and Vehaskari, V.M. (2002) Upregulation of renal BSC1 and TSC in prenatally programmed hypertension. *American Journal of Physiology Renal Physiology* 283, F202–F206.

McCalla, C.O., Nacharaju, V.L., Muneyyirci-Delale, O., Glasgow, S. and Feldman, J.G. (1998) Placental 11β-hydroxysteroid dehydrogenase activity in normotensive and pre-eclamptic pregnancies. *Steroids* 63, 511–515.

Merlet-Benichou, C., Gilbert, T., Muffat-Joly, M., Lelievre-Pegorier, M. and Leroy, B. (1994) Intrauterine growth retardation leads to a permanent nephron deficit in the rat. *Pediatric Nephrology* 8, 175–180.

Moritz, K.M. and Wintour, E.M. (1999) Functional development of the meso- and metanephros. *Pediatric Nephrology* 13, 171–178.

Moritz, K.M., Wintour, E.M. and Dodic, M. (2002) Fetal uninephrectomy leads to post-natal hypertension and compromised renal function. *Hypertension* 39, 1071–1076.

Nelson, R.G., Morgenstern, H. and Bennett, P.H. (1998) Birth weight and renal disease in Pima Indians with type 2 diabetes mellitus. *American Journal of Epidemiology* 148, 650–656.

Nishimura, H., Yerkes, E., Hohenfellner, K., Miyazaki, Y., Ma, J., Hunley, T.E., Yoshida, H., Ichiki, T., Threadgill, D., Phillips III, J.A., Hogan, B.M., Fogo, A., Brock III, J.W., Inagami, T. and Ichikawa, I. (1999) Role of the angiotensin type 2 receptor gene in congenital anomalies of the kidney and urinary tract, CAKUT, of mice and men. *Molecular Cell* 3, 1–10.

Nwagwu, M.O., Cook, A. and Langley-Evans, S.C. (2000) Evidence of progressive deterioration of renal function in rats exposed to a maternal low-protein diet *in utero*. *British Journal of Nutrition* 83, 79–85.

Nyengaard, J.R. and Bendtsen, T.F. (1992) Glomerular number and size in relation to age, kidney weight, and body surface in normal man. *Anatomical Record* 232, 194–201.

Ozaki, T., Nishina, H., Hanson, M.A. and Poston, L. (2001) Dietary restriction in pregnant rats causes gender-related hypertension and vascular dysfunction in offspring. *Journal of Physiology* 530, 141–152.

Poore, K.R., Forhead, A.J., Gardner, D.S., Giussani, D.A. and Fowden, A.L. (2002) The effects of birth weight on basal cardiovascular function in pigs at 3 months of age. *Journal of Physiology* 539, 969–978.

Reinisch, J.M., Simon, N.G., Karow, W.G. and Gandelman, R. (1978) Prenatal exposure to prednisone in humans and animals retards intrauterine growth. *Science* 202, 436–438.

Robinson, J.S., Kingston, E.J., Jones, C.T. and Thorburn, G.D. (1979) Studies on experimental growth retardation in sheep: the effect of removal of endometrial caruncles on fetal size and metabolism. *Journal of Developmental Physiology* 1, 379–398.

Rogerson, F.M., Kayes, K.M. and White, P.C. (1997) Variation in placental type 2 11β-hydroxysteroid dehydrogenase activity is not related to birth weight or placental weight. *Molecular and Cellular Endocrinology* 128, 103–109.

Rossing, P., Tarnow, L., Nielsen, F.S., Hansen, B.V., Brenner, B.M. and Parving, H.-H. (1995) Low birth weight: a risk factor for development of diabetic nephropathy? *Diabetes* 44, 1405–1407.

Shams, M., Kilby, M.D., Somerset, D.A., Howie, A.J., Gupta, A., Wood, P.J., Afnan, M. and Stewart, P.M. (1998) 11β-hydroxysteroid dehydrogenase type 2 in human pregnancy and reduced expression in intrauterine growth restriction. *Human Reproduction* 13, 799–804.

Smith, S., Laprad, P. and Grantham, J. (1985) Long-term effect of uninephrectomy on serum creatinine concentration and arterial blood pressure. *American Journal of Kidney Disease* 6, 143–148.

Stewart, P.M., Rogerson, F.M. and Mason, J.I. (1995) Type 2 11β-hydroxysteroid dehydrogenase messenger ribonucleic acid and activity in human placenta and fetal membranes: its relationship to birth weight and putative role in fetal adrenal steroidogenesis. *Journal of Clinical Endocrinology and Metabolism* 80, 885–890.

Tonkiss, J., Trzcinska, M., Galler, J.R., Ruiz-Opazo, N. and Herrera, V.L.M. (1998) Prenatal malnutrition-induced changes in blood pressure. Dissociation of stress and nonstress responses using radiotelemetry. *Hypertension* 32, 108–114.

Tufro-McReddie, A., Johns, D.W., Geary, K.M., Dagli, H., Everett, A.D., Chevalier, R.L., Carey, R.M. and Gomez, R.A. (1994) Angiotensin II type 1 receptor: role in renal growth and gene expression during normal development. *American Journal of Physiology* 266, F911–F918.

Tufro-McReddie, A., Romano, L.M., Harris, J.M., Ferder, L. and Gomez, R.A. (1995) Angiotensin II regulates nephrogenesis and renal vascular development. *American Journal of Physiology* 269, F110–F115.

Vehaskari, V.M., Aviles, D.H. and Manning, J. (2001) Prenatal programming of adult hypertension in the rat. *Kidney International* 59, 238–245.

Vincenti, F., Amend, W.J.C. Jr, Kaysen, G., Feduska, N., Birnbaum, J., Duca, R. and Salvatierra, O. (1983) Long-term renal function in kidney donors. Sustained compensatory hyperfiltration with no adverse effects. *Transplantation* 36, 626–629.

Woodall, S.M., Johnston, B.M., Breier, B.H. and Gluckman, P.D. (1996) Chronic maternal undernutrition in the rat leads to delayed postnatal growth and elevated blood pressure of offspring. *Pediatric Research* 40, 438–443.

Woods, L.L. (1999) Neonatal uninephrectomy causes hypertension in adult rats. *American Journal of Physiology* 276, R974–R978.

Woods, L.L. and Rasch, R. (1998) Perinatal ANGII programs adult blood pressure, glomerular number, and renal function in rats. *American Journal of Physiology* 275, R1593–R1599.

Woods, L.L. and Weeks, D.A. (2004a) Programming of adult hypertension by maternal high Na$^+$ diet: renal mechanisms (in press).

Woods, L.L. and Weeks, D.A. (2004b) Perinatal programming of adult blood pressure: role of maternal corticosteroids. *Hypertension* (in press).

Woods, L.L. and Weeks, D.A. (2004c) Inverse relationship between birthweight and adult blood pressure in rats. *Hypertension* (in press).

Woods, L.L., Ingelfinger, J.R., Nyengaard, J.R. and Rasch, R. (2001a) Maternal protein restriction suppresses the newborn renin–angiotensin system and programs adult hypertension in rats. *Pediatric Research* 49, 460–467.

Woods, L.L., Weeks, D.A. and Rasch, R. (2001b) Hypertension after neonatal uninephrectomy in rats precedes glomerular damage. *Hypertension* 38, 337–342.

Woods, L.L., Weeks, D.A. and Rasch, R. (2004a) Programming of adult blood pressure by maternal protein restriction: role of nephrogenesis. *Kidney International* (in press).

Woods, L.L., Ingelfinger, J.R. and Rasch, R. (2004b) Modest maternal protein restriction fails to program adult hypertension in female rats. *American Journal of Physiology (Regulatory, Integrative Comparative Physiology)* (in press).

Williams, S.L., Oler, J. and Jorkasky, D.K. (1986) Long-term renal function in kidney donors: a comparison of donors and their siblings. *Annals of Internal Medicine* 105, 1–8.

Zeman, F.J. (1968) Effects of maternal protein restriction on the kidney of the newborn young of rats. *Journal of Nutrition* 94, 111–116.

Zidar, N., Avgustin Cavic, M., Kenda, R.B., Koselj, M. and Ferluga, D. (1998) Effect of intrauterine growth retardation on the clinical course and prognosis of IgA glomerulonephritis in children. *Nephron* 79, 28–32.

Zimanyi, M.A., Bertram, J.F. and Black, J.M. (2000) Nephron number in the offspring of rats fed a low protein diet during pregnancy. *Image Analysis and Stereology* 19, 219–222.

12 Perinatal Determinants of Atopic Disease

Kitaw Demissie, Katherine D. Chung and
Bijal A. Balasubramanian

School of Public Health, University of Medicine and Dentistry of New Jersey, Piscataway, NJ 08854, USA

Introduction

Allergic diseases comprise a variety of clinical syndromes with manifestations of eczema, hay fever and asthma. Allergic disease is a growing medical and public health concern worldwide. The International Study of Asthma and Allergies in Childhood (ISAAC) employed a standard methodology to determine the prevalence rates of asthma and atopic diseases in 155 collaborating centres in 56 countries globally, and among 721,601 children aged 6–14 years (Anonymous, 1998a,b; Williams *et al.*, 1999). Prevalence rates for asthma, wheeze and atopic eczema reported from selected countries are shown in Table 12.1.

The highest prevalences of asthma symptoms, wheeze and atopic eczema were reported in New Zealand, Australia, the UK and the Republic of Ireland, whereas areas of low prevalence included Eastern Europe, Indonesia and Ethiopia. The large between-country variations in the prevalence of allergic diseases are not well understood. Known and putative determinants of allergic disease can be grouped under the general categories of host, environmental and lifestyle factors (see Table 12.2).

In the past few decades there has been an increase in the prevalence of allergic diseases globally, and this increase has been most striking in industrialized countries (Taylor *et al.*, 1984; Ninan and Russell, 1992; von Mutius *et al.*, 1992; Nakagomi *et al.*, 1994; Peat *et al.*, 1994; Anonymous, 1998a). It has been suggested that the observed increase is due to changes in diagnostic practices and/or criteria. However, studies that have documented prevalence rates in the same populations over time using comparable methodologies support the assertion that the increase is real (Ninan and Russell, 1992; Peat *et al.*, 1994). In Aberdeen, UK, 7-year-old schoolchildren were studied in 1964 and again in 1989, in the same school using a comparable instrument. During the interval, the prevalence of wheezing, diagnosed asthma, hay fever and eczema had almost doubled (Ninan and Russell, 1992).

Table 12.1. Prevalence (%) of asthma, wheezing and atopic eczema among children in the previous year for selected countries participating In ISAAC.

	Asthma		Wheeze		Atopic eczema
	6–7 years	13–14 years	6–7 years	13–14 years	6–7 years
UK	22.9	20.7	18.4	32.2	13.0
New Zealand	26.5	24.4	24.5	30.2	14.7
Australia	27.1	28.2	24.6	29.4	10.9
Republic of Ireland	–	15.2	–	29.1	–
Canada	14.7	16.5	17.6	28.1	8.5
USA	–	16.5	–	21.7	–
Chile	12.1	10.7	17.9	10.2	10.9
Singapore	18.5	20.9	15.7	9.7	2.8
Malaysia	10.4	10.9	6.1	9.6	8.5
Ethiopia	–	2.5	–	6.2	–
India	3.7	4.5	5.6	6.0	2.7
Greece	5.4	4.5	5.6	6.0	2.7
Georgia	3.1	3.1	7.6	3.6	4.6
Romania	–	3.7	–	3.0	–
Albania	3.1	1.6	7.6	2.6	2.5
Indonesia	6.6	1.6	4.1	2.1	–

Table 12.2. Known and putative determinants of allergic diseases.

Host	Environment	Lifestyle
• Genetic factors • Family history of allergies, in particular maternal history • Atopy • Race and/or ethnic origin	• Sustained exposure to indoor allergens, pre- and postnatal • Environmental exposure to tobacco smoke, pre- and postnatal • Community air pollution related to vehicle exhaust • Viral infections • Absence of certain infections in the first year of life • Certain home characteristics such as gas cooking, electric home heating, carpeting, dampness • Certain occupational exposures to sensitizing chemicals such as isocyanates • Socio-economic disadvantage	• Westernized lifestyle • Urban versus rural • Breastfeeding practices • Diet • Physical activity • Stress • Drugs

The reasons for this increase in allergic diseases have been debated. Changes in the gene pool of the population, or in the environment, or lifestyle, or the interaction among these factors can serve as a conceptual framework within which to examine the increase in the prevalence of allergic diseases. Changes in the genetic make-up of a stable population are an unlikely explanation, as the gene pool is not likely to change significantly in one century. The probable cause of the epidemic is more likely a change in individual and population susceptibility (i.e. a more susceptible host), or a change in environment (i.e. a more toxic environment), or a change in the lifestyle of the individual or population (i.e. an allergy-symptom-enhancing lifestyle). This chapter will largely review the evidence suggesting that exposure to certain factors during fetal life may produce a more susceptible host, and will also describe how exposure to a more toxic environment during critical periods in postnatal life may also contribute to allergic diseases.

A More Susceptible Host

Atopy is the genetic predisposition for mounting an immunoglobulin (predominantly IgE) response to common allergens. It is associated with increased levels of IgE in the circulation and tissues, and is believed to play a central role in the pathogenesis of allergic diseases (Pepys, 1986). Atopy is present in approximately 80% of children with childhood asthma (Nelson, 1985). In the population of Tucson, Arizona, asthma was found to be almost always associated with some type of IgE-mediated reaction (Burrows *et al.*, 1989). Similarly, in a longitudinal study of a birth cohort of 562 children (11 years old at the time of the study) in New Zealand (Sears *et al.*, 1991), the prevalence of bronchial hyper-responsiveness (an exaggerated bronchoconstriction response; Boushey *et al.*, 1980) to methacholine was strongly related to the serum IgE level. Most atopic subjects develop allergic rhinitis with conjunctivitis and atopic dermatitis (Magnan and Vervloet, 2000). Atopy may remain clinically silent in a good number of subjects and is only detected through a positive skin test or serum IgE to specific aeroallergens. Factors enhancing the translation of atopic status to clinically allergic syndromes remain unknown.

In the 1980s, a very useful framework was put forth that advocated the division of cytokine-producing T cells into T helper 1 (Th1) and T helper 2 (Th2) subsets, on the basis of cytokines they produced and their related functional activities (Mosmann *et al.*, 1986). This model has since evolved, and now Th1 cells are defined by their production of interleukin-2 (IL-2), interferon-γ (IFN-γ) and tumour necrosis factor-β (TNF-β). Th2 cells, on the other hand, are defined by their production of IL-4, IL-5, IL-6, IL-10 and IL-13. Both Th1 and Th2 cell types produce IL-3, TNF-α and granulocyte macrophage-colony stimulating factor (GM-CSF) (Kelso, 1995). Although the Th1/Th2 paradigm was first described in cloned lines of murine CD4+ T cells, the applicability of this model in human T-cell activation has been demonstrated (Romagnani, 1991).

This division of cytokine-producing T cells into Th1 and Th2 subsets has increasingly been called into question (Kelso, 1995). The current thinking on the regulatory role of T cells is that individual T cells display a remarkable diversity in their cytokine profiles and collectively form a continuous spectrum, in which Th1 and Th2 cells may be only two of the possible extreme phenotypes. Thus T-cell activation may result in a Th1-predominant pole (mostly Th1 cytokines) or a Th2-predominant pole (mostly Th2 cytokines) with the production of both types of cytokine responses at varying degrees between the poles (Magnan *et al.*, 2001).

The balance between the local level of IFN-γ, IL-4 and other cytokines is an important determinant of the Th1- or Th2-predominant response. There is substantial evidence demonstrating that IFN-γ and IL-4 exert opposite effects on various immune parameters (Kelso, 1995). The cytokine environment during early T-cell activation determines the dominant cytokine profile of the T-cell response. IFN-γ and IL-12 promote IFN-γ production, promoting the Th1-dominant cytokine response, and inhibiting the production of IL-4 and the Th2 response. On the other hand, IL-4 stimulates the Th2 cytokine response and inhibits the proliferation of the Th1 response. Often, the T-cell population is committed to either Th1 or Th2 dominance (Magnan *et al.*, 2001).

The Th1-dominant cytokine response is directed towards activating cytotoxicity and phagocytosis against viruses and intracellular pathogens. The Th2-dominant cytokine response is necessary for production of immunoglobulin E (IL-4) and eosinophil (IL-5), which are essential components of an allergic reaction (Magnan *et al.*, 2001) (Fig. 12.1).

Normal pregnancy has been characterized by a reduced maternal-cell-mediated anti-fetal immunity and a dominant hormonal immune response (Raghupathy, 1997). It has been suggested that Th1-type cytokines are detrimental to pregnancy and are incompatible with successful pregnancy, and there is a universal skewing towards a Th2 response that characterizes a successful pregnancy (Wegmann *et al.*, 1993; Bjorksten, 1999; Magnan *et al.*, 2001). However, this model appears to be an oversimplification of events occurring at the maternal–fetal interface during the course of a normal pregnancy (Athanassakis and Vassiliadis, 2002; Chaouat *et al.*, 2002; Sacks *et al.*, 2003). Data indicate a critical role of Th1-type cytokines, including IFN-γ, in the successful vascularization of the maternal–fetal interface. New evidence also suggests that the maternal–fetal interaction is not simply a matter of maternal tolerance to foreign

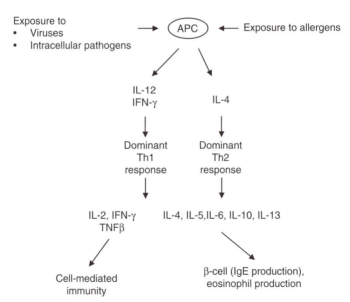

Fig. 12.1. Development of the Th1- or Th2-dominant response. Th, T helper; APC, antigen-presenting cell; IL, interleukin; IFN, interferon; TNF, tumour necrosis factor; IgE, immunoglobulin E.

tissue, but a delicate mutual cytokine interaction, with precise timing and tuning leading to successful implantation and vascularization (Chaouat *et al.*, 2002).

The Th1 cell response to antigens is not uniform among individuals. For example, *Mycobacterium leprae* causes tuberculoid leprosy (Th1-dominated response) in some and lepromatous leprosy (Th2-dominated response) in others (Salgame *et al.*, 1991). The pre- and postnatal evaluation of the immune system is therefore dependent on the genetic background (atopy) and several other factors (Table 12.3). A collection of factors may be required to act singly or in combination to determine the switch of the T cell to either the Th1 or Th2 direction. Among these factors, atopy (the genetic predisposition of the host to produce IgE) plays a central role. Between one-half and three-quarters of allergic patients have a family history of allergic diseases (Bousquet and Kjellman, 1986). Genetic studies have documented the risk of developing atopy based on family history of atopy.

Atopy is a complex polygenic hereditary trait with a high population prevalence. Possible loci of atopy genes have been identified on chromosome 11q (only through the maternal line), and chromosomes 14 and 5 (Cookson *et al.*, 1992; Wilkinson and Holgate, 1996; Sears, 1997). The genes coding for IL-4, IL-5 and IL-3 are also located on chromosome 5q, while chromosome 11q contains the gene coding for the β-chain of the high-affinity IgE receptor (Magnan *et al.*, 2001). The key enigma is to understand how these alternate forms of Th memory profiles are imprinted on the immune system, and what factors play a role in the selection of Th2-skewed memory in individuals who are genetically predisposed to atopy.

The shift of the T cell towards either Th1- or Th2-dominant cytokine expression may depend on the genetic background (atopy), on antigenic stimulation and on other host factors. Antigenic stimulation of a genetically susceptible host may result in Th2-dominant cytokine expression, but the expression of atopic phenotype may be modified by several identified and unidentified factors, including maternal smoking, birth order and maternal diet (Devereux *et al.*, 2002). The increase in the prevalence of allergic diseases in the past few decades is unlikely to be due to mutations in atopic genes, but may

Table 12.3. Factors favouring dominant Th1 or Th2 type of cytokine response (Williams *et al.*, 1999).

Th1 phenotype	Th2 phenotype
• Viral infections	• Genetically determined background (atopy)
• Tuberculosis, measles or hepatitis A infection	• Prenatal allergen exposure
	• Fetal infections
• Early exposure to day-care	Newborn's intestinal flora
• Presence of older siblings	• Maternal diet
• Rural environment	• Length of gestation
	• Maternal stress
	• Breastfeeding
	• Widespread use of antibiotics
	• Urban environment

be related to an increase in host factors that may play a role in the expression of the atopic phenotype. However, identification of genetic markers of atopy is important in screening a high-risk mother and child for possible intervention. Currently, parental history (in particular, maternal history) of allergies is the only available marker for use in screening high-risk individuals.

Prenatal allergen exposure

Priming is the functional enhancement of a given cell by cytokines, resulting in a number of cellular alterations, including morphological and physical cell changes (Kroegel et al., 2000). There is substantial evidence suggesting that the enhanced functional status of a primed cell spontaneously returns to the prepriming levels (depriming). Thus, priming is a reversible process, provided that sufficient time has elapsed without exposure to the priming agent (Kroegel et al., 2000). The fetus can encounter allergens in utero. The presence of a high degree of concordance in the concentrations of inhalant and nutritive allergens between the mother's blood and the amniotic fluid is direct evidence for the transamniotic and transplacental transfer of allergens (Holloway et al., 2000; Szepfalusi et al., 2000a). Allergen-specific immune responses may be detected in fetal blood and, therefore, cord blood can be used to evaluate the presence of in utero priming to allergens (Warner et al., 1996; Prescott et al., 1999; Barker et al., 2002). Cord-blood lymphocytes have been shown to exhibit proliferation after in utero stimulation with allergens (Kondo et al., 1992). Also, the serum IgE level can be determined from cord blood (Michel et al., 1980). Cord-blood mononuclear cells (CBMC) have been studied in order to determine whether prenatal allergen exposure stimulates the fetal immune system and thereby plays a role in the postnatal risk of developing atopic disease. In these studies, the CBMC proliferative and cytokine expressive responses were quantified and their associations with subsequent childhood atopic disease were evaluated. Similar assays have been performed on peripheral blood mononuclear cells (PBMC) obtained during infancy and childhood.

Longitudinal study results of CBMC and PBMC proliferative and cytokine responses after in vitro stimulation with allergens, and their association with atopic disease, are summarized in Tables 12.4 and 12.5. While most of the studies reported a positive association between increased CBMC proliferative responses and the development of atopic disease (Kondo et al., 1992; Warner et al., 1994; Miles et al., 1996; van der Velden et al., 2001), this association was not reported in some studies (Chan-Yeung et al., 1999; Prescott et al., 1999; Laan et al., 2000). On the other hand, studies of CBMC cytokine responses at birth provided more consistent results (Table 12.5). A study from The Netherlands (van der Velden et al., 2001) that followed 133 newborns at high risk of developing atopic symptoms, from birth until the first year of life, found a significantly decreased level of IFN-γ in atopic versus non-atopic infants. This finding suggests that the selective development of a Th2 cytokine profile in high-risk children who develop atopy may be the result of a regulatory defect leading to impaired IFN-γ production at birth. A lower level of IFN-γ production at birth in

Table 12.4. Studies relating CBMC proliferative responses to subsequent development of atopic disease.

Study	Ages	Population	Endpoint	Findings			
Kondo *et al.* (1992)	Birth to 1 year	37 term, general population	Atopic dermatitis, wheezy bronchitis	BSA OVA	↑ ↑		
Warner *et al.* (1994)	Birth to 1 year	34 high risk	Atopic eczema	Anti CD3 ↑ BLG ↑		CAT – OVA –	
van der Velden *et al.* (2001)	Birth to 1 year	133 high risk	Atopic diseases	CM ↑ Egg ↑		HDM ↑	
Miles *et al.* (1996)	Birth to 1 year	88 high risk, 12 no risk	Asthma, eczema	PHA – Anti CD3 ↑		OVA ↑ BLG ↑	
Prescott *et al.* (1999)	Birth to 2 years	18 high risk, 13 low risk	Atopic diseases	HDM – Fel d 1 –		OVA –	
Chan-Yeung *et al.* (1999)	Birth to 2 years	74 high risk	Possible asthma, probable asthma, rhinitis without colds	HDM –			
Laan *et al.* (2000)	Birth to 2 years	133 high risk	Atopic diseases, asthma-like disease, food allergy	HDM – CM – Egg white –			

CBMC, cord-blood mononuclear cells; OVA, ovalbumin; BSA, bovine serum albumin; CAT, cat allergen; BLG, betalactoglobulin; HDM, house dust mite antigen; Fel d 1, cat allergen; CM, cow's milk.

atopic versus non-atopic children was also reported from Australian (Tang *et al.*, 1994), Japanese (Kondo *et al.*, 1998) and British (Warner *et al.*, 1994) studies. At 6 and 12 months of age, a strong Th2 profile (characterized by increased levels of IL-4 and decreased levels of IFN-γ) was demonstrated in PBMC of children developing atopy (Prescott *et al.*, 1999; van der Velden *et al.*, 2001).

Taken together, the study findings discussed earlier suggest that intrauterine allergen exposure may trigger a switch in the fetal immune system towards a Th2 response, predisposing the fetus to development of atopy later in life. The implication of these observations is that allergen avoidance intervention during pregnancy may prevent the development of allergic diseases. If this is the case, then one would expect that the type of proliferative and cytokine responses would be directly related to the extent of maternal exposure to aeroallergens. The association between maternal exposure to seasonal allergens and CBMC proliferative responses supports this premise (Jones *et al.*, 1996; van der Velden *et al.*, 2001). However, findings from more recent studies do not lend support to this line of evidence. A study from Austria (Szepfalusi *et al.*, 2000b), after examining T-cell reactivity of cord-blood cells derived through cordocentesis from unborn and term babies, showed similar CBMC proliferative responses during the course of gestation that were not associated with maternal exposure to timothy grass and birch pollen. A Canadian study (Chan-Yeung *et al.*, 1999) also failed to demonstrate a relationship between maternal dust mite exposure and CBMC proliferative responses. Similarly, an Australian study (Marks *et al.*, 2002) was unable to demonstrate an association between house dust mite

Table 12.5. Studies relating CBMC cytokine responses to subsequent development of atopic disease.

Study	Ages	Sample size	Endpoint	Cytokine	Findings — Cytokines in atopic versus non-atopic				
					Birth	6 months	12 months	18 months	24 months
van der Velden et al. (2001)	Birth to 1 year	133 high risk	Atopic diseases, atopic dermatitis, asthma-like disease or food allergy	IL-4	↑	↑	↑		
				IL-5	Same	↑	↑		
				IL-13	Same	↑	↑		
				IFN-γ	→	→	→		
Tang et al. (1994)	Birth to 1 year	35 high risk	Atopic disease, eczema or MD-diagnosed asthma	IFN-γ	→				
Kondo et al. (1998)	Birth to 6 years	21 general	Atopic dermatitis, allergic rhinitis or bronchial asthma	IFN-γ	→				
				IL-2	Same				
Warner et al. (1994)	Birth to 1 year	34 high risk	Atopic eczema	IFN-γ	→				
Prescott et al. (1999)	Birth to 2 years	18 high risk, 13 low risk	Atopic eczema, recurrent wheezing, urticaria or rhinitis	IL-4	→	Same	↑	↑	Same
				IL-13	→	Same	↑	Same	↑
				IL-6	→	Same	Same	Same	Same
				IL-10	→	Same	Same	Same	Same
				IFN-γ	Same	→	→	→	Same

allergen concentrations collected from the maternal bed at 36 weeks' gestation and CBMC cytokine responses.

Although it is difficult to reconcile the findings of the longitudinal proliferative and cytokine expression studies with those obtained from maternal exposure studies, some unaccounted factors may explain some of the differences. A recent study (Devereux *et al.*, 2002) reported that parental atopy and *in utero* allergen sensitization are weak influences on CBMC responses, whereas maternal smoking, birth order and maternal dietary vitamin E play a more important role. We believe these factors may modulate or influence the interaction between genetic predisposition to atopy and allergen exposure *in utero*.

In sum, prenatal exposure to allergens may not be the sole determinant of the development of atopic disease later in life. However, along with genetic predisposition and other factors, it could play an important role in the pathogenesis of allergic diseases. Thus allergen avoidance measures during pregnancy may contribute to preventing priming, or to depriming, the primed T cells of the fetus.

Prenatal exposure to cigarette smoking

Transplacental transfer of cigarette constituents is known to occur during pregnancy (Perera *et al.*, 1999). Prenatal exposure to smoking has been linked with atopy and asthma-like illness in children. Asthma-like illness could be atopy related, or it could be wheezing illness without an element of allergy. The association between prenatal exposure to smoking and allergy-related diseases might derive from a direct influence of cigarette smoke on the developing thymus gland during fetal life. Rat studies have shown that exposure to nicotine leads to lasting deficiencies in the T-lymphocyte mitogenic response (Navarro *et al.*, 2001). Current evidence supports the assertion that exposure to smoking modulates the priming of the fetal T cells, favouring a shift towards a Th2-dominated response (Devereux *et al.*, 2002).

Cord blood of infants of mothers who smoked during pregnancy exhibited a higher proliferative mononuclear response when stimulated with house dust mite antigen (Devereux *et al.*, 2002). Further evidence for this observation came from an older study that looked at the rate of parental smoking on IgE levels in cord serum and the subsequent development of allergy during infancy (Magnusson, 1986). In that study, neonates of non-allergic parents had a more than threefold higher incidence of elevated cord blood IgE and a fourfold higher risk of developing atopic disease during infancy if the mother smoked during pregnancy. On the other hand, the association between cigarette smoking during pregnancy and childhood wheezing illness could be mediated through preterm birth. Cigarette smoking during pregnancy is a known risk factor for premature delivery (Shah and Bracken, 2000). Platelet activating factor is one of the most potent pro-inflammatory mediators and has been implicated in the pathophysiology of asthma (Narahara and Johnston, 1993). It has also been shown to be involved in parturition. Platelet activating factor of fetal lung and kidney origin has been detected in the amniotic fluid of women at term in labour, and in increased concentrations in amniotic fluid of women undergoing preterm labour.

Infants born preterm have smaller airways (Demissie *et al.*, 1997), and smaller airways during infancy predict wheezing illness later in childhood. This wheezing illness could be transient or could proceed to asthma, but is unlikely to be atopy related (Martinez *et al.*, 1995a).

Several large, prospective studies have examined the effect of cigarette smoking during pregnancy on subsequent development of atopy, bronchial hyper-responsiveness, respiratory symptoms and reduced lung function during childhood. In a cohort of 440 children in south Wales, maternal smoking during pregnancy was not associated with skin-prick test positivity at 7 years (Burr *et al.*, 1997). Two other studies also reported no association between prenatal smoking by the mother and skin-prick tests performed when the children were 5–8 years of age (Kuehr *et al.*, 1992; Schafer *et al.*, 1997). The lack of association persisted when skin-prick tests were performed when the children were 7–13 years of age (Henderson *et al.*, 1995; Soyseth *et al.*, 1995). A longer follow-up of children from birth to 35 years of age reported an inverse relationship between maternal smoking during pregnancy and skin-test positivity (Strachan *et al.*, 1997a). Similarly, maternal smoking was not associated with childhood airways responsiveness to carbachol, exercise and methacholine in studies from Italy, Germany and Norway, respectively (Martinez *et al.*, 1988; Frischer *et al.*, 1992a; Soyseth *et al.*, 1995).

Epidemiological studies of the association between maternal smoking during pregnancy and subsequent development of respiratory symptoms, such as persistent or current wheeze, have mostly produced consistent findings (Table 12.6). Longitudinal studies, from the USA (Gold *et al.*, 1999), New Zealand (Sears *et al.*, 1996) and the UK (Strachan *et al.*, 1996; Dezateux *et al.*, 1999), that followed infants reported a higher cumulative rate of wheezing during the first year of life in children of mothers who smoked during pregnancy. In the above and other longitudinal studies, the higher risk of wheezing illness associated with maternal smoking during pregnancy persisted when the children were followed through elementary school ages (Sears *et al.*, 1996; Gold *et al.*, 1999; Stein *et al.*, 1999). However, the effect of smoking during pregnancy diminished and disappeared when the children were followed into adolescence and adulthood (Lewis *et al.*, 1996; Strachan *et al.*, 1996; Tariq *et al.*, 2000). These findings reported from cohort studies were confirmed by several cross-sectional and case–control studies (Weitzman *et al.*, 1990; Cunningham *et al.*, 1996; Ehrlich *et al.*, 1996; Oliveti *et al.*, 1996; Agabiti *et al.*, 1999; Darlow *et al.*, 2000; Gilliland *et al.*, 2001; London *et al.*, 2001). Similarly, a reduction in lung-function measures has been demonstrated from several longitudinal and cross-sectional studies (Hanrahan *et al.*, 1992; Tager *et al.*, 1995; Stick *et al.*, 1996; Lodrup Carlsen *et al.*, 1997; Milner *et al.*, 1999; Young *et al.*, 2000) that examined prenatal exposure to tobacco smoke among infants. Although measurement of lung function during infancy is currently being performed, the validity of these measurements is controversial. However, using a reliable methodology, *in utero* exposure to cigarette smoke was associated with reduced lung function among schoolchildren (Cunningham *et al.*, 1994, 1995; Gilliland *et al.*, 2000; Li *et al.*, 2000).

One of the challenges in interpreting studies relating maternal smoking during pregnancy with subsequent development of allergies and wheezing illnesses

Table 12.6. Prospective studies on the association between maternal smoking during pregnancy and respiratory symptoms.

Study	Ages	Sample size	Outcomes	Findings
Gold *et al.* (1999)	Birth to 1 year	499	≥ 2 episodes of wheeze	RR (95% CI), 2.29 (1.44, 3.63)
Sears *et al.* (1996)	Birth to 18 years	880	Asthma symptoms at age 1, asthma symptoms at age 9	Significant correlation with smoking in third trimester; significant trend if mother smoked > 20 cigarettes/day in the first and second trimester
Strachan *et al.* (1996)	Birth to 33 years	5801	Wheezing illness	Age (years) OR (95% CI) 0–7 1.72 (1.11, 2.67) 8–16 0.94 (0.39, 2.25) 17–33 1.71 (0.97, 3.00)
Dezateux *et al.* (1999)	Birth to 1 year	101	Doctor-diagnosed asthma	OR (95% CI), 4 9 (1.6, 15.0)
Stein *et al.* (1999)	Birth to 11 years	956	Current wheeze	OR (95% CI), 2 3 (1.4, 3.8)
Lewis *et al.* (1996)	Birth to 16 years	20,528	Asthma or wheezy bronchitis	No significant relationship
Tariq *et al.* (2000)	Birth to 4 years	1218	Asthma or any respiratory symptoms	No significant relationship

RR, Relative risk; CI, confidence interval; OR, odds ratio.

in their offspring is distinguishing the effects of *in utero* exposure from exposure during the postnatal period. This is because it is difficult to identify mothers who smoke during the prenatal period only. More commonly, women smoke either prenatally and postnatally or in the postnatal period only (Gilliland *et al.*, 2000; Li *et al.*, 2000). Taken together, prenatal and postnatal exposure to tobacco smoke increases the likelihood of wheezing illnesses during childhood, but its role in atopy- and allergy-related asthma is not conclusive. Smoking cessation intervention studies may help to evaluate the independent effects of prenatal exposure to tobacco smoke and to more clearly define the modifying role of *in utero* exposure to tobacco smoke in the Th1 or Th2 expression profile.

Maternal nutrition during pregnancy

Changes in dietary habits have been suspected to contribute to the increasing prevalence of atopic disease (Arm *et al.*, 1989; Demissie and Ernst, 1994; Seaton *et al.*, 1994; Demissie *et al.*, 1996; Langley-Evans, 1997; Soutar *et al.*, 1997; Hodge *et al.*, 1998; Butland *et al.*, 1999; Beck *et al.*, 2000; Hijazi *et al.*, 2000; Seaton and Devereux, 2000). During the past few decades, the consumption of antioxidant-rich fresh fruits and vegetables has declined (Seaton *et al.*, 1994; Fogarty and Britton, 2000) and the intake of omega-6-polyunsaturated fatty acids has increased (Black and Sharpe, 1997; Weiland *et al.*, 1999). Moreover, fast-food eating behaviour and its associated contribution to a high body mass index has increased among low-income families (Kuczmarski *et al.*, 1994; Wechsler *et al.*, 1995; Jeffery and French, 1998; Diez-Roux *et al.*, 1999; Binkley *et al.*, 2000; Flegal *et al.*, 2002; McTigue *et al.*, 2002; Morland *et al.*, 2002a,b; Nielsen *et al.*, 2002), and in the same group the increase in prevalence of allergic diseases has been marked (Lewis and Britton, 1998a; Litonjua *et al.*, 1999; Lewis *et al.*, 2001; Koopman *et al.*, 2002; Strunk *et al.*, 2002). Interestingly, higher concentrations of cord serum IgE have been reported in Black relative to White infants (Thomas *et al.*, 1979). This shift in the population's dietary habits has a direct reflection on the diet of pregnant women and may affect the developing fetal immune system. Antioxidants are believed to prevent the development of inflammation by decreasing IL-4-dependent IgE production by β-cells (Warner and Warner, 2000). Diets rich in polyunsaturated fatty acids inhibit the synthesis of the Th-1 cytokines IL-2 and INF-γ and promote IL-4 production (Langley-Evans, 1997). Moreover, omega-6 fatty acids are precursors of arachidonic acid and hence the leukotrienes (Magnan *et al.*, 2001).

There is a paucity of data on the association between maternal diet during pregnancy and the development of allergic diseases in the offspring. A recent UK study (Devereux *et al.*, 2002) demonstrated a significantly higher CBMC proliferative response to timothy grass and house dust mite among neonates whose mothers had the lowest intakes of vitamin E during pregnancy, as determined by food frequency questionnaire. The findings suggest that maternal diet during pregnancy may influence the developing fetal immune system, rendering them liable to a higher risk of developing atopy. The Childhood Asthma Prevention Study (Mihrshahi *et al.*, 2001, 2003), a randomized controlled trial, evaluated whether the incidence of atopy and asthma could be reduced by a diet supplemented with omega-3 fatty acids. The dietary supplement started when the infants were 6 months of age. At 18 months of age the intervention provided a modest benefit in reducing wheezing symptoms but had no effect on serum IgE, atopy or doctors' diagnosis of asthma. It remains to be seen, when this study is followed up, whether maternal dietary intervention that starts during early pregnancy demonstrates a longer-term benefit among children at age 3 and 5 (persistent inhalant allergens will be established at follow-up) (van Asperen et al., 1984).

Fetal size (birthweight, length and head circumference) is, in part, a marker of fetal nutrition and has been studied in relation to the development of allergic diseases. However, most of these investigations have not separated the effect attributed to duration of gestation from that of fetal growth. For example, a low birthweight infant, although preterm, may have grown appropriately for that gestational age. Table 12.7 summarizes the results of studies that have examined the relationship between gestational age and atopic diseases. Preterm birth has been consistently associated with a higher prevalence of wheezing illness during infancy (Elder et al., 1996) and in childhood (von Mutius et al., 1993; Oliveti et al., 1996; Demissie et al., 1997; Gregory et al., 1999), but not in adulthood (Hagstrom et al., 1998; Pekkanen et al., 2001). Preterm birth is also linked with deficits in lung function measures in childhood (von Mutius et al., 1993; Demissie et al., 1997). These associations are consistent with the finding that preterm children have smaller airways, predisposing them to lower respiratory tract infections that lead to a higher incidence of recurrent respiratory symptoms in childhood, including wheeze. Most of these symptoms tend to resolve with age. Although the association between preterm birth and either atopy or bronchial hyper-responsiveness (BHR) is not consistent (von Mutius et al., 1993; Demissie et al., 1997), increasing gestational age was associated with atopy, as measured by skin-prick test or serum IgE, and the diagnosis of asthma (Gregory et al., 1999; Darlow et al., 2000; Pekkanen et al., 2001). Because most studies did not separate the effect of gestational age from that of birthweight, the effect observed with increasing gestational age could be attributable to increased fetal growth.

The results of the association between birthweight and childhood atopy, asthma and airway function are summarized in Table 12.8. Birthweight was shown to be consistently associated with decreased airway function in childhood (Chan et al., 1989; Frischer et al., 1992b; Demissie et al., 1997). However, in general, birthweight and respiratory symptoms, including the diagnosis of asthma and atopy, exhibit a U-shaped association. In other words, the prevalence of symptoms is higher in the extremes of birthweight distribution (Seidman et al., 1991; Frischer et al., 1992b; Oliveti et al., 1996; Gregory et al., 1999). Because most studies did not attempt to separate the effect of gestational age from that of birthweight, the findings may reflect the effect of preterm birth and increased fetal growth at the lower and higher end of the birthweight distribution respectively. On the other hand, increasing fetal size (measured after correcting for duration of gestation) was shown to be associated with increased incidence and prevalence of asthma, wheeze and atopy (Gregory et al., 1999; Leadbitter

Table 12.7. Studies describing the relationship between gestational age and atopic diseases.

Study, country	Study design	Follow-up	Number of subjects	Measurement of gestational age	Findings
Elder et al. (1996), Australia	Prospective cohort	Birth to 1 year	525 very preterm infants, 657 controls	Early ultrasound	Prevalence of recurrent wheeze requiring bronchodilator treatment
					Whole group Excluding parental history, BHR and passive smoke exposure
				Very preterm (< 33 weeks)	14.5% 5.3%
				Term infants	3% 3%
Demissie et al. (1997), Canada	Retrospective cohort	Birth to 5–13 years	327	Parental interview	Exercise-induced bronchospasm OR (95% CI)
				Term (≥ 37 weeks)	1.00 1.00
				Preterm (< 37 weeks)	1.8 (0.9, 3.4) 1.80 (0.9, 3.5)
					Change in methacholine dose–response ranking (95% CI)
				Term	0
				Preterm	12.7 (–18.3, 43.7)
Oliveti et al. (1996), USA	Case–control	Birth to 4–9 years	131 cases, 131 controls	Obstetric records	% Preterm births
					Children with asthma Children without asthma
				Preterm birth ≤ 37 weeks	24.6 13.7
Gregory et al. (1999), UK	Longitudinal	Birth to 6–23 years	239	Birth records	% Current wheeze % Asthma treatment % IgE > 150 IU IgE geometric mean Skin test > 3 mm
				< 37 weeks	16.7 16.7 50.0 145.8 33.3
				37–38 weeks	16.7 16.7 32.1 61.5 46.7
				39–40 weeks	22.6 18.8 38.1 87.4 46.2
				≥ 41 weeks	26.4 22.2 33.3 59.3 48.0

Study	Design	Age	N	Method
von Mutius et al. (1993), Germany	Retrospective cohort	Birth to 9–11 years	7445	Parental questionnaire; preterm birth defined as < 37 weeks of gestation and ≤ 2500 g
Pekkanen et al. (2001), Canada	Prospective cohort	Birth to 31 years	5192	Menstrual period
Hagstrom et al. (1998), Sweden	Case–control	Birth to 30 years	55 cases, 92 controls	Obstetric records
Darlow et al. (2000), New Zealand	Prospective cohort	Birth to 7–8 years	29	Obstetric records, gestational age

von Mutius et al. (1993), Germany

	OR (95% CI)	
	Males	Females
Current asthma	1.0 (0.4, 2.1)	2.6 (1.4, 4.7)
Recurrent wheeze	0.9 (0.5, 1.5)	1.7 (1.1, 2.7)

% Abnormal lung function among girls

	Term	Preterm No ventilatory support	Preterm Ventilatory support
PEFR	5.2	4.5	26.5
BHR	6.3	3.8	10.0
Atopy	34.3	28.6	19.5

Pekkanen et al. (2001), Canada

	OR (95% CI)	
	Atopy	Asthma
≤ 35 weeks	1.00	1.00
36–38 weeks	1.22 (0.87, 1.70)	0.90 (0.54, 1.49)
39–40 weeks	1.42 (1.02, 1.98)	0.81 (0.49, 1.33)
≥ 41 weeks	1.65 (1.16, 2.34)	0.94 (0.55, 1.61)

Hagstrom et al. (1998), Sweden

Gestational age (95% CI)	
Asthma	No asthma
39.4 (38.3, 40.0)	39.7 (39.4, 40.0)

Darlow et al. (2000), New Zealand

	% Asthma ever	% current asthma
< 26 weeks	56.3	43.8
26, 27 weeks	58.5	41.5
28, 29 weeks	48.5	29.1
30, 31 weeks	38.7	21.3
32+ weeks	59.6	42.3

BHR, bronchial hyper-responsiveness; PEFR, peak expiratory flow rate; OR, odds ratio; CI, confidence interval.

Table 12.8. Measures of fetal growth and the occurrence of allergy, atopy or asthma.

Study, country	Study design	Follow-up	Number of subjects	Measurement of growth at birth	Findings
Demissie et al. (1997), Canada	Retrospective cohort	Birth to 5–13 years	327	Per kilogram increase in birthweight	Change in methacholine response ranking (95% CI) -22.6 (-41, -4.2); % change in FEV_1 (95% CI) 4.4 (1.8, 7.2)
Frischer et al. (1992), Germany	Retrospective cohort	Birth to entry to primary school	1812	Birthweight	MD-diagnosed asthma (%) / PEFR before exercise (l/min) / Wheeze (%) / Cough after wheeze (%): Low 18 / 240 / 40 / 24; Normal 11 / 248 / 26 / 12
Chan et al. (1989), UK	Longitudinal	Birth to 7 years	130 low birthweight, 120 normal birthweight	Birthweight (g)	Mean (SD) — FVC (litres) / $FEV_{0.75}$ (litres) / MEF_{75} (l/s) / MEF_{50} (l/s): Low (< 2000) 1.39 (0.24) / 1.16 (0.19) / 2.69 (0.65) / 1.85 (0.54); Normal 1.41 (0.21) / 1.25 (0.17) / 3.01 (0.53) / 2.15 (0.49)
Oliveti et al. (1996), USA	Case–control	Birth to 4–9 years	131 cases, 131 controls	Birthweight (g)	% birthweight < 2500 g: Children with asthma 20.6; Children without asthma 9.9; < 2500
Sears et al. (1996), New Zealand	Prospective cohort	Birth to 18 years	1661	Birthweight (g)	% atopy at 13 years / % wheezing at 9 years / % asthmatic at 18 years: < 2500 37.1 / 21.4 / 8.7; 2500–2999 30.4 / 22.4 / 19.0; 3000–3499 44.2 / 29.6 / 26.2; 3500–3999 36.4 / 29.3 / 20.5; 4000–4499 30.7 / 34.9 / 19.8; ≥ 4500 0.0 / 44.4 / 15.4
Hagstrom et al. (1998), Sweden	Case–control	Birth to 30 years	55 asthmatic, 92 non-asthmatic	Mean birthweight (kg); Head circumference (cm); Placental weight (g); Ponderal index	Asthmatic adults (95% CI) / Non-asthmatic adults (95% CI): Mean birthweight 3.53 (3.38, 3.67) / 3.54 (3.34, 3.60); Head circumference 34.4 (34.0, 34.8) / 34.6 (34.3, 34.9); Placental weight 613 (580, 647) / 626 (601, 651); Ponderal index 2.77 (2.70, 2.84) / 2.75 (2.69, 2.80)

Pekkanen et al. (2001), Finland — Prospective cohort — Birth to 31 years — 5192 — Birthweight (g)

Birthweight (g)	Atopy OR (95% CI)	MD-diagnosed asthma OR (95% CI)
≤ 3090	1.00	1.00
3100–3390	1.02 (0.84, 1.25)	1.14 (0.81, 1.60)
3400–3620	0.99 (0.81, 1.22)	1.12 (0.79, 1.59)
3630–3900	0.87 (0.70, 1.07)	1.02 (0.71, 1.046)
≥ 3910	1.05 (0.85, 1.31)	1.07 (0.74, 1.55)

Seidman et al. (1991), Israel — Retrospective cohort — Birth to 17 years — 20,312 — Birthweight (g)

Birthweight (g)	Asthma at 17 years OR (95% CI)
< 2000	1.44 (0.79, 2.62)
2000–2499	1.49 (1.05, 2.12)
2500–2999	1.09 (0.89, 1.35)
3000–3499	1.00
3500–3999	0.97 (0.81, 1.17)
4000–4499	1.11 (0.83, 1.49)
≥ 4500	1.30 (0.73, 2.67)

Gregory et al. (1999), UK — Longitudinal — Birth to 6–23 years — 239 — Head circumference (cm)

Head circumference (cm)	Current wheeze (%)	Asthma treatment (%)	IgE ≥ 150 IU (%)	Skin test ≥ 3 mm (%)
< 34	17.9	21.4	33.3	40.7
34–34.9	11.3	15.1	27.7	39.6
35–35.9	36.4	23.6	38.3	47.2
36–36.9	22.9	11.4	34.4	52.8
≥ 37	26.3	26.3	62.5	57.9

Xu et al. (2000), Finland — Prospective cohort — Birth to 31 years — 5272 — Ponderal index

Ponderal index	Prevalence of atopy (%) BMI ≤ 24.8	Prevalence of atopy (%) BMI > 24.8
< 2.64	30.4	35.5
2.64–2.83	26.3	28.7
> 2.83	30.5	34.2

Leadbitter et al. (1999), New Zealand — Longitudinal — Birth to 13 years — 732 — Head circumference (cm)

Head circumference (cm)	Ever asthma OR (95% CI)	BHR OR (95% CI)	IgE ≥ 150 IU OR (95% CI)	SPT + OR (95% CI)
< 34	1.7 (0.8, 3.9)	1.0 (0.3, 2.7)	1.0 (0.5, 1.9)	0.5 (0.3, 1.0)
34–36.9	1.0	1.0	1.0	1.0
≥ 37	0.2 (0.1, 0.9)	0.9 (0.2, 4.3)	3.4 (1.4, 7.9)	1.2 (0.6, 2.8)

CI, confidence interval; SD, standard deviation; OR, odds ratio; PEFR, peak expiratory flow rate; FEV, forced expiratory volume; FVC, forced vital capacity; MEF, maximum expiratory flow; BMI, body mass index; BHR, bronchial hyper-responsiveness; SPT, skin-prick test.

et al., 1999; Xu *et al.*, 2000). In conclusion, the evidence on the association between maternal dietary habit and nutrition during pregnancy and the development of allergies, although promising, is in its infancy. Innovative studies on the measurement and characterization of deficiencies or excesses in maternal diet are required.

Maternal infections during pregnancy

The association between infection of the mother during pregnancy, as well as intrauterine infection, and allergic disease in the offspring is complex. Theoretically, intrauterine infections, such as chorioamnionitis, are believed to stimulate cell-mediated immunity and thus protect the infant from developing antibody-producing T-cells (Th2 response). A recent study that evaluated the cytokine expressions of cord blood in neonates born to mothers with and without uterine infection (chorioamnionitis) demonstrated more IFN-γ-producing T cells in the cord blood of infants born to mothers with uterine infection (Matsuoka *et al.*, 2001). However, infected neonates with the longest duration of ruptured membranes exhibited an increased percentage of IL-4-producing T cells (Matsuoka *et al.*, 2001). The results from epidemiological studies are in line with this finding.

A northern Finland birth cohort study that followed about 8000 children born in 1985/86 found that children at the age of 7 years had a higher risk of asthma if their mothers experienced vaginitis and febrile infections during pregnancy (Xu *et al.*, 1999). The adjusted odds ratios with 95% confidence intervals for infections were 2.08 (1.13, 3.82) during the first trimester, 1.73 (1.09, 2.75) during the second and 1.44 (0.97, 2.15) during the third trimester (Xu *et al.*, 1999). Respiratory tract infections during pregnancy were also shown to be associated with an increased risk of childhood asthma in a case–control study of 200 asthmatic and age-matched controls aged 5–16 years (Hughes *et al.*, 1999). A study from Tanzania also found the presence of malaria parasites in cord blood to confer six times the risk of developing wheezing illness at the age of 4 years, and increased total IgE levels (Sunyer *et al.*, 2001). Parasitaemia at birth was not related to total IgE in cord blood (Sunyer *et al.*, 2001). Maternal vaginal colonization with *Ureaplasma urealyticum* and staphylococci during pregnancy was associated with a twofold increased risk of wheezing during infancy in a cohort study from Finland involving about 3000 infants (Benn *et al.*, 2002). In that study, there was a 70% increased risk of asthma during the first year of life if the mother used antibiotics during pregnancy. The association between antibiotic use during pregnancy and increased risk of asthma in the child was confirmed by another cohort study of 25,000 children that showed a dose–response relationship (McKeever *et al.*, 2002). In another study from the UK, the use of paracetamol at 20–32 weeks of pregnancy was associated with risk of wheeze in the infant (OR 2.10; 95% CI 1.30, 3.41) (Shaheen *et al.*, 2002). Antibiotic and antipyretic use during pregnancy might be a marker of infection and the effect observed in these studies may reflect the effect of infection during pregnancy. More studies are needed to properly conceptualize the relationship between intrauterine infection, preterm birth, and their influences on the risk of developing allergic diseases during childhood.

Maternal stress during pregnancy

Psychosocial stress may impact upon immune function and, in particular, maternal stress-induced hormones may influence the T helper cell balance through neuroimmunomodulation (Herbert and Cohen, 1993; Chrousos, 2000; von Hertzen, 2002). There is evidence that corticosteroids and catecholamines, two major products of the stress response, tip the Th1/Th2 balance towards the Th2 type of immunity (Chrousos, 2000; von Hertzen, 2002). The effect of cortisol occurs largely through suppression of Th1 function as a result of inhibited IL-12 production and responsiveness (Chrousos, 2000). Cortisol is a challenging hormone to study during pregnancy, since it is essential to normal maturation of T cells, and an increase in cortisol, as well as corticotrophin releasing hormone (CRH), ACTH and β-endorphin, is a normal finding through gestation. Furthermore, there is a counterintuitive positive feedback loop whereby cortisol causes placental CRH to stimulate maternal and fetal adrenal cortisol production (Blumenfeld and Jaffe, 1986; Jones and Edwards, 1990; Goland et al., 1994).

Studies in rats (Zarrow et al., 1970) and in humans (Murphy et al., 1974; Gitau et al., 1998) provide evidence that cortisol levels in the mother may affect her offspring. Furthermore, several animal studies have shown that elevated prenatal stress in the mother impacts upon the immune function of the offspring (Henry et al., 1994; Kay et al., 1998; Coe et al., 2002). In humans, there have been several studies that demonstrate an association between prenatal stress of the mother and poor birth outcomes (Newton et al., 1979; Pagel et al., 1990; Wadhwa et al., 1993), yet direct evidence of an association between prenatal stress of the mother and immune function and Th1/Th2 balance determination in the offspring is lacking (von Hertzen, 2002).

In a prospective study of 490 families with a history of asthma or allergy, Wright et al. (2002) showed that perceived stress (over the past month) in caregivers, ascertained when infants were between 2 and 3 months of age, was associated with wheeze in the first 14 months of life (adjusted RR 1.4, 95% CI 1.1, 1.9). However, this study did not measure prenatal maternal stress, a factor for which determination of an association with asthma in offspring is yet to be made. At an ecological level, there has been a secular increase in stress, as measured through work-related conditions and pressures, stress symptoms and perceptions of stress (Kivimaki et al., 2000; von Hertzen, 2002)), while the prevalence of asthma has also increased (Peat et al., 1994; Seaton et al., 1994; Taylor et al., 1997; Anonymous, 1998a; Mannino et al., 2002). Individual-level data are needed to confirm the ecological association.

The potential association between stress and asthma may help our understanding of racial and ethnic disparities in asthma. In the past two decades, there has been a greater increase in the prevalence of asthma in African Americans relative to that in Whites. The prevalence rates of self-reported asthma in African-Americans and Whites in 1980 were 33.1 and 31.4 per 1000 respectively, and in 1999 the respective prevalence rates were 42.7 and 37.6 per 1000 (Mannino et al., 2002). Similar racial disparities were observed in mortality, hospitalizations, and emergency department (ED) visits due to asthma. The stress of living in urban settings, and in difficult and more socio-economically deprived neighbourhoods (Taylor et al., 1997; Williams, 1999), may be one of the contributing factors for the disproportionately higher rates of asthma in minority communities (Wright et al., 1998; von Hertzen, 2002). Researchers are beginning to examine the effects of factors such as perceived racism and stress on health outcomes (Williams, D.R., 1996; Kennedy et al., 1997; Schulz et al., 2000; Williams and Collins, 2001; Jones, 2002), and neuroimmunomodulation via the stress response provides a potential explanation.

Breastfeeding

There is significant controversy in the literature concerning the relationship between breastfeeding and the primary development of atopic disease in children. A review by Kramer (1988) summarized the literature up to 1988, using methodological and biological standards to rate the quality of published studies. The methodological standards included non-reliance on prolonged maternal recall of exposure, blind ascertainment of infant feeding history, strict diagnostic criteria, blind ascertainment of outcome, control for confounding, assessment of dose–response effects and adequate statistical power. The biological standards included sufficient duration of breastfeeding, sufficient exclusivity of breast-feeding, objective criteria for severity of outcome, assessment of age at onset of outcome and assessment of effect in children at high risk. Twenty-two studies on atopic eczema and 13 studies on asthma were reviewed. The study findings were inconsistent, in that there were both studies demonstrating and failing to demonstrate an association between breastfeeding and atopy. Generally, the studies that found a protective effect of breastfeeding were more likely to have higher ratings on the biological standards, while negative studies were more likely to have higher ratings on methodological standards. Kramer concluded that, based on the mixed results of the studies reviewed, as well as failure to meet important methodological and biological standards, no valid inferences could be made about the association between breastfeeding and atopy.

In an analysis of data from the Third National Health and Nutrition Examination Survey (NHANES III), 1988–1994, Chulada et al. (2003) demonstrated that, after adjusting for potential confounders, there was no statistically significant protective effect of breastfeeding on asthma up to 3 years of age. In that study, however, children who had been breastfed for any length of time had a lower risk of asthma diagnosis before the age of 24 months (OR 0.72, 95% CI 0.54, 0.95) and infants who were exposed to environmental tobacco smoke and who were breastfed had a lower risk of asthma relative to those who were not breastfed ($P < 0.05$). Another analysis of NHANES III data (Rust et al., 2001), which examined asthma risk in children aged 2 months to 6 years, failed to show the protective role of breastfeeding.

A prospective birth cohort of 2187 children in Western Australia (Oddy *et al.*, 1999) (1598 with skin-prick test (SPT)) demonstrated that children who were introduced to some other form of milk besides breast milk prior to 4 months of age, were more likely to have asthma diagnosed by a doctor and SPT ≥ 2 mm by the age of 6 years (OR asthma 1.25, 95% CI 1.02,1.52; OR positive SPT 1.30, 95% CI 1.04, 1.61). Similarly, in a New Zealand cohort of 1037 children (Sears *et al.*, 2002), breastfeeding appeared to increase the risk of SPT ≥ 2 mm to any allergen at age 13, and current asthma at age 9 (respective OR 1.94 (1.42, 2.65), 1.83 (1.35, 2.47)). Family history of atopy did not affect the results. This study met with significant criticism regarding its conclusion that breastfeeding may be a risk factor for atopy. The critiques focused on factors such as the 3-year recall period for ascertainment of breastfeeding history (Becquet *et al.*, 2003), failure to examine exclusive breastfeeding as an exposure (Murray, 2003), and the potential role of higher socio-economic status in explaining the increased risk of atopy in children who were breastfed (Boelens, 2003).

In a Tucson, Arizona, cohort of 1246 children (Wright *et al.*, 2001), exclusive breastfeeding for ≥ 4 months, in children of asthmatic mothers, was associated with an increased risk of asthma in the child by ages 6–13 years (adjusted OR 8.7, 95% CI 3.4, 22.2; adjusted for maternal education, maternal smoking in first year of life, gender, race, and siblings in the home or use of day-care). Exclusive breastfeeding ≥ 4 months was also associated with an increased risk of recurrent wheeze at ages 6–14 years (OR 5.7, 95% CI 2.3, 14.1). Exclusive breastfeeding yielded a statistically significant protection from recurrent wheeze at the age of 2 years (adjusted OR 0.45, 95% CI 0.2, 0.9), but this protection was no longer statistically significant by age 3. Maternal asthma or atopy had no effect on these results. In a Perth, Australia, cohort of 2187 children enrolled prenatally (Oddy *et al.*, 1999), introduction of milk other than breast milk before 4 months of age was associated with an increased risk for current asthma by age 6 and SPT ≥ 2 mm to at least one common allergen (current asthma-adjusted HR 1.25, 95% CI 1.02, 1.52; positive SPT-adjusted HR 1.30, 95% CI 1.04, 1.61).

In a cluster-randomized trial from the Republic of Belarus by Kramer *et al.* (2001), where intervention sites encouraged breastfeeding through a multi-faceted programme, and control sites had the usual infant feeding practices, breastfeeding was associated with a decreased risk of atopic eczema (OR 0.54, 95% CI 0.31, 0.95; adjusted for family history of atopy). In a dietary clinical trial in which mothers of newborns at risk for atopy were recommended to breastfeed for at least 4 months and to avoid solid foods (865 infants exclusively breastfed compared to 256 infants formula-fed) (Schoetzau *et al.*, 2002), breastfed infants were protected from development of atopic dermatitis by the age of 1 year (adjusted OR 0.47, 95% CI 0.30, 0.74).

A meta-analysis of prospective studies on the association between breastfeeding and atopic dermatitis (Gdalevich *et al.*, 2001) showed that the summary odds ratio for the effect of breastfeeding was 0.70, 95% CI 0.60, 0.81. In children with a family history of atopy, the summary OR was 0.52, 95% CI 0.35, 0.79. In studies of children with no family history of atopy there was no association between breastfeeding and atopic dermatitis (summary OR 0.99, 95% CI 0.48, 2.03). The authors concluded that breastfeeding is particularly protective against the development of atopy in infants with a family history of atopy.

In a meta-analysis of prospective studies of the association between allergic rhinitis and breastfeeding, Mimouni Bloch *et al.* (2002) demonstrated a non-statistically significant protective effect of breastfeeding on the risk of allergic rhinitis in general (OR 0.74, 95% CI 0.54, 1.01) and in those with a family history of atopy (OR 0.87, 95% CI 0.48, 1.58). In this analysis, breastfeeding seems less beneficial to children without a family history of atopy, which is opposite to the finding in the previous meta-analysis. Interestingly, the hypothesis that breastfeeding may be more protective against atopic disease in those without a family history of atopy, however, is corroborated by other studies that have demonstrated differences in the composition of breast milk of atopic and non-atopic women, as well as the relationship between the IgE level in the mother's breast milk and that in the child. For example, chemoattractants such as IL-8 and RANTES (regulated on activation, normal T cell expressed and secreted), have been found to exist in higher concentrations in the breast milk of allergic, relative to non-allergic, mothers (Bottcher *et al.*, 2000a). Similarly, the concentrations of IL-4, IL-5 and IL-13 may be higher in the colostrum of allergic relative to non-allergic mothers (Bottcher *et al.*, 2000b). Furthermore, in the 6-year-old children of non-atopic mothers, breastfeeding has been demonstrated to be associated with lower IgE levels, whereas in the children of atopic mothers, breastfeeding was associated with higher IgE levels (Wright *et al.*, 1999). These findings may account for an increase in allergic markers and symptoms in the offspring of mothers with allergy who breastfeed. That is, in breastfed children of mothers with allergy, there may be a greater activation of cells involved in the allergic process. Of course, a greater risk of atopy in the offspring of an atopic mother might be due to genetic factors, such that teasing apart the environmental and genetic influences remains an important challenge. In conclusion, due to the inconsistency of the evidence, it is not possible to make a definitive conclusion on the association between breastfeeding and atopy, based on the current literature.

Asthma during pregnancy

Asthma is a growing problem, and is the most frequent respiratory disorder complicating pregnancy. Estimates from the National Health Interview Survey indicate that asthma affects between 3.7 and 8.4% of pregnant women in the USA (Kwon *et al.*, 2003). The course of asthma during pregnancy varies, such that in one-third of patients asthma symptoms remain the same, in one-third they improve, and in one-third the symptoms worsen (Schatz, 1999; Kelsen, 2003). The majority of patients whose asthma changes course during pregnancy revert to their pre-pregnancy state during the postpartum period (Schatz, 1999; Kelsen, 2003). The severity of asthma peaks between 24 and 36 weeks of pregnancy (Schatz, 1999), at which time mothers are at greatest risk of developing pregnancy complications. This supports the reported associations between uncontrolled asthma and adverse infant and maternal outcomes. In various studies, maternal asthma during pregnancy has been linked to preterm births (Kramer *et al.*, 1995; Demissie *et al.*, 1998a, 1999; Liu *et al.*, 2001; Wen *et al.*, 2001; Sorensen *et al.*, 2003), pre-eclampsia (Dombrowski *et al.*, 1986; Demissie *et al.*, 1998a, 1999; Liu *et al.*, 2001; Wen *et al.*, 2001), placenta praevia (Alexander *et al.*, 1998; Demissie *et al.*, 1998a, 1999; Wen *et al.*, 2001), placental abruption (Alexander *et al.*, 1998; Liu *et al.*, 2001; Wen *et al.*, 2001), low birthweight (Demissie *et al.*, 1998a, 1999), very small and small for gestational age (Demissie *et al.*, 1998a., 1999; Liu *et al.*, 2001), large for gestational age (Liu *et al.*, 2001), transient tachypnoea of the newborn (Schatz *et al.*, 1991; Demissie *et al.*, 1998b) and gestational diabetes (Wen *et al.*, 2001). Asthmatic mothers also have an increased rate of Caesarean delivery and prolonged hospital stay (Demissie *et al.*, 1998a, 1999; Wen *et al.*, 2001).

Several mechanisms may operate in the association between maternal asthma and pregnancy complications. An underlying diathesis (atopy or triggers) in the mother may cause hyperactivity or irritability of both the bronchial and uterine smooth muscles. Thus conditions that cause hyper-responsiveness of the bronchial smooth muscles may, at the same time, lead to preterm births (Demissie *et al.*, 1998a). For transient tachypnea of the newborn, a genetic predisposition to β-adrenergic hyper-responsiveness, both in the mother and the child, have been suggested (Demissie *et al.*, 1998b). Fetal hypoxaemia in the setting of uncontrolled asthma may explain the association between asthma and fetal growth restriction and placenta praevia (Demissie *et al.*, 1998b). The latter is supported by the higher incidence of placenta preavia among women who live at higher altitudes (McClung, 1969). Medications used to treat asthma during pregnancy, particularly steroids, may be responsible for the excess gestational diabetes and large for gestational age (LGA) births among asthmatic mothers (Liu *et al.*, 2001). Constriction of airway smooth muscle during asthma attacks may be caused by local release of bioactive mediators, such as platelet activating factor, histamine, kinins and leukotrienes, which are implicated in the pathogenesis of pre-eclampsia (Drazen, 1992).

Many of the obstetric complications that are associated with maternal asthma also predispose the offspring to the development of asthma during early life. Studies in the past 2–3 years have reported that pregnancy complications, particularly uterine-related, are associated with the development of asthma in the offspring. A study from the UK (Annesi-Maesano *et al.*, 2001) reported threatened abortion, and malposition or malpresentation of the fetus, to be associated with the development of asthma in the child. Similarly, a Norwegian study showed that uterus-related complications, such as antepartum haemorrhage, preterm contractions and placental insufficiency, increased the risk of bronchial obstruction, asthma and allergic rhinitis when the child was 2–4 years of age (Nafstad *et al.*, 2000a).

The series of events that links maternal asthma with obstetric complications and the subsequent development of asthma in the child is complex, and distinct pathophysiological pathways may be involved. A child of an asthmatic mother is more likely to develop asthma because of genetic predisposition, irrespective of the pregnancy complications. Also, factors such as smoking during pregnancy and infections could be common causes for the obstetric complications and the development of asthma in the offspring. Alternatively, pregnancy complications, independent of genetic predisposition and smoking, may increase the likelihood of asthma in the child by acting on the developing immune system of the fetus. For example, Caesarean delivery may change the gut microflora and result in Th2 dominance in the child. In conclusion, it is entirely possible that a certain proportion of childhood asthma is attributable to asthma during pregnancy.

Intestinal flora

The microflora of the large intestine may play an important role in the development of allergic diseases. It has been suggested that ingestion of raw and unpasteurized milk containing lactobacilli may enhance Th1-dominated cytokine responses and protect the child from the development of allergic diseases (Kilpelainen et al., 2000; Riedler et al., 2000; von Ehrenstein et al., 2000; Warner and Warner, 2000). Differences in gut flora have been reported between infants from Estonia and Sweden (Sepp et al., 1997; Bjorksten et al., 1999), where the prevalence of allergies is low in Estonia and high in Sweden (Braback et al., 1995). Colonization with lactobacilli and *Eubacterium* were more common among Estonian children, whereas among Swedish infants, colonization with *Clostridium difficile* was more common.

Changes in the intestinal flora of infants occur following delivery by Caesarean section. As a result, the risk of allergies among children born by Caesarean section has been the focus of recent investigation. A Finnish study (Xu et al., 2001) examined the association between Caesarean delivery and the risk of developing allergic disease at 31 years of age. Caesarean delivery was strongly associated with current doctor-diagnosed asthma at the age of 31 years (adjusted OR 3.23; 95% CI 1.53, 6.80). No association was reported between Caesarean delivery and the later development of atopy, hay fever or atopic eczema. Similarly, a follow-up of children from birth to 7 years of age, through record linkage of various registries in Finland (Kero et al., 2002), demonstrated a significantly higher cumulative incidence of asthma at the age of 7 years in children born by Caesarean section (4.2%) than in those vaginally delivered (3.3%, OR 1.27; 95% CI 1.13, 1.42). In another cohort (Turku birth cohort), children born by Caesarean as compared with vaginal delivery were also reported to have more asthma symptoms (14.2% versus 9.4%), positive allergic skin test (41% versus 29%) and physician-confirmed asthma (12% versus 6%). However, these comparisons did not achieve statistical significance. Properly designed studies are needed to confirm the concurrent increases in Caesarean delivery rates and the prevalence of allergic diseases.

Infections

Recent studies have claimed that infections during childhood are found to be protective against asthma and allergic diseases. This finding is also linked to decreasing family size and increased likelihood of developing asthma. The observation that, over time, there is a declining family size and at the same time an increase in allergy and asthma, has led some investigators to propose what is termed 'the hygiene hypothesis'.

Studies that have examined the relationship between family size and atopic disease are summarized in Table 12.9. A number of studies have demonstrated that the risk of allergic diseases is significantly lower among children who grow up in large families. A landmark study conducted in the UK (Strachan, 1989), which studied 17,414 children born during 1 week in March 1958 and followed until the age of 23 years, showed an inverse relation between the occurrence of hay fever at 11 and 23 years of age and the number of children in the household at age 11. This association persisted after adjusting for the effects of potential confounders, such as father's social class, breastfeeding, region of birth and cigarette smoking at age 23. Similarly, a recent retrospective study from the UK (McKeever *et al.*, 2001), which followed 29,238 children from birth to 2.9 years of age, demonstrated a decreasing trend for the occurrence of eczema and hay fever with increasing number of older siblings in the household. However, that study did not show a similar trend for doctor-diagnosed asthma. The results obtained from cross-sectional studies of family size and the presence of hay fever and eczema consistently show a negative association (Jarvis *et al.*, 1997; Bodner *et al.*, 1998). However, the same is not true for wheeze and asthma (Jarvis *et al.*, 1997; Rona *et al.*, 1997; Bodner *et al.*, 1998).

The validity of studies where the outcome is the occurrence of symptoms of hay fever, eczema or asthma may be weakened because of recall bias, as well as inconsistencies in defining these allergic diseases. Therefore some investigators have used a more objective measure of sensitization, i.e. skin-prick test, to study the association between the number of siblings in the household and the presence of skin-prick test positivity to common aeroallergens. Cross-sectional studies of family size and allergic sensitization consistently demonstrate a decreasing trend in the occurrence of skin-prick test positivity with increasing number of siblings in the household (von Mutius *et al.*, 1994; Strachan *et al.*, 1997b; Matricardi *et al.*, 1998). However, the results from longitudinal studies are equivocal. Although a British study (Strachan *et al.*, 1997a) that followed 1369 children from birth to 35 years of age showed that subjects who had three or more older siblings were almost 50% less likely (OR 0.49, 95% CI 0.28, 0.86) to be skin-prick test positive, another study from the same country (Karmaus *et al.*, 2001) did not show such an association. Interestingly, when the pulmonary function of 677 school-age children was measured, the per cent predicted FVC and FEV_1 values became progressively larger as the number of siblings increased, indicating a reduced propensity for bronchial obstruction (Mattes *et al.*, 1999).

It has been postulated that the occurrence of fewer signs and symptoms of allergic diseases among children from large families could be explained by reduced cross-infection between siblings in smaller families (Strachan, 1989). This 'hygiene hypothesis' is thought to be mediated through immune modulation of the T-helper lymphocytes, whereby infectious agents induce the secretion of anti-allergic Th1 cytokines. Although the negative association between the occurrence of atopic diseases and family size has been attributed to the 'hygiene

Table 12.9. Studies examining the relationship between family size, birth order and atopic diseases.

Study, country	Study design	Ages (years)	N	Exposure	Findings		
Strachan et al. (1989), UK	Prospective cohort	Birth to 23	17,414	No. of older siblings	Prevalence of hay fever in previous year (%)	Prevalence of eczema in first year of life (%)	
				0	20.4	6.1	
				1	15.0	5.2	
				2	12.5	4.6	
				3	10.6	3.7	
				≥ 4	8.6	2.8	
McKeever et al. (2001), UK	Retrospective cohort	Birth to 2.9	29, 238	No. of older siblings	OR (95% CI)		
					Asthma	Eczema	Hay fever
				0	1.00	1.00	1.00
				1	1.13 (1.06–1.20)	0.89 (0.85–0.94)	0.82 (0.72–0.94)
				2	1.18 (1.09–1.27)	0.82 (0.76–0.87)	0.76 (0.63–0.91)
				> 2	1.17 (1.06–1.29)	0.70 (0.64–0.76)	0.67 (0.52–0.86)
Jarvis et al. (1997), UK	Cross-sectional	20–44	1159		OR (95% CI)		
					Hay fever	Wheeze without cold	Asthma
				Family size	0.84 (0.79–0.94)	0.86 (0.75–0.98)	0.77 (0.61–0.97)
				Birth order	0.87 (0.77–0.98)	0.90 (0.77–1.04)	0.81 (0.62–1.04)
Bodner et al. (1998), UK	Cross-sectional	10–14	2111	No. of siblings	OR (95% CI)		
					Asthma	Eczema	Hay fever
				0	1.0	1.0	1.0
				1	1.6 (0.7–4.0)	0.6 (0.3–1.2)	0.9 (0.4–2.0)
				2	1.8 (0.8–4.5)	0.6 (0.3–1.1)	0.6 (0.3–1.5)
				3	1.3 (0.5–3.3)	0.6 (0.3–1.2)	0.3 (0.1–0.9)
				4	0.6 (0.2–2.0)	0.2 (0.1–0.7)	0.6 (0.2–1.7)
				≥ 5	0.9 (0.3–2.7)	0.2 (0.05–0.6)	0.2 (0.04–1.0)
Rona et al. (1997), UK	Cross-sectional	Primary school-children	11,924	Family size	OR (95% CI)		
					Asthma and/or wheeze		
				1	1.00		
				2	0.71 (0.58, 0.86)		
				3	0.62 (0.51, 0.77)		
				> 3	0.50 (0.40, 0.62)		

Reference	Design	Age	No.	Variable	Category	Prevalence of atopy	
						West Germany	East Germany
von Mutius *et al.* (1994), Germany	Cross-sectional	9–11	2335	No. of siblings	0	36.1	19.4
					1	38.0	17.7
					2	36.5	15.5
					3	31.7	15.4
					4	28.6	16.7
					> 5	25.0	11.1
						OR (95% CI)	
						Any allergy	
Strachan *et al.* (1997), UK	Cross-sectional	14–45	11,042	No. of brothers	0	1.00	
					1	0.80 (0.72–0.90)	
					2	0.66 (0.57–0.76)	
					> 3	0.51 (0.47–0.56)	
				No. of sisters	0	1.00	
					1	0.98 (0.88–1.1)	
					2	0.88 (0.76–1.01)	
					> 3	0.93 (0.78–1.11)	
						OR (95% CI)	
						Atopy (assessed by elevated IgE)	
Matricardi *et al.* (1998), Italy	Cross-sectional	18–24	11,371	No. of older siblings	0	1.00	
					1	0.82 (0.73–0.92)	
					2	0.62 (0.52–0.74)	
					≥ 3	0.54 (0.42–0.70)	
				No. of younger siblings	0	1.00	
					1	0.87 (0.77–0.98)	
					2	0.71 (0.60–0.83)	
					≥ 3	0.63 (0.48–0.83)	

continued

Table 12.9. *Continued.*

Study, country	Study design	Ages (years)	N	Exposure	Findings	
Strachan *et al.* (1997), UK	Prospective cohort	Birth to 35	1369	No. of older siblings	OR (95% CI) Atopy (assessed by SPT)	
				0	1.00	
				1	0.71 (0.54–0.95)	
				2	0.53 (0.36–0.79)	
				≥3	0.49 (0.28–0.86)	
Karmaus *et al.* (2001), UK	Prospective	Birth to 4	857	Birth order	OR (95% CI) Atopy (assessed by SPT)	
				1	1.00	
				2	0.94 (0.63–1.39)	
				≥3	0.82 (0.52–1.30)	
Mattes *et al.* (1999), Germany	Prospective	Birth to 7–16	677	No. of younger siblings	FVC%(SE) †	FEV$_1$%(SE) †
				0	reference	reference
				1	+1.5 (1.1)	+1.8 (1.1)
				≥2	+2.6 (1.3)	+2.9 (1.3)
				No. of older siblings		
				0	reference	reference
				1	+2.3 (1.1)	+2.6 (1.1)
				≥2	+2.5 (1.4)	+2.4 (1.5)

†Expressed as a percentage of deviation from the predicted values.
OR, Odds ratio; CI, confidence interval; SPT, skin-prick test; FVC, forced vital capacity; FEV, forced expiratory volume; SE, standard error.

hypothesis', the results of studies investigating the relationship between childhood infections and atopy have been inconsistent. The Tucson cohort study (Martinez *et al.*, 1995b) demonstrated a reduced occurrence of skin-test reactivity among children with non-wheezing lower respiratory tract infections within the first 3 years of life. Another study from the UK (Illi *et al.*, 2001), which followed 1314 children from birth to 7 years of age, also demonstrated a reduced risk for doctor-diagnosed asthma at age 7 among children who had two or more episodes of runny nose (OR 0.52, 95% CI 0.29, 0.92) during infancy and one or more episodes of viral infection of the herpes type (OR 0.48, 95% CI 0.26, 0.89) during the first 3 years of life. However, an increasing number of lower respiratory tract infections in the first 3 years of life in that study was associated with an increasing risk for doctor-diagnosed asthma. Other investigators have also demonstrated a greater risk for atopy and asthma in the presence of respiratory tract infections during early life (Bodner *et al.*, 1998; Farooqi and Hopkin, 1998; Ponsonby *et al.*, 1999; Nafstad *et al.*, 2000b; Bager *et al.*, 2002; Celedon *et al.*, 2002).

Of the common childhood infections, the role of measles in the occurrence of allergic diseases has been studied extensively. However, the results obtained from such studies do not show a consistent pattern. Although some investigators found a negative association (Shaheen *et al.*, 1996; Bodner *et al.*, 1998, 2000; Wickens *et al.*, 1999), others showed either no risk (Farooqi and Hopkin, 1998; Lewis and Britton, 1998b; Matricardi *et al.*, 1998; Illi *et al.*, 2001) or, conversely, an increased risk for allergic diseases (Paunio *et al.*, 2000; Bager *et al.*, 2002) among those exposed to measles during childhood. Investigators also sought to examine the effect of measles immunization on the occurrence of allergic sensitization. A longitudinal study from Guinea-Bissau (Shaheen *et al.*, 1996) examined children who were infected with wild measles during an epidemic and compared them with those who did not contract measles during the epidemic and were subsequently immunized. In that study, those who received post-epidemic immunization had an increased prevalence of allergic sensitization as opposed to those who had been infected with the disease during the epidemic. One of the interpretations offered by the authors to explain these findings was that measles immunization may enhance the occurrence of atopy. However, a subsequent study of over 6000 British children showed no association between measles immunization and hay fever (Lewis and Britton, 1998b).

The possibility of an increased risk of atopy due to measles vaccination led to an investigation of the effect of pertussis immunization on the occurrence of atopy. The first study conducted to examine this effect recruited 1934 individuals from the 1975–1984 birth cohort at an Oxfordshire general practice (Farooqi and Hopkin, 1998). That study showed a 75% increase in the risk of atopic diseases among those who were vaccinated with whole-cell pertussis vaccines. After this study, a Swedish randomized trial (Nilsson *et al.*, 1998), conducted to study the effect of pertussis vaccines on atopic disease, showed no relationship between the two. Another prospective study from the UK also corroborated the findings of the Swedish trial (Henderson *et al.*, 1999).

Another childhood infectious agent, *Mycobacterium tuberculosis*, has generated considerable interest among researchers with respect to its preventive role in the occurrence of atopic diseases, because of its ability to stimulate the secretion of Th1 cytokines. Evidence in favour of an inverse association between mycobacterial infection and atopy came from a Japanese study (Shirakawa *et al.*, 1997) of 867 children who underwent routine tuberculin tests prior to BCG vaccination at ages 6 and 12 years. That study demonstrated a significant protective effect of delayed hypersensitivity to *M. tuberculosis* on the occurrence of atopy at the age of 12 years. On the other hand, a recent Norwegian study (Omenaas *et al.*, 2000) showed no significant relationship between tuberculin reactivity and atopy among young adults routinely vaccinated with BCG at age 14. Furthermore, other studies also failed to demonstrate any association between exposure to *M. tuberculosis* and subsequent development of atopy (von Hertzen *et al.*, 1999; von Mutius *et al.*, 2000).

It can be hypothesized that if infection with mycobacteria reduces the risk of atopy, then BCG vaccination in early life may have a protective effect on the occurrence of subsequent atopy. Several studies have attempted to investigate this hypothesis. A retrospective cohort study of 3- to 14-year-old children from Guinea-Bissau (Aaby *et al.*, 2000) showed a reduced occurrence of atopy among children who were vaccinated with BCG (21% versus 40%). On the other hand, a Swedish study (Alm *et al.*, 1997), which enrolled 216 children with a strong family history of atopy who had received BCG vaccination and 358 age-matched controls who had not been vaccinated, showed that there was no significant difference in the occurrence of atopy and symptoms of allergic disease between the two groups. Contrary to that study, Marks *et al.* (2003) found a significant inverse relationship between BCG vaccination and atopy only among children with a positive family history of atopy (RR 0.46, 95% CI 0.22, 0.95). Other studies reported either no relationship (Krause *et al.*, 2003) or a weak protective effect (Gruber *et al.*, 2002).

Most studies have attempted to explain the inverse association between family size and atopy by an increased propensity for infection in early childhood, which may be transmitted by contact with siblings. However, Varner (2002) proposed an interesting alternative hypothesis for this inverse relationship. He hypothesized that the atopic predisposition (Th2 immune response) may confer an evolutionary advantage to the atopic infant by reducing the severity and frequency of respiratory infections early in life. He, further, elaborates his viewpoint by citing literature that demonstrates that the Th2 immune response not only ensures successful pregnancy and term birth, but also provides the infant protection against infections by common pathogens in early life (Sporik *et al.*, 1990).

In sum, the findings of studies relating exposure to common infections and vaccines in childhood and the occurrence of atopy and asthma are not consistent in supporting the hygiene hypothesis. It is entirely possible that exposures occurring *in utero* may have influenced the results of these studies.

A More Toxic Environment

Children today spend more of their time indoors relative to outdoors and, as such, indoor pollutants are believed to be more important. Indoor exposures include aeroallergens (dust mite, cat and cockroach allergens) and irritants (particulate matter PM_{10}, $PM_{2.5}$, NO_2, SO_4). Exposure to indoor irritants in early life has not been linked directly to the incidence of atopy or asthma (Samet *et al.*, 1993; Garrett *et al.*, 1998). On the other hand, exposure to these indoor aeroallergens has been associated with the development of atopy and asthma (Sporik *et al.*, 1990; Perzanowski *et al.*, 1999; Custovic *et al.*, 2002).

The first strong evidence for the association between exposure to house dust mite (HDM) during the first 6 months of life and subsequent development of asthma came from a prospective study of 67 children from the UK (Sporik *et al.*, 1990). In that study, a greater degree of exposure to HDM allergen (Der p1) was associated with an increasing trend of sensitization at the age of 11 years. The relative risk of asthma in children exposed to more than 10 µg of Der p1 per gram of dust during infancy was approximately 5.0. The results of this and several other studies (Sears *et al.*, 1993; Sporik *et al.*, 1993; Peat *et al.*, 1996; Rosenstreich *et al.*, 1997; Lau *et al.*, 2000) laid the foundation for the paradigm for the pathogenesis of asthma that has been widely accepted since the 1990s. This paradigm is that genetically susceptible individuals upon exposure to allergen will be sensitized (atopy). Subsequent exposure to the same allergens will result in degranulation of mast cells through anamnestic response, leading to inflammation and asthma.

Based on this framework, four large randomized trials were mounted in order to assess the efficacy of allergen avoidance measures in preventing the development of asthma and allergies (Arshad *et al.*, 1992, 2003; Hide *et al.*, 1994, 1996; Chan-Yeung *et al.*, 2000; Custovic *et al.*, 2001; Mihrshahi *et al.*, 2003) (Table 12.10).

Arshad *et al.* (1992) prenatally randomized pregnant women into prophy-lactic and control groups and evaluated the occurrence of asthma, eczema and food intolerance among their infants at 1 year of age. In the prophylactic group, mothers and children were asked to follow a strict diet, which excluded allergenic foods. The infants' mattresses were covered with polyvinyl and the head areas were vented. In addition, an acaricidal preparation was used to treat the infants' bedrooms, the living room and all upholstered furniture. The prophylactic group was found to have a reduced incidence of asthma, eczema and food intolerance. However, the diagnosis of asthma at 1 year of age is questionable. Furthermore, introducing inclusion or exclusion criteria after randomization may have intro-duced bias. The Canadian randomized trial (Chan-Yeung *et al.*, 2000) reported a borderline statistically significant protection for probable asthma at 1 year with a 90% confidence limit. The results of another UK randomized trial (Custovic *et al.*, 2001), with similar intervention, showed borderline protection for wheeze, but not for asthma or eczema. Similarly, an Australian randomized trial (Mihrshahi *et al.*, 2003) did not show any significant benefit from allergen avoidance measures on the occurrence of wheeze and eczema. In a further follow-up of infants at 2 years in the study by Arshad and colleagues, the protection for eczema persisted, while that for asthma disappeared. When the same group of infants was evaluated at 4 and 8 years of age (Hide *et al.*, 1994, 1996), the prophylactic group still had a lower risk of eczema, but not asthma.

Table 12.10. Randomized controlled trials for primary prevention of allergies and asthma among high-risk infants.

Study, country	Randomization	Endpoint	Loss to follow-up Prophylactic (%)	Loss to follow-up Control (%)	Study size Prophylactic	Study size Control	Outcome	Findings (control is reference category)
Arshad *et al.* (1992), UK	Prenatal	12 months	19	8	58	62		OR (95% CI)
							Asthma	0.24 (0.06, 0.91)
							Eczema	0.28 (0.08, 1.00)
							Food intolerance	0.30 (0.06, 1.67)
							Allergic disorder	0.16 (0.05, 0.50)
Chan-Yeung *et al.* (2000), Canada	Prenatal	12 months	11	10	251	242		RR (90% CI)
							Probable asthma	0.54 (0.29, 0.98)
							Possible asthma	0.80 (0.49, 1.31)
							Rhinitis	0.51 (0.35, 0.74)
Custovic *et al.* (2001), UK	Prenatal	12 months	6	14	145	146		RR (95% CI)
							Severe wheeze	0.44 (0.20–1.00)
							Wheeze medication	0.58 (0.36–0.95)
							MD-diagnosed asthma	0.48 (0.19–1.27)
							Eczema	1.07 (0.78–1.46)
Mihrshahi *et al.* (2003), Australia	Prenatal	18 months	N/A	N/A	276	278		% difference (95% CI)
							Wheeze/breathlessness	0.9 (−5.5, 7.2)
							Visit to ER for wheeze	0.6 (−4.7, 5.7)
							Eczema	8.2 (0.6, 15.8)
Hide *et al.* (1994), UK	Prenatal	24 months	19	8	58	62		OR (95% CI)
							Asthma	0.46 (0.17, 1.23)
							Eczema	0.11 (0.02, 0.56)
							Food intolerance	0.80 (0.17, 3.33)
							Allergic disorder	0.10 (0.03, 0.37)
Hide *et al.* (1996), UK	Prenatal	48 months	19	8	58	62		OR (95% CI)
							Asthma	Not significant
							Eczema	0.29 (0.10, 0.83)
							Atopy	0.27 (0.1, 0.77)
							Allergic disorders	0.37 (0.16, 0.83)
Arshad *et al.* (2003), UK	Prenatal	8 years	19	8	58	62		OR (95% CI)
							Asthma	0.11 (0.01, 1.02)
							Atopy	0.21 (0.07, 0.62)

OR, Odds ratio; CI, confidence interval; RR, relative risk; N/A, not available; ER, Emergency Room.

The findings from these randomized trials challenge the sensitization, airway responsiveness, inflammation and asthma paradigm that is widely accepted. This challenge is further sustained by a recent study (Pearce *et al.*, 1999) that scrutinized all observational studies of atopy and asthma. The proportion of asthmatic cases attributable to atopy varied from 25% to 63% with a weighted mean of 38% in children, and from 8% to 55% with a weighted mean of 37% in adults.

Study results from developing countries and from some isolated communities also revealed a lack of association between atopy and asthma (Hemmelgarn and Ernst, 1997; Yemaneberhan *et al.*, 1997; Sunyer *et al.*, 2000). A study conducted in the western part of Ethiopia showed a dissociation in the rate of atopy, as measured by skin-test positivity, and symptoms of wheeze (in rural areas the prevalence of atopy and wheeze were 11.8% and 1.2%, respectively, while in the urban area they were 4% and 3.7% respectively) (Yemaneberhan *et al.*, 1997). Another study from Tanzania also failed to find a relationship between atopy, as measured by serum IgE to Der p1 and cockroach, and asthma diagnosis (Sunyer *et al.*, 2000). In this study, Der p1 and cockroach were highly prevalent. Similarly, among Inuit primary school children in far northern Quebec, atopy, as measured by skin-prick test, was not found to be associated with either exercise-induced bronchospasm or $FEV_1/FVC < 0.75$ (Hemmelgarn and Ernst, 1997). In these communities, lifestyle factors that require more vigorous physical activity may have played a role in the lack of translation from atopy to allergic symptoms. In sum, asthma is a heterogeneous disease and investigators need to be open-minded to understand the risk indicators for both atopy-related and atopy-unrelated asthma.

Air pollution may aggravate existing disease by triggering symptoms. For example, exposure to a higher concentration of ozone has been suggested to increase the sensitivity of asthmatic patients to allergens (Weinmann, 1996). A recent study also found an association between outdoor pollution (particulate matter, SO_2 and NO_2) and wheeze among children who exhibited bronchial hyper-responsiveness and, at the same time, had high serum total IgE levels (Boezen *et al.*, 1999). However, for the most part, outdoor air pollution has not been associated with the development of atopy or asthma (Dockery *et al.*, 1989; Bates, 1995; Donaldson *et al.*, 2000) and is not the main explanation for the increasing incidence of allergic diseases (Seaton *et al.*, 1994).

German investigators (von Mutius *et al.*, 1992) compared the prevalences of allergies and asthma in two cities of Germany (Leipzig and Munich) with homogeneous genetic make-up. Leipzig is a highly polluted city in the former East Germany and Munich is a relatively clean city in West Germany. The prevalence of positive skin-tests and asthma was higher in the West than the East. Their findings suggest that lifestyle factors (e.g. carpeted Western-style buildings) rather than air pollution are more important in the occurrence of allergic diseases (Cookson and Moffatt, 1997).

Fetal Origins of Allergic Disease

The proposition that various adult chronic diseases may have their origin in fetal and infant life (Forsdahl, 1977; Kermack *et al.*, 2001) has been an active area of research in the past two decades (Barker and Osmond, 1986a,b, 1987) (Barker *et al.*, 1989a,b, 1991, 1993, 1995; Osmond *et al.*, 1990; Law *et al.*, 1993; Godfrey *et al.*, 1994; Fall *et al.*, 1995). The University of Southampton investigators published several reports linking fetal and early childhood growth to adult chronic diseases such as coronary heart disease, stroke, hypertension, diabetes and chronic obstructive lung disease. On the basis of the findings, the same group of investigators proposed the 'fetal origins' hypothesis, which postulates that physiological or metabolic programming occurs when a stimulus or insult operates during a critical period of the fetal development that results in permanent structural and functional alterations (Rasmussen, 2001). The validity of the fetal programming hypothesis, although supported by several investigators, has been questioned by others (Joseph and Kramer, 1996; Seckl, 1998).

The framework described in this chapter on the link between perinatal factors and allergic diseases does not completely fall into the classical fetal programming arena. However, there is some overlap with respect to selected factors. Langley-Evans (1997) discussed the role of nutritional factors during fetal life in programming the immune function. Increased head circumference at birth in disproportion to the growth of other organs, including those involved in the immune system (spleen, thymus), may permanently reduce the number of lymphocytes. Factors such as exposure to prenatal allergens, *in utero* exposure to cigarette smoke, change in intestinal flora and others may shift the Th1/Th2 immunological balance towards Th2, but the permanency of these changes is uncertain at this time. Even if we assume that these changes persist until adolescence, at which time a good proportion of children grow out of allergies and asthma, the proportion of subjects who develop chronic obstructive lung disease in adulthood will be small and the public health impact of the fetal programming hypothesis is modest. However, a thorough understanding of the association between perinatal factors and childhood allergic diseases is important to design interventions that reduce the very high disease burden during childhood.

Conclusion

Perinatal factors play an important role in the aetiology of allergies at birth and early childhood. Whether these factors will persist into late childhood and adolescence is unknown at this time. Clearly, the field is in its infancy and more data are needed to better understand the complex interplay between these factors. The translation of atopy to asthma symptoms, particularly the role of lifestyle-enhancing physical activity, warrants further examination. Furthermore, asthma is a very heterogeneous disease and the risk indicators for non-allergic asthma as opposed to allergic asthma should be one of the areas of future research. Collectively, the evidence presented on prenatal factors in the aetiology of allergic diseases is very promising. However, due to the paucity of information in this area, prenatal intervention is not warranted at this time.

References

Aaby, P., Shaheen, S.O., Heyes, C.B., Goudiaby, A., Hall, A.J., Shiell, A.W., Jensen, H. and Marchant, A. (2000) Early BCG vaccination and reduction in atopy in Guinea-Bissau. *Clinical and Experimental Allergy* 30, 644–650.

Agabiti, N., Mallone, S., Forastiere, F., Corbo, G.M., Ferro, S., Renzoni, E., Seshni, P., Rusconi, F., Ciccone, G., Viegi, C., Chellini, E. and Pfiffer, S. (1999) The impact of parental smoking on asthma and wheezing. SIDRIA Collaborative Group. Studi Italiani sui Disturbi Respiratori nell'Infanzia e l'Ambiente. *Epidemiology* 10, 692–698.

Alexander, S., Dodds, L. and Armson, B.A. (1998) Perinatal outcomes in women with asthma during pregnancy. *Obstetrics and Gynecology* 92, 435–440.

Alm, J.S., Lilja, G., Pershagen, G. and Scheynius, A. (1997) Early BCG vaccination and development of atopy. *Lancet* 350, 400–403.

Annesi-Maesano, I., Moreau, D. and Strachan, D. (2001) *In utero* and perinatal complications preceding asthma. *Allergy* 56, 491–497.

Anonymous (1998a) Worldwide variations in the prevalence of asthma symptoms: the International Study of Asthma and Allergies in Childhood (ISAAC). *European Respiratory Journal* 12, 315–335.

Anonymous (1998b) Worldwide variation in prevalence of symptoms of asthma, allergic rhinoconjunctivitis, and atopic eczema: ISAAC. The International Study of Asthma and Allergies in Childhood (ISAAC) Steering Committee. *Lancet* 351, 1225–1232.

Arm, J.P., Horton, C.E., Spur, B.W., Mencia-Huerta, J.M. and Lee, T.H. (1989) The effects of dietary supplementation with fish oil lipids on the airways response to inhaled allergen in bronchial asthma. *American Review of Respiratory Disease* 139, 1395–1400.

Arshad, S.H., Matthews, S., Gant, C. and Hide, D.W. (1992) Effect of allergen avoidance on development of allergic disorders in infancy. *Lancet* 339, 1493–1497.

Arshad, S.H., Bateman, B. and Matthews, S.M. (2003) Primary prevention of asthma and atopy during childhood by allergen avoidance in infancy: a randomised controlled study. *Thorax* 58, 489–493.

Athanassakis, I. and Vassiliadis, S. (2002) Interplay between T helper type 1 and type 2 cytokines and soluble major histocompatibility complex molecules: a paradigm in pregnancy. *Immunology* 107, 281–287.

Bager, P., Westergaard, T., Rostgaard, K., Hjalgrim, H. and Melbye, M. (2002) Age at childhood infections and risk of atopy. *Thorax* 57, 379–382.

Barker, D.J. and Osmond, C. (1986a) Infant mortality, childhood nutrition, and ischaemic heart disease in England and Wales. *Lancet* 1, 1077–1081.

Barker, D.J. and Osmond, C. (1986b) Childhood respiratory infection and adult chronic bronchitis in England and Wales. *British Medical Journal (Clinical Research Edition)* 293, 1271–1275.

Barker, D.J. and Osmond, C. (1987) Death rates from stroke in England and Wales predicted from past maternal mortality. *British Medical Journal (Clinical Research Edition)* 295, 83–86.

Barker, D.J., Osmond, C. and Law, C.M. (1989a) The intrauterine and early postnatal origins of cardiovascular disease and chronic bronchitis. *Journal of Epidemiology and Community Health* 43, 237–240.

Barker, D.J., Winter, P.D., Osmond, C., Margetts, B. and Simmonds, S.J. (1989b) Weight in infancy and death from ischaemic heart disease. *Lancet* 2, 577–580.

Barker, D.J., Godfrey, K.M., Fall, C., Osmond, C., Winter, P.D. and Shaheen, S.O. (1991) Relation of birth weight and childhood respiratory infection to adult lung function and death from chronic obstructive airways disease. *British Medical Journal* 303, 671–675.

Barker, D.J., Osmond, C., Simmonds, S.J. and Wield, G.A. (1993) The relation of small head circumference and thinness at birth to death from cardiovascular disease in adult life. *British Medical Journal* 306, 422–426.

Barker, D.J., Osmond, C., Rodin, I., Fall, C.H. and Winter, P.D. (1995) Low weight gain in infancy and suicide in adult life. *British Medical Journal* 311, 1203.

Barker, R.N., Erwig, L.P., Hill, K.S., Devine, A., Pearce, W.P. and Rees, A.J. (2002) Antigen presentation by macrophages is enhanced by the uptake of necrotic, but not apoptotic, cells. *Clinical and Experimental Immunology* 127, 220–225.

Basta, P.V., Navarro, H.H., Seidler, F.J. and Slotkin, T.A. (2001) Adolescent nicotine: deficits in immune function. *Developmental Brain Research* 130, 253–256.

Bates, D.V. (1995) Observations on asthma. *Environmental Health Perspectives* 103(suppl. 6), 243–247.

Beck, M., Zelczak, G. and Lentze, M.J. (2000) Abnormal fatty acid composition in umbilical cord blood of infants at high risk of atopic disease. *Acta Paediatrica* 89, 279–284.

Becquet, R., Leroy, V. and Salmi, L.R. (2003) Breastfeeding, atopy and asthma. *Lancet* 361, 174.

Benn, C.S., Thorsen, P., Jensen, J.S., Kjaer, B.B., Bisgaard, H., Andersen, M., Rostgaard, K., Bjorksten, B. and Melbye, M. (2002) Maternal vaginal microflora during pregnancy and the risk of asthma hospitalization and use of antiasthma medication in early childhood. *Journal of Allergy and Clinical Immunology* 110, 72–77.

Binkley, J.K., Eales, J. and Jekanowski, M. (2000) The relation between dietary change and rising US obesity. *International Journal of Obesity and Related Metabolic Disorders* 24, 1032–1039.

Bjorksten, B. (1999) The intrauterine and postnatal environments. *Journal of Allergy and Clinical Immunology* 104, 1119–1127.

Bjorksten, B., Naaber, P., Sepp, E. and Mikelsaar, M. (1999) The intestinal microflora in allergic Estonian and Swedish 2-year-old children. *Clinical and Experimental Allergy* 29, 342–346.

Black, P.N. and Sharpe, S. (1997) Dietary fat and asthma: is there a connection? *European Respiratory Journal* 10, 6–12.

Blumenfeld, Z. and Jaffe, R.B. (1986) Hypophysiotropic and neuromodulatory regulation of adrenocorticotropin in the human fetal pituitary gland. *Journal of Clinical Investigation* 78, 288–294.

Bodner, C., Godden, D. and Seaton, A. (1998) Family size, childhood infections and atopic diseases. The Aberdeen WHEASE Group. *Thorax* 53, 28–32.

Bodner, C., Anderson, W.J., Reid, T.S. and Godden, D.J. (2000) Childhood exposure to infection and risk of adult onset wheeze and atopy. *Thorax* 55, 383–387.

Boelens, J.J. (2003) Breastfeeding, atopy and asthma. *Lancet* 361, 174–175.

Boezen, H.M., van der Zee, S.C., Postma, D.S., Vonk, J.M., Gerritsen, J., Hoek, G., Brunekreef, B., Rijcken, B. and Schoneten, J.P. (1999) Effects of ambient air pollution on upper and lower respiratory symptoms and peak expiratory flow in children. *Lancet* 353, 874–878.

Bottcher, M.F., Jenmalm, M.C., Bjorksten, B. and Garofalo, R.P. (2000a) Chemo-attractant factors in breast milk from allergic and nonallergic mothers. *Pediatric Research* 47, 592–597.

Bottcher, M.F., Jenmalm, M.C., Garofalo, R.P. and Bjorksten, B. (2000b) Cytokines in breast milk from allergic and nonallergic mothers. *Pediatric Research* 47, 157–162.

Boushey, H.A., Holtzman, M.J., Sheller, J.R. and Nadel, J.A. (1980) Bronchial hyper-reactivity. *American Review of Respiratory Disease* 121, 389–413.

Bousquet, J. and Kjellman, N.I. (1986) Predictive value of tests in childhood allergy. *Journal of Allergy Clinical Immunology* 78, 1019–1022.

Braback, L., Breborowicz, A., Julge, K. *et al.* (1995) Risk factors for respiratory symptoms and atopic sensitisation in the Baltic area. *Archives of Disease in Childhood* 72, 487–493.

Burr, M.L., Merrett, T.G., Dunstan, F.D. and Maguire, M.J. (1997) The development of allergy in high-risk children. *Clinical and Experimental Allergy* 27, 1247–1253.

Burrows, B., Martinez, F.D., Halonen, M., Barbee, R.A. and Cline, M.G. (1989) Association of asthma with serum IgE levels and skin-test reactivity to allergens. *New England Journal of Medicine* 320, 271–277.

Butland, B.K., Strachan, D.P. and Anderson, H.R. (1999) Fresh fruit intake and asthma symptoms in young British adults. confounding or effect modification by smoking? *European Respiratory Journal* 13, 744–750.

Celedon, J.C., Litonjua, A.A., Ryan, L., Weiss, S.T. and Gold, D.R. (2002) Day care attendance, respiratory tract illnesses, wheezing, asthma, and total serum IgE level in early childhood. *Archives of Pediatric and Adolescent Medicine* 156, 241–245.

Chan, K.N., Noble-Jamieson, C.M., Elliman, A., Bryan, E.M. and Silverman, M. (1989) Lung function in children of low birth weight. *Archives of Disease in Childhood* 64, 1284–1293.

Chan-Yeung, M., Ferguson, A., Chan, H., *et al.* (1999) Umbilical cord blood mono-nuclear cell proliferative response to house dust mite does not predict the development of allergic rhinitis and asthma. *Journal of Allergy and Clinical Immunology* 104, 317–321.

Chan-Yeung, M., Manfreda, J., Dimich-Ward, H., Ferguson, A., Watson, W. and Becker, A. (2000) A randomized controlled study on the effectiveness of a multifaceted intervention program in the primary prevention of asthma in high-risk infants. *Archives of Pediatric and Adolescent Medicine* 154, 657–663.

Chaouat, G., Zourbas, S., Ostojic, S., Lappree-Delage, G., Dubanet, S., Ledee, N. and Martel, J. (2002) A brief review of recent data on some cytokine expressions at the materno-foetal interface which might challenge the classical Th1/Th2 dichotomy. *Journal of Reproductive Immunology* 53, 241–256.

Chrousos, G.P. (2000) The stress response and immune function: clinical implications. The 1999 Novera H. Spector Lecture. *Annals of the New York Academy of Sciences* 917, 38–67.

Chulada, P.C., Arbes, S.J. Jr, Dunson, D. and Zeldin, D.C. (2003) Breast-feeding and the prevalence of asthma and wheeze in children: analyses from the Third National Health and Nutrition Examination Survey, 1988–1994. *Journal of Allergy and Clinical Immunology* 111, 328–336.

Coe, C.L., Kramer, M., Kirschbaum, C., Netter, P. and Fuchs, E. (2002) Prenatal stress diminishes the cytokine response of leukocytes to endotoxin stimulation in juvenile rhesus monkeys. *Journal of Clinical Endocrinology and Metabolism* 87, 675–681.

Cookson, W.O. and Moffatt, M.F. (1997) Asthma: an epidemic in the absence of infection? *Science* 275, 41–42.

Cookson, W.O., Young, R.P., Sandford, A.J., Moffatt, M.F., Shirakawa, T., Sharp, P.A., Faux, J.A., Julier, C., Nakumuura, Y. and Nakumura, Y. (1992) Maternal inheritance of atopic IgE responsiveness on chromosome 11q. *Lancet* 340, 381–384.

Cunningham, J., Dockery, D.W. and Speizer, F.E. (1994) Maternal smoking during pregnancy as a predictor of lung function in children. *American Journal of Epidemiology* 139, 1139–1152.

Cunningham, J., Dockery, D.W., Gold, D.R. and Speizer, F.E. (1995) Racial differences in the association between maternal smoking during pregnancy and lung function in children. *American Journal of Respiratory and Critical Care Medicine* 152, 565–569.

Cunningham, J., O'Connor, G.T., Dockery, D.W. and Speizer, F.E. (1996) Environmental tobacco smoke, wheezing, and asthma in children in 24 communities. *American Journal of Respiratory and Critical Care Medicine* 153, 218–224.

Custovic, A., Simpson, B.M., Simpson, A., Kissen, P. and Woodcock, A. (2001) Effect of environmental manipulation in pregnancy and early life on respiratory symptoms and atopy during first year of life: a randomised trial. *Lancet* 358, 188–193.

Custovic, A., Murray, C.S., Gore, R.B. and Woodcock, A. (2002) Controlling indoor allergens. *Annals of Allergy, Asthma and Immunology* 88, 432–441.

Darlow, B.A., Horwood, L.J. and Mogridge, N. (2000) Very low birthweight and asthma by age seven years in a national cohort. *Pediatric Pulmonology* 30, 291–296.

Demissie, K. and Ernst, P. (1994) Is increased dietary salt intake a cause of increased airway responsiveness or a marker of an unhealthy life style? *Respiratory Medicine* 88, 79–81.

Demissie, K., Ernst, P., Gray Donald, K. and Joseph, L. (1996) Usual dietary salt intake and asthma in children: a case-control study. *Thorax* 51, 59–63.

Demissie, K., Ernst, P., Joseph, L. and Becklake, M.R. (1997) Birthweight and preterm birth in relation to indicators of childhood asthma. *Canadian Respiratory Journal* 4, 91–97.

Demissie, K., Breckenridge, M.B. and Rhoads, G.G. (1998a) Infant and maternal outcomes in the pregnancies of asthmatic women. *American Journal of Respiratory and Critical Care Medicine* 158, 1091–1095.

Demissie, K., Marcella, S.W., Breckenridge, M.B. and Rhoads, G.G. (1998b) Maternal asthma and transient tachypnea of the newborn. *Pediatrics* 102, 84–90.

Demissie, K., Breckenridge, M.B. and Rhoads, G.G. (1999) Infant and maternal outcomes in the pregnancies of asthmatic women. *Obstetrical and Gynecological Survey* 54, 355–356.

Devereux, G., Barker, R.N. and Seaton, A. (2002) Antenatal determinants of neonatal immune responses to allergens. *Clinical and Experimental Allergy* 32, 43–50.

Dezateux, C., Stocks, J., Dundas, I. and Fletcher, M.E. (1999) Impaired airway function and wheezing in infancy: the influence of maternal smoking and a genetic predisposition to asthma. *American Journal of Respiratory and Critical Care Medicine* 159, 403–410.

Diez-Roux, A.V., Nieto, F.J., Caulfield, L., Tyroler, H.A., Watson, R.L. and Szklo, M. (1999) Neighbourhood differences in diet: the Atherosclerosis Risk in Communities (ARIC) Study. *Journal of Epidemiology and Community Health* 53, 55–63.

Dockery, D.W., Speizer, F.E., Stram, D.O., Ware, J.H., Spengler, J.D. and Ferris, B.G. Jr (1989) Effects of inhalable particles on respiratory health of children. *American Review of Respiratory Disease* 139, 587–594.

Dombrowski, M.P., Bottoms, S.F., Boike, G.M. and Wald, J. (1986) Incidence of pre-eclampsia among asthmatic patients lower with theophylline. *American Journal of Obstetrics and Gynecology* 155, 265–267.

Donaldson, K., Gilmour, M.I. and MacNee, W. (2000) Asthma and PM10. *Respiration Research* 1, 12–15.

Drazen, J. (1992) Asthma. In: Wyngaarden, J., Smith, L. and Bennett, J. (eds) *Cecil Textbook of Medicine*. W.B. Saunders, Philadelphia, Pennsylvania, pp. 381–386.

Ehrlich, R.I., Du Toit, D., Jordaan, E., Zuarenstein, M., Potter, P., Volmink, Z.A. and Weinsberg, E. (1996) Risk factors for childhood asthma and wheezing. Importance of maternal and household smoking. *American Journal of Respiratory and Critical Care Medicine* 154, 681–688.

Elder, D.E., Hagan, R., Evans, S.F., Benninger, H.R. and French, N.P. (1996) Recurrent wheezing in very preterm infants. *Archives of Disease in Childhood. Fetal and Neonatal Edition* 74, F165–171.

Fall, C.H., Vijayakumar, M., Barker, D.J., Osmond, C. and Duggleby, S. (1995) Weight in infancy and prevalence of coronary heart disease in adult life. *British Medical Journal* 310, 17–19.

Farooqi, I.S. and Hopkin, J.M. (1998) Early childhood infection and atopic disorder. *Thorax* 53, 927–932.

Flegal, K.M., Carroll, M.D., Ogden, C.L. and Johnson, C.L. (2002) Prevalence and trends in obesity among US adults, 1999–2000. *Journal of the American Medical Association* 288, 1723–1727.

Fogarty, A. and Britton, J. (2000) The role of diet in the aetiology of asthma. *Clinical and Experimental Allergy* 30, 615–627.

Forsdahl, A. (1977) Are poor living conditions in childhood and adolescence an important risk factor for arteriosclerotic heart disease? *British Journal of Preventive and Social Medicine* 31, 91–95.

Frischer, T., Kuehr, J., Meinert, R., Karmusens, W., Barth, R., Hermann-Kunze, E. and Urbanek, R. (1992a) Maternal smoking in early childhood: a risk factor for bronchial responsiveness to exercise in primary-school children. *Journal of Pediatrics* 121, 17–22.

Frischer, T., Kuehr, J., Meinert, R., Karmusens, W., Barth, R., Hermann-Kunze, E. and Urbanek, R. (1992b) Relationship between low birth weight and respiratory symptoms in a cohort of primary school children. *Acta Paediatrica* 81, 1040–1041.

Garrett, M.H., Hooper, M.A., Hooper, B.M. and Abramson, M.J. (1998) Respiratory symptoms in children and indoor exposure to nitrogen dioxide and gas stoves. *American Journal of Respiratory and Critical Care Medicine* 158, 891–895.

Gdalevich, M., Mimouni, D., David, M. and Mimouni, M. (2001) Breast-feeding and the onset of atopic dermatitis in childhood: a systematic review and meta-analysis of prospective studies. *Journal of the American Academy of Dermatology* 45, 520–527.

Gilliland, F.D., Berhane, K., McConnell, R., Gauderman, W.J., Vora, H., Rappaport, E.P., Avol, E. and Peters, J.M. (2000) Maternal smoking during pregnancy, environmental tobacco smoke exposure and childhood lung function. *Thorax* 55, 271–276.

Gilliland, F.D., Li, Y.F. and Peters, J.M. (2001) Effects of maternal smoking during pregnancy and environmental tobacco smoke on asthma and wheezing in children. *American Journal of Respiratory and Critical Care Medicine* 163, 429–436.

Gitau, R., Cameron, A., Fisk, N.M. and Glover, V. (1998) Fetal exposure to maternal cortisol. *Lancet* 352, 707–708.

Godfrey, K.M., Barker, D.J. and Osmond, C. (1994) Disproportionate fetal growth and raised IgE concentration in adult life. *Clinical and Experimental Allergy* 24, 641–648.

Goland, R.S., Jozak, S. and Conwell, I. (1994) Placental corticotropin-releasing hormone and the hypercortisolism of pregnancy. *American Journal of Obstetrics and Gynecology* 171, 1287–1291.

Gold, D.R., Burge, H.A., Carey, V., Milton, D.K., Platts-Mills, T. and Weiss, S.T. (1999) Predictors of repeated wheeze in the first year of life: the relative roles of cockroach, birth weight, acute lower respiratory illness, and maternal smoking. *American Journal of Respiratory and Critical Care Medicine* 160, 227–236.

Gregory, A., Doull, I., Pearce, N. *et al.* (1999) The relationship between anthropometric measurements at birth: asthma and atopy in childhood. *Clinical and Experimental Allergy* 29, 330–333.

Gruber, C., Meinlschmidt, G., Bergmann, R., Wahn, U. and Stark, K. (2002) Is early BCG vaccination associated with less atopic disease? An epidemiological study in German preschool children with different ethnic backgrounds. *Pediatric Allergy and Immunology* 13, 177–181.

Hagstrom, B., Nyberg, P. and Nilsson, P.M. (1998) Asthma in adult life – is there an association with birth weight? *Scandinavian Journal of Primary Health Care* 16, 117–120.

Hanrahan, J.P., Tager, I.B., Segal, M.R., Tosteson, T.D., Castle, R.G., van Vunaka, S.H., Weiss, S.T. and Speizer, F.E. (1992) The effect of maternal smoking during pregnancy on early infant lung function. *American Review of Respiratory Disease* 145, 1129–1135.

Hemmelgarn, B. and Ernst, P. (1997) Airway function among Inuit primary school children in far northern Quebec. *American Journal of Respiratory and Critical Care Medicine* 156, 1870–1875.

Henderson, F.W., Henry, M.M., Ivins, S.S., Morris, R., Neebe, E.C., Leu, S.Y. and Devlin, R.B. (1995) Correlates of recurrent wheezing in school-age children. The Physicians of Raleigh Pediatric Associates. *American Journal of Respiratory and Critical Care Medicine* 151, 1786–1793.

Henderson, J., North, K., Griffiths, M., Harvey, I. and Golding, J. (1999) Pertussis vaccination and wheezing illnesses in young children: prospective cohort study. The Longitudinal Study of Pregnancy and Childhood Team. *British Medical Journal* 318, 1173–1176.

Henry, C., Kabbaj, M., Simon, H., Le Moal, M. and Maccari, S. (1994) Prenatal stress increases the hypothalamo-pituitary–adrenal axis response in young and adult rats. *Journal of Neuroendocrinology* 6, 341–345.

Herbert, T.B. and Cohen, S. (1993) Stress and immunity in humans: a meta-analytic review. *Psychosomatic Medicine* 55, 364–379.

Hide, D.W., Matthews, S., Matthews, L., Stevens, M., Ridout, S., Twistleton, R., Gant, C. and Arshad, S.H. (1994) Effect of allergen avoidance in infancy on allergic manifestations at age two years. *Journal of Allergy and Clinical Immunology* 93, 842–846.

Hide, D.W., Matthews, S., Tariq, S. and Arshad, S.H. (1996) Allergen avoidance in infancy and allergy at 4 years of age. *Allergy* 51, 89–93.

Hijazi, N., Abalkhail, B. and Seaton, A. (2000) Diet and childhood asthma in a society in transition: a study in urban and rural Saudi Arabia. *Thorax* 55, 775–779.

Hodge, L., Salome, C.M., Hughes, J.M., Liu-Brennan, D., Rimmer, J., Allman, M., Pang, D., Armour, C. and Woolcock, A.J. (1998) Effect of dietary intake of omega-3 and omega-6 fatty acids on severity of asthma in children. *European Respiratory Journal* 11, 361–365.

Holloway, J.A., Warner, J.O., Vance, G.H., Diaper, N.D., Warner, J.A. and Jones, C.A. (2000) Detection of house-dust-mite allergen in amniotic fluid and umbilical-cord blood. *Lancet* 356, 1900–1902.

Hughes, C.H., Jones, R.C., Wright, D.E. and Dobbs, F.F. (1999) A retrospective study of the relationship between childhood asthma and respiratory infection during gestation. *Clinical and Experimental Allergy* 29, 1378–1381.

Illi, S., von Mutius, E., Lau, S., Bergmann, R., Niggemann, B., Sommerfeld, C. and Wahn, U. (2001) Early childhood infectious diseases and the development of asthma up to school age: a birth cohort study. *British Medical Journal* 322, 390–395.

Jarvis, D., Chinn, S., Luczynska, C. and Burney, P. (1997) The association of family size with atopy and atopic disease. *Clinical and Experimental Allergy* 27, 240–245.

Jeffery, R.W. and French, S.A. (1998) Epidemic obesity in the United States: are fast foods and television viewing contributing? *American Journal of Public Health* 88, 277–280.

Jones, A.C., Miles, E.A., Warner, J.O., Colwell, B.M., Bryant, T.N. and Warner, J.A. (1996) Fetal peripheral blood mononuclear cell proliferative responses to mitogenic and allergenic stimuli during gestation. *Pediatric Allergy and Immunology* 7, 109–116.

Jones, C. (2002) The impact of racism on health. *Ethnicity and Disease* 12, S2–10–3

Jones, C.T. and Edwards, A.V. (1990) Adrenal responses to corticotrophin-releasing factor in conscious hypophysectomized calves. *Journal of Physiology* 430, 25–36.

Joseph, K.S. and Kramer, M.S. (1996) Review of the evidence on fetal and early childhood antecedents of adult chronic disease. *Epidemiologic Reviews* 18, 158–174.

Karmaus, W., Arshad, H. and Mattes, J. (2001) Does the sibling effect have its origin *in utero*? Investigating birth order, cord blood immunoglobulin E concentration, and allergic sensitization at age 4 years. *American Journal of Epidemiology* 154, 909–915.

Kay, G., Tarcic, N., Poltyrev, T. and Weinstock, M. (1998) Prenatal stress depresses immune function in rats. *Physiology and Behavior* 63, 397–402.

Kelsen, S.G. (2003) Asthma and pregnancy. *Journal of Allergy and Clinical Immunology* 112, 268–270.

Kelso, A. (1995) Th1 and Th2 subsets: paradigms lost? *Immunology Today* 16, 374–379.

Kennedy, B.P., Kawachi, I., Lochner, K., Jones, C. and Prothrow-Stith, D. (1997) (Dis)respect and black mortality. *Ethnicity and Disease* 7, 207–214.

Kermack, W.O., McKendrick, A.G. and McKinlay, P.L. (2001) Death-rates in Great Britain and Sweden. Some general regularities and their significance. *International Journal of Epidemiology* 30, 678–683.

Kero, J., Gissler, M., Gronlund, M.M. *et al.* (2002) Mode of delivery and asthma – is there a connection? *Pediatric Research* 52, 6–11.

Kilpelainen, M., Terho, E.O., Helenius, H. and Koskenvuo, M. (2000) Farm environment in childhood prevents the development of allergies. *Clinical and Experimental Allergy* 30, 201–208.

Kivimaki, M., Vahtera, J., Pentti, J. and Ferrie, J.E. (2000) Factors underlying the effect of organisational downsizing on health of employees: longitudinal cohort study. *British Medical Journal* 320, 971–975.

Kondo, N., Kobayashi, Y., Shinoda, S., Kashara, K., Kameyama, T., Iwasa, S. and Orii, T. (1992) Cord blood lymphocyte responses to food antigens for the prediction of allergic disorders. *Archives of Disease in Childhood* 67, 1003–1007.

Kondo, N., Kobayashi, Y., Shinoda, S., Takenaka, R., Teramoto, T., Kaneko, H., Fukao, T., Matsui, E., Kashara, K. and Yokoyama, Y. (1998) Reduced interferon gamma production by antigen-stimulated cord blood mononuclear cells is a risk factor of allergic disorders – 6-year follow-up study. *Clinical and Experimental Allergy* 28, 1340–1344.

Koopman, L.P., Wijga, A., Smit, H.A., De Jongste, J.C., Kerkhof, M., Gerritsen, J., Vos, A.D., van Strien, R.T., Brunekreef, B. and Neijens, H.J. (2002) Early respiratory and skin symptoms in relation to ethnic background: the importance of socioeconomic status; the PIAMA study. *Archives of Disease in Childhood* 87, 482–488.

Kramer, M.S. (1988) Does breast feeding help protect against atopic disease? Biology, methodology, and a golden jubilee of controversy. *Journal of Pediatrics* 112, 181–190.

Kramer, M.S., Coates, A.L., Michoud, M.C., Dugenaus, S., Mostonas, D., Davis, G.M., Hamilton, G.F., Nuwayhid, B., Joshi, A.K. and Papageorgiou, A. (1995) Maternal asthma and idiopathic preterm labor. *American Journal of Epidemiology* 142, 1078–1088.

Kramer, M.S., Chalmers, B., Hodnett, E.D. and the PROBIT Study Group (2001) Promotion of Breastfeeding Intervention Trial (PROBIT): a randomized trial in the Republic of Belarus. *Journal of the American Medical Association* 285, 413–420.

Krause, T.G., Hviid, A., Koch, A., Friborg, J., Hjuber, T., Wohlfahrt, J., Olsen, R., Kristensen, B. and Melbye, M. (2003) BCG vaccination and risk of atopy. *Journal of the American Medical Association* 289, 1012–1015.

Kroegel, C., Foerster, M., Hafner, D., Grahmann, P.R., Warner, J.A. and Braun, R. (2000) Putting priming into perspective – from cellular heterogeneity to cellular plasticity. *Immunology Today* 21, 218–222.

Kuczmarski, R.J., Flegal, K.M., Campbell, S.M. and Johnson, C.L. (1994) Increasing prevalence of overweight among US adults. The National Health and Nutrition Examination Surveys, 1960 to 1991. *Journal of the American Medical Association* 272, 205–211.

Kuehr, J., Frischer, T., Karmaus, W., Meinert, R., Barth, R., Hermann-Kunz, E., Forster, J. and Urbanek, R. (1992) Early childhood risk factors for sensitization at school age. *Journal of Allergy and Clinical Immunology* 90, 358–363.

Kwon, H.L., Belanger, K. and Bracken, M.B. (2003) Asthma prevalence among pregnant and childbearing-aged women in the United States: estimates from national health surveys. *Annals of Epidemiology* 13, 317–324.

Laan, M.P., Baert, M.R., Bijl, A.M., Vredendall, A.E., De Waard-van der Spekt, B., Oranje, A.P., Savelkoul, H.F. and Neijens, H.J. (2000) Markers for early sensitization and inflammation in relation to clinical manifestations of atopic disease up to 2 years of age in 133 high-risk children. *Clinical and Experimental Allergy* 30, 944–953.

Langley-Evans, S. (1997) Fetal programming of immune function and respiratory disease. *Clinical and Experimental Allergy* 27, 1377–1379.

Lau, S., Illi, S., Sommerfeld, C., Niggemann, B., Bergmann, R., von Mutius, E. and Wahn, U. (2000) Early exposure to house-dust mite and cat allergens and development of childhood asthma: a cohort study. Multicentre Allergy Study Group. *Lancet* 356, 1392–1397.

Law, C.M., de Swiet, M., Osmond, C., Fayers, P.M., Barker, D.J., Cruddas, A.M. and Fall, C.H. (1993) Initiation of hypertension *in utero* and its amplification throughout life. *British Medical Journal* 306, 24–27.

Leadbitter, P., Pearce, N., Cheng, S., Sears, M.R., Holdaway, M.D., Flannagen, E.M., Herbison, G.P. and Beasley, R. (1999) Relationship between fetal growth and the development of asthma and atopy in childhood. *Thorax* 54, 905–910.

Lewis, S.A. and Britton, J.R. (1998a) Consistent effects of high socioeconomic status and low birth order, and the modifying effect of maternal smoking on the risk of allergic disease during childhood. *Respiratory Medicine* 92, 1237–1244.

Lewis, S.A. and Britton, J.R. (1998b) Measles infection, measles vaccination and the effect of birth order in the aetiology of hay fever. *Clinical and Experimental Allergy* 28, 1493–1500.

Lewis, S., Butland, B., Strachan, D., Bynner, J., Richards, D., Butler, N. and Britton, J. (1996) Study of the aetiology of wheezing illness at age 16 in two national British birth cohorts. *Thorax* 51, 670–676.

Lewis, S.A., Weiss, S.T., Platts-Mills, T.A., Syring, M. and Gold, D.R. (2001) Association of specific allergen sensitization with socioeconomic factors and allergic disease in a population of Boston women. *Journal of Allergy and Clinical Immunology* 107, 615–622.

Li, Y.F., Gilliland, F.D., Berhane, K., *et al.* (2000) Effects of *in utero* and environmental tobacco smoke exposure on lung function in boys and girls with and without asthma. *American Journal of Respiratory and Critical Care Medicine* 162, 2097–2104.

Litonjua, A.A., Carey, V.J., Weiss, S.T. and Gold, D.R. (1999) Race, socioeconomic factors, and area of residence are associated with asthma prevalence. *Pediatric Pulmonology* 28, 394–401.

Liu, S., Wen, S.W., Demissie, K., Marcoux, S. and Kramer, M.S. (2001) Maternal asthma and pregnancy outcomes: a retrospective cohort study. *American Journal of Obstetrics and Gynecology* 184, 90–96.

Lodrup Carlsen, K.C., Jaakkola, J.J., Nafstad, P. and Carlsen, K.H. (1997) *In utero* exposure to cigarette smoking influences lung function at birth. *European Respiratory Journal* 10, 1774–1779.

London, S.J., James Gauderman, W., Avol, E., Rappaport, E.B. and Peters, J.M. (2001) Family history and the risk of early-onset persistent, early-onset transient, and late-onset asthma. *Epidemiology* 12, 577–583.

Magnan, A. and Vervloet, D. (2000) [Natural history of atopy]. *Revue des Maladies Respiratoires* 17, 235–244.

Magnan, A., Boniface, S., Mely, L., Romanet, S., Mamessier, E. and Vervloet, D. (2001) Cytokines, from atopy to asthma: the Th2 dogma revisited. *Cellular and Molecular Biology* 47, 679–687.

Magnusson, C.G. (1986) Maternal smoking influences cord serum IgE and IgD levels and increases the risk for subsequent infant allergy. *Journal of Allergy and Clinical Immunology* 78, 898–904.

Mannino, D.M., Homa, D.M., Akinbami, L.J., Moorman, J.E., Gwynn, C. and Redd, S.C. (2002) Surveillance for asthma – United States, 1980–1999. *MMWR CDC Surveillance Summaries* 51, 1–13.

Marks, G.B., Zhou, J., Yang, H.S., Joshi, P.A., Bishop, G.A. and Britton, W.J. (2002) Cord blood mononuclear cell cytokine responses in relation to maternal house dust mite allergen exposure. *Clinical and Experimental Allergy* 32, 355–360.

Marks, G.B., Ng, K., Zhou, J., Toelle, B.G., Xuan, W., Belousova, E.G. and Britton, W.J. (2003) The effect of neonatal BCG vaccination on atopy and asthma at age 7 to 14 years: an historical cohort study in a community with a very low prevalence of tuberculosis infection and a high prevalence of atopic disease. *Journal of Allergy and Clinical Immunology* 111, 541–549.

Martinez, F.D., Antognoni, G., Macri, F., Bonci, E., Midula, F., De Castro, G. and Ronchetti, R. (1988) Parental smoking enhances bronchial responsiveness in nine-year-old children. *American Review of Respiratory Disease* 138, 518–523.

Martinez, F.D., Wright, A.L., Taussig, L.M., Holberg, C.J., Halonen, M. and Morgan, W.J. (1995a) Asthma and wheezing in the first six years of life. The Group Health Medical Associates. *New England Journal of Medicine* 332, 133–138.

Martinez, F.D., Stern, D.A., Wright, A.L., Taussig, L.M. and Halonen, M. (1995b) Association of non-wheezing lower respiratory tract illnesses in early life with persistently diminished serum IgE levels. Group Health Medical Associates. *Thorax* 50, 1067–1072.

Matricardi, P.M., Franzinelli, F., Franco, A., Caprio, G., Murru, F., Cioffi, D., Ferrigho, L., Palermo, A., Cicccarelli, N. and Rosmini, F. (1998) Sibship size, birth order, and atopy in 11,371 Italian young men. *Journal of Allergy and Clinical Immunology* 101, 439–444.

Matsuoka, T., Matsubara, T., Katayama, K., Takeda, K., Koga, M. and Furukawa, S. (2001) Increase of cord blood cytokine-producing T cells in intrauterine infection. *Pediatrics International* 43, 453–457.

Mattes, J., Karmaus, W., Storm van's Gravesande, K., Moseler, M., Forster, J. and Kuehr, J. (1999) Pulmonary function in children of school age is related to the number of siblings in their family. *Pediatric Pulmonology* 28, 414–417.

McClung, J. (1969) *Effects of High Altitude on Human Birth: Observations on Mothers, Placentas, and the Newborn in Two Peruvian Populations.* Harvard University Press, Cambridge, Massachusetts, pp. 76–139.

McKeever, T.M., Lewis, S.A., Smith, C. and Hubbard, R. (2001) Siblings, multiple births, and the incidence of allergic disease: a birth cohort study using the West Midlands general practice research database. *Thorax* 56, 758–762.

McKeever, T.M., Lewis, S.A., Smith, C. and Hubbard, R. (2002) The importance of prenatal exposures on the development of allergic disease: a birth cohort study using the West Midlands General Practice Database. *American Journal of Respiratory and Critical Care Medicine* 166, 827–832.

McTigue, K.M., Garrett, J.M. and Popkin, B.M. (2002) The natural history of the development of obesity in a cohort of young U.S. adults between 1981 and 1998. *Annals of Internal Medicine* 136, 857–864.

Michel, F.B., Bousquet, J., Greillier, P., Robinet-Levy, M. and Coulomb, Y. (1980) Comparison of cord blood immunoglobulin E concentrations and maternal allergy for the prediction of atopic diseases in infancy. *Journal of Allergy and Clinical Immunology* 65, 422–430.

Mihrshahi, S., Peat, J.K., Webb, K., Tovey, E.R., Marks, G.B., Mellis, C.M. and Leeder, S.R. (2001) The childhood asthma prevention study (CAPS): design and research protocol of a randomized trial for the primary prevention of asthma. *Controlled Clinical Trials* 22, 333–354.

Mihrshahi, S., Peat, J.K., Marks, G.B., Mellis, C.M., Tovey, E.R., Webb, K., Britton, W.J. and Leeder, S.R. (2003) Eighteen-month outcomes of house dust mite avoidance and dietary fatty acid modification in the Childhood Asthma Prevention Study (CAPS). *Journal of Allergy and Clinical Immunology* 111, 162–168.

Miles, E.A., Warner, J.A., Jones, A.C., Colwell, B.M., Bryant, T.N. and Warner, J.O. (1996) Peripheral blood mononuclear cell proliferative responses in the first year of life in babies born to allergic parents. *Clinical and Experimental Allergy* 26, 780–788.

Milner, A.D., Marsh, M.J., Ingram, D.M., Fox, G.F. and Susiva, C. (1999) Effects of smoking in pregnancy on neonatal lung function. *Archives of Disease in Childhood Fetal and Neonatal Edition* 80, F8–14.

Mimouni Bloch, A., Mimouni, D., Mimouni, M. and Gdalevich, M. (2002) Does breastfeeding protect against allergic rhinitis during childhood? A meta-analysis of prospective studies. *Acta Paediatrica* 91, 275–279.

Morland, K., Wing, S. and Diez Roux, A. (2002a) The contextual effect of the local food environment on residents' diets: the atherosclerosis risk in communities study. *American Journal of Public Health* 92, 1761–1767.

Morland, K., Wing, S., Diez Roux, A. and Poole, C. (2002b) Neighborhood characteristics associated with the location of food stores and food service places. *American Journal of Preventive Medicine* 22, 23–29.

Mosmann, T.R., Cherwinski, H., Bond, M.W., Giedlin, M.A. and Coffman, R.L. (1986) Two types of murine helper T cell clone. I. Definition according to profiles of lymphokine activities and secreted proteins. *Journal of Immunology* 136, 2348–2357.

Murphy, B.E., Clark, S.J., Donald, I.R., Pinsky, M. and Vedady, D. (1974) Conversion of maternal cortisol to cortisone during placental transfer to the human fetus. *American Journal of Obstetrics and Gynecology* 118, 538–541.

Murray, E. (2003) Breastfeeding, atopy and asthma. *Lancet* 361, 174.

Nafstad, P., Magnus, P. and Jaakkola, J.J. (2000a) Risk of childhood asthma and allergic rhinitis in relation to pregnancy complications. *Journal of Allergy and Clinical Immunology* 106, 867–873.

Nafstad, P., Magnus, P. and Jaakkola, J.J. (2000b) Early respiratory infections and childhood asthma. *Pediatrics* 106, E38.

Nakagomi, T., Itaya, H., Tominaga, T., Yamaki, M., Hisamatsu, S. and Nakagomi, O. (1994) Is atopy increasing? *Lancet* 343, 121–122.

Narahara, H. and Johnston, J.M. (1993) Smoking and preterm labor: effect of a cigarette smoke extract on the secretion of platelet-activating factor-acetylhydrolase by human decidual macrophages. *American Journal of Obstetrics and Gynecology* 169, 1321–1326.

Nelson, H.S. (1985) The Bela Schick lecture for 1985. The atopic diseases. *Annals of Allergy* 55, 441–447.

Newton, R.W., Webster, P.A., Binu, P.S., Maskrey, N. and Phillips, A.B. (1979) Psychosocial stress in pregnancy and its relation to the onset of premature labour. *British Medical Journal* 2, 411–413.

Nielsen, S.J., Siega-Riz, A.M. and Popkin, B.M. (2002) Trends in food locations and sources among adolescents and young adults. *Preventive Medicine* 35, 107–113.

Nilsson, L., Kjellman, N.I. and Bjorksten, B. (1998) A randomized controlled trial of the effect of pertussis vaccines on atopic disease. *Archives of Pediatrics and Adolescent Medicine* 152, 734–738.

Ninan, T.K. and Russell, G. (1992) Respiratory symptoms and atopy in Aberdeen schoolchildren: evidence from two surveys 25 years apart. *British Medical Journal* 304, 873–875.

Oddy, W.H., Holt, P.G., Sly, P.D., Read, A.W., Landau, L.I., Stanley, F.J., Kendall, G.E. and Burton, P.R. (1999) Association between breast feeding and asthma in 6-year-old children: findings of a prospective birth cohort study. *British Medical Journal* 319, 815–819.

Oliveti, J.F., Kercsmar, C.M. and Redline, S. (1996) Pre- and perinatal risk factors for asthma in inner city African-American children. *American Journal of Epidemiology* 143, 570–577.

Omenaas, E., Jentoft, H.F., Vollmer, W.M., Buist, A.S. and Gulsvik, A. (2000) Absence of relationship between tuberculin reactivity and atopy in BCG vaccinated young adults. *Thorax* 55, 454–458.

Osmond, C., Barker, D.J. and Slattery, J.M. (1990) Risk of death from cardiovascular disease and chronic bronchitis determined by place of birth in England and Wales. *Journal of Epidemiology and Community Health* 44, 139–141.

Pagel, M.D., Smilkstein, G., Regen, H. and Montano, D. (1990) Psychosocial influences on new born outcomes: a controlled prospective study. *Social Science and Medicine* 30, 597–604.

Paunio, M., Heinonen, O.P., Virtanen, M., Leinikki, P., Patja, A. and Peltola, H. (2000) Measles history and atopic diseases: a population-based cross-sectional study. *Journal of the American Medical Association* 283, 343–346.

Pearce, N., Pekkanen, J. and Beasley, R. (1999) How much asthma is really attributable to atopy? *Thorax* 54, 268–272.

Peat, J.K., van den Berg, R.H., Green, W.F., Mellis, C.M., Leeder, S.R. and Woolcock, A.J. (1994) Changing prevalence of asthma in Australian children. *British Medical Journal* 308, 1591–1596.

Peat, J.K., Tovey, E., Toelle, B.G., *et al.* (1996) House dust mite allergens. A major risk factor for childhood asthma in Australia. *American Journal of Respiratory and Critical Care Medicine* 153, 141–146.

Pekkanen, J., Xu, B. and Jarvelin, M.R. (2001) Gestational age and occurrence of atopy at age 31 – a prospective birth cohort study in Finland. *Clinical and Experimental Allergy* 31, 95–102.

Pepys, J. (1986) Natural history of 'atopy'. *Journal of Allergy and Clinical Immunology* 78, 959–961.

Perera, F.P., Jedrychowski, W., Rauh, V. and Whyatt, R.M. (1999) Molecular epidemiologic research on the effects of environmental pollutants on the fetus. *Environmental Health Perspectives* 107(suppl. 3), 451–460.

Perzanowski, M.S., Ronmark, E., Nold, B., Lundback, B. and Platts-Mills, T.A. (1999) Relevance of allergens from cats and dogs to asthma in the northernmost province of Sweden: schools as a major site of exposure. *Journal of Allergy and Clinical Immunology* 103, 1018–1024.

Ponsonby, A.L., Couper, D., Dwyer, T., Carmichael, A. and Kemp, A. (1999) Relationship between early life respiratory illness, family size over time, and the development of asthma and hay fever: a seven year follow up study. *Thorax* 54, 664–669.

Prescott, S.L., Macaubas, C., Smallacombe, T., Holt, B.J., Sly, P.D. and Holt, P.G. (1999) Development of allergen-specific T-cell memory in atopic and normal children. *Lancet* 353, 196–200.

Raghupathy, R. (1997) Th1-type immunity is incompatible with successful pregnancy. *Immunology Today* 18, 478–482.

Rasmussen, K.M. (2001) The 'fetal origins' hypothesis: challenges and opportunities for maternal and child nutrition. *Annual Review of Nutrition* 21, 73–95.

Riedler, J., Eder, W., Oberfeld, G. and Schreuer, M. (2000) Austrian children living on a farm have less hay fever, asthma and allergic sensitization. *Clinical and Experimental Allergy* 30, 194–200.

Romagnani, S. (1991) Human TH1 and TH2 subsets: doubt no more. *Immunology Today* 12, 256–257.

Rona, R.J., Duran-Tauleria, E. and Chinn, S. (1997) Family size, atopic disorders in parents, asthma in children, and ethnicity. *Journal of Allergy and Clinical Immunology* 99, 454–460.

Rosenstreich, D.L., Eggleston, P., Kattan, M., Baker, D., Slavin, R.G., Gergen, P., Mitchel, H., McNiff-Mortimer, K., Lynn, H., Ownby, D. and Malveaux, F. (1997) The role of cockroach allergy and exposure to cockroach allergen in causing morbidity among inner-city children with asthma. *New England Journal of Medicine* 336, 1356–1363.

Rust, G.S., Thompson, C.J., Minor, P., Davis-Mitchell, W., Holloway, K. and Murray, V. (2001) Does breastfeeding protect children from asthma? Analysis of NHANES III survey data. *Journal of the National Medical Association* 93, 139–148.

Sacks, G.P., Redman, C.W. and Sargent, I.L. (2003) Monocytes are primed to produce the Th1 type cytokine IL-12 in normal human pregnancy: an intracellular flow cytometric analysis of peripheral blood mononuclear cells. *Clinical and Experimental Immunology* 131, 490–497.

Salgame, P., Abrams, J.S., Clayberger, C., Goldstein, H., Convit, J., Modlin, R.L. and Bloom, B.R. (1991) Differing lymphokine profiles of functional subsets of human CD4 and CD8 T cell clones. *Science* 254, 279–282.

Samet, J.M., Lambert, W.E., Skipper, B.J., Cushing, A.H., Hunt, W.C., Young, S.A., McLaren, L.C., Schwab, M. and Spengler, G.P. (1993) Nitrogen dioxide and respiratory illness in children. Part I: Health outcomes. *Research Report/ Health Effects Institute* 1–32; discussion 51–80.

Schafer, T., Dirschedl, P., Kunz, B., Ring, J. and Uberla, K. (1997) Maternal smoking during pregnancy and lactation increases the risk for atopic eczema in the offspring. *Journal of the American Academy of Dermatology* 36, 550–556.

Schatz, M. (1999) Interrelationships between asthma and pregnancy: a literature review. *Journal of Allergy and Clinical Immunology* 103, S330–S336.

Schatz, M., Zeiger, R.S., Hoffman, C.P., Saunders, B.S., Harden, K.M. and Forsythe, A.B. (1991) Increased transient tachypnea of the newborn in infants of asthmatic mothers. *American Journal of Diseases of Childhood* 145, 156–158.

Schoetzau, A., Filipiak-Pittroff, B., Franke, K., Koletzko, S., Von Berg, A., Gruebl, A., Bauer, C.P., Berdel, D., Reinhardt, D. and Wichmann, H.E. (2002) Effect of exclusive breast-feeding and early solid food avoidance on the incidence of atopic dermatitis in high-risk infants at 1 year of age. *Pediatric Allergy and Immunology* 13(4), 234–242.

Schulz, A., Israel, B., Williams, D., Parker, E., Becker, A. and James, S. (2000) Social inequalities, stressors and self reported health status among African American and white women in the Detroit metropolitan area. *Social Science and Medicine* 51, 1639–1653.

Sears, M.R. (1997) Epidemiology of childhood asthma. *Lancet* 350, 1015–1020.

Sears, M.R., Burrows, B., Flannery, E.M., Herbison, G.P., Hewitt, C.J. and Holdaway, M.D. (1991) Relation between airway responsiveness and serum IgE in children with asthma and in apparently normal children. *New England Journal of Medicine* 325, 1067–1071.

Sears, M.R., Burrows, B., Flannery, E.M., Herbison, G.P. and Holdaway, M.D. (1993) Atopy in childhood. I. Gender and allergen related risks for development of hay fever and asthma. *Clinical and Experimental Allergy* 23, 941–948.

Sears, M.R., Holdaway, M.D., Flannery, E.M., Herbison, G.P. and Silva, P.A. (1996) Parental and neonatal risk factors for atopy, airway hyper-responsiveness, and asthma. *Archives of Disease in Childhood* 75, 392–398.

Sears, M.R., Greene, J.M., Willan, A.R., Taylor, R., Flannery, E.M., Cowan, J.O., Herbison, G.P. and Poulton, R. (2002) Long-term relation between breastfeeding and development of atopy and asthma in children and young adults: a longitudinal study. *Lancet* 360, 901–907.

Seaton, A. and Devereux, G. (2000) Diet, infection and wheezy illness: lessons from adults. *Pediatric Allergy and Immunology* 11(suppl. 13), 37–40.

Seaton, A., Godden, D.J. and Brown, K. (1994) Increase in asthma: a more toxic environment or a more susceptible population? *Thorax* 49, 171–174.

Seckl, J.R. (1998) Physiologic programming of the fetus. *Clinics in Perinatology* 25, 939–962, vii.

Seidman, D.S., Laor, A., Gale, R., Stevenson, D.K. and Danon, Y.L. (1991) Is low birth weight a risk factor for asthma during adolescence? *Archives of Disease in Childhood* 66, 584–587.

Sepp, E., Julge, K., Vasar, M., Naaber, P., Bjorksten, B. and Mikelsaar, M. (1997) Intestinal microflora of Estonian and Swedish infants. *Acta Paediatrica* 86, 956–961.

Shah, N.R. and Bracken, M.B. (2000) A systematic review and meta-analysis of prospective studies on the association between maternal cigarette smoking and preterm delivery. *American Journal of Obstetrics and Gynecology* 182, 465–472.

Shaheen, S.O., Aaby, P., Hall, A.J., Barker, D.J., Heyes, C.B., Shiell, A.W. and Goudiaby, A. (1996) Measles and atopy in Guinea-Bissau. *Lancet* 347, 1792–1796.

Shaheen, S.O., Newson, R.B., Sherriff, A., Henderson, A.J., Heron, J.E., Burney, P.G., Golding, J. and the ALSPAC study team (2002) Paracetamol use in pregnancy and wheezing in early childhood. *Thorax* 57, 958–963.

Shirakawa, T., Enomoto, T., Shimazu, S. and Hopkin, J.M. (1997) The inverse association between tuberculin responses and atopic disorder. *Science* 275, 77–79.

Sorensen, T.K., Dempsey, J.C., Xiao, R., Frederick, I.O., Luthy, D.A. and Williams, M.A. (2003) Maternal asthma and risk of preterm delivery. *Annals of Epidemiology* 13, 267–272.

Soutar, A., Seaton, A. and Brown, K. (1997) Bronchial reactivity and dietary antioxidants. *Thorax* 52, 166–170.

Soyseth, V., Kongerud, J. and Boe, J. (1995) Postnatal maternal smoking increases the prevalence of asthma but not of bronchial hyperresponsiveness or atopy in their children. *Chest* 107, 389–394.

Sporik, R., Holgate, S.T., Platts-Mills, T.A. and Cogswell, J.J. (1990) Exposure to house-dust mite allergen (Der p I) and the development of asthma in childhood. A prospective study. *New England Journal of Medicine* 323, 502–507.

Sporik, R., Platts-Mills, T.A. and Cogswell, J.J. (1993) Exposure to house dust mite allergen of children admitted to hospital with asthma. *Clinical and Experimental Allergy* 23, 740–746.

Stein, R.T., Holberg, C.J., Sherrill, D., Wright, A.L., Morgan, W.J., Tuussig, L. and Martinez, F.D. (1999) Influence of parental smoking on respiratory symptoms during the first decade of life: the Tucson Children's Respiratory Study. *American Journal of Epidemiology* 149, 1030–1037.

Stick, S.M., Burton, P.R., Gurrin, L., Sly, P.D. and LeSouef, P.N. (1996) Effects of maternal smoking during pregnancy and a family history of asthma on respiratory function in newborn infants. *Lancet* 348, 1060–1064.

Strachan, D.P. (1989) Hay fever, hygiene, and household size. *British Medical Journal* 299, 1259–1260.

Strachan, D.P., Butland, B.K. and Anderson, H.R. (1996) Incidence and prognosis of asthma and wheezing illness from early childhood to age 33 in a national British cohort. *British Medical Journal* 312, 1195–1199.

Strachan, D.P., Harkins, L.S., Johnston, I.D. and Anderson, H.R. (1997a) Childhood antecedents of allergic sensitization in young British adults. *Journal of Allergy and Clinical Immunology* 99, 6–12.

Strachan, D.P., Harkins, L.S. and Golding, J. (1997b) Sibship size and self-reported inhalant allergy among adult women. ALSPAC Study Team. *Clinical and Experimental Allergy* 27, 151–155.

Strunk, R.C., Ford, J.G. and Taggart, V. (2002) Reducing disparities in asthma care: priorities for research – National Heart, Lung, and Blood Institute workshop report. *Journal of Allergy and Clinical Immunology* 109, 229–237.

Sunyer, J., Torregrosa, J., Anto, J.M., Menendez, C., Acosta, C., Schellenberg, D., Alonso, P.L. and Kahigwa, E. (2000) The association between atopy and asthma in a semirural area of Tanzania (East Africa). *Allergy* 55, 762–766.

Sunyer, J., Mendendez, C., Ventura, P.J., Aponte, K.K., Schellenberg, D., Kahigwa, E., Acosta, C., Anto, J.M. and Alonso, P.L. (2001) Prenatal risk factors of wheezing at the age of four years in Tanzania. *Thorax* 56, 290–295.

Szepfalusi, Z., Loibichler, C., Pichler, J., Reisenberger, K., Ebner, C. and Urbanek, R. (2000a) Direct evidence for transplacental allergen transfer. *Pediatric Research* 48, 404–407.

Szepfalusi, Z., Pichler, J., Elsasser, S., *et al.* (2000b) Transplacental priming of the human immune system with environmental allergens can occur early in gestation. *Journal of Allergy and Clinical Immunology* 106, 530–536.

Tager, I.B., Ngo, L. and Hanrahan, J.P. (1995) Maternal smoking during pregnancy. Effects on lung function during the first 18 months of life. *American Journal of Respiratory and Critical Care Medicine* 152, 977–983.

Tang, M.L., Kemp, A.S., Thorburn, J. and Hill, D.J. (1994) Reduced interferon-gamma secretion in neonates and subsequent atopy. *Lancet* 344, 983–985.

Tariq, S.M., Hakim, E.A., Matthews, S.M. and Arshad, S.H. (2000) Influence of smoking on asthmatic symptoms and allergen sensitisation in early childhood. *Postgraduate Medical Journal* 76, 694–699.

Taylor, B., Wadsworth, J., Wadsworth, M. and Peckham, C. (1984) Changes in the reported prevalence of childhood eczema since the 1939–45 war. *Lancet* 2, 1255–1257.

Taylor, S.E., Repetti, R.L. and Seeman, T. (1997) Health psychology: what is an unhealthy environment and how does it get under the skin? *Annual Review of Psychology* 48, 411–447.

Thomas, J., Abrishami, M.A., Chehreh, M.N. and Walters, C.S. (1979) Neonatal IgE values in the black population. *Annals of Allergy* 43, 144–145.

Van Asperen, P.P., Kemp, A.S. and Mellis, C.M. (1984) Skin test reactivity and clinical allergen sensitivity in infancy. *Journal of Allergy and Clinical Immunology* 73, 381–386.

van der Velden, V.H., Laan, M.P., Baert, M.R., de Waal Malefyt, R., Neijens, H.J. and Savelkoul, H.F. (2001). Selective development of a strong Th2 cytokine profile in high-risk children who develop atopy: risk factors and regulatory role of IFN-gamma, IL-4 and IL-10. *Clinical and Experimental Allergy* 31, 997–1006.

Varner, A.E. (2002) The increase in allergic respiratory diseases: survival of the fittest? *Chest* 121, 1308–1316.

Von Ehrenstein, O.S., Von Mutius, E., Illi, S., Baumann, L., Bohm, O. and von Kries, R. (2000) Reduced risk of hay fever and asthma among children of farmers. *Clinical and Experimental Allergy* 30, 187–193.

von Hertzen, L.C. (2002) Maternal stress and T-cell differentiation of the developing immune system: possible implications for the development of asthma and atopy. *Journal of Allergy and Clinical Immunology* 109, 923–928.

von Hertzen, L., Klaukka, T., Mattila, H. and Haahtela, T. (1999) *Mycobacterium tuberculosis* infection and the subsequent development of asthma and allergic conditions. *Journal of Allergy and Clinical Immunology* 104, 1211–1214.

von Mutius, E., Fritzsch, C., Weiland, S.K., Roll, G. and Magnussen, H. (1992) Prevalence of asthma and allergic disorders among children in united Germany: a descriptive comparison. *British Medical Journal* 305, 1395–1399.

von Mutius, E., Nicolai, T. and Martinez, F.D. (1993) Prematurity as a risk factor for asthma in preadolescent children. *Journal of Pediatrics* 123, 223–229.

von Mutius, E., Martinez, F.D., Fritzsch, C., Nicolai, T., Reitmeir, P. and Thiemann, H.H. (1994) Skin test reactivity and number of siblings. *British Medical Journal* 308, 692–695.

von Mutius, E., Pearce, N., Beasley, R., Cheng, S., von Ehrenstein, O., Bjorksten, B. and Weiland, S. (2000) International patterns of tuberculosis and the prevalence of symptoms of asthma, rhinitis, and eczema. *Thorax* 55, 449–453.

Wadhwa, P.D., Sandman, C.A., Porto, M., Dunkel-Schetter, C. and Garite, T.J. (1993) The association between prenatal stress and infant birth weight and gestational age at birth: a prospective investigation. *American Journal of Obstetrics and Gynecology* 169, 858–865.

Warner, J.A. and Warner, J.O. (2000) Early life events in allergic sensitisation. *British Medical Bulletin* 56, 883–893.

Warner, J.A., Miles, E.A., Jones, A.C., Quint, D.J., Colwell, B.M. and Warner, J.O. (1994) Is deficiency of interferon gamma production by allergen-triggered cord blood cells a predictor of atopic eczema? *Clinical and Experimental Allergy* 24, 423–430.

Warner, J.A., Jones, A.C., Miles, E.A. and Warner, J.O. (1996) Prenatal sensitisation. *Pediatric Allergy and Immunology* 7, 98–101.

Wechsler, H., Basch, C.E., Zybert, P., Lantigua, R. and Shea, S. (1995) The availability of low-fat milk in an inner-city Latino community: implications for nutrition education. *American Journal of Public Health* 85, 1690–1692.

Wegmann, T.G., Lin, H., Guilbert, L. and Mosmann, T.R. (1993) Bidirectional cytokine interactions in the maternal–fetal relationship: is successful pregnancy a TH2 phenomenon? *Immunology Today* 14, 353–356.

Weiland, S.K., von Mutius, E., Husing, A. and Asher, M.I. (1999) Intake of trans fatty acids and prevalence of childhood asthma and allergies in Europe. ISAAC Steering Committee. *Lancet* 353, 2040–2041.

Weinmann, G.G. (1996) An update on air pollution. *Current Opinion in Pulmonary Medicine* 2, 121–128.

Weitzman, M., Gortmaker, S. and Sobol, A. (1990) Racial, social, and environmental risks for childhood asthma. *American Journal of Diseases in Childhood* 144, 1189–1194.

Wen, S.W., Demissie, K. and Liu, S. (2001) Adverse outcomes in pregnancies of asthmatic women: results from a Canadian population. *Annals of Epidemiology* 11, 7–12.

Wickens, K.L., Crane, J., Kemp, T.J., Lewis, S.J., D'Souza, W.J., Sawyer, G.M., Stone, M.L., Tohill, S.J., Kennedy, J.C., Slater, T.M. and Pearce, N.E. (1999) Family size, infections, and asthma prevalence in New Zealand children. *Epidemiology* 10, 699–705.

Wilkinson, J. and Holgate, S.T. (1996) Candidate gene loci in asthmatic and allergic inflammation. *Thorax* 51, 3–8.

Williams, D.R. (1996) Racism and health: a research agenda. *Ethnicity and Disease* 6, 1–8.

Williams, D.R. (1999) Race, socioeconomic status, and health. The added effects of racism and discrimination. *Annals of the New York Academy of Science* 896, 173–188.

Williams, D.R. and Collins, C. (2001) Racial residential segregation: a fundamental cause of racial disparities in health. *Public Health Reports* 116, 404–416.

Williams, H., Robertson, C., Stewart, A., Ait-Khaled, N., Anabwani, G., Anderson, R., Asher, I., Beasley, R., Bjorksten, B., Burr, M., Clayton, T., Crane, J., Ellwood, P., Keil, U., Lai, C., Mallol, J., Martinez, F., Mitchell, E., Montefort, S., Pearce, N., Shah, J., Sibbald, B., Strachan, D., von Mutius, E. and Weiland, S.K. (1999) Worldwide variations in the prevalence of symptoms of atopic eczema in the International Study of Asthma and Allergies in Childhood. *Journal of Allergy and Clinical Immunology* 103, 125–138.

Wright, A.L., Sherrill, D., Holberg, C.J., Halonen, M. and Martinez, F.D. (1999) Breast-feeding, maternal IgE, and total serum IgE in childhood. *Journal of Allergy and Clinical Immunology* 104, 589–594.

Wright, A.L., Holberg, C.J., Taussig, L.M. and Martinez, F.D. (2001) Factors influencing the relation of infant feeding to asthma and recurrent wheeze in childhood. *Thorax* 56, 192–197.

Wright, R.J., Rodriguez, M. and Cohen, S. (1998) Review of psychosocial stress and asthma: an integrated biopsychosocial approach. *Thorax* 53, 1066–1074.

Wright, R.J., Cohen, S., Carey, V., Weiss, S.T. and Gold, D.R. (2002) Parental stress as a predictor of wheezing in infancy: a prospective birth-cohort study. *American Journal of Respiratory and Critical Care Medicine* 165, 358–365.

Xu, B., Pekkanen, J., Jarvelin, M.R., Olsen, P. and Hartikainen, A.L. (1999) Maternal infections in pregnancy and the development of asthma among offspring. *International Journal of Epidemiology* 28, 723–727.

Xu, B., Jarvelin, M.R. and Pekkanen, J. (2000) Body build and atopy. *Journal of Allergy and Clinical Immunology* 105, 393–394.

Xu, B., Pekkanen, J., Hartikainen, A.L. and Jarvelin, M.R. (2001) Caesarean section and risk of asthma and allergy in adulthood. *Journal of Allergy and Clinical Immunology* 107, 732–733.

Yemaneberhan, H., Bekele, Z., Venn, A., Lewis, S., Parry, E. and Britton, J. (1997) Prevalence of wheeze and asthma and relation to atopy in urban and rural Ethiopia. *Lancet* 350, 85–90.

Young, S., Sherrill, D.L., Arnott, J., Diepeveen, D., LeSouef, P.N. and Landau, L.I. (2000) Parental factors affecting respiratory function during the first year of life. *Pediatric Pulmonology* 29, 331–340.

Zarrow, M.X., Philpott, J.E. and Denenberg, V.H. (1970) Passage of ^{14}C-4-corticosterone from the rat mother to the foetus and neonate. *Nature* 226, 1058–1059.

13 Fetal Programming of Immune Function

THOMAS W. MCDADE AND CHRISTOPHER W. KUZAWA

Northwestern University, Department of Anthropology, Evanston, IL 60208–1310, USA

Introduction

Evidence continues to mount in support of the hypothesis that many chronic degenerative diseases in adulthood have prenatal or early postnatal origins, probably due to programming of cardiovascular and endocrine systems early in development. However, the implications of early environments for the development and function of the immune system in adulthood are less well understood (Moore, 1998). This is an important area of enquiry, in that immunological processes are centrally involved in infectious, neoplastic, atopic and autoimmune diseases, and may, in some cases, contribute to cardiovascular disease. This chapter will review a range of research relevant to the immune programming hypothesis, and discuss attempts to investigate the long-term immunological effects of early environments in an ongoing, prospective study in the Philippines (McDade *et al.*, 2001a,b, 2004).

The Early Life Origins of Immune Function

Compelling circumstantial evidence for the relevance of early environments to adult immunocompetence comes from recent research in the Gambia. In this region, the annual cycle of climate introduces marked seasonal variation in nutritional status, with the annual rains contributing to periods of significant hunger. Analysis of demographic records indicates that being born during the hungry season – itself associated with lower birthweight and higher postnatal disease exposure – increases the risk of premature death in young adulthood by a factor of 3.7 after the age of 14.5 years, and by a factor of 10.3 after 25 years (Moore *et al.*, 1999). The majority of these premature deaths were infectious in aetiology, suggesting impairment in some aspect of immune function. Although direct support for this link in human populations is currently limited, a number of convergent lines of evidence suggest that this is an important area of enquiry.

Early research with murine models documented alterations in offspring immune function following maternal nutritional deficiencies (both macro- and micro-nutrient) that last into adulthood and into the next generation, despite *ad libitum* feeding of both F_1 and F_2 generations (Chandra, 1975a; Beach *et al.*, 1982). There is evidence that the hypothalamic–pituitary–adrenal axis may be involved in these associations. Injection of pregnant rat dams with dexamethasone, a cortisol agonist, has been associated with lymphoid atrophy and impaired immunity in offspring (Eishi *et al.*, 1983), while rats born to undernourished mothers demonstrate reduced hypothalamic–pituitary–adrenal (HPA) and tumour necrosis factor (TNF)-α responsiveness to endotoxaemia, compared to offspring of well-nourished mothers (Chisari *et al.*, 2001). A similar pattern of results is emerging from research conducted among non-human primates: gestational stress, as well as injections of adrenocorticotrophic hormone (ACTH) or dexamethasone during pregnancy, are associated with lasting irregularities in immune function and HPA activity in juvenile offspring (Coe *et al.*, 1992, 1996; Clarke *et al.*, 1994; Coe and Lubach, 2000).

The immediate effects of protein–energy malnutrition on immune function in infancy and early childhood have been well documented. Postnatal undernutrition is associated with deficits in several components of cell-mediated immunity, involution of the thymus and reduced antibody response to vaccination (Chandra, 1988; Gershwin *et al.*, 2000; Suskind and Tontisirin, 2001). Less intensively investigated are the immunological implications of prenatal undernutrition, although a relatively limited number of studies suggest that there are significant impairments in aspects of immunity following intrauterine growth retardation (IUGR) (Table 13.1) (Chandra, 1975b, 1981; Moscatelli *et al.*, 1976; Chandra *et al.*, 1977; Ferguson, 1978; Saha *et al.*, 1983; Pittard *et al.*, 1984; Mussi-Pinhata *et al.*, 1993; Chatrath *et al.*, 1997; Moore *et al.*, 1999). These findings are consistent with the fourfold increase in neonatal mortality risk, and the twofold increase in postneonatal mortality risk, for infants born small for gestational age (SGA, full term, less than 2500 g) compared to infants born appropriate for gestational age (AGA, full term, > 2500 g) (Ashworth, 1998). Similarly, SGA infants have been shown to be at increased risk of infectious morbidity in infancy and early childhood (Kebede and Larson, 1994; Lira *et al.*, 1996). Deficits in immune function following prenatal undernutrition persist for weeks, and in some cases years, but their long-term implications for immunocompetence beyond childhood have not been previously reported.

Gestational age is a potential confounder of the association between low birthweight and immune function, and in a number of studies it is not possible to separate the effects of preterm delivery from fetal undernutrition and growth restriction. This may be an important distinction, since Chandra (1981) has shown that by 3 months of age, pre-term AGA infants (30–34 weeks' gestation) recover normal T lymphocyte percentage and proliferative responsiveness to phytohaemagglutinin (PHA), whereas full-term, SGA infants (37–41 weeks) continue to demonstrate impairment at 12 months. Similarly, SGA infants have reduced thymic hormone activity at 1 month, while pre-term AGA infants do not

Table 13.1. Prior research on the effects of prenatal undernutrition on human immune function in infancy and childhood.

Participants (gestational age)	Age at assessment	Main outcomes	Reference
26 SGA (29–42 weeks), 26 AGA (not reported)	Birth, 1 month, 3 months	SGA = reduced DTH response at 1 month; reduced lymphocyte response to PHA at birth; reduced % T lymphocytes at birth, 1 month, 3 months; reduced bactericidal capacity at birth; reduced response to polio vaccine	Chandra (1975b)
19 SGA (38–41 weeks), 30 AGA (not reported)	Birth to 3 months	SGA = reduced % and number of T and B lymphocytes at birth; no difference in lymphocyte response to PHA	Moscatelli et al. (1976)
50 SGA (not reported)	3 months to 5 years	SGA = reduced % T lymphocyte, DTH response	Chandra et al. (1977)
17 SGA (35–41 weeks), 31 AGA (31–41 weeks)	< 4 days	SGA = reduced DTH response; reduced number total and T lymphocytes; no difference in lymphocyte response to PHA	Ferguson (1978)
8 children born SGA (not reported), 11 'healthy' age-matched controls (not reported)	1–5 years	SGA = reduced DTH response; reduced % T lymphocytes; reduced lymphocyte response to PHA	
9 SGA (37–41 weeks), 7 AGA (30–34 weeks), 7 AGA (37–41 weeks)	Birth, 1, 3 and 12 months	SGA = reduced thymic hormone activity at 1 month; reduced number T lymphocytes at all ages; reduced PHA response at birth, 3 months, 12 months	Chandra (1987)
20 AGA (38 ± 1.0), 15 AGA (32.8 ± 1.4), 15 SGA (38.0 ± 0.8)	Birth, 3 and 6 months	SGA = reduced DTH response, reduced IgA and IgM production at 3 and 6 months; reduced number total lymphocytes at 3 months	Saha et al. (1983)
29 SGA (33–42 weeks), 120 AGA (33–42 weeks)	Birth	No difference in lymphocyte response to PHA, PWM, ConA, SpA	Pittard et al. (1984)
57 SGA (37–41 weeks), 52 AGA (37–41 weeks)	3 months, 6 months or 9 months	No difference in DTH or lymphocyte response to BCG vaccination given 12–14 weeks prior to assessment	Mussi-Pinhata et al. (1993)
25 SGA ('full-term'), 25 AGA ('full-term')	Birth	SGA = reduced number and % lymphocytes, reduced CD4:CD8 ratio, reduced IgG and C3	Chatrath et al. (1997)
472 children in the Gambian Intervention group: maternal dietary supplementation for 20 weeks before delivery; control group: maternal supplementation for 20 weeks after delivery	6–9 years	Maternal supplementation before delivery associated with improved DTH response; supplementation after delivery associated with improved response to rabies vaccine; no associations with birthweight	Moore et al. (1999)

AGA, appropriate for gestational age; SGA, small for gestational age; DTH, delayed type hypersensitivity; PHA, phytohaemagglutinin; PWM, pokeweed mitogen; ConA, concanavalin A; SpA, serotype c-specific polysaccharide antigen; BCG, bacille Calmette-Guérin.

differ substantially from healthy full-term infants. However, mortality statistics in a range of populations do not suggest a dramatic difference in neonatal and post-neonatal mortality risk between fullterm, SGA infants, and preterm infants of the same birthweight (Ashworth, 1998).

Prior to our research in the Philippines (see below), only two studies had reported an association between fetal growth and a measure of immune activity beyond childhood. In a sample of 280 men and women aged 47–55 years from the UK, a larger head circumference at birth was associated with an increased likelihood of elevated immunoglobulin E (IgE) in adulthood (Godfrey et al., 1994). A larger birthweight was also associated with increased IgE, but this association disappeared when the associations were adjusted for head circumference. In a different UK sample of 305 women aged 60–71 years, lower birthweights were associated with increased likelihood of thyroglobulin and thyroid peroxidase autoantibody production in adults (Phillips et al., 1993). These findings suggest that fetal environments may programme immune function in adulthood, with potentially important implications for the development of allergic and autoimmune disease.

In both these studies, as well as those from the Gambia (Moore et al., 1999, 2001), impaired thymic development has been proposed as a key mediator of the association between early environments and later immunocompetence. The thymus is a primary lymphoid organ critical for normal T-lymphocyte maturation and function, and for the production of thymic hormones with wide-ranging immuno-regulatory properties (Steinman 1986; Schulof et al., 1987). Lymphoid tissues are acutely sensitive to undernutrition in infancy and early childhood, to the extent that severe malnutrition may lead to what has been described as a nutritional 'thymectomy', with significant and lasting impairments in cell-mediated immunity (Naeye et al., 1971; Dutz et al., 1976; Dourov, 1986). Recent sonographic analyses indicate that thymic size in infancy is positively associated with birthweight and body length, suggesting that prenatal nutrition or fetal growth influence thymic development (Hasselbalch et al., 1999). Since lymphoid tissues begin to develop in the second and third month of gestation, and since prenatal undernutrition appears to have a disproportionate impact on these tissues, the effects of early nutritional insults may be even greater than those endured postnatally (Xanthou, 1985; Owens et al., 1989).

A parallel line of enquiry has indicated that exposure to infectious disease early in life may have significant long-term consequences for immunity. Findings from Guinea-Bissau suggest that measles infection in early infancy increases the risk of death before 5 years of age by a factor of 3.8 (Aaby et al., 1993), and that measles infection in childhood more than doubles the risk of suppressed cell-mediated immunity 3 years later (Shaheen et al., 1996a). In addition, earlier research has shown that gastroenteritis in the first 6 months of life – but not after – is associated with thymic atrophy and impaired cell-mediated immunity up to 5 years later (Dutz et al., 1976; Ghavami et al., 1979).

Similarly, proponents of the 'hygiene hypothesis' suggest that infectious morbidity early in life has long-term consequences for immune function by biasing lymphocyte maturation toward the Th1 phenotype. Atopic immune processes associated with Th2 lymphocytes are therefore reduced, protecting against the development of atopic disease in adulthood (Shaheen *et al.*, 1996b; Shirakawa *et al.*, 1997; Matricardi *et al.*, 2000; Illi *et al.*, 2001). A relative absence of infectious disease early in life is thereby hypothesized as accounting for the rising rates of allergy and asthma in developed nations (Rook and Stanford, 1998).

In sum, research to date suggests that both prenatal and early postnatal environments are important for immune development and may have long-term implications for infectious, atopic and autoimmune disease. Although the fetal origins hypothesis focuses attention on prenatal conditions, early postnatal environments are also critical in shaping immune development, and should be given serious consideration. Few studies have been able to simultaneously evaluate the effects of prenatal and postnatal environments, even though it is likely that they play independent, and perhaps interactive, roles in the development of immunocompetence. A unique opportunity to explore these issues is provided by a dataset collected from a small cohort in the Philippines. Data from this sample have been collected prospectively from the third trimester of pregnancy through adolescence, and allow examination of the interaction between factors in fetal life, infancy and childhood as determinants of immune development and function.

Early Origins of Immune Function in the Philippines

Research participants and protocol

The early origins of immune function were evaluated in the Cebu Longitudinal Health and Nutrition Study (CLHNS). This ongoing population-based survey of maternal and child health in the Philippines began in 1983 with the recruitment of 3327 pregnant women (Cebu Study Team, 1989). As in many countries in the developing world, IUGR (defined as birthweight for gestational age below a reference 10th percentile; Hoffman *et al.*, 1974) is common in the Philippines, most likely due to high rates of maternal undernutrition during pregnancy associated with poverty. In the CLHNS, the prevalence of IUGR is 20.9% (Adair, 1989).

Home visits were made prior to birth, immediately following birth, and every 2 months for 2 years, to collect in-depth data on child and maternal health, anthropometry, patterns of breastfeeding, dietary intake, rates of diarrhoea and respiratory disease, household socio-economic status and demographics, and environmental quality (Popkin *et al.*, 1990). Follow-up surveys were conducted in 1991, 1994–1995 and 1998–1999. The prospective design of this study, as well as the detailed information collected at multiple time points, provides a unique opportunity to evaluate a number of variables that may confound, mediate or moderate the association between IUGR and later immune function. The immune studies reported here are part of a broader research agenda focused on elucidating the role of prenatal and early postnatal environments on growth, maturation and risk for chronic and infectious disease in childhood and adolescence (Adair, 1999, 2001; Adair *et al.*, 2001; Adair and Cole, 2003; Kuzawa and Adair, 2003).

In 1998–1999, 2089 CLHNS participants, 14–15 years of age at the time, were contacted for follow-up data collection. From these remaining participants, a subsample of 103 girls and boys was recruited based on the following criteria: fullterm birth (≥ 37 weeks), currently healthy, and small for gestational age (SGA: defined as $< 10th$ percentile of birthweight for gestational age) versus appropriate for gestational age (AGA: $\geq 10th$ percentile) (Hoffman *et al.*, 1974). By restricting the sample to fullterm births, the potentially confounding effects of preterm delivery were eliminated. The study therefore focused upon small size, assumed to be related to fetal undernutrition. The subsample of SGA individuals recruited for this study was representative of all SGA individuals in the larger CLHNS cohort, except that the average birthweight was significantly lower than the average of 2494 g for all SGA individuals in the CLHNS ($P < 0.001$).

Upon enrolment in the immune study, EDTA plasma was collected and immediately frozen, followed by immunization against typhoid fever with a 25 µg dose of purified Vi cell-surface polysaccharide extracted from *Salmonella typhi*, delivered in 500 µl sterile solution via intramuscular injection (Pasteur Merieux, Lyon, France). Two weeks and 3 months later, follow-up blood was drawn. Participants had not been previously immunized against typhoid.

Measures of immune function

A range of complementary immune measures was investigated to illuminate the possible role of early environments in shaping resistance to infectious disease, thymic development and function, and risk for atopic disease.

Anti-typhoid antibody titre

The humoral-mediated response to vaccination was assessed by comparing anti-typhoid antibody titres in baseline samples to those drawn 2 weeks and 3 months following vaccination. This method provides an *in vivo*, functional measure of immunocompetence that mimics the real-world process of pathogen exposure and immune response that is critical in defining resistance to infectious disease.

Thymopoietin

The thymus produces a range of thymic hormones with important roles in T-lymphocyte maturation and peripheral T-lymphocyte function (Dardenne and Bach, 1988; Goss and Flye, 1993). Thymopoietin – a 49-amino-acid poly-peptide produced primarily by thymic epithelial cells – is among the best characterized, and is involved in early T-lymphocyte differentiation and the peripheral regulation of mature T-lymphocyte function (Goldstein *et al.*, 1979; Ranges *et al.*, 1982; Singh *et al.*, 1998). Serum thymopoietin concentrations show a pattern of age-related decline that parallel declines in thymic volume: levels are highest at 15–30 years and drop with age (Lewis *et al.*, 1978). Since the thymus may be an important link between early environments and later immunocompetence, thymopoietin was measured as an indicator of thymic activity.

Immunoglobulin E

Asthma, allergy and other atopic diseases are mediated by IgE responses to primarily innocuous, common environmental allergens, and elevated total IgE concentrations are consistently found in atopic individuals (Wittig *et al.*, 1980; Magnusson, 1988). A number of studies have reported significant associations between measures of fetal growth and later risk for allergy, asthma and obstructive airways disease (Barker *et al.*, 1991; Seidman *et al.*, 1991; Godfrey *et al.*, 1994; Fergusson *et al.*, 1997; Gregory *et al.*, 1999; Shaheen *et al.*, 1999; Lopuhaa *et al.*, 2000). IgE is also significant in that early postnatal exposure to infectious disease has been associated with reduced IgE production, and reduced risk for allergy and asthma later in life (Martinez *et al.*, 1995; Shaheen *et al.*, 1996b; Shirakawa *et al.*, 1997; Matricardi *et al.*, 2000; Illi *et al.*, 2001).

Data analysis

Maximum likelihood logistic regression (Stata Corporation, College Station, Texas, USA) was used to model the likelihood of responding to the vaccine with at least a fourfold increase in antibody titre, and least squares regression was used to evaluate predictors of log-transformed thymopoietin and of log-transformed IgE. Intrauterine growth retardation was the primary independent variable of interest, but aspects of the prenatal environment (maternal nutritional status during pregnancy, parity and season of birth), postnatal environment (household socio-economic status, pattern of breastfeeding, pathogen exposure and infectious morbidity) and growth (length, weight) and current status (pubertal status, nutritional status) were also considered as potential confounders or covariates in these analyses (see Table 13.2).

It was hypothesized that SGA individuals would differ significantly from AGA individuals in our markers of immune function. The model-building strategy outlined by Lucas *et al.* (1999) was applied to increase confidence that any association between IUGR and later immune function was due to the quality of the prenatal environment, rather than correlated aspects of postnatal experience. The crude association between SGA and later immune function was first evaluated. Measures of current nutritional status, as well as variables representing multiple aspects of postnatal growth and morbidity, were then added. Interactions between SGA and these variables were considered where appropriate. If adjustment for postnatal factors was found to attenuate the effect of SGA, we concluded that postnatal rather than prenatal environments were more likely to be causally related to adolescent immune function. If adjustment for postnatal factors amplified the effect of SGA, it was concluded that both prenatal and postnatal influences were relevant. Significant interactions between SGA and postnatal factors were assumed to indicate that SGA modified the effect of later environments.

Prenatal and postnatal influences on adolescent immune function

Characteristics of SGA and AGA individuals in the sample are presented in Table 13.2. As expected, SGA individuals had significantly lower birthweights, and were significantly shorter and lighter in adolescence as well. In addition, SGA individuals were more likely to come from households with lower incomes, and to be born to mothers with lower body mass index (BMI), who were pregnant for the first time.

Table 13.3 presents the mean unadjusted differences in the three measures of immunity. It was immediately apparent that prenatal undernutrition did not have a dramatic main effect on immune function. Although differences were in

Table 13.2. Descriptive statistics for small-for-gestational age (SGA) and appropriate-for-gestational age (AGA) girls and boys. Mean (SD) values are presented for continuous variables.

	SGA (N = 55)	AGA (N = 48)
Female (%)	52.7	62.5
Prenatal environment		
Gestational age (weeks)	39.4 (1.9)	40.1 (1.9)
Birthweight (g)	2369 (211)**	3301 (376)
Ponderal index	2.15 (0.30)***	2.59 (0.38)
Maternal BMI (kg/m^2)	21.1 (2.2)*	22.3 (2.6)
First pregnancy (%)	30.9**	8.5
Born in wet season (%)	41.8	35.4
Weekly HH income (pesos)	194 (192)*	280 (228)
Birth to 1 year		
Growth in length (cm)	21.1 (2.8)	20.4 (2.6)
Weight gain, 1st year (kg)	5.0 (0.9)*	4.6 (1.06)
Duration of exclusive breastfeeding (days)	50.5 (32.8)	46.6 (43.3)
Episodes of diarrhoea[a]	1.4 (1.1)	1.0 (1.0)
Episodes of respiratory infection[a]	4.6 (1.1)	4.7 (1.3)
Unsanitary food storage area (%)	44.8	30.0
Adequate excreta disposal (%)	39.1	64.6
Crowding, persons/room	3.0 (1.8)	3.2 (1.9)
Age 10 or 11 years		
Height (cm)	132.0 (7.3)**	136.0 (6.2)
Weight (kg)	26.5 (5.3)**	29.8 (5.7)
BMI (kg/m^2)	15.1 (1.7)	16.0 (2.1)
Age 14 or 15 years		
Height (cm)	132.0 (7.3)**	136.0 (6.2)
Weight (kg)	26.5 (5.3)**	29.8 (5.7)
BMI (kg/m^2)	15.1 (1.7)*	16.0 (2.1)
Weekly HH income (pesos)	2635 (1783)***	4487 (3329)
Unsanitary food storage area (%)	32.1	25.5

[a]As assessed at six bimonthly intervals. Scores can range from 0 to 6.
*$P < 0.05$ (Student's t-test for continuous variables); **$P < 0.01$; ***$P < 0.001$.
BMI, body mass index; HH, household.

the hypothesized direction, they were not statistically significant. However, multivariate analyses revealed that prenatal undernutrition was significantly associated with each immune marker when considered in interaction with aspects of the postnatal environment. Table 13.4 demonstrates the importance of considering such interactions.

Predictors of antibody response to typhoid vaccination

Current nutritional status is an important factor in shaping one's ability to mount an adequate immune response to vaccination, but in this sample responders and non-responders did not differ significantly in BMI (18.4 and 18.5 kg/m^2, respectively, $P = 0.80$ for Student's t-test). However, current nutritional status interacted significantly with prenatal undernutrition to predict antibody

Table 13.3. Measures of immune function for adolescents born small-for-gestational age (SGA) and appropriate-for-gestational age (AGA).

	SGA	AGA	P value[a]
Adequate vaccine response	45.5%	51.2%	0.78
	($N = 55$)	($N = 41$)	
Thymopoietin (pmol/l)	31.1 (33.5)	35.5 (32.0)	0.31
	($N = 48$)	($N = 45$)	
IgE (IU/ml)	146.5 (219.1)	99.0 (117.7)	0.47
	($N = 55$)	($N = 48$)	

[a]Student's t-tests were used to evaluate the difference in log-transformed thymopoietin and IgE concentrations for SGA and AGA individuals. The χ^2 test for independence of categorical variables was used to evaluate vaccine responsiveness.

Table 13.4. Measures of immune function for adolescents born small-for-gestational age (SGA) and appropriate-for-gestational age (AGA) in interaction with significant postnatal factors.

			SGA	AGA	P value[a]
Probability of adequate	BMI:	< sex-specific median	0.32	0.71	< 0.05
vaccine response[b]		≥ sex-specific median	0.52	0.49	
Thymopoietin (log pmol/l)[c]	Exclusive breastfeeding:	< 51 days	1.59	1.54	< 0.01
		≥ 51 days	1.53	1.77	
IgE (log IU/ml)[d]	Household hygiene:	poor	2.11	1.88	< 0.01
		good	1.88	1.90	

[a]Significance level for the interaction term with birthweight-for-gestational-age.
[b]Adjusted for sex, pubertal status, duration of exclusive breastfeeding and diarrhoeal morbidity in first year.
[c]Adjusted for sex.
[d]Adjusted for sex and current household income.
BMI, body mass index.

responsiveness (Table 13.4). Adolescents born SGA, and who were currently below the sex-specific median value for BMI, stood out as those who were least likely to respond to the vaccination. With other covariates held constant, the probability of an adequate response was 0.32 for SGA/low current BMI adolescents, compared to a range of 0.49–0.70 for adolescents born AGA, with high current BMI or both (McDade et al., 2001b).

Aspects of the early postnatal environment were also found to be significant predictors of adolescent immune function. The presence of at least one episode of diarrhoea in the first year of life (as assessed at six bimonthly home visits) more than doubled the likelihood of an adequate antibody response, while rapid weight gain in the first 6 months and prolonged exclusive breastfeeding were also associated with improved responsiveness. The combined effects of significant prenatal and postnatal exposures is presented in Fig. 13.1. In the best-case scenario – AGA, high current BMI, rapid weight gain in the first 6 months and prolonged breastfeeding – the predicted probability of mounting an adequate antibody response to vaccination in adolescence was more than three times greater than in the worst-case scenario of SGA, low current BMI, slow postnatal weight gain and abbreviated breastfeeding.

Recent work on cardiovascular disease (CVD) risk factors has revealed sex differences in relationships with prenatal nutrition or birth outcome (Adair et al., 2001; Adair and Cole, 2003; Kuzawa and Adair, 2003). Poor maternal energy status during pregnancy (low adiposity) is a stronger predictor of future CVD risk

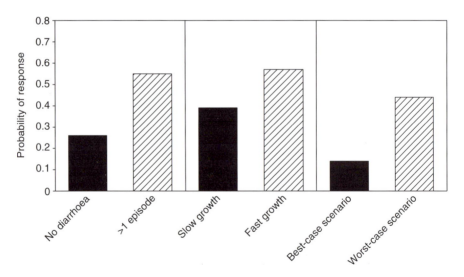

Fig. 13.1. Probability of mounting an adequate antibody response in relation to significant prenatal and postnatal exposures: diarrhoea in the first year of life, rate of weight gain in the first 6 months, and the combined effects of birthweight for gestational age, current body mass index (BMI), rate of weight gain and duration of exclusive breastfeeding. The 'worst-case' scenario represents adolescents born small for gestational age (SGA), low current BMI, slow weight gain and short duration of breastfeeding. (Data from McDade et al., 2001b.)

than is low birthweight, and this association is independent of birthweight status. Similar relationships with immune function were considered in the CLHNS cohort. There was a significant sex-by-SGA interaction in logistic regression models predicting antibody response to typhoid vaccination (Fig. 13.2). Males who were SGA had a *higher* response rate than males who were AGA, while the opposite trend by birth-outcome status was apparent among females. Building from these models, maternal third-trimester arm fat area was modestly positively related to vaccine responsiveness, and both associations were strengthened to borderline significance ($P < 0.10$) once the child's own adiposity was added to the model (not shown). In contrast to the association with SGA, there were no sex differences in the relationship between maternal pregnancy adiposity and offspring immunity.

Predictors of thymopoietin concentration

Individuals born SGA were found to have lower concentrations of thymopoietin in adolescence than AGA individuals, but this difference was only statistically significant when prenatal undernutrition was considered in interaction with the duration of exclusive breastfeeding. Individuals were classified as short or long breastfeeders if they were below or above the median duration of exclusive breastfeeding in this population (51 days). Thymopoietin production was reduced in adolescents born SGA, regardless of the duration of breast-feeding. For AGA individuals, short breastfeeding was associated with compara-bly low concentrations, while thymopoietin was significantly elevated in long breastfeeders (Table 13.4) (McDade *et al.*, 2001a).

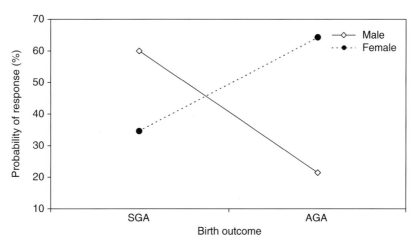

Fig. 13.2. Interaction between male sex and birthweight for gestational age in predicting the likelihood of an adequate antibody response to typhoid vaccination. Parameters from logistic regression model including maturational status, male sex, small for gestational age (SGA) and male × SGA; odds ratio (95% confidence interval): male 0.15 (0.03, 0.67) *P* < 0.02; SGA, 0.29 (0.10, 0.90) *P* < 0.04; male × SGA 18.7 (2.86, 122.1) *P* < 0.002.

Postnatal growth in the first year of life was an equally important predictor of adolescent thymopoietin production: adolescents one standard deviation above the mean in first-year length increment (23.4 cm) had thymopoietin concentrations that were 1.5 times higher than those one standard deviation below the mean (18.0 cm). Growth during the first 6 months appeared to be particularly important, showing a stronger positive association with adolescent thymopoietin than growth between 6 and 12 months. Sex was also an important factor, with boys having median thymopoietin concentrations (35.8 pmol/l) that were more than twice those for girls (14.9 pmol/l).

Predictors of total IgE

Consistent with previous work suggesting an association between impaired fetal growth and subsequent IgE production, individuals born SGA had elevated IgE concentrations in adolescence, although this elevation was not statistically significant. However, a significant effect of IUGR emerged in interaction with the pathogenicity of the postnatal environment. For both boys and girls born SGA, adolescent IgE production was positively associated with a relatively unsanitary household environment in the first year of life (presence of domestic animals under the house, unhygienic food storage area, unsanitary infant food preparation practices) (Table 13.4). For AGA girls, a similar, but weaker association was found, whereas the opposite pattern was found for AGA boys: unsanitary conditions in the first year were associated with slightly reduced levels of adolescent IgE (McDade et al., 2004).

In addition, consistent with previous reports of a protective effect of early infection on later risk for atopy, respiratory and/or diarrhoeal disease in the first 6 months of life was associated with reduced IgE production in adolescence. For adolescents who had only one reported episode of morbidity in early infancy (recorded at 2 months, 4 months and 6 months of age), average IgE concentrations were nearly four times higher than those of adolescents who had four morbidity episodes (114.8 IU/ml versus 32.4 IU/ml). Similar associations were found when respiratory and diarrhoeal morbidity were considered separately, and infectious morbidity in the second 6 months of life was not significantly associated with IgE. Weight velocity in the first 6 months was positively associated with adolescent IgE, and current household income was negatively related to IgE. Lastly, as with thymopoietin, boys were found to have significantly higher IgE concentrations than girls (72.8 and 43.2 IU/ml, respectively).

Associations between immune measures

Since it was hypothesized that IUGR would be associated with reduced antibody responsiveness to vaccination, reduced thymopoietin concentration and increased IgE concentration, it was anticipated that vaccine responsiveness and thymopoietin should be positively related, and that IgE should be negatively related to both these measures. Physiologically, it is reasonable to expect these relationships to be at least in part causal – rather than merely correlational – since the thymus plays an important role in processes of T-cell development and function that have implications for IgE production and antibody responsiveness to pathogen challenge.

Since thymopoietin and IgE concentrations differed significantly for boys and girls, separate analyses were performed for each. No significant associations among the immune measures were found, although there was a trend toward reduced IgE in boys who did not respond to typhoid vaccination. The opposite pattern was found in girls, although this difference was not statistically significant. In addition, for girls, a trend toward the expected negative association between thymopoietin and IgE (Pearson $R = -0.22$, $P = 0.09$, $N = 57$) was noted. A weak positive association was found for boys (Pearson $R = 0.23$, $P = 0.18$, $N = 36$). The small sample size – particularly with boys – was an obvious limitation here, and these associations should be interpreted with caution.

Leptin

Immune defences – particularly antigen-specific defences – are energetically expensive, and a growing number of investigators are applying an evolutionary, cost–benefit approach to the study of immunology (McDade and Worthman, 1999; Buttgereit et al., 2000; Read and Allen, 2000). Scaffolded in an adaptationist framework, this perspective recognizes that organisms have limited energy, and that investment in immune defences consumes energy that cannot be used for other purposes. The physiological mechanisms through which these trade-offs are mediated are far from clear, but leptin is a likely candidate.

Leptin is similar in structure to IL-2, and is produced primarily by adipocytes. Its role as an endocrine indicator of energy status has been probed intensively, and a number of studies with animal models have indicated that leptin is critical to normal cell-mediated immune processes (Howard et al., 1999; Lord, 2002), although a recent study of Gambian children did not detect an in vivo association (Moore et al., 2002). In the Filipino sample, prenatal undernutrition was not related to leptin concentrations independent of adiposity. However, because leptin signals energy reserves, it was assessed as a potential mediator of the long-term effects of early environments on later immuno-competence. Since leptin concentrations showed the expected sexual dimorphism, with levels considerably higher in females compared to males, separate analyses were performed for each. Prenatal undernutrition was not associated with leptin concentration in adolescence. However, consistent with leptin's role as an indicator of energy status, current BMI was positively associated with leptin for both boys (Pearson $R = 0.58$, $P < 0.001$) and girls (Pearson $R = 0.50$, $P < 0.001$).

Antibody responsiveness to typhoid vaccination was not associated with leptin: for both boys and girls, responders and non-responders did not differ in their mean leptin concentrations (boys: 0.22 versus 0.20 log ng/ml; girls: 0.59 versus 0.59 log ng/ml). Controlling for current BMI did not alter this pattern of associations.

In contrast, a positive association between leptin and thymopoietin was noted in girls (Fig. 13.3). The crude association between these measures was weak (Pearson $R = 0.20$, $P = 0.15$, $N = 55$), but was strengthened considerably when the effect of current BMI was taken into account (partial $R = 0.30$, $P = 0.029$). A positive association between leptin and thymopoietin makes sense from an energetic perspective, and it is consistent with previous research in starved mice, indicating that leptin administration protects against cell-mediated immune suppression and thymic involution that would normally follow undernutrition (Howard *et al.*, 1999). However, this finding needs to be interpreted with caution given the small sample size, and the absence of a significant association between leptin and thymopoietin in boys (partial $R = -0.12$, $P = 0.50$, $N = 32$).

For both boys and girls, lower concentrations of leptin were associated with increased IgE production (Fig. 13.4). Partial correlations – controlling again

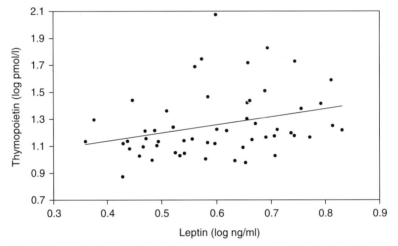

Fig. 13.3.   The partial correlation between thymopoietin and leptin in adolescent girls ($N = 55$), controlling for current body mass index (BMI).

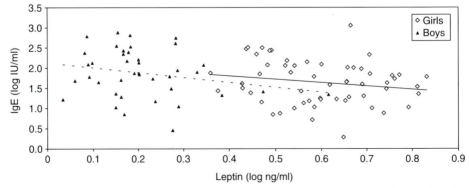

Fig. 13.4.   The partial correlation between IgE and leptin in adolescent girls ($N = 57$) and boys ($N = 40$), controlling for current body mass index (BMI).

for current BMI – approached statistical significance (boys: partial $R = -0.23$, $P = 0.16$, $N = 40$; girls: partial $R = -0.19$, $P = 0.17$, $N = 57$). However, for the entire sample, the negative relationship between leptin and IgE was significant (controlling for BMI and sex, partial $R = -0.21$, $P = 0.037$, $N = 97$). Although negative associations between leptin and IgE have not been reported, this pattern is consistent with previous research in mice indicating that leptin promotes activity associated with Th1 lymphocytes, rather than Th2 activity linked to IgE production (Matarese *et al.*, 2001; Lord, 2002).

For the most part, the Filipino study found a pattern of associations among leptin, thymopoietin and IgE that was consistent with current research in this area. However, these analyses must be regarded as preliminary, and suggestive for future research into the potential mechanisms associated with immune programming.

Current Perspectives on the Programming of Immunity

Research on the programming of immune function is in its early stages, but it is clear that this is an important area of enquiry. Future work with animal models and clinical human samples will be necessary to clarify the physiological processes through which early environments exert long-term immunological effects. Complementing this approach, additional population-based research will be necessary to explore the ecological contexts within which these processes operate, and the factors that moderate their expression. More specifically, future research should consider the following: definitions of prenatal environmental quality, interactions between pre- and postnatal environments, physiological mechanisms and clinical implications.

In a sample of adolescents from the Philippines, prenatal undernutrition was associated with reduced thymopoietin production, reduced antibody response to typhoid vaccination and elevated total IgE. We now have consistent evidence in this population, using three different parameters of immunity, that provides support for the hypothesis that human immune function is, at least in part, programmed by early environments. These findings underscore the importance of accounting for interactions between prenatal and postnatal environments when studying early-life influences on immune function. For each immune marker, the main effect of prenatal undernutrition was not statistically significant, but emerged only in interaction with aspects of postnatal experience: The duration of exclusive breastfeeding was found to moderate the effect of prenatal undernutrition on adolescent thymopoietin concentration; adolescents born SGA were less likely to respond to typhoid vaccination only if they were also below the median for BMI at the time of inoculation; and a relatively unhygienic household environment in the first year of life was associated with significant elevations in IgE only for adolescents born SGA. This pattern of results suggests that the long-term immunological effects of prenatal environments are not over-determined, and may in fact be largely contingent.

While the prenatal nutritional environment is an important predictor of later immune function, the Filipino findings also underscore the role of the early postnatal environment in shaping immune development. Vaccine responsiveness, thymopoietin concentration and IgE concentration in adolescence were all positively associated with growth in length and/or weight during the first 6 months of life. Early episodes of infectious morbidity were associated with reduced IgE and increased vaccine responsiveness in adolescence. Since early infancy is a critical period for immune development in general, and the thymus in particular, it is not surprising that postnatal factors programme immunity in significant ways (Lewis and Wilson, 1995; Hasselbalch et al., 1999).

It is likely that significant correlations exist between prenatal and postnatal environments, thereby increasing the challenges associated with separating their relative contributions to immune development. For example, in the Filipino study population, prenatal undernutrition reduced antibody responsiveness to vaccination in adolescence, whereas diarrhoeal morbidity in the first year of life increased antibody responsiveness. Since SGA infants are more likely to suffer from diarrhoea in the first year of life (Table 13.2) (Ashworth, 1998), the long-term immunological effects of prenatal undernutrition may in part be attenuated by postnatal infectious disease experience. This situation, as well as the failure to explicitly consider interactions between pre- and postnatal environments, may obscure significant long-term effects of prenatal undernutrition and lead to an underestimation of their importance.

Birthweight alone is a poor indicator of the prenatal nutritional environment, and prior research emphasizes the importance of distinguishing between infants born small for gestational age and those born preterm, but with a comparable birthweight. For the former, immunological impairment in infancy may be more severe, whereas preterm AGA infants demonstrate recovery (Chandra, 1981). Similarly, disproportionate fetal growth (as indicated by an increase in head circumference) has been shown to be a better predictor of adult IgE concentration than birthweight, perhaps revealing an impoverished prenatal environment that favours brain growth at a cost to the development of lymphoid tissues (Godfrey et al., 1994).

Moreover, because birthweight follows a normal distribution among even well-nourished and healthy populations, size at birth per se may not always be a reliable indicator of prenatal nutritional sufficiency (Chard et al., 1993). The limitations of birthweight as a marker of relevant prenatal exposures are illustrated by research into the early life predictors of adolescent blood pressure and cholesterol metabolism, both of which relate most strongly to maternal energy status during pregnancy and are independent of variation in birthweight (Adair et al., 2001; Kuzawa and Adair, 2003). Observation of a borderline positive association between third-trimester maternal energy status and offspring antibody response that was independent of SGA status is consistent with these findings. Thus, as has been demonstrated for CVD risk factors, using a birth outcome such as birthweight as the sole marker of fetal nutrition is likely to miss important associations between the prenatal environment and postnatal immune function.

It is also interesting that measures of current environmental quality do not appear to be significantly related to measures of adolescent immunity. Exceptions include a negative association between current household income and IgE, and a moderating role for current BMI with respect to vaccine responsiveness. Measures of pre- and postnatal environmental quality were the primary predictors of adolescent immunity, despite the wide range of measures of childhood and adolescent environmental quality available in the CLHNS dataset. The relative importance of early environments in setting the long-term trajectory of immune development is further evidence in support of the programming hypothesis.

The long-term immunological effects of early environments may, however, be largely contingent upon conditions experienced after birth, and interactions between prenatal, postnatal and current environments should be considered explicitly. Research to date indicates that large main effects of prenatal under-nutrition on immune function may not be evident beyond infancy and early childhood. Findings such as ours suggest that effects may emerge only in a subset of individuals who are exposed to specific combinations of prenatal and postnatal environments.

The physiological mechanisms linking early experience to later immuno-competence require further elucidation. Likely candidates that have been explored in previous research include impaired development of lymphoid tissues (the thymus in particular), and lasting irregularities in hypothalamus–pituitary–adrenal function. Preliminary findings from our research also suggest that leptin – as an indicator of energetic status with immunoregulatory properties – may be an important mediator of early environments. In addition, we have found a number of sex differences in immune outcomes, and instances suggestive of sex differences in relationships between early exposures and later immune function, perhaps indicating a role for other hormones, such as sex steroids. It is likely that a range of experimental, clinical and population-level research designs will be necessary to reveal the mechanisms associated with immune programming.

The health implications of immune programming remain to be explored. Prior research suggests that prenatal undernutrition increases the risk of premature death from infectious disease (Moore *et al.*, 1999), as well as the risk of atopic and autoimmune disease in adulthood (Phillips *et al.*, 1993; Godfrey *et al.*, 1994; Moore *et al.*, 1999), and that early exposure to infectious disease reduces adult risk of atopy (Shaheen *et al.*, 1996b; Shirakawa *et al.*, 1997; Matricardi *et al.*, 2000; Illi *et al.*, 2001). With respect to infectious disease morbidity and mortality, the impact of immune programming is likely to be most evident in impoverished settings, where pathogen exposure is relatively high. In addition, to the extent that inflammatory processes are related to the patho-physiology of cardiovascular disease, cancers and other chronic conditions (Kalayoglu *et al.*, 2002; Ryu, 2003), immune programming may be a critical factor mediating the association between prenatal undernutrition and adult chronic disease processes that has been reported in a large range of populations, from both developed and developing nations (Yajnik, 2000; Gill, 2001).

References

Aab, P., Andersen, M. and Knudsen, K. (1993) Excess mortality after early exposure to measles. *International Journal of Epidemiology* 22, 156–162.

Adair, L.S. (1989) Low birth weight and intra-uterine growth retardation in Filipino infants. *Pediatrics* 84, 613–622.

Adair, L.S. (1999) Filipino children exhibit catch-up growth from age 2 to 12 years. *Journal of Nutrition* 129, 1140–1148.

Adair, L.S. (2001) Size at birth predicts age at menarche. *Pediatrics* 107, E59.

Adair, L. and Cole, T. (2003) Rapid child growth raises blood pressure in adolescent boys who were thin at birth. *Hypertension* 41, 451–456.

Adair, L.S., Kuzawa, C.W. and Borja, J. (2001) Maternal energy stores and diet composition during pregnancy program adolescent blood pressure. *Circulation* 104, 1034–1039.

Ashworth, A. (1998) Effects of intrauterine growth retardation on mortality and morbidity in infants and young children. *European Journal of Clinical Nutrition* 52, S34–S42.

Barker, D.J., Godfrey, K.M., Osmond, C., Winter, P.D. and Shaheen, S.O. (1991) Relations of birth weight and childhood respiratory infection to adult lung function and death from chronic obstructive airways disease. *British Medical Journal* 303, 671–675.

Beach, R.S., Gershwin, M.E. and Hurley, L.S. (1982) Gestational zinc deprivation in mice: Persistence of immunodeficiency for three generations. *Science* 281, 469–471.

Buttgereit, F., Burmester, G.R. and Brand, M.D. (2000) Bioenergetics of immune functions: fundamental and therapeutic aspects. *Immunology Today* 21, 192–199.

Cebu Study Team (1989) Underlying and proximate determinants of child health: the Cebu Longitudinal Health and Nutrition Study. *American Journal of Epidemiology* 133, 185–201.

Chandra, R.K. (1975a) Antibody formation in first and second generation offspring of nutritionally deprived rats. *Science* 190, 289–290.

Chandra, R.K. (1975b) Fetal malnutrition and postnatal immunocompetence. *American Journal of Diseases of Childhood* 129, 450–454.

Chandra, R.K. (1981) Serum thymic hormone activity and cell-mediated immunity in healthy neonates, preterm infants, and small-for-gestational age infants. *Pediatrics* 67, 407–411.

Chandra, R.K. (1988) *Nutrition and Immunology*. Alan R. Liss, New York.

Chandra, R.K., Ali, S.K., Kutty, K.M. and Chandra, S. (1977) Thymus-dependent lymphocytes and delayed hypersensitivity in low birth weight infants. *Biology of the Neonate* 31, 15–18.

Chard, T., Yoong, A. and Macintosh, M. (1993) The myth of fetal growth retardation at term. *British Journal of Obstetrics and Gynaecology* 100, 1076–1081.

Chatrath, R., Saili, A., Jain, M. and Dutta, A.K. (1997) Immune status of full-term small-for-gestational age neonates in India. *Journal of Tropical Pediatrics* 43, 345–348.

Chisari, A.N., Giovambattista, A., Perello, M., Gaillard, R.C. and Spinedi, E.S. (2001) Maternal undernutrition induces neuroendocrine immune dysfunction in male pups at weaning. *Neuroimmunomodulation* 9, 41–48.

Clarke, A.S., Wittwer, D.J., Abbott, D.H. and Schneider, M.L. (1994) Long-term effects of prenatal stress on HPA axis activity in juvenile rhesus monkeys. *Developmental Psychobiology* 27, 257–269.

Coe, C.L. and Lubach, G.R. (2000) Prenatal influences on neuroimmune set points in infancy. *Annals of the New York Academy of Sciences* 917, 468–477.

Coe, C.L., Lubach, G.R., Schneider, M.L., Dierschke, D.J. and Ershler, W.B. (1992) Early rearing conditions alter immune responses in the developing infant primate. *Pediatrics* 90, 505–509.

Coe, C., Lubach, G., Karaszewski, J. and Ershler, W. (1996) Prenatal endocrine activation alters postnatal cellular immunity in infant monkeys. *Brain, Behavior, and Immunity* 10, 221–234.

Dardenne, M. and Bach, J.F. (1988) Functional biology of thymic hormones. *Thymus Update* 1, 101–116.

Dourov, N. (1986) Thymic atrophy and immune deficiency in malnutrition. *Current Topics in Pathology* 75, 127–150.

Dutz, W., Rossipal, E., Ghavami, H., Vessal, K., Kohout, E. and Post, C. (1976) Persistent cell mediated immune-deficiency following infantile stress during the first 6 months of life. *European Journal of Pediatrics* 122, 117–130.

Eishi, Y., Hirokawa, K. and Hatakeyama, S. (1983) Long-lasting impairment of immune and endocrine systems of offspring induced by injection of dexamethasone into pregnant mice. *Clinical Immunology and Immunopathology* 26, 335–349.

Ferguson, A.C. (1978) Prolonged impairment of cellular immunity in children with intrauterine growth retardation. *Journal of Pediatrics* 93, 52–56.

Fergusson, D.M., Crane, J., Beasley, R. and Horwood, L.J. (1997) Perinatal factors and atopic disease in childhood. *Clinical and Experimental Allergy* 27, 1394–1401.

Gershwin, M.E., German, J.B. and Keen, C.L. (eds) (2000) *Nutrition and Immunology.* Humana Press, Totowa, New Jersey.

Ghavami, H., Dutz, W., Mohallattee, M., Rossipal, E. and Vessal, K. (1979) Immune disturbances after severe enteritis during the first six months of life. *Israel Journal of Medical Science* 15, 364–368.

Gill, T.P. (2001) Cardiovascular risk in the Asia–Pacific region from a nutrition and metabolic point of view: abdominal obesity. *Asia–Pacific Journal of Clinical Nutrition* 10, 85–89.

Godfrey, K.M., Barker, D.J.P. and Osmond, C. (1994) Disproportionate fetal growth and raised IgE concentration in adult life. *Clinical and Experimental Allergy* 24, 641–648.

Goldstein, G., Scheid, M.P., Boyse, E.A., Schlesinger, D.H. and Van Wauwe, J. (1979) A synthetic pentapeptide with biological activity characteristic of the thymic hormone thymopoietin. *Science* 204, 1309–1310.

Goss, J.A. and Flye, M.W. (1993) *The Thymus – Regulator of Cellular Immunity.* R.G. Landes Company, Austin, Texas.

Gregory, A., Doull, I., Pearce, N., Cheng, S., Leadbitter, P., Holgate, S. and Beasley, R. (1999) The relationship between anthropometric measurements at birth: asthma and atopy in childhood. *Clinical and Experimental Allergy* 29, 330–333.

Hasselbalch, H., Ersboll, A.K., Jeppesen, D.L. and Nielsen, M.B. (1999) Thymus size in infants from birth until 24 months of age evaluated by ultrasound. *Acta Radiologica* 40, 41–44.

Hoffman, H.J., Stark, C.R., Lundin, F.E. and Ashbrook, J.D. (1974) Analyses of birth weight, gestational age and fetal viability, U.S. births, 1968. *Obstetrical and Gynecological Survey* 29, 651–681.

Howard, J.K., Lord, G.M., Matarese, G., Vendetti, S., Ghatei, M.A., Ritter, M.A., Lechler, R.I. and Bloom, S.R. (1999) Leptin protects mice from starvation-induced lymphoid atrophy and increases thymic cellularity in ob/ob mice. *Journal of Clinical Investigation* 104, 1051–1059.

Illi, S., von Mutius, E., Lau, S., Bergmann, R., Niggemann, B., Sommerfeld, C. and Wahn, U. (2001) Early childhood infectious diseases and the development of asthma up to school age: A birth cohort study. *British Medical Journal* 322, 390–395.

Kalayoglu, M.V., Libby, P. and Byrne, G.I. (2002) *Chlamydia pneumoniae* as an emerging risk factor in cardiovascular disease. *Journal of the American Medical Association* 288, 2724–2731.

Kebede, A. and Larson, C. (1994) The health consequences of intrauterine growth retardation in southwestern Ethiopa. *Tropical Doctor* 24, 64–69.

Kuzawa, C. and Adair, L. (2003) Lipid profiles in adolescent Filipinos: relationship to birth weight and maternal energy status during pregnancy. *American Journal of Clinical Nutrition* 77, 960–966.

Lewis, D. and Wilson, C. (1995) Developmental immunology and the role of host defenses in neonatal susceptibility. In Remington, J. and Klein, J. (eds) *Infectious Diseases of the Fetus and Newborn Infant*, 4th edn. W.B. Saunders, Philadelphia, Pennsylvania, pp. 108–139.

Lewis, V.M., Twomey, J.J., Bealmear, P., Goldstein, G. and Good, R.A. (1978) Age, thymic involution, and circulating thymic hormone activity. *Journal of Clinical Endocrinology and Metabolism* 47, 145–150.

Lira, P.I.C., Ashworth, A. and Morris, S.S. (1996) Low birth weight and morbidity from diarrhea and respiratory infection in northeast Brazil. *Journal of Pediatrics* 128, 497–504.

Lopuhaa, C.E., Roseboom, T.J., Osmond, C., Barker, D.J.P., Ravelli, A.C.J., Bleker, O.P., van der Zee, J.S. and van der Meulen, J.H.P. (2000) Atopy, lung function, and obstructive airways disease after prenatal exposure to famine. *Thorax* 55, 555–561.

Lord, G.M. (2002) Role of leptin in immunology. *Nutrition Reviews* 60, S35–S38.

Lucas, A., Fewtrell, M.S. and Cole, T.J. (1999) Fetal orgins of adult disease – the hypothesis revisited. *British Medical Journal* 319, 245–249.

Magnusson, C.G.M. (1988) Cord serum IgE in relation to family history and as predictor of atopic disease in early infancy. *Allergy* 43, 241–251.

Martinez, F.D., Stern, D.A., Wright, A.L., Taussig, L.M. and Halonen, M. (1995) Association of non-wheezing lower respiratory tract illnesses in early life with persistently diminished serum IgE levels. *Thorax* 50, 1067–1072.

Matarese, G., Di Giacomo, A., Sanna, V., Lord, G.M., Howard, J.K., Di Tuoro, A., Bloom, S.R., Lechler, R.I., Zappacosta, S. and Fontana, S. (2001) Requirement for leptin in the induction and progression of autoimmune encephalomyelitis. *Journal of Immunology* 166, 5909–5916.

Matricardi, P.M., Rosmini, F., Riondino, S., Fortini, M., Ferrigno, L., Rapicetta, M. and Bonini, S. (2000) Exposure to foodborne and orofecal microbes versus airborne viruses in relation to atopy and allergic asthma: epidemiological study. *British Medical Journal* 320, 412–417.

McDade, T.W. and Worthman, C.M. (1999) Evolutionary process and the ecology of human immune function. *American Journal of Human Biology* 11, 705–717.

McDade, T.W., Beck, M.A., Kuzawa, C.W. and Adair, L.S. (2001a) Prenatal undernutrition and postnatal growth are associated with adolescent thymic function. *Journal of Nutrition* 131, 1225–1235.

McDade, T.W., Beck, M.A., Kuzawa, C.W. and Adair, L.S. (2001b) Prenatal undernutrition, postnatal environments, and antibody response to vaccination in adolescence. *American Journal of Clinical Nutrition* 74, 543–548.

McDade, T.W., Kuzawa, C.W., Beck, M.A. and Adair, L.S. (2004) Prenatal and early postnatal environments are significant predictors of IgE concentration in Filipino adolescents. *Clinical and Experimental Allergy* 34, 44–50.

Moore, S.E. (1998) Nutrition, immunity and the fetal and infant origins of disease hypothesis in developing countries. *Proceedings of the Nutrition Society* 57, 241–247.

Moore, S.E., Cole, T.J., Collinson, A.C., Poskitt, E.M., McGregor, I.A. and Prentice, A.M. (1999) Prenatal or early postnatal events predict infectious deaths in young adulthood in rural Africa. *International Journal of Epidemiology* 28, 1088–1095.

Moore, S.E., Collinson, A.C. and Prentice, A.M. (2001) Immune function in rural Gambian children is not related to season of birth, birth size, or maternal supplementation status. *American Journal of Clinical Nutrition* 74, 840–847.

Moore, S.E., Morgan, G., Collinson, A.C., Swain, J.A., O'Connell, M.A. and Prentice, A.M. (2002) Leptin, malnutrition, and immune response in rural Gambian children. *Archives of Disease in Childhood* 87, 192–197.

Moscatelli, P., Bricarelli, F.D., Piccinini, A., Tomatis, C. and Dufour, M.A. (1976) Defective immunocompetence in foetal undernutrition. *Helvetica Paediatrica Acta* 31, 241–247.

Mussi-Pinhata, M.M., Goncalves, A.L. and Foss, N.T. (1993) BCG vaccination of full-term infants with chronic intrauterine malnutrition: influence of immunization age on development of post-vaccination, delayed tuberculin hypersensitivity. *Bulletin of the World Health Organization* 71, 41–48.

Naeye, R.L., Diener, M.M., Harcke, H.T. and Blanc, W.A. (1971) Relation of poverty and race to birth weight and organ and cell structure in the newborn. *Pediatric Research* 5, 17–22.

Owens, J.A., Owens, P.C. and Robinson, J.S. (1989) Experimental fetal growth retardation: metabolic and endocrine aspects. In: Gluckman, P.D., Johnston, B.M. and Nathanielsz, P.W. (eds) *Advances in Fetal Physiology*. Perinatology Press, Ithaca, New York, pp. 263–286.

Phillips, D.I.W., Cooper, C., Fall, C., Prentice, L., Osmond, C., Barker, D.J.P. and Rees Smith, B. (1993) Fetal growth and autoimmune thyroid disease. *Quarterly Journal of Medicine* 86, 247–253.

Pittard, W.B., Miller, K. and Sorensen, R.U. (1984) Normal lymphocyte responses to mitogens in term and premature neonates following normal and abnormal intrauterine growth. *Clinical Immunology and Immunopathology* 30, 178–187.

Popkin, B.M., Adair, L.S., Akin, J.S., Black, R., Briscoe, J. and Flieger, W. (1990) Breast-feeding and diarrheal morbidity. *Pediatrics* 86, 874–882.

Ranges, G.E., Goldstein, G., Boyse, E.A. and Scheid, M.P. (1982) T-cell development in normal and thymopoietin treated nude mice. *Journal of Experimental Medicine* 156, 1057–1064.

Read, A.F. and Allen, J.E. (2000) The economics of immunity. *Science* 290, 1104–1105.

Rook, G.A.W. and Stanford, J.L. (1998) Give us this day our daily germs. *Immunology Today* 19, 113–116.

Ryu, W.S. (2003) Molecular aspects of hepatitis B viral infection and the viral carcinogenesis. *Journal of Biochemistry and Molecular Biology* 36(1), 138–143.

Saha, K., Kaur, P., Srivastava, G. and Chaudhury, D.S. (1983) A six-months' follow-up study of growth, morbidity and functional immunity in low birth weight neonates with special reference to intrauterine growth retardation in small-for-gestational-age infants. *Journal of Tropical Pediatrics* 29, 278–282.

Schulof, R.S., Naylor, P.H., Sztein, M.B. and Goldstein, A.L. (1987) Thymic physiology and biochemistry. *Advances in Clinical Chemistry* 26, 203–292.

Seidman, D.S., Laor, A., Gale, R., Stevenson, K.K. and Danon, Y.L. (1991) Is low birth weight a risk factor for asthma during adolescence? *Archives of Disease in Childhood* 66, 584–587.

Shaheen, S.O., Aaby, P., Hall, A.J., Barker, D.J., Heyes, C.B., Shiell, A.W. and Goudiaby, A. (1996a) Cell mediated immunity after measles in Guinea-Bissau: historical cohort study. *British Medical Journal* 313, 969–974.

Shaheen, S.O., Aaby, P., Hall, A.J., Barker, D.J., Heyes, C.B., Shiell, A.W. and Goudiaby, A. (1996b) Measles and atopy in Guinea-Bissau. *Lancet* 347, 1792–1796.

Shaheen, S.O., Sterne, J.A., Montgomery, S.M. and Azima, H. (1999) Birth weight, body mass index and asthma in young adults. *Thorax* 54, 396–402.

Shirakawa, T., Enomoto, T., Shimazu, S. and Hopkin, J.M. (1997) The inverse association between tuberculin responses and atopic disorder. *Science* 275, 77–79.

Singh, V.K., Biswas, S., Mathur, K.B., Haq, W., Garg, S.K. and Agarwal, S.S. (1998) Thymopentin and splenopentin as immunomodulators. *Immunology Research* 17, 345–368.

Steinman, G.G. (1986) Changes in the human thymus during aging. *Current Topics in Pathology* 75, 43–88.

Suskind, R.M. and Tontisirin, K. (eds) (2001) *Nutrition, Immunity, and Infection in Infants and Children*. Lippincott, Williams and Wilkins, Philadelphia, Pennsylvania.

Wittig, H.J., Belloit, J., De Fillipi, I. and Royal, G. (1980) Age-related serum immunoglobulin E levels in healthy subjects and in patients with allergic disease. *Journal of Allergy and Clinical Immunology* 66, 305–313.

Xanthou, M. (1985) Immunologic deficiencies in small-for-dates neonates. *Acta Paediatrica Scandinavica. Supplementum* 319, 143–149.

Yajnik, C. (2000) Interactions of perturbations in intrauterine growth and growth during childhood on the risk of adult-onset disease. *Proceedings of the Nutrition Society* 59, 257–265.

14 Programming in the Pre-implantation Embryo

LORRAINE E. YOUNG,[1] WILLIAM D. REES[2] AND KEVIN D. SINCLAIR[3]

[1]University of Nottingham, School of Human Development, Division of Obstetrics and Gynaecology, Queen's Medical Centre, Nottingham NH7 2UH, UK; [2]Rowett Research Institute, Bucksburn, Aberdeen AB21 9SB, UK; [3]School of Biosciences, University of Nottingham, Sutton Bonington Campus, Loughborough LE12 5RD, UK

Heritable DNA Methylation Changes as a Means to Induce Nutritional Programming in the Pre-implantation Embryo: Overview

This chapter will outline the hypothesis that maternal nutritional effects in developing oocytes, and in procedures used in assisted reproduction, can programme fetal development and adult health, via heritable epigenetic changes in DNA methylation at specific gene loci. This hypothesis arises from a range of diverse experimental evidence, including studies in the sheep and rat. Imbalances in nitrogen metabolism during sheep oocyte growth, for example, have been demonstrated to increase the incidence and severity of aberrant conceptus development that can arise following *in vitro* embryo culture (Sinclair *et al.*, 1999, 2000a). These developmental defects are associated with DNA methylation changes in an imprinted gene key to fetal growth and organ development (Young, 2001; Young *et al.*, 2001). Rat studies suggest that, rather than a general restriction of amino acid supply in the low-protein diets typically used to model poor nutrition (see Chapters 6 and 8, this volume), it is likely to be the metabolism of sulphur-containing amino acids that induces an increase in DNA methylation in specific fetal tissues (Rees, 2002).

By combining these data with parallels of epigenetic reprogramming in studies of cancer, we will develop the evidence that embryo technologies can result in fetal programming and effects that provide clues to the mechanisms underlying the fetal/embryonic origins of adult disease. The hypotheses will be advanced that a range of diets offered during the period of oocyte growth and maturation and pre-implantation embryo development can alter subsequent conceptus and postnatal development, while a range of nutrients and metabolites may alter the availability of methyl groups available within cells for DNA methylation. Imprinted genes are particularly vulnerable to DNA methylation changes during pre-implantation development, and polymorphisms in methyl metabolism enzymes may provide a genetic link to fetal programming.

Background and Significance

Although it is now widely accepted that metabolic responses to diet and suscepti- bility to age-related diseases in adult humans are influenced by nutritional status *in utero* (Barker and Osmond, 1986; Hales and Barker, 1992; Barker, 1998), more recent studies with animals have shown that very early events can also influence clinically relevant outcomes in the offspring (Young *et al.*, 1998; Sinclair *et al.*, 2000a; McEvoy *et al.*, 2001). However, the mechanisms by which molecular events within the oocyte and/or early embryo can programme much later development have not been established. Heritable epigenetic change (i.e. change in the conformation of chromatin without a change in DNA sequence) provides a strong potential mechanism, with DNA methylation being the most likely candidate (Bird, 2002). Here we suggest that specific dietary inadequacies, superovulation regimes and/or oocyte/embryo culture conditions can influence the availability of the methyl groups necessary for the epigenetic methylation of DNA. Identification of DNA methylation alterations at specific loci in the oocyte would provide measurable characteristics indicative of the future development of specific phenotypes.

Assisted reproduction

Recent evidence suggests that the incidence of birth defects and low birthweights among singleton pregnancies achieved by clinically assisted reproduction technology (ART) may be twice as high as that in the general population (Hansen *et al.*, 2002; Schieve *et al.*, 2002; Moll *et al.*, 2003). At present it is uncertain what factors may contribute to low birthweights following ART, but studies in mice indicate that ovarian stimulation prior to *in vitro* fertilization (IVF) can delay embryo development and retard fetal development (van der Auwera and D'Hooghe, 2001). Even in naturally mated mice, superovulation reduces the implantation rate by 50% and lowers birthweight (Ertzeid and Storeng, 2001). We and others have suggested that since both superovulation and *in vitro* maturation recover oocytes from some small or medium antral follicles (from which they would not naturally have completed development and been ovu- lated), factors required for the normal control of development post-fertilization may be deficient in a subset of oocytes used for ART (Young and Fairburn, 2000; Gandolfi and Gandolfi, 2001). We have now demonstrated that this principle is correct, where single-oocyte RT-PCR analysis of the *IGF2R* gene revealed expression in bovine oocytes from large, but not small or medium, antral follicles (K. Georgadaki and L. Young, unpublished and Fig. 14.1).

Considerable experience gained from studies with farm animals suggests that adoption of new procedures, such as *in vitro* maturation and extended *in*

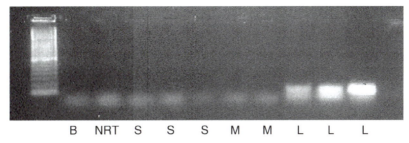

B   NRT   S   S   S   M   M   L   L   L

Fig. 14.1. RT-PCR detection of *IGF2R* in single oocytes from bovine antral follicles of varying size. B, No cDNA, blank control; NRT, no reverse-transcriptase; S, small (< 5 mm); M, medium (5–8 mm); L, large (> 8 mm).

vitro (blastocyst) culture, may introduce additional problems, including *in utero* overgrowth and a varied range of congenital abnormalities that persist into adulthood (Sinclair *et al.*, 2000a). Exposure to unusual culture environments in both sheep and mice leads to developmental defects associated with methylation alterations in imprinted genes (Khosla *et al.*, 2001; Young *et al.*, 2001) as well as with genome-wide defects in DNA methylation (Shi and Haaf, 2002). In addition, many reports exist of altered gene expression associated with specific embryo culture conditions, although it is more difficult to associate these with a specific developmental outcome (Taylor *et al.*, 2003). Although there may well be species differences in terms of the effect of a particular oocyte/embryo culture environment or in the specific genes affected, mechanistic understanding of any perturbation provides an important tool for predicting, testing and avoiding its initiation in any new procedure.

Large offspring syndrome (LOS) and human imprinting syndromes

Unusually large offspring, presenting a broad range of congenital abnormalities, have been born in ruminant species following the transfer of embryos that have been exposed to an artificial, *in vitro*, environment during the periods of oocyte maturation, fertilization and/or culture (Young *et al.*, 1998), or manipulated in some way, e.g. by nuclear transfer (Wilmut *et al.*, 2002). A characteristic of LOS is its sporadic occurrence both within and between laboratories using similar protocols and media for *in vitro* maturation, fertilization and culture (Sinclair *et al.*, 2000a). This has been attributed to differences between batches of somatic support cells and sera typically used in these studies, and to the predisposition of batches of oocytes used in *in vitro* embryo production. Nevertheless, its sporadic occurrence has rendered this a rather difficult phenomenon for many groups to study. By contrast, we have developed a system for the *in vitro* culture of sheep embryos that results in the highest reported incidence of aberrant conceptus development (around one in two pregnancies) (Sinclair *et al.*, 2000a), allowing statistical differences at the molecular level to be identified. At present we are uncertain as to what components of this system may contribute to this high incidence, but suspect that animal genotype, the process of ovarian stimulation and the presence or absence of key constituents within the culture media (of which serum is one) play a part. In addition, there is mounting evidence that maternal nutrition plays an important role.

The extreme phenotypes observed with ART-associated LOS in cattle and sheep share many common features with naturally occurring fetal overgrowth syndromes in humans, such as Beckwith–Wiedemann Syndrome (BWS) and Simpson–Golabi–Behmel syndrome, including polyhydramnios, visceromegaly, renal dysplasia and neoplasia (Young *et al.*, 1998; Sinclair *et al.*, 2000a). The great majority of BWS cases occur sporadically, either as a result of paternal trisomy or paternal uniparental disomy, involving a cluster of fetal growth-related imprinted genes on chromosome 11 (11p15.5), including *H19*, *p57KIP2*, *KvLQT1* and *IGF2*. Three independent studies of children affected with BWS have reported a three- to sixfold increase in the incidence amongst children conceived using either IVF or intra-cytoplasmic sperm injection (ICSI), compared with the general population (Maher *et al.*, 2003). In both BWS and in another imprinting syndrome, Angelmann syndrome, the incidence of ART-related cases associated with epigenetic DNA methylation changes in imprinted gene loci, rather than to chromosomal defects, is unusually high (Maher *et al.*, 2003), further suggesting a mechanistic link. Furthermore, direct effects of embryo or murine embryonic stem (ES) cell culture on methylation changes in imprinted genes have been established from a variety of studies (Dean *et al.*, 1998; Doherty *et al.*, 2000; Khosla *et al.*, 2001; Young *et al.*, 2001).

Maternal nutrition and LOS

More recently it has been observed that the nature of the diet offered to zygote donor sheep during the period of ovarian stimulation with follicle-stimulating hormone (FSH) can greatly influence both the incidence and severity of aberrant conceptus development following the transfer of *in vitro*-cultured embryos (Sinclair *et al.*, 2003). The data depicted in Fig. 14.2 relate the heart:fetal weight ratio (×100) of Day 125 fetuses (gestation = 146 days) to blood urea concentrations. Evidence from a number of studies investigating the effects of nitrogen metabolism on fertility in ruminant species indicates a threshold concentration of plasma urea of around 7.5 mmol/l, beyond which embryo development and fertility are compromised (Sinclair *et al.*, 2000b). Data points above the 3 standard deviation line (3 SD) are more than 3 SD above the mean of *in vivo* control fetuses (Fig. 14.2). Numbers in parentheses are fetal weights more than 3 SD above the mean of controls. It is quite apparent that there is a cluster of animals in the top right-hand quadrant that exhibit both aberrant patterns of growth and of development, and these data highlight the importance of maternal nitrogen metabolism around the time of conception.

Lane *et al.* (2001) have also recently provided direct evidence for nitrogen metabolic effects on the murine embryo. High levels of ammonium in the culture media (either through supplementation or spontaneous degradation of amino acids) reduce blastocyst cell number, impair metabolism and pH regulation, increase apoptosis, alter expression of the *H19* imprinted gene and result in

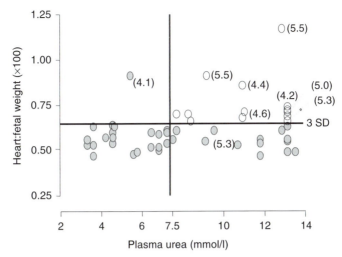

Fig. 14.2. The relationship between heart:fetal weight ratio (×100) in Day 125 fetuses and plasma urea concentrations in donor sheep at the time of zygote recovery and *in vitro* culture. Data in parentheses represent fetal weights > three standard deviations (3 SD) above the mean of the controls. (Sinclair *et al.*, 2003.)

impaired fetal growth. The mechanism by which nitrogen metabolism can affect this programming response in ruminants and mice is not known.

Nutrient provision during early development

Studies in sheep have demonstrated that mothers initiating pregnancy with low nutritional body stores suffer marked impairment of fetal and placental growth if exposed to a further period of undernutrition during mid-pregnancy, whereas mothers well-nourished at conception respond to mid-term dietary restriction by inducing placental hypertrophy (Robinson *et al.*, 1999). More specific evidence of a peri-conceptual effect was obtained in sheep when maternal undernutrition both before and for 7 days after conception resulted in an increase in arterial blood pressure in the late-gestation fetus (Edwards and McMillen, 2002a,b).

Peri-conceptual nutritional effects in rodents have been demonstrated by the widely used 'low-protein rat model', 50% protein restriction supplemented with methionine (to satisfy the high demand for sulphur-containing amino acids for fur production) (Langley-Evans and Jackson, 1996). This dietary treatment has now been shown, in both rats and mice, to result in hypertensive offspring, even when applied for only the first 4 days of pregnancy (Kwong *et al.*, 2000; Jackson *et al.*, 2002; Petrie *et al.*, 2002). In rats and mice this diet induces elevated maternal levels of homocysteine and abnormal growth of the lung, kidney and brain. A low-protein diet in the rat can also permanently alter the function of the developing liver (Byrne and Philips, 2000; Rees *et al.*, 2000). Furthermore, pregnant rats fed a low-protein diet produced offspring with high blood pressure compared to the control group (Langley-Evans, 2001). As discussed below, more defined studies now suggest that an overall deficiency in protein or protein nitrogen is not the cause of programming induced by a low-protein diet; rather, effects of specific amino acids, such as methionine and glycine, may underlie the mechanism (Rees *et al.*, 2000; Jackson *et al.*, 2002; Petrie *et al.*, 2002).

DNA methylation

It is likely that many of the effects of altered nutrition and of the pre-implantation environment arise as a consequence of reprogrammed gene expression, and the favoured mechanism underlying stably inherited changes in gene expression is an epigenetic one. The first evidence that adult phenotype in mice could be affected by epigenetic events in the early embryo came from a study by Wolf Reik and his colleagues in 1993, where zygotic nucleocytoplasmic hybrid embryos were created using nuclear transfer of female pronuclei into a recipient egg from a different strain (Reik *et al.*, 1993). The hybrid mouse pups showed DNA methylation and transcriptional repression of major urinary protein genes in their liver, as well as fetal growth deficiency.

The epigenetic process of DNA methylation is a strong candidate for inducing early programming effects, as it is associated with silenced, heterochromatic DNA and is environmentally influenced by the local availability of methyl groups (Bird, 2002; Friso and Choi, 2002; Rees, 2002). Genomes are organized into regions of dense heterochromatin that are transcriptionally silent, and compartments of more open euchromatin, the sites of gene expression. This bimodal pattern is established early in pre-implantation development. Once set up in a lineage-specific manner, the heterochromatic compartment is then stably inherited through subsequent cell divisions by maintaining the methylation of DNA on the newly replicated strand by the maintenance methyltransferase, DNA methyltransferase 1 (DNMT1). Methyl groups are needed to methylate replicated DNA and to promote cell division, and so sufficient methyl-group donors are required to support the rapid growth of the embryo and conceptus. While early pre-implantation development in the mouse is associated with low levels of DNA methylation (Dean *et al.*, 2001), this is not the case in the sheep (Wilmut *et al.*, 2002; N. Beaujean, R. Meehan and L. Young, unpublished data) and the situation in humans is unknown. However, the inner cell mass of both sheep and mouse embryos (from which the fetus forms and ES cells are derived) shows considerable levels of methylation.

Metabolism of methyl groups

Methyl groups are needed to produce new DNA and to promote cell division, and so sufficient methyl-group donors are required to support the rapid growth of the conceptus. The basic metabolic cycles that supply methyl groups are complicated and involve interactions between a number of different nutrients, as shown in Fig. 14.3. DNA methyltransferases utilize *S*-adenosyl methionine

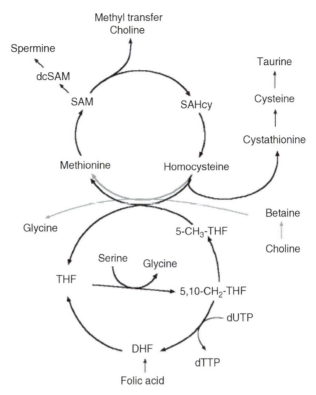

Fig. 14.3. The methionine and folic acid cycles. SAM, *S*-adenosyl methionine; SAHcy, *S*-adenosyl homocysteine; 5-CH$_3$-THF, methyl tetrahyrofolate; 5,10-CH$_2$-THF, methylene tetrahydrofolate; DHF, dihydrofolate; THF, tetrahydrofolate; dUTP, deoxyuridine triphosphate; TTP, thymidine triphosphate; dcSAM, decarboxylated *S*-adenosyl methionine.

(SAM), produced from the amino acid methionine, as the substrate to provide the methyl groups for the modification of DNA. In addition to a range of biosynthetic methylation reactions, SAM is also an important precursor for the synthesis of the polyamines spermine and spermidine, which play a vital role in dividing cells. The current model of SAM action on DNA methylation suggests that an increase in the concentration of SAM alters the kinetics of the DNA methyltransferase reaction, triggering hypermethylation of the site being modified (Detich *et al.*, 2003).

After SAM has donated its methyl group to an acceptor, it is converted to *S*-adenosyl homocysteine (SAHcy) which subsequently loses the adenosine residue to form the non-protein amino acid, homocysteine. This non-protein amino acid is a central intermediate in the metabolism of sulphur in all animals. SAHcy inhibits DNA methyltransferases and therefore its accumulation may lead to hypomethylation of DNA (Chiang, 1998). As the precursor for the bio-synthesis of cysteine, homocysteine can be used to supplement the dietary cysteine supply through biosynthesis. This pathway also produces another non-protein sulphur-containing amino acid, taurine, which has also been shown to be important for fetal development. Feeding a diet containing an excess of methionine increases the conversion of methionine to cystathionine (Rees *et al.*, 1999, 2000).

The remaining homocysteine, not destined for cysteine synthesis, is re-methylated to form methionine. In mammals, two separate enzymes catalyse this step to complete the series of reactions, known as the methionine cycle, shown in the upper part of Fig. 14.3. One enzyme, methionine synthase, utilizes a derivative of folic acid, N^5-methyltetrahydrofolate (MTHF), as the methyl donor. The reaction is mediated by the coenzyme, methylcobalamin, derived from dietary vitamin B_{12}. The activity of this reaction is therefore determined by the availability of two vitamins, folic acid and vitamin B_{12}. A second metabolic cycle, the folate cycle, regenerates N^5-methyltetrahydrofolate using the amino acid serine as the methyl donor (shown in the lower part of Fig. 14.3).

An alternative re-methylation reaction using betaine as the cofactor is also available to convert homocysteine to methionine. Betaine is derived from the breakdown of choline, so the activity of the enzyme homocysteine-betaine methyl transferase is partly determined by the availability of choline in the diet. However, it is important to note that there are large species differences in the relative activity of this enzyme (Snoswell and Xue, 1987). Therefore species with a low homocysteine-betaine methyl transferase activity are more reliant on the folate-dependent reactions, whereas choline plays a very important role in species with a high enzyme activity, such as rodents. When choline is deficient, SAM can be used to synthesize it, further increasing the demand for SAM at a time when betaine is not available to supplement the re-methylation of homocysteine. In ruminants, exogenous methionine is not derived directly from dietary protein but largely from microbial proteins passing from the rumen, and only a very small amount of methionine is derived from the diet. Under these circumstances single-carbon metabolism is modified and *de novo* methylneogenesis increased, with a significant elevation in homocysteine-betaine methyl transferase activity (Snoswell and Xue, 1987). Consequently the vitamin B_{12} deficiency resulting from a restricted dietary intake of cobalt reduces homocysteine-betaine methyl transferase activity in a variety of tissues (Kennedy *et al.*, 1992).

DNA methylation and disease

A wide range of studies has now shown that diets that are low in folate, methionine, glycine and choline, known generically as 'methyl-deficient diets', can promote cancer and other diseases (Choi and Mason, 2000; Ehrlich, 2000; Kimura *et al.*, 2001). Often, human diets are likely to be deficient in methionine and folate, leading to a low availability of methyl groups (Choi and Mason, 2000). This is particularly important for humans as they have a low homocysteine-betaine methyl transferase activity, therefore diets low in folate increase plasma homocysteine concentrations. In adults, elevated plasma homocysteine is now widely considered as a correlate of elevated cardiovascular disease risk. Elevated homocysteine is also associated with persistent miscarriage, pre-eclampsia and the development of neural tube defects (Nelen et al., 2000).

Supplementation with vitamins B_6, B_{12}, folic acid and betaine have all been shown effectively to lower homocysteine levels in human blood. In the Physicians Health Study undertaken in Harvard, the risk of myocardial infarction was threefold higher in those patients with the highest 5% of homocysteine levels. The homocyteine-associated risk was strongly enhanced by hypertension. However, it is not yet clear whether elevated homocysteine is a direct cause of cardiovascular problems (although it is toxic to cells lining blood vessels) or an indicator of an indirect pathogenic process, such as epigenetically programmed alterations in gene expression. The association of DNA methylation changes with disease is an emerging field. The association with cancer has long been well documented (Ehrlich, 2000); however, the development of genome wide methylation profiling assays now makes the study of other diseases more feasible.

One disease of interest in the fetal origins of adult disease context is type 2 diabetes. Non-insulin-dependent diabetes is the subject of a current DNA methylation profiling study undertaken by the German biotechnology company, Epigenomics, using combined-array- and mass-spectrometry-based analysis technologies that allow the analysis of up to 50,000 methylation positions per day (Maier and Olek, 2002). Diabetic disease progression has recently been found to be associated with decreased blood concentrations of SAM and altered MTHF activity (Poirier et al., 2001). It is suggested that aberrant DNA methylation patterns are laid down early in the development of insulin target tissues and may thus lead to insulin resistance in adult life (Maier and Olek, 2002). In terms of the pre-implantation embryo, Moley (1999) also demonstrates significant developmental effects of maternal diabetes on the GLUT1 transporter gene at the blastocyst stage in mice. The down-regulation of this gene resulted in decreased glucose transport into the blastocyst, lowering glucose levels within the embryonic cells at a time when glucose is the key energy substrate. The current challenge is to establish whether there is a mechanistic link between early nutrition and altered DNA methylation.

DNA methylation and nutrition

Initial clues to a potential mechanism linking nutrient provision and fetal programming arose from murine dams fed with high levels of methyl donors (folate, choline, betaine and vitamin B_{12}), resulting in altered gene expression of the agouti locus and coat colour (Wolff et al., 1998). This has recently been confirmed to be caused by an epigenetic increase in transposable element DNA methylation within the agouti locus (Waterland and Jirtle, 2003). This transposable element contains a promoter-like sequence, which stimulates expression of the gene and determines the coat colour of the offspring. Thus, in this experimental paradigm, the adult phenotype is dependent on the provision of methyl supplements in the maternal diet and is independent of the genotype.

In the more widely used rat models of nutritional programming, a number of observations suggest a link with methyl-group metabolism. For example, dietary excess of methionine leads to an increase in plasma homocysteine in rat dams during early gestation (Petrie *et al.*, 2002). There are also changes in the ratio of SAM:S-adenosyl homocysteine (SAH; an inhibitor of DNA methylation) in the maternal liver. The effects of these changes on the early stages of embryonic and fetal development are as yet unknown. It is clear, however, that later in gestation the excess of methionine increases global DNA methylation in the fetal liver and, in extreme cases, leads to neonatal mortality, probably as a result of liver and kidney damage (Fontanier-Razzaq *et al.*, 2002). These changes in organ growth appear to be the result of changes in cellularity, reflected by a lower DNA content. Furthermore, these changes in the growth of the organs may be consistent with the observation that there is an increase in blood pressure in the offspring of dams exposed to these diets early in the postconception period (Kwong *et al.*, 2000). Changes in adiposity and glucose tolerance reported for the offspring of rats fed the low-protein diets are a result of interactions with other dietary components, and are not believed to be associated with the excess of methionine. The maternal low-protein diet in rats permanently alters the structure and function of the fetal liver, reducing anabolic glucokinase and glutamine synthase and increasing catabolic enzyme activities (Burns *et al.*, 1997). This may predispose the liver to produce, rather than use, glucose.

The observation that glycine supplementation can prevent the hypertensive effects of a low-protein diet (Jackson *et al.*, 2002) provides further evidence for the methyl cycle effect, since glycine metabolism drives the further production of SAM. Since the low-protein diet is associated with excess methionine, degraded methionine would increase glycine utilization. Thus Jackson *et al.* (2002) suggest that the effects of glycine supplementation may limit the damaging effects of methionine or its metabolic products, such as homocysteine, on the maternal, fetal or placental compartments. Rats have a high requirement for sulphur-containing amino acids for fur formation. If excess to requirements, degraded methionine would increase glycine utilization. We suggest that the observed increases in homocysteine in low-protein dietary experiments are likely to be due to its production when excess methionine is metabolized to cysteine (Petrie *et al.*, 2002). Elevated plasma homocysteine elevates SAH, inhibits methyl donation from SAM, reduces DNA methylation and correlates with developmental abnormalities (Chen *et al.*, 2001). In our low-protein-diet studies, maternal, but not fetal, glycine concentration was increased (Rees *et al.*, 1999). Jackson *et al.* (2002) have suggested that increased maternal glycine might increase the drive to cross the placenta. Marginal glycine levels may be available during human pregnancies on low-protein diets (Jackson *et al.*, 1996) and it is interesting to note that folate deficiency can further limit glycine availability (Arnstein and Stankovic, 1956). Homocysteine clearance by re-methylation to methionine can also occur using the enzyme methyltetrahydrofolate reductase but, in the process, folate deficiency is incurred, providing an alternative means of inducing early pregnancy loss and fetal defects.

Methyl-deficient diets are not commonly studied during pregnancy in the sheep, where methyl groups are usually provided by rumen microorganisms, rather than from direct nutrition. However, dietary deficiency in vitamin B_{12} can be induced in adults by dietary cobalt deficiency, resulting in appetite reduction and weight gain (Marston, 1970). By imposing cobalt-deficiency-induced vitamin B_{12} deficiency in lambs, Kennedy *et al.* (1992) found that methionine synthase activity (catalysing the transfer of methyl groups from 5-methyltetrahydrofolate to homocysteine) was significantly reduced in the liver, kidney and spinal cord. The SAM:SAH ratio was reduced in liver, suggesting that activity of SAM-dependent methyltransferase enzymes would be impaired, and the plasma homocysteine concentrations were also elevated. Thus natural dietary deficiencies in sheep, as in rats and humans, can alter components of the methyl cycle, providing an experimental means for direct application of fetal or embryonic programming studies in this organism. This is a major focus of our current research.

Role of DNA Methylation in Programming the Embryo

During pre-implantation development, when the embryo is free-living in the oviduct and uterus, maternal nutrients may have a much more direct effect on development than postplacentation. In addition, the extensive chromatin remodelling occurring during pre-implantation development, when the structurally diverse sperm and oocyte chromatin structures combine, means that DNA methylation reprogramming is highly dynamic (Young and Fairburn, 2000; Reik *et al.*, 2001; Li, 2002) and may induce particularly severe programming effects at this time. For this brief period, transposable elements incorporated into mammalian genomes through the course of evolution can be temporarily expressed through loss of DNA methylation-mediated silencing (Walsh *et al.*, 1998) and perturbation of this process by methyl-donor nutrients has been demonstrated, at least at the agouti locus in mice (Waterland and Jirtle, 2003). Since the human genome comprises over 35% transposable elements, and 4% of these are found within genes, such sequences may be more susceptible to dietary alteration early in development and thus are prime candidates for the programming mechanism. Other candidates include imprinted gene loci, as discussed below.

Imprinted genes

The genes most likely to be involved in nutritional programming during early development remain to be clarified. Several imprinted genes are potent determinants of birthweight and specific genes can affect development of specific organs and the placenta, making this group of monallelically expressed genes strong candidates for mediating disease programming (Jirtle *et al.*, 2000; Young, 2001). As candidate mediators of the proposed epigenetic basis for nutritionally programmed effects leading to impaired fetal development and adult disease, imprinted genes may be particularly vulnerable to disruptions in DNA methylation during oogenesis and pre-implantation embryogenesis, when methylation imprints are established and maintained (Young, 2001; Kiersenbaum, 2002).

Around 60 imprinted genes have been identified in the mouse genome and, of those so far examined, around half are expressed in the placenta (Reik *et al.*, 2003). In the mouse, most imprinted genes are not monoallelically expressed until after implantation. In contrast, the *IGF2* gene is already monoallelically expressed by the blastocyst stage in the human embryo (Lighten *et al.*, 1997) and is also monoallelically expressed prior to implantation in the sheep embryo (McLaren and Montgomery, 1999). These observations highlight the importance of choosing the best available model for human embryo studies, on the basis of similarities in biology. Working with sheep, we have recently demonstrated that imprinted genes can be disrupted in the pre-implantation embryo by *in vitro* culture and somatic cell nuclear transfer, and that this can lead to aberrations in conceptus growth and development (Young *et al.*, 2001, 2003). Whether nutrition can induce a similar effect now requires a direct test.

Effects of *in vitro* culture on methyl cycle activity

Serum is a rather poorly defined media constituent, known to result in epigenetic alterations in gene expression in both the mouse and sheep embryo (Doherty *et al.*, 2000; Young *et al.*, 2001). Serum added to embryo culture also increases both the incidence and severity of aberrant fetal phenotypes in cattle, sheep and mice (Sinclair *et al.*, 1999, 2000a; Khosla *et al.*, 2001). Working with a similar batch of serum to that used in earlier LOS studies (Sinclair *et al.*, 1999; Young *et al.*, 2001), we have recently begun to investigate the effects of serum on the methylation status of blastocysts (Rooke *et al.*, 2003). Bovine oocytes were matured, fertilized and then cultured in our standard synthetic oviductal fluid medium (SOF; Tervit *et al.*, 1972), either in the presence or absence of serum, according to the method of Sinclair *et al.* (2000b). SAM and SAHcy were measured in bovine blastocysts (two blastocysts per assay) by pulse labelling (2 h) with (^{35}S)methionine. Including steer serum in the medium used to culture blastocysts increased the incorporation of label into SAM compared to our basal medium of SOF plus albumin (2278 versus 899 pmol per two blastocysts per 2 h, $P < 0.01$), and also tended to reduce incorporation into SAHcy (126 versus 205 pmol per two blastocysts per 2 h, $P < 0.1$). As a result, the ratio of SAM to SAHcy was increased from 8 to 26 when cow serum was included in SOF ($P < 0.05$). Therefore serum, known to perturb epigenetic markers during *in vitro* culture (Young *et al.*, 2001), changed the methyl-group availability in bovine blastocysts.

Genetic and programmed variability

The high degree of variability in the expression of aberrant fetal development in the LOS study of Young *et al.* (2001) and related studies, even for full-sibling fetuses derived from embryos cultured in the same micro-drop environment, suggests a variable predisposition of the oocyte prior to embryo culture (Sinclair *et al.*, 2000a). This variability may have arisen as a consequence of the inherent genetic variability that exists between oocytes from a single donor animal (Young, 2001). Oocyte cytoplasmic influences on DNA methylation, resulting in growth deficiency, have been observed in mouse experiments with zygotes of mixed genotype (Reik et al., 1993). The extent of DNA methylation in fetal tissues depends on methyl enzyme polymorphisms that act to determine the abundance of methyl groups (Friso and Choi, 2002). Genes for methyl-group metabolizing enzymes such as methyltetrahydrofolate reductase, methionine synthase and cystathione β-synthetase, have specific alleles that predispose to cancer and cardiovascular disease in adults through elevated plasma homo-cysteine, a determinant of methyl-group availability (Ueland et al., 2001). It is part of our working hypothesis, therefore, that nutritional challenges that compromise DNA methylation will be exacerbated in fetuses and/or mothers exhibiting such genetic traits. The most common MTHF mutation affects around 12% of the population and so can create significant variability in nutritional response. Gillman (2002) has pointed out that what is genetic for the mother is environmental for the fetus, citing that the maternal thermolabile allele of methyltetrahydrofolate reductase may confer risk of neural tube defects even in a fetus with normal genotype (Wenstrom, 2002).

DNA methyltransferases

The functional DNA methyltransferases direct methyl groups directly on to the DNA (Bird, 2002). DNMT3L has been identified recently as specifically influenc-ing the methylation of imprinted genes during oogenesis (Hata et al., 2002). Alterations in the expression of the methyltransferases have been observed in a wide variety of human tumours, where alterations in DNA methylation are a common feature (Reid et al., 2002). Thus, in addition to methyl-group availabil-ity induced by experimental diets, DNA methylation is also dependent on the expression of the DNA methyltransferase enzymes. As DNMT1, 3a, 3b and 3L are all expressed in mature oocytes (H. Fairburn, J. Taylor and L. Young, unpublished data), their deposition during oogenesis may be incomplete in some smaller antral follicles prematurely ovulated after FSH stimulation. Such variable expression of the DNA methyltransferases may provide a further variable determining the ultimate extent of methylation in the oocyte and pre-implantation embryo. Since gene expression is more easily, quickly and inexpensively determined than DNA methylation in routine assays, differences may provide the basis of more routine screening methods for use in oocytes/pre-implantation embryos.

The most accepted current model of SAM action on DNA methylation is that an increased concentration of SAM stimulates DNA methyltransferase action, triggering hypermethylation, and that this protects the genome against cancer risk by preventing global hypomethylation and activation of oncogenes (Detich et al., 2003). SAH, on the other hand, inhibits DNA methyltransferases (Chiang, 1998). However, it has recently been suggested that SAM also results in hyper-methylation of DNA by inhibiting the action of the methyl DNA binding protein 2 (Mbd2) 'demethylase' (Detich et al., 2003), an enzyme whose functionality has been the subject of recent controversy (Bhattacharya _et al._, 1999; Ng _et al._, 1999; Ramchandani _et al._, 1999). In addition to _in vitro_ demethylation assays, support may be given to this mechanism by the observation that methyl-deficient diets hypermethylated liver DNA although most liver cells are postmitotic and do not undergo replication (Poirier _et al._, 2001). This is a prerequisite for maintenance of DNA methylation.

Clinical relevance

In addition to dietary restriction, nutritional supplements commonly taken during pregnancy, especially folate and vitamin B_{12}, are potent regulators of methyl-group availability and hence may be very effective in determining embryonic and fetal epigenetic programming. As folate supplementation is only common-place within women actively intending pregnancy, lack of supplementation may induce previously uninvestigated changes that are less dramatic than the well-investigated neural tube defects. Alteration in DNA methylation by dietary methyl supplementation throughout pregnancy in the agouti mouse altered the phenotype to one that enjoyed increased adult health and longevity (Cooney _et al._, 2002), suggesting the possibility for nutritional intervention. Studies providing an insight into the efficacy of dietary influences on methyl-group availability in programming oocyte quality, and ultimately promoting adult health, are now timely. Elucidation of the importance of interactions with genotype, and exploring the possible influence of heterogeneity in DNA methyltransferase expression between oocytes, are also key elements that may provide novel potential markers of oocyte quality and developmental potential. In addition, definition of the mechanisms by which methyl-group availability to the oocyte can be altered (e.g. nutrition, superovulation or embryo culture) would provide an important route for developing improved assisted reproduction procedures.

Embryonic stem cells: a model for the future?

The application of assisted reproduction technologies, such as _in vitro_ fertilization and embryo culture, may also programme development through a similar mechanism to that proposed here for methyl-donor-related nutrients. Since the availability of a controlled, normal population of human embryos is not available for investigation of these questions, we now propose that human embryonic stem cells (hESC) provide an ideal system in which to model and test the pre-implantation effects of specific nutrients/_in vitro_ culture environments on DNA methylation, and to assess their phenotypic effects on relevant differenti-ated tissues in the fetus. In order to establish directly the metabolic events medi-ating nutrient–gene interactions by epigenetic programming, cultures of hESC could be assayed for key components of the methyl cycle and tested for the influence of various methyl-donor enzyme polymorphisms. The programmed effects on DNA methylation after _in vitro_ differentiation of hESC into fetal cell types could then be investigated. This approach will allow the first test of the hypothesis outlined in this chapter in a human embryonic system.

Conclusion

Although compelling evidence exists from a variety of sources that DNA methylation can be programmed in ways that can induce adult disease phenotypes, the strong suggestion that this mechanism may also variably programme the oocyte and pre-implantation embryo, depending on the dietary effect on methyl-group metabolism, remains to be evaluated. Newer evidence that histone methylation may also be a heritable epigenetic modification also merits study of nutritional effects on this process. We suggest that the health implications for human pregnancy and infertility now merit testing of these hypotheses.

References

Arnstein, H.R.V. and Stankovic, V. (1956) The effect of certain vitamin deficiencies on glycine biosynthesis. *Biochemical Journal* 62, 190–198.

Barker, D.J. (1998) *In utero* programming of chronic disease. *Clinical Science* 95, 115–128.

Barker, D.J. and Osmond, C. (1986) Infant mortality, childhood nutrition, and ischaemic heart disease in England and Wales. *Lancet* I, 1077–1081.

Bhattacharya, S.K., Ramchandani, S., Cervoni, N. and Szyf, M. (1999) A mammalian protein with specific demethylase activity for mCpG DNA. *Nature* 397, 579–583.

Bird, A. (2002) DNA methylation patterns and epigenetic memory. *Genes and Development* 16, 6–21

Burns, S.P., Desai, M., Cohen, R.D., Hales, C.N., Iles, R.A., Germain, J.P., Going, T.C.H. and Bailey, R.A. (1997) Gluconeogenesis, glucose handling, and structural changes in livers of the adult offspring of rats partially deprived of protein during pregnancy and lactation. *Journal of Clinical Investigation* 100, 1768–1774.

Byrne, C.D. and Philips, D.I. (2000) Fetal origins of adult disease: epidemiology and mechanisms. *Journal of Clinical Pathology* 53, 822–828.

Chen, Z.T., Karaplis, A.C., Ackerman, S.L., Pogribny, I.P., Melnyk, S., Lussier-Cacan, S., Chen, M.F., Pai, A., John, S.W.M., Smith, R.S., Bottiglieri, T., Bagley, P., Selhub, J., Rudnicki, M.A., James, S.J. and Rozen, R. (2001) Mice deficient in methylenetetra-hydrofolate reductase exhibit hyperhomocysteinemia and decreased methylation capacity, with neuropathology and aortic lipid deposition. *Human Molecular Genetics* 10, 433–443.

Chiang, P.K. (1998) Biological effects of inhibitors of S-adenosylhomocysteine hydrolase. *Pharmacology and Therapeutics* 77, 115–134.

Choi, S.W. and Mason, J.B. (2000) Folate and carcinogenesis: an integrated scheme. *Journal of Nutrition* 130, 129–132.

Cooney, C.A., Dave, A.A. and Wolff, G.L. (2002) Maternal methyl supplements in mice affect epigenetic variation and DNA methylation of offspring. *Journal of Nutrition* 132, 2393S–2400S.

Dean, W., Bowden, L., Aitchison, A., Klose, J., Moore, T., Meneses, J.J., Reik, W. and Feil, R. (1998) Altered imprinted gene methylation and expression in completely

ES-cell derived mouse fetuses: association with aberrant phenotypes. *Development* 125, 2273–2282.

Dean, W., Santos, F., Stojkovic, M., Zakhartchenko, V., Walter, J., Wolf, E. and Reik, W. (2001) Conservation of methylation reprogramming in mammalian development: aberrant reprogramming in cloned embryos. *Proceedings of the National Academy of Sciences USA* 98, 13734–13738.

Detich, N., Hamm, S., Just, G., Knox, J.D. and Szyf, M. (2003) The methyl donor *S*-adenosylmethionine inhibits active demethylation of DNA: a candidate novel mechanism for the pharmacological effects of *S*-adenosylmethionine. *Journal of Biological Chemistry* 278, 20812–20820.

Doherty, A.S., Mann, M.R., Tremblay, K.D., Bartolomei, M.S. and Schultz, R.A. (2000) Differential effects of culture on imprinted H19 expression in the preimplantation mouse embryo. *Biology of Reproduction* 62, 1526–1535.

Edwards, L.J. and McMillen, I.C. (2002a) Impact of maternal undernutrition during the periconceptional period, fetal number, and fetal sex on the development of the hypothalamo-pituitary adrenal axis in sheep during late gestation. *Biology of Reproduction* 66, 1562–1569.

Edwards, L.J. and McMillen, I.C. (2002b) Periconceptional nutrition programs development of the cardiovascular system in the fetal sheep. *American Journal of Physiology* 283, R669–R679.

Ehrlich, M. (2000) DNA hypomethylation and cancer. In: Ehrlich, M. (ed.) *DNA Alterations in Cancer*. Eaton Publishing, Natick, Massachusetts, pp. 273–291.

Ertzeid, G. and Storeng, R. (2001) The impact of ovarian stimulation on implantation and fetal development in mice. *Human Reproduction* 16, 221–225.

Fontanier-Razzaq, N., Harries, D.N., Hay, S.M. and Rees, W.D. (2002) Amino acid deficiency up-regulates specific mRNAs in murine embryonic cells. *Journal of Nutrition* 132, 2137–2142.

Friso, S. and Choi, S.W. (2002) Gene–nutrient interactions and DNA methylation. *Journal of Nutrition* 132, 2382S–2387S.

Gandolfi, T.A. and Gandolfi, F. (2001) The maternal legacy to the embryo: cytoplasmic components and their effects on early development. *Theriogenology* 55, 1255–1276.

Gillman, M.W. (2002) Breast-feeding and obesity. *Journal of Pediatrics* 141, 749–757.

Hales, C.N. and Barker, D.J. (1992) Type 2 (non-insulin-dependent) diabetes mellitus: the thrifty phenotype hypothesis. *Diabetologia* 35, 595–601.

Hansen, M., Kurinczuk, J.J., Bower, C. and Webb, S. (2002) The risk of major birth defects after intracytoplasmic sperm injection and *in vitro* fertilization. *New England Journal of Medicine* 346, 725–730.

Hata, K., Okano, M., Lei, H. and Li, E. (2002) Dnmt3L cooperates with the Dmbt3 family of *de novo* DNA methyltransferases to establish maternal imprints in mice. *Development* 129, 1983–1993.

Jackson, A.A., Persaud, C., Meakins, T.S. and Bundy, R. (1996) Urinary excretion of 5-L-oxoproline (pyroglutamic acid) is increased in normal adults consuming vegetarian or low protein diets. *Journal of Nutrition* 126, 2813–2822.

Jackson, A.A., Dunn, R.L., Marchand, M.C. and Langley-Evans, S.C. (2002) Increased systolic blood pressure in rats induced by maternal low-protein diet is reversed by dietary supplementation with glycine. *Clinical Science* 103, 633–639.

Jirtle, R.L., Sander, M. and Barrett, J.C. (2000) Genomic imprinting and environmental disease susceptibility. *Environmental Health Perspectives* 108, 271–278.

Kennedy, D.G., Blanchflower, W.J., Scot, J.M., Weir, D.G., Molloy, A.M., Kennedy, S. and Young, P.B. (1992) Cobalt–vitamin B-12 deficiency decreases methionine synthase activity and phospholipid methylation in sheep. *Journal of Nutrition* 122, 1384–1390.

Khosla, S., Dean, W., Brown, D., Reik, W. and Feil, R. (2001) Culture of preimplantation mouse embryos affects fetal development and the expression of imprinted genes. *Biology of Reproduction* 64, 918–926.

Kiersenbaum, A.L. (2002) Genomic imprinting and epigenetic reprogramming: unearthing the garden of forking paths. *Molecular Reproduction and Development* 63, 269–272.

Kimura, F., Florl, A.R., Steinhoff, C., Golka, K., Willers, R., Seifert, H.-H. and Schulz, W.A. (2001) Polymorphic methyl group metabolism genes in patients with transitional cell carcinoma of the urinary bladder. *Mutation Research and Genomics* 458, 49–54.

Kwong, W.Y., Wild, A.E., Roberts, P., Willis, A.C. and Fleming, T.P. (2000) Maternal undernutrition during the preimplantation period of rat development causes blastocyst abnormalities and programming of postnatal hypertension. *Development* 127, 4195–4202.

Lane, M., Hooper, K. and Gardner, D.K. (2001) Effect of essential amino acids on mouse embryo viability and ammonium production. *Journal of Assisted Reproduction and Genetics* 18, 519–525.

Langley-Evans, S.C. (2001) Fetal programming of cardiovascular function through exposure to maternal undernutrition. *Proceedings of the Nutrition Society* 60, 505–513.

Langley-Evans, S.C. and Jackson, A.A. (1996) Rats with hypertension induced by *in utero* exposure to maternal low-protein diets fail to increase blood pressure in response to a high salt intake. *Annals of Nutrition and Metabolism* 40, 1–9.

Li, E. (2002) Chromatin modification and epigenetic reprogramming in mammalian development. *Nature Reviews Genetics* 3, 662–673.

Lighten, A.D., Hardy, K., Winston, R.M. and Moore, G.E. (1997) IGF2 is parentally imprinted in human preimplantation embryos. *Nature Genetics* 15, 122–123.

Maher, E.R., Brueton, L.A., Bowdin, S.C., Luharia, A., Cooper, W., Cole, T.R., Macdonald, F., Sampson, J.R., Barratt, C.L., Reik, W. and Hawkins, M.M. (2003) Beckwith–Wiedemann syndrome and assisted reproduction technology (ART) *Journal of Medical Genetics* 40, 62–64.

Maier, S. and Olek, A. (2002) Diabetes: a candidate disease for efficient DNA methylation profiling. *Journal of Nutrition* 132(suppl. 8), 2440S–2443S.

Marston, H.R. (1970) The requirement of sheep for cobalt or for vitamin B-12. *British Journal of Nutrition* 24, 615–633.

McEvoy, T.G., Robinson, J.J. and Sinclair, K.D. (2001) Developmental consequences of embryo and cell manipulation in mice and farm animals. *Reproduction* 122, 507–518.

McLaren, R.J. and Montgomery, G.W. (1999) Genomic imprinting of the insulin-like growth factor 2 gene in sheep. *Mammalian Genome* 10, 588–591.

Moley, K.H. (1999) Diabetes and preimplantation events of embryogenesis. *Seminars in Reproduction and Endocrinology* 17, 137–151.

Moll, A.C., Imhof, S.M., Schouten-van Meeteren, A.Y. and van Leeuwen, F.E. (2003) *In vitro* fertilisation and retinoblastoma in human ART. *Lancet* 361, 1392.

Nelen, W.L.D.M., Blom, H.J., Steegers, E.A., den Heijer, M., Thomas, C.M. and Eskes, T.K. (2000) Homocysteine and folate levels as risk factors for recurrent early pregnancy loss. *Obstetrics and Gynaecology* 4, 519–524.

Ng, H.H., Zhang, Y., Hendrich, B., Johnson, C.A., Turner, B.M., Erdjument-Bromage, H., Tempst, P., Reinberg, D. and Bird, A. (1999) MBD2 is a transcriptional repressor belonging to the MeCP1 histone deacetylase complex. *Nature Genetics* 23, 58–61.

Petrie, L., Duthie, S.J., Rees, W.D. and McConnell, J.M.L. (2002) Serum concentrations of homocysteine are elevated during early pregnancy in rodent models of fetal programming. *British Journal of Nutrition* 88, 471–477.

Poirier, L.A., Brown, A.T., Fink, L.M., Wise, C.K., Randolph, C.J., Delongchamp, R.R. and Fonseca, V.A. (2001) Blood S-adenosylmethionine concentrations and lymphocyte methylenetetrahydrofolate reductase activity in diabetes mellitus and diabetic nephropathy. *Metabolism* 50, 1014–1018.

Ramchandani, S., Bhattacharya, S.K., Cervoni, N. and Szyf, M. (1999) DNA methylation is a reversible biological signal. *Proceedings of the National Academy of Sciences USA* 96, 6107–6112.

Rees, W.D. (2002) Manipulating the sulphur amino acid content of the early diet and its implications for long term health. *Proceedings of the Nutrition Society* 61, 1–7.

Rees, W.D., Hay, S.M., Fontanier-Razzaq, N.C., Antipatis, C. and Harries, D.N. (1999) Expression of the growth arrest genes (gas and gadd) changes during organogenesis in the rat fetus. *Journal of Nutrition* 129, 1532–1536.

Rees, W.D., Hay, S.M., Brown, D.S., Antipatis, C. and Palmer, R.M. (2000) Hyper-methylation of DNA in the liver of rat fetuses is a result of maternal protein deficiency. *Journal of Nutrition* 130, 1821–1826.

Reid, G.K., Besterman, J.M. and MacLeod, A.R. (2002) Selective inhibition of DNA methyltransferase enzymes as a novel strategy for cancer treatment. *Current Opinion in Molecular Therapy* 4, 130–137.

Reik, W., Romer, I., Barton, S.C., Surani, M.A., Howlett, S.K. and Klose, J. (1993) Adult phenotpye in the mouse can be affected by epigenetic events in the early embryo. *Development* 119, 933–942.

Reik, W., Dean, W. and Walter, J. (2001) Epigenetic reprogramming in mammalian development. *Science* 293, 1089–1093.

Reik, W., Constancia, M., Fowden, A., Anderson, N., Dean, W., Ferguson-Smith, A., Tycko, B. and Sibley, C. (2003) Regulation of supply and demand for maternal nutrients in mammals by imprinted genes. *Journal of Physiology* 547, 35–44.

Robinson, J.J., Sinclair, K.D. and McEvoy, T.G. (1999) Nutritional effects on foetal growth. *Animal Science* 68, 315–331.

Rooke, J.A., Anderson, J., Staines, M.E. and Sinclair, K.D. (2003) Quantification of S-adenosylmethionine (SAM) and S-adenosyl homocysteine (SAH) in bovine granulose cells (BGC) and blastocysts under differing cultural conditions. *Reproduction Abstract Series* July, p. 54.

Schieve, L.A., Meikle, S.F., Ferre, C., Peterson, H.B., Jeng, G. and Wilcox, L.S. (2002) Low and very low birth weight in infants conceived with the use of assisted reproductive technology. *New England Journal of Medicine* 346, 731–737.

Shi, W. and Haaf, T. (2002) Aberrant methylation patterns at the two-cell stage as an indicator of early developmental failure. *Molecular Reproduction and Development* 63, 329–334.

Sinclair, K.D., McEvoy, T.G., Maxfield, E.K., Maltin, C.A., Young, L.E., Wilmut, I., Broadbent, P.J. and Robinson, J.J. (1999) Aberrant fetal growth and development following *in vitro* culture of sheep zygotes. *Journal of Reproduction and Fertility* 116, 177–186.

Sinclair, K.D., Young, L.E., Wilmut, I. and McEvoy, T.G. (2000a) *In utero* overgrowth in ruminants following embryo culture: lessons from mice and a warning to men. *Human Reproduction* 15(suppl. 5), 68–86.

Sinclair, K.D., Kuran, M., Gebbie, F.E., Webb, R. and McEvoy, T.G. (2000b) Nitrogen metabolism and fertility in cattle: II. Development of oocytes recovered from heifers offered diets differing in their rate of nitrogen release in the rumen. *Journal of Animal Science* 78, 2670–2680.

Sinclair, K.D., Powell, K.A., McEvoy, T.G., Ashworth, C.J., Rooke, J.A., Young, L.E., Wilmut, I. and Robinson, J.J. (2003) Zygote donor nutrition affects ovine fetal development following *in vitro* embryo culture. *Reproduction, Abstract Series* 30, 55–56.

Snoswell, A.M. and Xue, G.P. (1987) Methyl group metabolism in sheep. *Comparative Biochemistry and Physiology* 88B, 383–394.

Taylor, J., Fairburn, H., Beaujean, N., Meehan, R. and Young, L.E. (2003) Gene expression in the developing embryo and fetus. *Reproduction Suppl.* 61, 151–165.

Tervit, H.R., Whittingham, D.G. and Rowson, L.E.A. (1972) Successful culture *in vitro* of sheep and cattle ova. *Journal. Reproduction and Fertility* 30, 493–497.

Ueland, P.M., Hustad, S., Schneede, J., Refsum, H. and Vollset, S.E. (2001) Biological and clinical implications of the MTHFR C677T polymorphism. *Trends in Pharmacological Sciences* 22, 195–201.

Van der Auwera, I. and D'Hooghe, T. (2001) Superovulation of female mice delays embryonic and fetal development. *Human Reproduction* 16, 1237–1243.

Walsh, C.P., Chaillet, J.R. and Bestor, T.H. (1998) Transcription of IAP endogenous retroviruses is constrained by cytosine methylation. *Nature Genetics* 20, 116–117.

Waterland, R.A. and Jirtle, R.L. (2003) Transposable elements: targets for early nutritional effects on epigenetic gene regulation. *Molecular and Cellular Biology* 23, 5293–5300.

Wenstrom, K.D. (2002) Fragile X and other trinucleotide repeat diseases. *Obstetrics and Gynecology Clinics of North America* 29, 367–388.

Wilmut, I., Beaujean, N., de Sousa, P.A., Dinnyes, A., King, T.J., Paterson, L.A., Wells, D.N. and Young, L.E. (2002) Somatic cell nuclear transfer. *Nature* 419, 583–586.

Wolff, G.L., Kodell, R.L., Moore, S.R. and Cooney, G.A. (1998) Maternal epigenetics and methyl supplements affect *agouti* gene expression in A^{vy}/a mice. *FASEB Journal* 12, 949–957.

Young, L.E. (2001) Imprinting of genes and the Barker hypothesis. *Twin Research* 4, 307–317.

Young, L.E. and Fairburn, H.R. (2000) Improving the safety of embryo technologies: possible role of genomic imprinting. *Theriogenology* 53, 627–648.

Young, L.E., Sinclair, K.D. and Wilmut, I. (1998) Large offspring syndrome in ruminants. *Reviews of Reproduction* 3, 155–163.

Young, L.E., Fernandes, K., McEvoy, T.G., Butterwith, S.C., Guttierez, C., Carolan, C., Broadbent, P.J., Robinson, J.J., Wilmut, I. and Sinclair, K.D. (2001) Epigenetic change in *IGF2R* is associated with fetal overgrowth after sheep embryo culture. *Nature Genetics* 27, 153–154.

Young, L.E., Schnieke, A.E., McCreath, K.J., Wieckowski, S., Konfortova, G., Fernandes, K., Ptak, G., Kind, A., Wilmut, I., Loi, P. and Feil, R. (2003) Conservation of *IGF2-H19* and *IGF2R* imprinting in sheep: effects of somatic cell nuclear transfer. *Mechanisms in Development* 120, 1433–1442.

15 Endocrine Responses to Fetal Undernutrition: the Growth Hormone–Insulin-like Growth Factor Axis

MICHAEL E. SYMONDS, DAVID S. GARDNER, SARAH PEARCE AND TERENCE STEPHENSON

Academic Division of Child Health, School of Human Development, Queen's Medical Centre, University Hospital, Nottingham NG7 2UH, UK

Introduction

Growth hormone (GH) and insulin-like growth factors (IGFs) are members of either the class I, cytokine-receptor superfamily that encompasses other fetal hormones, including prolactin, or tyrosine kinase/mannose-6-phosphate receptors, all of which are implicated in the growth and maturation of the fetus (Symonds *et al.*, 2001a). Each hormone may have a direct and indirect role in regulating fetal responsiveness to undernutrition.

During pregnancy, the overall control of GH and IGF secretion resides primarily within the placenta and the fetal liver (Anthony *et al.*, 1995). A more important regulatory role for the placenta in modulating the programming effects of nutrient restriction is therefore predicted prior to the establishment of central control mechanisms within the fetus during late gestation. In contrast, during the embryonic period the maternal nutritional environment will have an overriding influence in regulating endocrine exposure and sensitivity of the conceptus. Within the fetal GH–IGF system, the magnitude of fetal response is dependent on the degree of maturity of the hypothalamic–pituitary–adrenal axis. For species in which this axis is immature at birth, such as rodents, a minimal fetal response to undernutrition would be expected.

In terms of reviewing our current knowledge of the fetal endocrine responses to undernutrition, it is important to have an established developmental framework which then enables us to understand why the fetal consequences can vary substantially. The stage of gestation will have a substantial influence on the mechanisms involved and the extent to which the mother, placenta or fetus are the primary sites of endocrine responsiveness (Fig. 15.1). It is also critical to remember that many consequences of fetal undernutrition are manifest in the absence of any gross change in fetal body or organ weights (Symonds *et al.*,

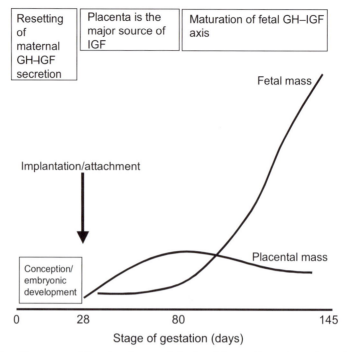

| Resetting of maternal GH–IGF secretion | Placenta is the major source of IGF | Maturation of fetal GH–IGF axis |

Fetal mass

Implantation/attachment

Conception/ embryonic development

Placental mass

| 0 | 28 | 80 | 145 |

Stage of gestation (days)

Fig. 15.1. Summary of the developmental role of the mother, placenta and fetus in determining the response of the insulin-like growth factor (IGF) and growth hormone (GH) axis to nutrient restriction.

2001b). Only under conditions of extreme fluctuations in maternal dietary intake (Antonov, 1947), or alterations in placental size, is fetal body weight normally restricted in a disproportionate fashion.

Timing of Maternal Nutritional Manipulation and Fetal Outcomes

An increasing number of epidemiological and animal-based studies provides support for the concept that the timing of nutritional restriction has a profound influence on the outcome in terms of sensitivity to adult cardiovascular disease. The most frequently cited examples come from the Dutch famine of 1944/1945. During the 5-month period of the famine, mean energy intake was 3.2 MJ/day, compared with 6.3 MJ/day immediately afterwards (Roseboom, 2000). Dietary restriction during early gestation had the greatest effect on the ratio of placental size to birthweight (Lumey, 1998). As a consequence, a normal-sized term infant with a disproportionately larger placenta is born, and such infants are proposed to have a much greater risk of adult coronary heart disease and obesity (Roseboom *et al.*, 2000a,b) (Fig. 15.2). In contrast, famine exposure in later gestation produced modest reductions of both placental and birthweights that are accompanied by glucose intolerance in the resulting offspring as adults (Ravelli *et al.*, 1998).

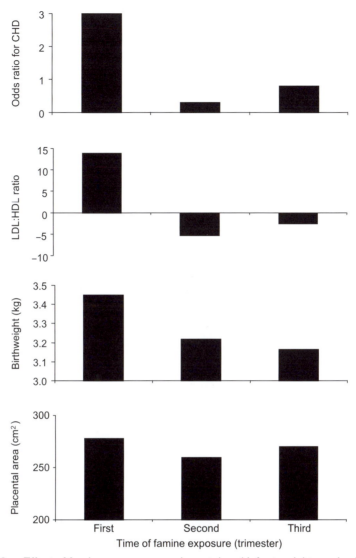

Fig. 15.2. Effect of famine exposure on placental and infant weights and subsequent predisposal to obesity and coronary heart disease (CHD). LDL, low-density lipoprotein; HDL, high-density lipoprotein. (Adapted from Roseboom *et al.*, 2000a,b.)

The sheep is perhaps an ideal animal model for studying these types of developmentally targeted nutritional interventions, and will be the primary focus for the rest of this chapter. Like humans, sheep have a long gestation, and normally produce a single fetus that is born with a mature hypothalamic–pituitary axis. It is interesting to note that when using sheep models of undernutrition, at the same magnitude of nutrient restriction imposed under the Dutch famine, there is seldom any effect on birthweight, but a pronounced effect on placental mass can occur (Fig. 15.3). The consistent finding that a 50% variation in

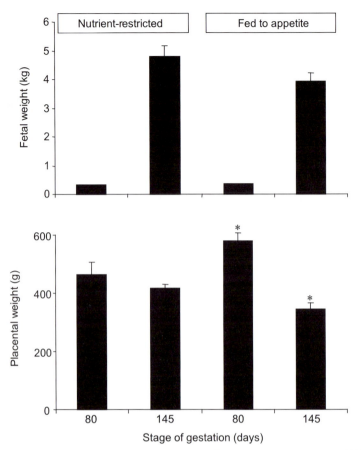

Fig. 15.3. Effect of maternal nutrient restriction (i.e. consuming 3.2–3.8 MJ/day of metabolizable energy) or feeding to appetite (i.e. consuming 8.7–9.9 MJ/day) up to 80 days' gestation followed by feeding to fully meet maintenance requirements (i.e. consuming 6.7–7.5 MJ/day) on fetal and placental mass at mid-gestation and near to term (145 days, term ~ 147 days) in sheep. Placental weights significantly different from nutrient-restricted groups: *$P < 0.05$. (Adapted from Clarke *et al.*, 1998; Heasman *et al.*, 1998.).

maternal food intake can determine placental mass may have further relevance to contemporary human populations, for which a similar range in the upper and lower quartiles for estimated maternal energy intake is found in both early and late gestation (Godfrey *et al.*, 1996).

A further important consideration, when determining how long-term adverse health outcomes can occur, is whether a population that is subjected to famine conditions, in addition to enemy wartime occupation, will exhibit an enhanced or prolonged stress response during pregnancy. Would this then significantly compromise fetal organ development in the absence of any pronounced effect on size at birth? (See Chapter 16, this volume.) In the case of the Leningrad siege, a halving of an already restricted subsistence ration resulted in a pronounced decrease in birthweight (Fig. 15.4).

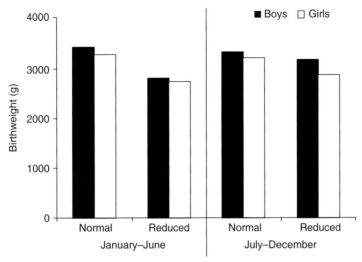

Fig. 15.4. Effect of the severe reduction in food intake that occurred during the Leningrad siege of 1941/42 on weight at birth. A normal ration was 500 g/day, compared with a reduced ration of 250–400 g/day. (Adapted from Antonov, 1947.)

Differential effects on metabolism of counter-regulatory hormones depending on stage of the life cycle

In terms of nutritional mediators of endocrine responses to undernutrition, it is necessary to consider other established metabolic counter-regulatory hormones, i.e. cortisol, thyroid hormones and prolactin, in addition to those within the GH–IGF axis. This is because of the close interactions in metabolic control between each and, in the case of GH and prolactin, the potential cross-reactivity in ligand–receptor binding. To identify how each hormone may act independently or synergistically on the embryo, placenta or fetus, emphasis should be placed on the very different effect each can elicit in comparison with established metabolic roles in the adult.

The majority of metabolic hormones have been studied under conditions of global nutrient restriction. In this state, changes in plasma concentrations act to ensure normal metabolic function is maintained (Bauer *et al.*, 1995). It is not therefore unexpected that the placenta or fetal organs exhibit a range of permanent compensatory responses to reduced nutrient availability, depending on which is growing faster during the period of nutrient restriction. As a consequence, hormone receptor abundance and/or sensitivity will be up- or down-regulated, thereby placing that individual at increased risk of metabolic impairment in later life (Whorwood *et al.*, 2001).

It is not only the stage of gestation during nutritional manipulation that will determine fetal outcome: maternal age and parity have a large influence on size at birth and the mother's ability to respond to nutritional interventions. For most species, the weight of their offspring will be smallest in their first pregnancy (e.g. Fig. 15.5). This is due to lower maternal body weight as well as to the competition between maternal tissues, the placenta and fetus for the available nutrition when both are growing. This is a state that occurs in pregnant adolescents but not in adults. In the overfed juvenile animal, pronounced placental and fetal growth retardation occurs (Wallace, 2000). Under these abnormal conditions it is not surprising that increasing maternal food intake results in intrauterine growth retardation. Consequently, this represents a very different range of maternal metabolic and endocrine adaptations than are found in nutrient-restricted adults with growth-retarded fetuses (Table 15.1). These very different outcomes are likely to have important implications for the interpretation

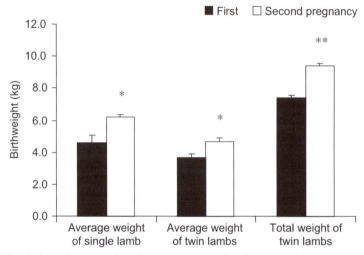

Fig. 15.5. Effect of maternal parity on weight at birth in sheep. Mean birthweights from sheep in their first and second pregnancies, with significant differences in birthweight with parity: $*P < 0.05$, $**P < 0.01$.

Table 15.1. Comparison of the maternal metabolic and hormonal environments that accompany intrauterine growth retardation (IUGR) following nutritional manipulation of the mother.

Maternal metabolite/ hormone	Maternal nutritional adaptation associated with IUGR		References
	Overfeeding of juvenile	Nutrient restriction of adult	
Glucose	↑	↓	Bauer *et al.* (1995), Wallace *et al.* (2000)
Insulin-like growth factor-I	↑	↓	Bauer *et al.* (1995), Wallace *et al.* (1997)
Insulin	↑	↓	Bauer *et al.* (1995), Wallace *et al.* (2000)
Growth hormone	↓	↑	Bauer *et al.* (1995), Wallace *et al.* (1997)
Thyroxine	↑	↓	Symonds *et al.* (1995), Wallace *et al.* (1997)
Tri-iodothyronine	↑	↓	Symonds *et al.* (1995), Wallace *et al.* (1997)

↑, Increased; ↓, decreased.

of pregnant rat studies, in which the majority of work has been conducted on young, growing mothers that are experiencing their first pregnancy (Gardner et al., 1998; Nwagwu et al., 2000).

Fetal Ontogeny and Responsiveness to Nutritional Enhancement of the GH–IGF System

Tissue responsiveness to GH, IGF and related hormones is determined by bioavailability of the hormone and receptor abundance. Relative expression, ontogeny and nutritional responsiveness vary greatly between tissues. Each receptor is most abundant in those tissues in which they have the greatest impact on metabolic regulation. In the liver, for the majority of ligands and receptors studied to date, abundance, when determined as either mRNA or protein, gradually increases with gestational age, to peak at term (Fig. 15.6). The notable exception to this is IGF-II (Li et al., 1993). This developmental process ensures that organ function attains maturity at around the time of birth, which is perhaps the most challenging point of any individual's life span. In the liver, birth is associated with the rapid onset of gluconeogenesis, non-essential amino acid synthesis and waste product removal, as well as haematopoiesis, a function performed primarily in bone marrow in later life. Hepatic function dramatically increases after birth, when nutritional supply to the offspring is no longer subjected to the constraints of both maternal and placental requirements, hence whole-body growth rate rapidly doubles. This is then followed by the appearance of adult forms of the GH receptor and gradual transition from insulin- to GH-dependent growth (Li et al., 1999).

Nutritional adaptations within the fetal GH–IGF axis become apparent at the time of birth in the liver, as mRNA abundance for IGF-I, and additionally receptors for GH and prolactin, all peak (Fig. 15.6). These developmental changes are mediated in part by an increase in fetal plasma cortisol concentration (Li et al., 1996, 1999; Phillips et al., 1997), but are also paralleled by higher plasma prolactin (Phillips et al., 1997). However, the ovine fetal GH receptor is considered unresponsive to circulating GH (McMillen et al., 2001), for which the plasma concentration remains high through late gestation. This poses the question as to the functional relevance of any change in plasma GH concentration with respect to fetal organ sensitivity to GH.

Endocrine Regulation of Fetal Growth

Many hormones in the fetal circulation, including IGF-I, have been shown to be positively correlated with birthweight, using large data sets that cover the full biological range of normal, small and large offspring (Owens, 1991). However, in order to identify the primary endocrine mediators involved in tissue growth, this type of strategy is not ideal. For example, fetal plasma concentrations of the catabolic hormone cortisol are not directly related to size at birth, but cortisol infusion into the fetus reduces growth rate, whereas adrenalectomy is associated with enhanced fetal growth (Fowden *et al.*, 1996).

In the case of intrauterine growth retardation resulting from placental insufficiency, the fetus is subjected to prolonged hypoxia as well as hypoglycaemia. This is a very different challenge compared with undernutrition alone, in which oxygen supply to the fetus would not necessarily be compromised. Placental

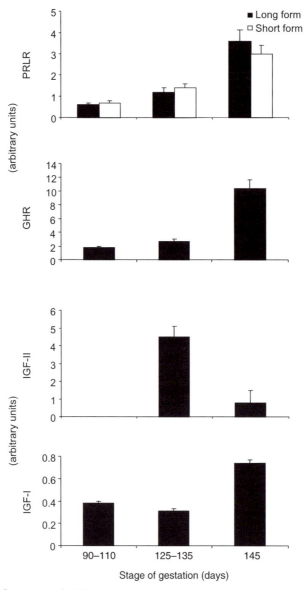

Fig. 15.6. Ontogeny of mRNA abundance for insulin-like growth factors (IGF-I and -II), growth hormone receptor (GHR) and long and short forms of the prolactin receptor (PRLR) in the fetal liver of sheep. (Adapted from Li *et al.*, 1996; Phillips *et al.*, 1997.)

restriction and the resulting hypoxia therefore has a very different effect on the fetal GH–IGF axis in late gestation compared to even severe nutrient restriction (Fig. 15.7). In the late-gestation, placentally restricted and growth-retarded sheep fetus, plasma IGF-I and GH are both reduced, whereas GH is raised during maternal nutrient restriction (Harding et al., 1985; Owens et al., 1994). The high plasma concentrations of IGF-II are unaltered by either manipulation, although, as discussed below, it is IGF-II receptor abundance that may be more important in determining tissue responsiveness.

Despite the pronounced rise in plasma GH during maternal nutrient restriction, there is no change in the specific binding of GH to its hepatic receptor (Bauer et al., 1995). A less severe, but longer, period of maternal nutrient restriction does, however, result in a sustained down-regulation in mRNA for both the GH and prolactin receptors (Fig. 15.8). These adaptations are not accompanied by any immediate effect on whole-body or liver growth. They may have important consequences when GH-dependent growth becomes dominant.

The extent to which IGF-II directly mediates nutritionally related effects on fetal growth has not been ascertained. IGF-I infusion into the late-gestation fetus results in increased mass of a range of organs, including the liver, lungs, heart, kidneys, spleen and adrenal glands, in conjunction with preventing the normal decrease in individual placentome weight seen with gestational age (Lok et al., 1996).

IGF-II as a regulator of fetal growth

Increases in fetal organ growth can accompany tissue-specific enhancements of either growth factor ligand or receptor abundance, although there is some overlap between complementary components of the IGF system. In the fetus, IGF-II is dominant over IGF-I, and its effects on fetal growth are mediated by both the IGF-I and -II receptors. The bioavailability of IGF-II is partly dependent on the abundance of its receptor, which acts to inactivate its anabolic effects. Intrauterine growth retardation arising as a consequence of placental insufficiency is accompanied by an increase in placental IGF-II mRNA (Abu-Amero et al., 1998), but a greater rise in receptor abundance (Fig. 15.9). In contrast, the fetal overgrowth that accompanies in vitro fertilization in sheep results in tissue-specific decreases in IGF-II receptor mRNA and protein abundance, for which the greatest effect is within the liver (Young et al., 2001). This has led to the hypothesis that reduced fetal methylation and expression of IGF-II receptor greatly promotes fetal growth.

Interestingly there is no change in the plasma concentration or tissue mRNA abundance of IGF-II between overgrown (in vitro-fertilized) and normal fetuses measured at 125 days' gestation (Young et al., 2001). No correlation has been demonstrated between fetal weight and any indices of IGF-II. Whether this example of fetal overgrowth is confined to sheep embryos produced in culture, or whether it may be replicated using a diet that would act to promote DNA methylation, e.g. by increasing methionine availability (Petrie et al., 2002), has yet to be confirmed.

GH and prolactin as endocrine regulators of fetal growth

The precise role(s) of GH and prolactin in regulating fetal growth remain a matter of debate. Prolactin could be more important than GH in terms of

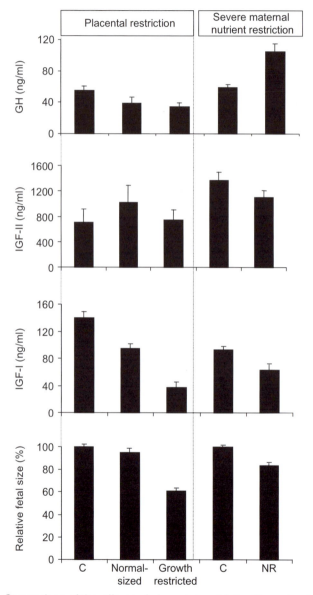

Fig. 15.7. Comparison of the effects of placental restriction throughout gestation with a severe period of maternal nutrient restriction (NR; 25% of *ad libitum* intake from 100 to 125 days' gestation) on fetal growth and the insulin-like growth factor (IGF) and growth hormone (GH) axis. C indicates control. (Adapted from Harding *et al.*, 1985; Owens *et al.*, 1994; Bauer *et al.*, 1995.)

promoting liver growth. GH secretion remains high through late gestation. In contrast, prolactin secretion is pulsatile and maintained by a tonic stimulatory, rather than inhibitory, drive from the hypothalamus (Houghton *et al.*, 1995; McMillen *et al.*, 2001) and its concentration increases during late gestation. A close temporal relationship between the pulsatility of GH and prolactin secretion exists in the fetal sheep (Albers *et al.*, 1993).

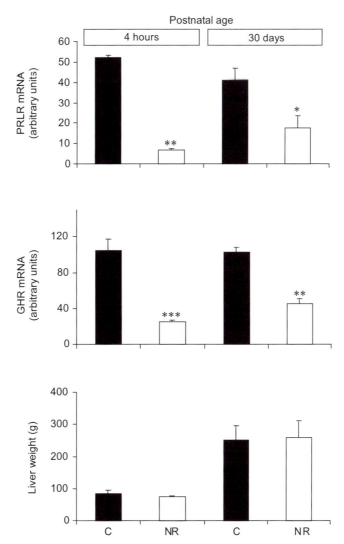

Fig. 15.8. Effect of maternal nutrient restriction (NR; 50% of calculated meta-bolizable energy requirements necessary to produce a 4.5 kg lamb) from 110 days gestation up to term on mRNA abundance for the growth hormone receptor (GHR) and prolactin receptor (PRLR) in the livers of young sheep. Significant differences between nutritional groups at the same postnatal age: *$P < 0.05$, **$P < 0.01$, ***$P < 0.001$. C indicates control. (Adapted from Hyatt *et al.*, 2002.)

The active promotion of fetal prolactin secretion suggests an important developmental role during late gestation, the plasma concentration being increased by increasing maternal nutrition (Stephenson *et al.*, 2001), thereby promoting adipose tissue maturation in preparation for life after birth (Budge *et al.*, 2000). In contrast, GH may normally have an overriding negative influence on fetal organ development, particularly adipose tissue. Fetal hypophysectomy results in a pronounced increase in adipose tissue deposition, which is overcome by GH replacement within the fetus (Stevens and Alexander,

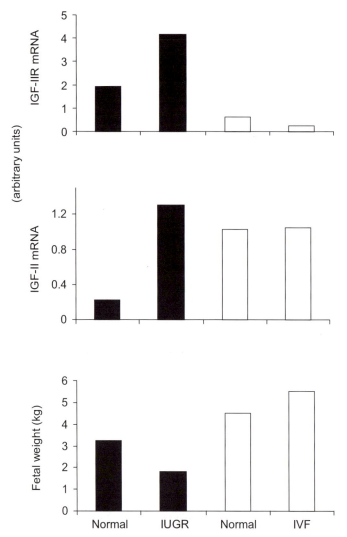

Fig. 15.9. Comparison of the relationship between fetal growth restriction or promotion and the insulin-like growth factor-II (IGF-II) axis; R, receptor. Data for intrauterine growth retardation (IUGR) are for the term human placenta (Abu-Amero *et al.*, 1998) and for *in vitro*-fertilized (IVF) 'overgrown' sheep fetuses, from which the livers were sampled at 125 days' gestation (Young *et al.*, 2001).

1986). At the same time, there is a pronounced increase in fetal body weight (Fig. 15.10). An inhibitory influence of GH on fetal growth is supported by the recent finding that chronic pulsatile infusion of GH into growth-retarded fetal sheep did not improve growth despite restoring fetal plasma IGF-I (Bauer *et al.*, 2003). At the same time, this procedure resulted in reduced fetal intestine and kidney weights.

The potential direct anabolic effects of prolactin on fetal growth have not been studied to date. There is an established seasonal influence on placental and fetal mass (Jenkinson *et al.*, 1994) that could be mediated by reciprocal increases in maternal and fetal plasma prolactin (Bassett *et al.*, 1989)

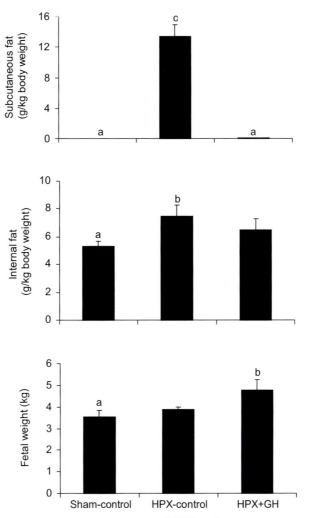

Fig. 15.10. Effect of fetal hypophysectomy (HPX) and growth hormone (GH) replacement on fetal weight and adiposity in the sheep. Significant differences between groups are indicated by different superscripts: a versus b, $P < 0.05$; a versus c, $P < 0.001$. (Adapted from Stevens and Alexander, 1986.)

(Fig. 15.11). However, maternal and fetal plasma prolactin is also under positive nutritional regulation (Koritnik *et al.*, 1981; Stephenson *et al.*, 2001), so any confounding effects of maternal nutrition in these studies of seasonality require clarification. A direct role for the prolactin receptor (PRLR) in determining fetal growth, as a result of changes in receptor abundance within the liver, could provide an explanation as to why the *Aa* heterozygote polymorphism (of the *a* allele of the PRLR locus) for the PRLR gene has recently been shown to be positively correlated with uterine length and placental mass in pigs (van Rens *et al.*, 2003).

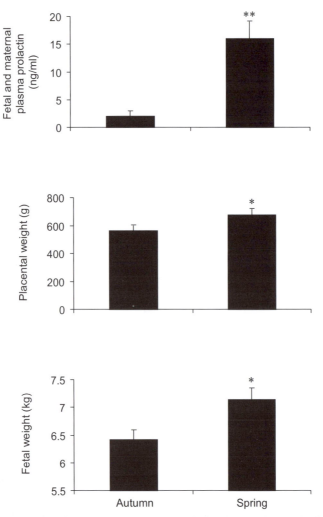

Fig. 15.11.   Influence of time of year on placental and fetal weights of twin pregnancies near to term and fetal plasma prolactin concentrations in sheep. Significant differences between seasonal groups: *$P < 0.05$, **$P < 0.01$. (Adapted from Bassett *et al.*, 1989; Jenkinson *et al.*, 1994.)

Composition and Amount of Food Intake as Determinants of Fetal Growth and Placental Morphology

The extent to which perturbations in maternal nutrition can directly influence fetal growth is not, as yet, fully quantified. This is due, in part, to the very different models of dietary manipulation that have been most widely published. When using historical epidemiological findings to gain insights into fetal programming, it must be noted that most individuals or populations are likely to have been subjected to a restricted diet in comparison to contemporary populations (Table 15.2). Energy intake also differs markedly between publications despite little, if any, effect on birthweight. Furthermore, within and between geographically adjacent groups of pregnant women, very large variations in recorded maternal food intake have been illustrated (Godfrey *et al.*, 1996; Mathews *et al.*, 1999).

Similar issues affect the interpretation of results from animal studies. For example, a failure to allow experimental animals to feed on their more natural diet, which for sheep, includes a high proportion of roughage, could have important consequences for the fetal GH–IGF axis. Allowing sheep to feed to appetite rather than an arbitrary amount calculated on a predetermined lamb birthweight (i.e. to 100% of Agriculture and Fisheries Research Council recommendations, taking into account requirements for both ewe maintenance and growth of the conceptus, in order to produce a 4.5 kg lamb at term; Agricultural Research Council, 1980), results in larger offspring for which liver size is enhanced (Fig. 15.12). Under these different nutritional conditions, fetal hepatic IGF-II, but not IGF-I, mRNA abundance is only significantly up-regulated in previously nutrient-restricted fetuses when the mothers are then fed to appetite (Brameld *et al.*, 2000). It is therefore not only the level of nutrient restriction, but also the subsequent amount of feed that is critical in determining the magnitude of adaptation within the GH–IGF axis. Conversely, feeding pregnant sheep a diet of pellets twice daily which are very rapidly consumed, but allowing *ad libitum* (and unrecorded) intake of a low-quality roughage, i.e. straw, appears to result in very different placental and fetal growth patterns than are found under more normal dietary regimes (Fig. 15.13).

Feeding a complete pelleted diet through pregnancy prevents the normal decline in placental weight with advancing gestational age observed in sheep,

Table 15.2. Comparison of published food intake for contemporary epidemiological studies with retrospective data from the time of the Dutch famine (1944/45).

Location	Maternal food intake (MJ/day)	Birthweight (g)	Reference
The Netherlands – not exposed to the famine	6.2	3383	Roseboom (2000)
Aberdeen, UK	10.1	3186	Campbell *et al.* (1996)
Southampton, UK	9.78 (early)/ 9.72 (late)	3527 (boys)/ 3444 (girls)	Godfrey *et al.* (1996)
Portsmouth, UK	8.58 (early)/ 9.23 (late)	3425 (boys)/ 3281 (girls)	Mathews *et al.* (1999)

and results in a complete loss of inverted, i.e. A-type, placentomes (Osgerby *et al.*, 2002). A loss of A-type and predominance of D-type placentomes is also associated with an adverse maternal environment earlier in gestation, e.g. when pregnant sheep are fed to 60% of calculated total metabolizable energy requirements with a mixed diet of hay and concentrate, compared with *ad libitum* hay and a fixed amount of concentrate, regardless of nutrient intake during the

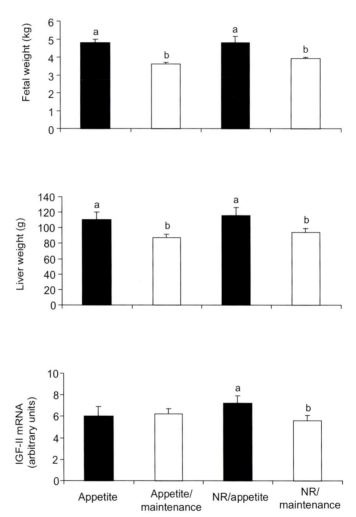

Fig. 15.12. Influence of increased maternal nutrition in the second half of gestation on the responsiveness of the fetal liver insulin-like growth factor-II (IGF-II) mRNA abundance near to term in sheep. Mothers were either fed to appetite through gestation (i.e. consuming 8.7–9.9 MJ/day) or nutrient restricted (NR) between 28 and 80 days' gestation (i.e. consuming 3.03–3.8 MJ/day) and then either fed to appetite or to fully meet maintenance requirements (i.e. consuming 6.7–7.5 MJ/day). Significant differences between nutritional groups are indicated by different superscripts: a versus b, *P* < 0.05. (Adapted from Brameld *et al.*, 2000; Heasman *et al.*, 2000.)

second half of gestation (Heasman *et al.*, 1998; Dandrea *et al.*, 2001). Similarly, chronic exposure of pregnant sheep to the hypobaric hypoxia of high altitude also produces such a placental phenotype (Penninga and Longo, 1998).

Abnormalities in placental development leading to the complete loss of inverted placentomes may explain the reduction in fetal and placental weights that are only found when nutrient restriction is imposed using a

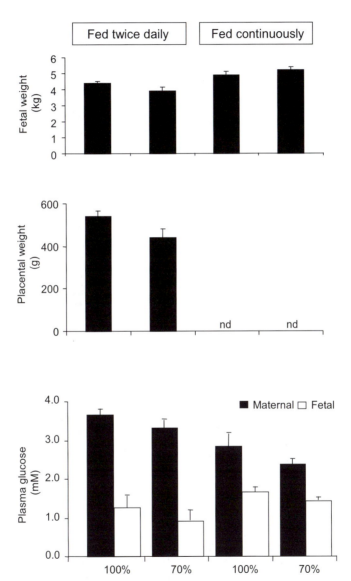

Fig. 15.13. Effect of frequency of maternal feeding on placental and fetal weight near to term and the maternal–fetal plasma glucose gradient. nd, data not available; % values relate to metabolizable energy intake with respect to values calculated to produce a 4.5 kg newborn sheep. Adapted from Osgerby *et al.* (2002) (twice-daily feeding) and Edwards and McMillen (2002) (feed continuously available).

high-concentrate, pellet-only diet (Fig. 15.13). Under these conditions, restricted fetal growth is accompanied by a lower plasma concentration of IGF-I and glucose, despite significantly higher maternal plasma glucose (Osgerby *et al.*, 2002). This comparison provides good evidence of the large effects that the frequency of feeding, compared with the absolute amount of feed intake, may have on fetal nutrition. Taken together, these findings indicate a marked divergence in the close correlation usually found between maternal and fetal plasma glucose concentrations, when restricted energy availability persists throughout a 24 h period (Fig. 15.13). Feeding the bulk of any diet only once or twice daily can have a substantial influence on the nutrient flux between the mother and fetus (Simonetta *et al.*, 1991). This may be a direct consequence of producing much greater fluctuations in fetal glucose and cortisol than are the norm when regular feeding patterns are adopted (Fig. 15.14). The extent to which transient daily rises in fetal plasma cortisol may be sufficient to reprogramme organ development and/or its sensitivity to later cortisol exposure has not been explored.

Cortisol as an Endocrine Regulator of the GH–IGF System?

Cortisol is of major importance in the regulation of hormone receptor abundance in preparation for life after birth. This, together with the assumption

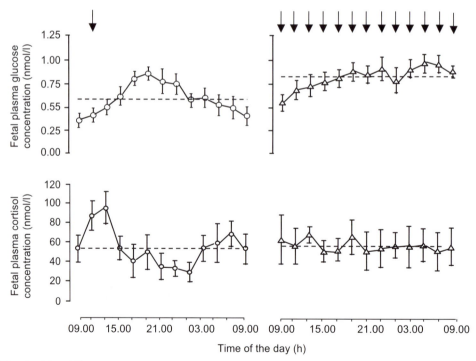

Fig. 15.14. Effect of frequency of maternal feeding on hourly changes in fetal plasma glucose and cortisol concentration. ↓ indicates time of feeding. (Adapted from Simonetta *et al.*, 1991, with permission.)

that undernutrition is a stressful experience for the fetus, has led to the wide acceptance that the primary candidate for mediating fetal tissue responses to undernutrition is cortisol.

The evidence that the programming effects of fetal nutrient restriction are mediated by cortisol, originates in part from developmental changes in IGF, GH and prolactin receptors in late gestation that can be induced by cortisol infusion into the fetus (Fig. 15.15). It has also been shown that maternal dexamethasone administration between 26 and 29, but not between 59 and 66, days' gestation can result in hypertension in the resulting offspring (Dodic *et al.*, 1998). A similar finding has been observed using cortisol at a dose sufficient to increase maternal

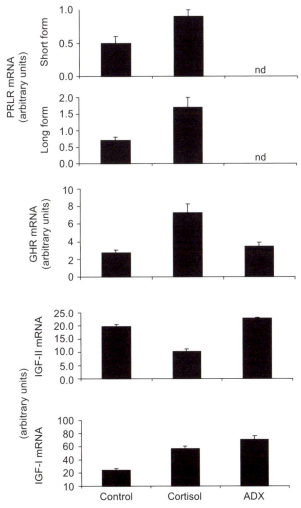

Fig. 15.15. Effect of fetal glucocorticoid status on the abundance of insulin-like growth factors-I (IGF-I), -II (IGF-II), and growth hormone (GHR) and prolactin (PRLR) receptors, in the late-gestation sheep fetus. ADX, adrenalectomized; nd, data not available. (Adapted from Li *et al.*, 1993, 1996; Phillips *et al.*, 1997.)

plasma concentrations eightfold (Fig. 15.16). This increase is appreciably higher than the transient doubling of maternal cortisol during nutrient restriction in late gestation (Edwards and McMillen, 2001). However, in contrast, when maternal nutrient restriction is imposed between 30 and 80 days' gestation, a marked reduction in plasma cortisol occurs (Bispham *et al.*, 2003). Irrespective of the timing of maternal nutrient restriction, no consistent effect on fetal plasma cortisol has been reported (Brameld *et al.*, 2000; Edwards and McMillen, 2001). Maternal cortisol infusion in late gestation sufficient to transiently double maternal and fetal plasma cortisol can, however, raise fetal blood pressure (Jenson *et al.*, 2002).

Interestingly, it has also been shown that administration of dexamethasone in late gestation results in a marked reduction in maternal food intake, with a 50% decline in maternal plasma thyroxine (Fig. 15.17). Similarly, in rats, a decrease in maternal food intake over the final week of gestation occurs following maternal dexamethasone administration (Holness and Sugden, 2001). No data have been published in sheep relating to maternal food intake or to the metabolic and hormonal environment, either at the time of, or following, dexamethasone or cortisol administration in early gestation.

Maternal nutrient restriction targeted at the time of maximal placental growth can have pronounced effects on liver development that are related to glucocorticoid sensitivity. Thus, in the livers of neonatal offspring, these include an increase in glucocorticoid receptor mRNA abundance and decreased 11β-hydroxysteroid dehydrogenase type 2 mRNA abundance or enzyme activity, which could be interpreted as enhancing tissue sensitivity to cortisol (Whorwood *et al.*, 2001). These hepatic adaptations are accompanied by higher GH receptor and IGF-I mRNA in the absence of any change in organ mass (Fig. 15.18). There is, however, a pronounced loss of the normal linear relationship between plasma IGF-I and liver weight at term in nutrient-restricted offspring compared to

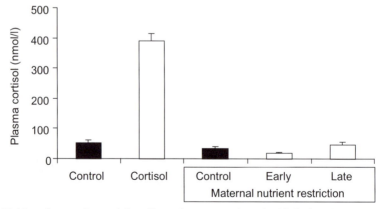

Fig. 15.16. Comparison of the effect of a maternal cortisol infusion that results in hypertensive offspring (Cortisol), with the changes in maternal plasma cortisol during nutrient restriction (i.e. 50% of calculated metabolizable energy requirements necessary to produce a 4.5 kg lamb) during early or late gestation. (Adapted from Edwards and McMillen, 2001; Dodic *et al.*, 2002; Bispham *et al.*, 2003.)

controls (Heasman *et al.*, 2000). Adaptations of this type may subsequently act to compromise hepatic expression of IGFs in later life, as well as liver growth.

Maternal Nutrient Restriction and Thyroid Hormones as Mediators of Fetal Reprogramming?

Other probable endocrine regulators of the fetal GH–IGF axis in addition to, or instead of, cortisol include the thyroid hormones. Reduced plasma thyroid hormones within both the mother and fetus are a consistent adaptation to maternal nutrient restriction that persists for the duration of the reduced caloric intake (Clarke *et al.*, 1998; Rae *et al.*, 2002). Following the restoration of maternal nutrition to appetite, maternal plasma thyroid hormones increase significantly. This is predicted to have important consequences for early fetal development prior to the formation of the fetal thyroid gland, as the only source of thyroid hormones for the conceptus is from the maternal circulation (St Germain, 1999). Thyroid hormones have a role in regulating the growth and/or development of nearly all fetal tissues and organs (Symonds, 1995). Abnormalities in tissue metabolism following reduced thyroid hormone secretion in adults include reduced oxygen uptake (Clausen *et al.*, 1991) for which a similar relationship is apparent in the late-gestation fetus. Tri-iodothyronine has also been implicated

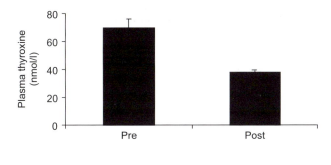

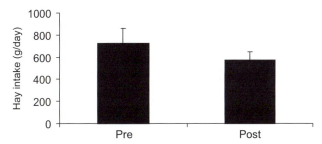

Fig. 15.17. Effect of maternal dexamethasone administration between 138 and 140 days' gestation on maternal food intake and plasma thyroid hormone concentration. Pre, before, and post, after dexamethasone treatment. (Adapted from Clarke and Symonds, 2003.)

in the prepartum down-regulation of IGF-II mRNA in the fetal liver, which may account for the hepatic overgrowth that accompanies fetal hypothyroidism (Forhead *et al.*, 1998).

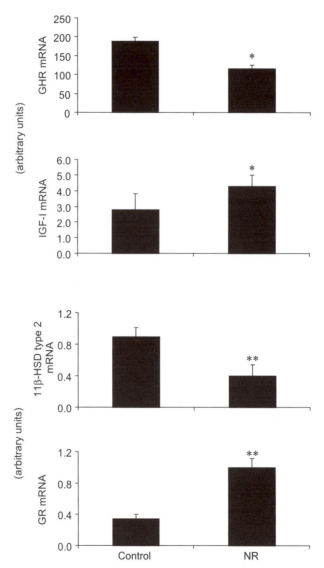

Fig. 15.18. Effect of maternal nutrient restriction (NR, i.e. consuming 3.2–3.8 MJ/ day of metabolizable energy) or feeding to appetite (i.e. consuming 8.7–9.9 MJ/ day) up to 80 days' gestation, followed by feeding to fully meet maintenance requirements (i.e. 6.7–7.5 MJ/day) on the fetal insulin-like growth factor (IGF)/ growth hormone (GH) axis, glucocorticoid (GR) receptor and 11β-hydroxysteroid dehydrogenase (HSD) type 2 mRNA in the near-term fetal sheep liver. Significant differences between nutritional groups: *$P < 0.05$; **$P < 0.01$. (Adapted from Brameld *et al.*, 2000; Whorwood *et al.*, 2001.)

Divergent effects of Hypoglycaemia on the Liver and Hypothalamic–Pituitary Axis

It is possible that transient fluctuations in fetal glucose mediated through chronic maternal undernutrition over the final month of gestation (Edwards *et al.*, 2001) may be sufficient to reset the fetal hypothalamic–pituitary–adrenal axis. In fetuses of nutrient-restricted ewes there is a precocious rise in ACTH in response to insulin-induced hypoglycaemia. At the same time, fetal glucose is negatively correlated to ACTH in nutrient-restricted fetuses only, whereas the established negative correlation with insulin is present in all fetuses, irrespective of maternal nutrition.

The extent to which a threshold concentration of glucose may exist with respect to the increase in GH during undernutrition has not been investigated. It is possible that ghrelin (a GH-releasing acylated peptide) released from the placenta near to term could have a direct involvement (Gualillo *et al.*, 2001). In adults it acts to increase plasma GH (Kojima *et al.*, 1999). A gestationally related rise in pituitary sensitivity to glucose could, in this way, be the signal for the increase in hypothalamic neuropeptide Y (NPY) content (Warnes *et al.*, 1998), thereby providing a nutritionally mediated signal for the onset of parturition (Fig. 15.19). This emphasizes the divergent sensitivity to fluctuations in plasma glucose concentration between peripheral tissues and the hypothalamic–pituitary axis as term approaches.

Inadequate substrate supply to the liver is unlikely to compromise fetal survival compared with a reduction in glucose supply to the brain. A resetting of IGF synthesis and/or receptor abundance will be sufficient to ensure liver metabolism is matched to nutrient availability. The brain has a much higher rate of metabolism than the liver, which, together with an obligatory requirement for glucose, would be predicted to promote glycaemic sensitivity. Growth of the brain is normally spared at the expense of other fetal tissues. In the mother an

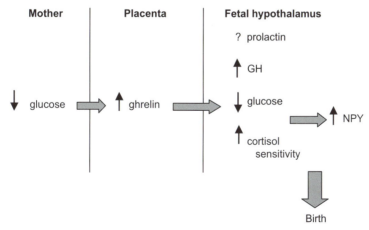

Fig. 15.19. Summary of the mechanism by which maternal nutrient restriction in late gestation enhances the sensitivity of the fetal hypothalamus to hypoglycaemia. GH, growth hormone; NPY, neuropeptide Y.

increase in GH acts to spare maternal glucose utilization by peripheral tissues, thereby maximizing its availability for the fetus. For the fetus, an increased capacity to sense and respond to a decrease in plasma glucose could be a critical trigger for initiating parturition. A failure to make this type of response, even in normally growing fetuses in the face of a further nutritional challenge, may contribute, at worst, to fetal death, or, more likely, to compromised fetal development and subsequent tissue functions. This susceptibility would be particularly pronounced towards the end of gestation, when the fetus is insensitive to GH, as a result of receptor insensitivity and the prevailing high concentrations (Bauer *et al.*, 1995).

Conclusion

It is apparent that the nutritional regulation of the fetal GH–IGF axis is highly complex. At any given stage of gestation, its activity and sensitivity is coordinated by both the current and previous nutritional experiences. A large number of anabolic and catabolic hormones can up- or down-regulate the ability of peripheral tissues and the brain to adapt effectively to an increase or decrease in nutrient supply. The consequences of these adaptations may become apparent immediately and lead to a reduction in fetal growth and/or precipitate parturition, or, more likely, will manifest much later in an individual's life span as a range of metabolic complications which contribute towards adult cardiovascular disease, including hypertension, diabetes and syndrome X (Barker, 1998).

References

Abu-Amero, S.N., Ali, Z., Bennett, P., Vaughan, J.I. and Morre, G.E. (1998) Expression of the insulin-like growth factors and their receptors in term placentas: a comparison between normal and IUGR births. *Molecular Reproduction and Development* 49, 229–235.

Agricultural Research Council (1980) Requirements for energy. In: *The Nutritional Requirements of Ruminant Livestock*. Commonwealth Agricultural Bureaux, Slough, UK, pp. 115–119.

Albers, N., Bettendorf, M., Herrmann, H., Kaplan, S.L. and Grumbach, M.M. (1993) Hormone ontogeny in the ovine fetus. XXVII. Pulsatile and copulsatile secretion of luteinizing hormone, follicle-stimulating hormone, growth hormone, and prolactin in late gestation: a new method for the analysis of copulsatility. *Endocrinology* 132, 701–709.

Anthony, R.V., Liang, R., Kayl, E.P. and Pratt, S.L. (1995) The growth hormone/prolactin gene family in ruminant placentae. *Journal of Reproduction and Fertility, Suppl.* 49, 83–95.

Antonov, A.N. (1947) Children born during the siege of Leningrad in 1942. *Journal of Pediatrics* 30, 250–259.

Barker, D.J.P. (1998) *In utero* programming of chronic disease. *Clinical Science* 95, 115–128.

Bassett, J.M., Curtis, N., Hanson, C. and Weeding, C.M. (1989) Effects of altered photoperiod or maternal melatonin administration on plasma prolactin concentrations in fetal lambs. *Journal of Endocrinology* 122, 633–643.

Bauer, M.K., Breier, B.H., Harding, J., Veldhuis, J.D. and Gluckman, P.D. (1995) The fetal somatotrophic axis during long term maternal undernutrition in sheep; evidence of nutritional regulation *in utero*. *Endocrinology* 136, 1250–1257.

Bauer, M.K., Breier, B.B., Bloomfield, F.H., Jensen, E.C., Gluckman, P.D. and Harding, J.E. (2003) Chronic pulsatile infusion of growth hormone to growth-restricted fetal sheep increases circulating fetal insulin-like growth factor-I levels but not fetal growth. *Journal of Endocrinology* 177, 83–92.

Bispham, J., Gopalakrishnan, G.S., Dandrea, J., Wilson, V., Budge, H., Keisler, D.H., Broughton Pipkin, F., Stephenson, T. and Symonds, M.E. (2003) Maternal endocrine adaptation throughout pregnancy to nutritional manipulation: consequences for maternal plasma leptin and cortisol and the programming of fetal adipose tissue development. *Endocrinology* 144, 3575–3585.

Brameld, J.M., Mostyn, A., Dandrea, J., Stephenson, T.J., Dawson, J., Buttery, P.J. and Symonds, M.E. (2000) Maternal nutrition alters the expression of insulin-like growth factors in fetal sheep liver and skeletal muscle. *Journal of Endocrinology* 167, 429–437.

Budge, H., Bispham, J., Dandrea, J., Evans, L., Heasman, L., Ingleton, P., Sullivan, C., Wilson, V., Stephenson, T. and Symonds, M.E. (2000) Effect of maternal nutrition on brown adipose tissue and prolactin receptor status in the fetal lamb. *Pediatric Research* 47, 781–786.

Campbell, D.M., Hall, M.H., Barker, D.J., Cross, J., Shiell, A.W. and Godfrey, K.M. (1996) Diet in pregnancy and the offspring's blood pressure 40 years later. *British Journal of Obstetrics and Gynaecology* 103, 273–280.

Clarke, L. and Symonds, M.E. (2003) Effect of maternal dexamethasone administration on maternal metabolism and food intake. *Pediatric Research* 53(suppl.), 35A.

Clarke, L., Heasman, L., Juniper, D.T. and Symonds, M.E. (1998) Maternal nutrition in early–mid gestation and placental size in sheep. *British Journal of Nutrition* 79, 359–364.

Clausen, T., Van Hardeveld, C. and Everts, M.E. (1991) Significance of cation transport in control of energy metabolism and thermogenesis. *Physiological Reviews* 71, 733–774.

Dandrea, J., Wilson, V., Gopalakrishnan, G., Heasman, L., Budge, H., Stephenson, T. and Symonds, M.E. (2001) Maternal nutritional manipulation of placental growth and glucose transporter-1 abundance in sheep. *Reproduction* 122, 793–800.

Dodic, M., May, C.N., Wintour, E.M. and Coghlan, J.P. (1998) An early prenatal exposure to excess glucocorticoid leads to hypertensive offspring in sheep. *Clinical Science* 94, 149–155.

Dodic, M., Hantzis, V., Duncan, J., Rees, S., Koukoulas, I., Johnson, K., Wintour, E.M. and Moritz, K. (2002) Programming effects of short prenatal exposure to cortisol. *FASEB Journal* 16, 1017–1026.

Edwards, L.J. and McMillen, I.C. (2001) Maternal undernutrition increases arterial blood pressure in the sheep fetus during late gestation. *Journal of Physiology, London* 533, 561–570.

Edwards, L.J. and McMillen, I.C. (2002) Impact of maternal undernutrition during the periconceptional period, fetal number, and fetal sex on the development of the hypothalamo-pituitary adrenal axis in sheep during late gestation. *Biology of Reproduction* 66, 1562–1569.

Edwards, L.J., Symonds, M.E., Warnes, K., Owens, J.A., Butler, T.G., Jurisevic, A. and McMillen, I.C. (2001) Responses of the fetal pituitary–adrenal axis to acute and chronic hypoglycaemia during late gestation in the sheep. *Endocrinology* 142, 1778–1785.

Forhead, A.J., Li, J., Gilmour, R.S. and Fowden, A.L. (1998) Control of hepatic insulin-like growth factor II gene expression by thyroid hormones in the fetal sheep near term. *American Journal of Physiology* 275, E149–E156.

Fowden, A.L., Szemere, J., Hughes, P., Gilmour, R.S. and Forhead, A.J. (1996) The effects of cortisol on the growth rate of the sheep fetus during late gestation. *Journal of Endocrinology* 151, 97–105.

Gardner, D.S., Jackson, A.A. and Langley-Evans, S.C. (1998) The effect of prenatal diet and glucocorticoids upon growth and systolic blood pressure in the rat. *Proceedings of the Nutrition Society* 57, 235–240.

Godfrey, K., Robinson, S., Barker, D.J.P., Osmond, C. and Cox, V. (1996) Maternal nutrition in early and late pregnancy in relation to placental and fetal growth. *British Medical Journal* 312, 410–414.

Gualillo, O., Caminos, J., Blanco, M., Garcia-Caballero, T., Kojima, M., Kangawa, K., Dieguez, C. and Casanueva, F. (2001) Ghrelin, a novel placental-derived hormone. *Endocrinology* 142, 788–794.

Harding, J.E., Jones, C.T. and Robinson, J.S. (1985) Studies on experimental growth retardation in sheep. The effects of a small placenta in restricting transport to and growth of the fetus. *Journal of Developmental Physiology* 7, 427–442.

Heasman, L., Clarke, L., Firth, K., Stephenson, T. and Symonds, M.E. (1998) Influence of restricted maternal nutrition in early to mid gestation on placental and fetal development at term in sheep. *Pediatric Research* 44, 546–551.

Heasman, L., Brameld, J.M., Mostyn, A., Budge, H., Dawson, J., Buttery, P.J., Stephenson, T. and Symonds, M.E. (2000) Maternal nutrient restriction during early to mid gestation alters the relationship between IGF-I and body size at term in fetal sheep. *Reproduction, Fertility, and Development* 12, 345–350.

Holness, M.J. and Sugden, M.C. (2001) Dexamethasone during late gestation exacerbates peripheral insulin resistance and selectively targets glucose-sensitive functions in β cell and liver. *Endocrinology* 142, 3742–3748.

Houghton, D.C., Young, I.R. and McMillen, I.C. (1995) Response of prolactin to different photoperiods after surgical disconnection of the hypothalamus and pituitary in sheep fetuses. *Journal of Reproduction and Fertility* 104, 199–206.

Hyatt, M., Bispham, J., Dandrea, J., Walker, D., Symonds, M.E. and Stephenson, T. (2002) Effect of maternal nutrient restriction during late-gestation on growth hormone (GH) and prolactin (PRL) receptor abundance in neonatal lambs. *Proceedings of the Nutrition Society* 61, 119A.

Jenkinson, C.M.C., Peterson, S.W., MacKenzie, D.D.S. and McCutcheon, S.N. (1994) The effects of season on placental development and fetal growth in sheep. *Proceedings of the New Zealand Society of Animal Production* 54, 227–230.

Jenson, E.C., Gallaher, B.W., Breier, B.H. and Harding, J.E. (2002) The effect of chronic maternal cortisol infusion on the late-gestation fetal sheep. *Journal of Endocrinology* 174, 27–36.

Kojima, M., Hosoda, H., Date, Y., Nakazato, M., Matsuo, H. and Kanagawa, K. (1999) Ghrelin is a growth-homone-releasing acylated peptide from stomach. *Nature* 402, 656–660.

Koritnik, D.R., Humphrey, W.D., Kaltenbach, C.C. and Dunn, T.G. (1981) Effects of maternal undernutrition on the development of the ovine fetus and associated changes in growth hormone and prolactin. *Biology of Reproduction* 24, 125–137.

Li, J., Saunders, J.C., Gilmour, R.S., Silver, M. and Fowden, A.L. (1993) Insulin-like growth factor-II messenger ribonucleic acid expression in fetal tissues of the sheep during late gestation: effects of cortisol. *Endocrinology* 132, 2083–2089.

Li, J., Owens, P.C., Owens, J.C., Saunders, J.C., Gilmour, R.S. and Fowden, A.L. (1996) The ontogeny of hepatic growth hormone receptor and insulin-like growth factor I gene expression in the sheep fetus during late gestation: developmental regulation by cortisol. *Endocrinology* 137, 1650–1657.

Li, J., Gilmour, R.S., Saunders, J.C., Dauncey, M.J. and Fowden, A.L. (1999) Activation of the adult mode of ovine growth hormone receptor gene expression by cortisol during late fetal development. *FASEB Journal* 13, 545–552.

Lok, F., Owens, J.A., Mundy, L., Robinson, J.S. and Owens, P.C. (1996) Insulin-like growth factor I promotes growth selectively in fetal sheep in late gestation. *American Journal of Physiology* 270, R1148–R1155.

Lumey, L.H. (1998) Compensatory placental growth after restricted nutrition in early pregnancy. *Placenta* 19, 105–112.

Mathews, F., Yudkin, P. and Neil, A. (1999) Influence of maternal nutrition on outcome of pregnancy: prospective cohort study. *British Medical Journal* 319, 339–343.

McMillen, I.C., Houghton, D.C. and Phillips, I.D. (2001) Maturation of cytokine-receptors in preparation for birth. *Biochemical Society Transactions* 29, 63–68.

Nwagwu, M.O., Cook, A. and Langley-Evans, S.C. (2000) Evidence of progressive deterioration of renal function in rats exposed to a maternal low-protein diet *in utero*. *British Journal of Nutrition* 83, 79–85.

Osgerby, J.C., Wathes, D.C., Howard, D. and Gadd, T.S. (2002) The effect of maternal undernutrition on fetal growth. *Journal of Endocrinology* 173, 131–141.

Owens, J.A. (1991) Endocrine and substrate control of fetal growth: placental and maternal influences and insulin-like growth factors. *Reproduction, Fertility, and Development* 3, 505–517.

Owens, J.A., Kind, K.L., Carbone, F., Robinson, J.S. and Owens, P.C. (1994) Circulating insulin-like growth factors-I and -II and substrates in fetal sheep following restriction of placental growth. *Journal of Endocrinology* 140, 5–13.

Penninga, L. and Longo, L.D. (1998) Ovine placental morphology: effect of high altitude, long-term hypoxia. *Placenta* 19, 187–193.

Petrie, L., Duthie, S.J., Rees, W.D. and McConnell, M.L. (2002) Serum concentrations of homocysteine are elevated during early pregnancy in rodent models of fetal programming. *British Journal of Nutrition* 88, 471–477.

Phillips, I.D., Anthony, R.V., Butler, T.G., Ross, J.T. and McMillen, I.C. (1997) Hepatic prolactin receptor gene expression increases in the sheep fetus before birth and after cortisol infusion. *Endocrinology* 138, 1351–1354.

Rae, M.T., Rhind, S.M., Kyle, C.E., Miller, D.W. and Brooks, A.N. (2002) Maternal undernutrition alters triiodothyronine concentrations and pituitary response to GnRH in fetal sheep. *Journal of Endocrinology* 173, 449–455.

Ravelli, A.C.J., van der Meulin, J.H.P., Michels, R.P.J., Osmond, C., Barker, D.J.P., Hales, C.N. and Bleker, O.P. (1998) Glucose tolerance in adults after *in utero* exposure to the Dutch famine. *Lancet* 351, 173–177.

Roseboom, T.J. (2000) *Prenatal Exposure to the Dutch Famine and Health in Later Life*. The University of Amsterdam.

Roseboom, T.J., van der Meulen, J.H.P., Osmond, C., Barker, D.J.P., Ravelli, A.C., Schroeder-Tanka, J.M., van Montfrans, G.A., Michels, R.P.J. and Blecker, O.P. (2000a) Coronary heart disease in adults after perinatal exposure to famine. *Heart* 84, 595–598.

Roseboom, T.J., van der Meulen, J.H.P., Osmond, C., Barker, D.J.P., Ravelli, A.C.J. and Blecker, O.P. (2000b) Plasma lipid profile in adults after perinatal exposure to famine. *American Journal of Clinical Nutrition* 72, 1101–1106.

Simonetta, G., Walker, D.W. and McMillen, I.C. (1991) Effect of feeding on the diurnal rhythm of plasma cortisol and adrenocorticotrophic hormone concentrations in the pregnant ewe and sheep fetus. *Experimental Physiology* 76, 219–229.

St Germain, D.L. (1999) Developmental effects of thyroid hormone: the role of deiodinases in regulatory control. *Biochemical Society Transactions* 27, 83–88.

Stephenson, T., Budge, H., Mostyn, A., Pearce, S., Webb, R. and Symonds, M.E. (2001) Fetal and neonatal adipose tissue maturation: a primary site of cytokine and cytokine-receptor action. *Biochemical Society Transactions* 29, 80–85.

Stevens, D. and Alexander, G. (1986) Lipid deposition after hypophysectomy and growth hormone treatment in the sheep fetus. *Journal of Developmental Physiology* 8, 139–145.

Symonds, M.E. (1995) Pregnancy, parturition and neonatal development – interactions between nutrition and thyroid hormones. *Proceedings of the Nutrition Society* 54, 329–343.

Symonds, M.E., Bird, J.A., Clarke, L., Gate, J.J. and Lomax, M.A. (1995) Nutrition, temperature and homeostasis during perinatal development. *Experimental Physiology* 80, 907–940.

Symonds, M.E., Mostyn, A. and Stephenson, T. (2001a) Cytokines and cytokine-receptors in fetal growth and development. *Biochemical Society Transactions* 29, 33–37.

Symonds, M.E., Budge, H., Stephenson, T. and McMillen, I.C. (2001b) Fetal endocrinology and development – manipulation and adaptation to long term nutritional and environmental challenges. *Reproduction* 121, 853–862.

van Rens, B.T., Evans, G.J. and van der Lende, T. (2003) Components of litter size in gilts with different prolactin receptor genotypes. *Theriogenology* 59, 915–926.

Wallace, J.M. (2000) Nutrient partitioning during pregnancy: adverse gestational outcome in overnourished adolescent dams. *Proceedings of the Nutrition Society* 59, 107–117.

Wallace, J.M., Da Silva, P., Aitken, R.P. and Cruickshank, M.A. (1997) Maternal endocrine status in relation to outcome in rapidly growing adolescent sheep. *Journal of Endocrinology* 155, 359–368.

Wallace, J.M., Bourke, D.A., Aitken, R.P., Palmer, R.P., Da Silva, P. and Cruickshank, M.A. (2000) Relationship between nutritionally mediated placental growth restriction and fetal growth, body composition and endocrine status during late gestation. *Placenta* 21, 100–108.

Warnes, K., Morris, M.J., Symonds, M.E., Phillips, I.D., Owens, J.A. and McMillen, I.C. (1998) Effects of gestation, cortisol and maternal undernutrition on hypothalamic neuropeptide Y mRNA levels in the sheep fetus. *Journal of Neuroendocrinology* 10, 51–57.

Whorwood, C.B., Firth, K.M., Budge, H. and Symonds, M.E. (2001) Maternal undernutrition during early to mid-gestation programmes tissue-specific alterations in the expression of the glucocorticoid receptor, 11β-hydroxysteroid dehydrogenase isoforms and type 1 angiotensin II receptor in neonatal sheep. *Endocrinology* 142, 1778–1785.

Young, L., Fernandes, K., McEvoy, T., Butterwith, S., Gutierrez, C., Carolan, C., Broadbent, P., Robinson, J., Wilmut, I. and Sinclair, K. (2001) Epigenetic change in IGF2R is associated with fetal overgrowth after embryo culture. *Nature Genetics* 27, 153–154.

16 Impact of Intrauterine Exposure to Glucocorticoids upon Fetal Development and Adult Pathophysiology

AMANDA J. DRAKE AND JONATHAN R. SECKL

Endocrinology Unit, School of Molecular and Clinical Medicine, University of Edinburgh, Molecular Medicine Centre, Western General Hospital, Edinburgh EH4 2XU, UK

Epidemiological Overview

Numerous epidemiological studies in distinct populations in the UK and the rest of the world have demonstrated a link between low birthweight and the subsequent development of hypertension, insulin resistance, type 2 diabetes and cardiovascular disease (Barker, 1991; Barker *et al.*, 1993a,b; Fall *et al.*, 1995; Yajnik *et al.*, 1995; Curhan *et al.*, 1996a,b; Leon *et al.*, 1996; Lithell *et al.*, 1996; Moore *et al.*, 1996; Forsen *et al.*, 1997; Rich-Edwards *et al.*, 1997). Even the smaller of twins at birth has higher blood pressure in later life (Levine *et al.*, 1994), although this has not been a consistent finding (Baird *et al.*, 2001). The association between birthweight and later cardio-metabolic disease appears to be largely independent of classical lifestyle risk factors such as smoking, adult weight, social class, alcohol and lack of exercise, which are additive to the effect of birthweight (Barker *et al.*, 1993b). The relationships are apparently continuous and represent birthweights within the normal range, rather than severe intrauterine growth retardation, multiple births or very premature babies (Barker, 1991, 1994; Curhan *et al.*, 1996a,b), although premature babies also have increased cardiovascular risk factors in adulthood (Irving *et al.*, 2000). Additionally, postnatal catch-up growth may also be predictive of later risk of cardiovascular disease (Barker, 1991; Osmond *et al.*, 1993; Levine *et al.*, 1994; Leon *et al.*, 1996; Bavdekar *et al.*, 1999; Eriksson *et al.*, 1999; Forsen *et al.*, 2000; Law *et al.*, 2002), suggesting that it is the restriction of intrauterine growth rather than smallness itself which is important.

These early life effects seem to be important predictors of later disease, increasing the risk of adult disease by 40–300% (Barker *et al.*,

1990; Curhan et al., 1996a,b). In the Preston study, a small baby with a large placenta had three times the relative risk of adult hypertension compared with a large baby with a normal placenta (Barker et al., 1990). In a study of 22,000 US men, those that were born lighter than 5.5 lb had a relative risk of adult hypertension of 1.26, and of type 2 diabetes of 1.75, compared with those of average birthweight (Curhan et al., 1996b). The relative risk of hypertension in light normal babies was 1.43 in 71,000 female American nurses (Curhan et al., 1996a). However, despite the large body of data describing such early life associations, there is still considerable debate as to the importance of birthweight in determining later disease (Huxley et al., 2002), and the magnitude of any such effect. It has been suggested that some studies linking lower birthweight with higher adult blood pressure fail to take into account the impact of random error, and may involve inappropriate adjustment for confounding factors (Huxley et al., 2002). Despite this caveat, the mass of human epidemiological data and the production of animal models showing that early life environmental manipulations produce persisting adult effects suggest that discrete prenatal events *can* have permanent effects on adult physiology and pathology.

The Concept of Fetal Programming

To explain the apparent association of fetal growth and later disease, the idea of early life physiological 'programming' or 'imprinting' has been proposed (Barker et al., 1993a; Edwards et al., 1993; Seckl, 1998). Such programming occurs in a variety of systems and reflects the action of a factor during sensitive periods or 'windows' of development to exercise organizational effects that persist throughout life. Two major environmental hypotheses have been proposed to explain the mechanism by which low birthweight is associated with adult disease: fetal undernutrition, and overexposure of the fetus to glucocorticoids. A third hypothesis suggests that genetic factors may lead to both low birthweight and subsequent risk of cardiovascular disease (Fig. 16.1). Indeed, genetic loci have been described which may link smallness at birth with adult disease (Dunger et al., 1998; Hattersley et al., 1998; Vaessen et al., 2001). Although the loci implicated relate to insulin, insulin-like growth factors and their cognate signalling pathways, making them biologically plausible candidates, there remains debate as to the reproducibility of the findings to date (Frayling et al., 2002), perhaps because studies have been underpowered (Frayling and Hattersley, 2001). Thus, the relative importance of genetic and environmental factors in programming phenomena remains unknown. However, the occurrence of associations between early life environmental manipulations and later physiology and disease risk in isogenic rodent models, and, less certainly, the birthweight–adult disease associations in human twins, strongly implicate environmental factors at least partly in the causation of the epidemiological findings. Here we address the specific issue of hormonal programming by glucocorticoids.

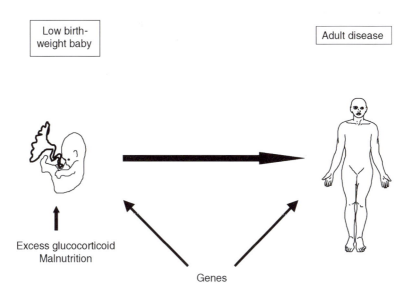

Low birth-
weight baby

Adult disease

Excess glucocorticoid
Malnutrition

Genes

Fig. 16.1. Two major environmental hypotheses have been proposed to explain the mechanism by which low birthweight is associated with adult disease: fetal undernutrition and overexposure of the fetus to glucocorticoids. A third hypothesis suggests that genetic factors may lead to both low birthweight and subsequent risk of cardiovascular disease: for example, a genetically mediated insulin resistance may lead to both reduced insulin-mediated fetal growth and later disease.

Prenatal Glucocorticoids as Mediators of Programming

Steroid hormones are typically associated with long-term organizational effects. For example, neonatal exposure to androgens programmes the expression of hepatic steroid-metabolizing enzymes and the development of sexually dimorphic structures in the anterior hypothalamus, as well as sexual behaviour (Arai and Gorski, 1968; Gustafsson *et al.*, 1983). Oestrogens also exert organizational effects on the developing CNS (Simerly, 2002). Critically, these effects can only be exerted during specific perinatal periods, but they then persist throughout life, largely irrespective of any subsequent sex steroid manipulations. The mechanisms may reflect the influences of sex steroids on the growth, maturation and remodelling of organs during the perinatal period. In the rat, the sexually dimorphic nucleus of the hypothalamic preoptic area is larger in males. Testosterone, selectively in this nucleus, inhibits apoptosis specifically between postnatal days 6 and 10, thus producing the male adult phenotype (Davis *et al.*, 1996).

Fetal glucocorticoid overexposure may have a role in the early-life programming of adult disease. Glucocorticoid receptors (GRs), members of the nuclear hormone receptor superfamily of ligand-activated transcription factors, are expressed in most fetal tissues from the early embryonal stages (Cole *et al.*, 1995). Expression of the closely related, higher-affinity mineralocorticoid receptor (MR) has a more limited tissue distribution and is only present at a later gestational stage (Brown *et al.*, 1996a,b). Additionally, GRs are highly expressed in the placenta (Sun et al., 1997). Perinatal glucocorticoids alter the rate of maturation of various organs, such as the lung (Ward, 1994), heart (Bian et al., 1992, 1993), kidney (Celsi et al., 1997) and gut. This maturing effect of glucocorticoids underpins their widespread use in obstetric and neonatal practice in accelerating fetal lung maturation when preterm labour threatens or occurs.

Glucocorticoid effects on birthweight

Glucocorticoid treatment during pregnancy has been shown to reduce birthweight in animals, including non-human primates (Reinisch et al., 1978; Ikegami et al., 1997; Nyirenda and Seckl, 1998; Nyirenda et al., 1998; French et al., 1999; Newnham et al., 1999; Newnham and Moss, 2001). Glucocorticoids are widely used in the management of women at risk of preterm delivery to enhance fetal lung maturation, and in the antenatal management of fetuses at risk of congenital adrenal hyperplasia. Human studies have confirmed that antenatal glucocorticoids are associated with a reduction in birthweight (French et al., 1999; Bloom et al., 2001), although normal birthweight has been reported in infants at risk of congenital adrenal hyperplasia receiving low-dose dexamethasone in utero from the first trimester (Forest et al., 1993; Mercado et al., 1995). Furthermore, in a recent study of pregnant women with asthma, use of daily inhaled and/or periodic oral glucocorticoid resulted in no changes in birthweight compared with a control non-asthmatic group. In contrast, a lack of glucocorticoid treatment in asthmatic women was found to be associated with a reduction in offspring birthweight (Murphy et al., 2002). However, these apparently paradoxical findings may be explained by an adverse effect of poorly controlled asthma on fetal growth, in particular due to the effects of inflammatory mediators on placental function. In addition, the route of steroid administration may be important: steroids were predominantly administered by inhalation, and, when oral steroids were given, prednisolone was used, which is rapidly inactivated by placental 11β-hydroxysteroid dehydrogenase type 2 (see below). Fetal cortisol levels are increased in human fetuses with intrauterine growth retardation or in pregnancies complicated by pre-eclampsia, implicating endogenous cortisol in retarded fetal growth (Goland et al., 1993, 1995). Cortisol also affects placental size, the effect being dependent on the dose and timing of exposure (Gunberg, 1957).

Prenatal glucocorticoid effects on the brain

Glucocorticoids are also essential for normal brain development, exerting a number of effects in most regions of the developing brain. During fetal development, the hippocampus and the hypothalamic–pituitary–adrenal (HPA) axis are particularly sensitive to endogenous and exogenous glucocorticoids. Perinatal glucocorticoids, or stress, programme specific effects in the brain, notably the HPA axis and dopaminergic-motor systems (Welberg and Seckl, 2001).

Prenatal glucocorticoid effects on blood pressure

Other glucocorticoid-sensitive systems are affected by early-life programming. Glucocorticoids are known to increase blood pressure in adults. Cortisol elevates the blood pressure in fetal sheep when infused directly *in utero* (Tangalakis *et al.*, 1992) and at birth in humans (Kari *et al.*, 1994) and in sheep (Berry *et al.*, 1997). The administration of betamethasone to pregnant baboons elevates fetal blood pressure (Koenen *et al.*, 2002). Antenatal glucocorticoid exposure also leads to permanently elevated blood pressure in later life. Rats treated with dexamethasone *in utero* have elevated blood pressure in adulthood (Benediktsson *et al.*, 1993; Sugden *et al.*, 2001), as do sheep exposed to excess glucocorticoid *in utero*, either as maternally administered dexamethasone or as a maternal cortisol infusion (Dodic *et al.*, 1998, 2002a,b; Jensen *et al.*, 2002). The timing of glucocorticoid exposure appears to be important; exposure to glucocorticoids during the final week of pregnancy in the rat is sufficient to produce permanent adult hypertension (Levitt *et al.*, 1996), whereas the sensitive window for such effects in sheep is earlier in gestation (Gatford *et al.*, 2000). Such differences may be due to the complex species-specific patterns of expression of GR, MR and the isoenzymes of 11β-hydroxysteroid dehydrogenase, which are crucial in both the regulation of maternal glucocorticoid transfer to the fetus, and in modulating glucocorticoid action at the tissue level.

Prenatal glucocorticoid effects on glucose homeostasis

Maternal glucocorticoid administration has an effect on cord glucose and insulin levels in the ovine fetus (Sloboda *et al.*, 2002a) and on glucose homeostasis in the adult offspring. In an ovine model, antenatal glucocorticoid exposure with or without fetal growth restriction altered glucose metabolism (Moss *et al.*, 2001). Maternal, but not fetal, injections of betamethasone restricted fetal growth (Newnham *et al.*, 1999); however, offspring of both groups had altered glucose metabolism postnatally (Moss *et al.*, 2001). The important implication of this study is that the programming effects on glucose homeostasis in this model are related to the exposure of the fetus to excess glucocorticoid *in utero*, rather than to an effect of intrauterine growth retardation. In rats, last-trimester glucocorticoid exposure programmes permanent hyperglycaemia and hyperinsulinaemia in the adult offspring (Nyirenda *et al.*, 1998). Indeed, the combination of hypertension, glucose intolerance and HPA axis activation in this animal model resembles the human 'metabolic syndrome', an important feature of the fetal origins observations. Again, the timing of exposure is important; earlier treatment does not result in glucose intolerance in the adult offspring.

Placental 11β-Hydroxysteroid Dehydrogenase Type 2

Glucocorticoids rapidly cross the placenta; however, fetal glucocorticoid levels are much lower than maternal levels (Beitins *et al.*, 1973). This is thought to be due to the enzyme 11β-hydroxysteroid dehydrogenase type 2 (11β-HSD-2) which is present in the placenta and catalyses the rapid metabolism of cortisol and corticosterone to the inert 11-keto steroids, cortisone and 11-dehydrocorticosterone (Brown *et al.*, 1996b) (Fig. 16.2). However, the enzyme is not a complete barrier to maternal steroids (Benediktsson *et al.*, 1997), and dexamethasone is a poor substrate (Albiston *et al.*, 1994). In addition, the efficiency of placental 11β-HSD-2 near term varies in both humans and rats (Benediktsson *et al.*, 1993; Stewart *et al.*, 1995). A relative deficiency of 11β-HSD-2, with consequent reduced inactivation of maternal steroids, may lead to overexposure of the fetus to glucocorticoids, retard fetal growth and programme responses leading to later disease (Edwards *et al.*, 1993). Studies in rats have demonstrated that lower placental 11β-HSD-2 activity is seen in the smallest fetuses with the largest placentas (Benediktsson *et al.*, 1993). Similar associations between placental 11β-HSD-2 activity and birthweight have been noted in humans (Stewart *et al.*, 1995; Shams *et al.*, 1998; McTernan *et al.*, 2001), although not all studies confirm this (Rogerson *et al.*, 1996, 1997). These babies are the ones predicted to have the highest adult blood pressures. Additionally, markers of fetal exposure to glucocorticoids, such as cord-blood levels of osteocalcin (a glucocorticoid-sensitive osteoblast gene product that

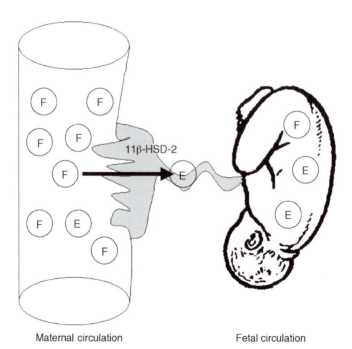

Maternal circulation   Fetal circulation

Fig. 16.2.   11β-Hydroxysteroid dehydrogenase-2 (11β-HSD-2) acts as a 'barrier' to maternal corticosteroids. 11β-HSD-2 is present in the placenta and many fetal tissues until mid-gestation, and inactivates cortisol (F) (corticosterone in rats and mice) to cortisone (E) (11-dehydrocorticosterone in rats and mice). The fetus therefore has much lower circulating levels of active glucocorticoid.

does not cross the placenta), also correlate with placental 11β-HSD-2 function (Benediktsson *et al.*, 1995).

Further evidence for the importance of 11β-HSD-2 as a placental barrier to maternal glucocorticoids comes from studies of individuals with the rare autosomal recessive syndrome of apparent mineralocorticoid excess. Individuals with this disorder are homozygous (or compound heterozygous) for mutations in the 11β-HSD-2 gene and are of low birthweight (1.2 kg less than unaffected siblings) (Dave-Sharma *et al.*, 1998). Thus, a lack of 11β-HSD-2 in the fetus or placenta causes growth retardation in humans. In contrast, 11β-HSD-2 null mice have normal birthweight (Kotelevtsev *et al.*, 1999). However, the crossed genetic background of the original 11β-HSD-2 null mouse may have obscured effects specific to the loss of 11β-HSD-2; indeed preliminary data suggest that in isogenic mice, 11β-HSD-2 nullizygosity lowers birthweight (Holmes *et al.*, 2002). Additionally, there may also be species differences here. Thus, the mouse shows mid-gestational loss of placental 11β-HSD-2 gene expression (Brown *et al.*, 1996a), whereas in humans, placental 11β-HSD-2 activity increases through gestation (Stewart *et al.*, 1995).

Inhibition of 11β-HSD-2 by treatment of pregnant rats with carbenoxolone has effects similar to those of dexamethasone, leading to offspring of reduced birthweight and adult hypertension and hyperglycaemia (Benediktsson *et al.*, 1993; Lindsay *et al.*, 1996a,b). These effects of carbenoxolone are independent of changes in maternal blood pressure or electrolytes, but do require the presence of maternal glucocorticoids; the offspring of adrenalectomized pregnant rats treated with carbenoxolone are protected from these effects. However, it must be noted that carbenoxolone is non-selective and inhibits other 11β-HSD isozymes and other related dehydrogenases.

A common mechanism may underlie fetal programming through maternal undernutrition and glucocorticoid exposure. Dietary protein restriction during rat pregnancy selectively attenuates 11β-HSD-2, but apparently not other placental enzymes (Langley-Evans *et al.*, 1996a; Bertram *et al.*, 2001; Lesage *et al.*, 2001). Indeed, in the maternal protein restriction model, offspring hypertension can be prevented by treating the pregnant dam with glucocorticoid synthesis inhibitors, and can be recreated by concurrent administration of corticosterone, at least in female offspring (Langley-Evans, 1997).

Because maternal glucocorticoid levels are much higher than those of the fetus, subtle changes in placental 11β-HSD-2 activity may have profound effects on fetal glucocorticoid exposure. A relative deficiency of placental 11β-HSD-2 therefore has far greater potential consequences in terms of the fetal glucocorticoid load than any alteration in fetal adrenal steroid production, once the capacity of the fetal HPA axis to suppress fetal adrenal output has been overwhelmed.

11β-HSD-2 and the Fetus

There may also be complex developmental windows of fetal tissue glucocorticoid sensitivity, the implications of which are uncertain. Many fetal tissues express 11β-HSD-2 until mid-gestation, at least in rodents, but probably also in humans (Stewart *et al.*, 1994; Brown *et al.*, 1996a). Glucocorticoids interact with both glucocorticoid and mineralocorticoid receptors (GRs and MRs), which are also widely expressed from mid-gestation. Dexamethasone and carbenoxolone may therefore exert effects directly on fetal tissues in addition to, or rather than, acting via the placenta. The time windows for glucocorticoid action are not fully determined, although for dexamethasone, treatment restricted to the last week of gestation in rats shows clear effects (Levitt *et al.*, 1996). However, fetal mouse tissues show striking silencing of the 11β-HSD-2 gene at mid-gestation, which presumably allows crucial developmental and maturational actions of glucocorticoids to occur before birth (Brown *et al.*, 1996a). The complex ontogeny of the 11β-HSD isozymes and corticosteroid receptors indicates intricate developmental control of glucocorticoid action at the cellular level (Brown *et al.*, 1996b; Diaz *et al.*, 1998), and may explain the developmental windows of tissue sensitivity to glucocorticoid programming. In human fetal tissues, 11β-HSD-2 also appears to be silenced. This probably occurs between weeks 19 and 26, since before this time enzyme activity is widespread (Stewart *et al.*, 1994), whereas later 11β-HSD-2 mRNA is not detected, except in kidney (and presumably other aldosterone target tissues). The implications of these complex developmental windows of tissue glucocorticoid sensitivity for fetal programming remain unexplored.

Regulation of 11β-HSD-2

If placental 11β-HSD-2 plays an important role in modulating maternal environmental actions upon fetal and placental development, then its regulation is of considerable interest. Placental 11β-HSD-2 is not apparently regulated by environmental factors such as ethanol or nicotine (Waddell and Atkinson, 1994). Nitric oxide selectively attenuates 11β-HSD-2 in human syncytiotrophoblasts *in vitro* (Sun *et al.*, 1997). Thus, nitric oxide-mediated placental vasodilatation might be counteracted by glucocorticoid vasoconstriction, which is enhanced by nitric oxide attenuation of glucocorticoid inactivation by 11β-HSD-2 (Sun *et al.*, 1997). However, the effect of exogenous glucocorticoid administration on placental and umbilical vessel resistance remains unknown; studies report conflicting effects of betamethasone administration in pregnancies complicated by intrauterine growth retardation and increased placental vascular resistance (Adamson and Kingdom, 1999; Wallace and Baker, 1999; Wijnberger *et al.*, 1999).

Recent studies have demonstrated that 11β-HSD-2 in the human placenta is regulated by oxygen concentrations (Alfaidy *et al.*, 2002). Pre-eclampsia is a condition causing significant maternal and perinatal morbidity and is associated with reduced fetal growth. The genesis of pre-eclampsia is related to deficient trophoblast invasion of maternal spiral arteries, which might result in a reduction of placental oxygen (Alfaidy *et al.*, 2002). In placental tissue from pre-eclamptic pregnancies, 11β-HSD-2 is reduced, and the activity and expression of 11β-HSD-2 in placental tissues is oxygen dependent throughout gestation

(Alfaidy *et al.*, 2002). These changes in 11β-HSD-2 may occur in response to the vascular abnormalities in pre-eclampsia and result in increased glucocorticoid action in the placenta and transfer to the fetus.

In pregnancies complicated by asthma, placental 11β-HSD-2 activity is significantly reduced in those women not taking inhaled glucocorticoid treatment (Murphy *et al.*, 2002). There is also an association between reduced placental 11β-HSD-2 activity, reduced birthweight and increased fetal cortisol concentrations in these pregnancies (Murphy *et al.*, 2002), suggesting that inflammatory mediators in uncontrolled asthma may have important deleterious effects on placental 11β-HSD-2 activity and placental function.

In the rat, placental 11β-HSD-2 activity is not regulated by maternal or fetal glucocorticoids or other adrenal steroids (Waddell *et al.*, 1998), although high progesterone levels inhibit 11β-HSD-2 (Baggia *et al.*, 1990; Brown *et al.*, 1996b), of potential relevance to the placenta near term. In contrast, in the baboon, oestrogens maintain placental 11β-HSD-2 (Baggia *et al.*, 1990). Intrauterine growth retardation in humans is also associated with reduced fetal adrenal androgen production (Goland *et al.*, 1993), which may then attenuate placental 11β-HSD-2, increasing materno-fetal glucocorticoid transfer. In the sheep, cortisol inhibits placental 11β-HSD-2 expression (Clarke *et al.*, 2002), suggesting it may increase further glucocorticoid action, contributing perhaps to the cortisol amplification cascade that triggers parturition in this species.

Maternal or fetal stress and glucocorticoids stimulate placental secretion of corticotrophin-releasing hormone (CRH), in contrast to their typical inhibition of CRH in the hypothalamus. CRH is elevated in the neonatal circulation in association with intrauterine growth retardation (Goland *et al.*, 1993) or maternal hypertension (Goland *et al.*, 1995). This might stimulate the fetal HPA axis to secrete glucocorticoids, amplifying fetal glucocorticoid excess. Thus, a cascade of effects may increase glucocorticoid levels in the growth-retarded fetus (Edwards *et al.*, 1993; Seckl, 1994). This fetal glucocorticoid excess may achieve a short-term benefit by increasing the availability of glucose and other fuels; however, the longer term consequences of such measures would be the programming of elevated glucocorticoid levels, higher blood pressure and hyperglycaemia. These responses may be useful to support a predicted increased level of environmental challenges after birth (the thrifty phenotype hypothesis); however, in the absence of such conditions the exaggerated set-point of offspring physiology and homeostasis may promote disease.

Tissue Targets of Glucocorticoid Programming

Liver and pancreas

Several important hepatic processes are regulated by glucocorticoids, including key enzymes of carbohydrate metabolism such as phosphenolpyruvate carboxykinase (PEPCK), a rate-limiting enzyme in gluconeogenesis. In rats, exposure to excess glucocorticoid *in utero* leads to offspring with permanent elevations in PEPCK transcription and activity in the gluconeogenic periportal region of the hepatic acinus (Nyirenda *et al.*, 1998). GR expression is also increased in adult rats exposed to antenatal dexamethasone, again only in the hepatic periportal zone. This increase in GR may be crucial, since animals exposed to dexamethasone *in utero* have potentiated plasma glucose responses to exogenous corticosterone (Nyirenda *et al.*, 1998).

Glucocorticoid exposure late in rat pregnancy predisposes the offspring to glucose intolerance in adulthood. Adult offspring of rats exposed to dexamethasone in late pregnancy have fasting hyperglycaemia, reactive hyperglycaemia and hyperinsulinaemia (Nyirenda *et al.*, 1998). Overexpression of PEPCK in a rat hepatoma cell line impairs suppression of gluconeogenesis by insulin (Rosella *et al.*, 1993), and transgenic mice with overexpression of hepatic PEPCK have impaired glucose tolerance (Valera *et al.*, 1994). Thus, the observed glucose intolerance in rats exposed to excessive glucocorticoids *in utero* may be explained in part by programmed hepatic PEPCK overexpression leading to increased gluconeogenesis. Additionally, this may be mediated by increased GR.

11β-Hydroxysteroid dehydrogenase type 1 (11β-HSD-1) is the predominant form of the enzyme found in liver, and is responsible for the reactivation of cortisol (corticosterone in rodents) from cortisone (11-dehydrocorticosterone in rodents). 11β-HSD-1 and GR have been co-localized in the rat liver (Whorwood *et al.*, 1992), suggesting that 11β-HSD-1 may regulate ligand access to GR (Whorwood *et al.*, 1992; Seckl and Chapman, 1997; Jamieson *et al.*, 2000). Glucocorticoids, in turn, regulate 11β-HSD-1 activity (Voice *et al.*, 1996). Studies have shown that increasing levels of plasma cortisol are associated with increases in the activity of PEPCK and other gluconeogenic enzymes in the fetus (Fowden *et al.*, 1993). Additionally, the activity of gluconeogenic enzymes is decreased in the 11β-HSD-1 knockout mouse (Kotelevtsev *et al.*, 1997), suggesting that local glucocorticoid concentrations are important in the regulation of hepatic gluconeogenesis. Changes in hepatic 11β-HSD-1 may therefore influence metabolic processes. Both maternal and fetal exposure to excess glucocorticoid result in an increase in hepatic 11β-HSD-1 mRNA and protein in fetal sheep (Yang *et al.*, 1995; Sloboda *et al.*, 2002a). Such changes in 11β-HSD-1 increase the potential to regenerate active glucocorticoids, and may further influence the expression of glucocorticoid-dependent hepatic enzymes involved in glucose homeostasis and HPA feedback. Hepatic 11β-HSD-1 mRNA levels in adult rats have been reported as unchanged in response to antenatal dexamethasone exposure (Nyirenda *et al.*, 1998) and decreased in response to antenatal carbenoxolone exposure (Saegusa *et al.*, 1999).

Administration of betamethasone to pregnant ewes, as single or multiple doses, reduces offspring birthweight and alters their glucose metabolism. Intriguingly, administration of betamethasone directly to the ovine fetus leads to offspring with normal birthweight, but again is associated with altered glucose metabolism (Moss *et al.*, 2001). Additionally, maternal betamethasone treatment in this model elevates cord plasma glucose levels (Sloboda *et al.*, 2002a,b). These findings indicate altered fetal glucose homeostasis, perhaps as a result of increases in intrahepatic glucocorticoid levels consequent on the increased hepatic 11β-HSD-1 activity and/or increased GR signalling (see below).

In utero undernutrition impairs rat pancreatic β-cell development (Garofano *et al.*, 1997, 1998), resulting in reduced β-cell mass and subsequent glucose intolerance, and recent evidence suggests that glucocorticoids may play an important part in this (Blondeau *et al.*, 2001). In rats with normal nutrition, fetal pancreatic insulin content is negatively correlated with fetal corticosterone levels, and β-cell mass increases when fetal steroid production is impaired (Blondeau *et al.*, 2001). Maternal malnutrition in the rat is associated with elevated maternal and fetal corticosterone levels, in addition to decreased fetal pancreatic insulin content and β-cell mass. Preventing the corticosterone increase in food-restricted dams, by adrenalectomy with corticosterone replacement, restores β-cell mass (Blondeau *et al.*, 2001). The mechanisms by which glucocorticoids modulate pancreatic development are unclear, but may include a direct effect of glucocorticoids on β-cells (Sharma *et al.*, 1997), or an effect on the developing exocrine pancreas (McEvoy and Hegre, 1976; Rall *et al.*, 1977). Further, gluco-corticoids influence the expression of insulin-like growth factor-II (IGF-II), a key peptide growth factor in pancreatic development, in addition to the IGF receptor and several insulin-like growth factor binding proteins (IGFBPs) (Hill and Duvillie, 2000).

Blood pressure

In rats, prenatal dexamethasone affects a number of organs related to blood pressure control and maintenance, in particular the heart, vasculature, kidney and brain. Effects include permanent induction of the pattern and balance of α- and β-adrenergic receptor expression and potentiation of adenylate cyclase (Huff *et al.*, 1991; Bian *et al.*, 1992), either of which might alter subsequent vascular responsivity to vasoconstrictors.

Fetal sheep become hypertensive and show increased pressor responses to angiotensin II when directly infused with cortisol (Tangalakis *et al.*, 1992). Additionally, chronic low-dose maternal cortisol infusions reduce fetal growth rate, increase heart weight and ventricular wall thickness and increase blood pressure in fetal sheep (Jensen *et al.*, 2002). Brief prenatal exposure to glucocorticoids *in utero* leads to hypertension in adult sheep of both sexes, in association with a permanent increase in angiotensin (AT) type 1 receptors in the hypothalamus, and increased MR and GR mRNA in the hippocampus prenatally (Dodic *et al.*, 2002a,b). Maternal dexamethasone treatment also programmes alterations in the renin–angiotensin system of the ovine fetal kidney (Moritz *et al.*, 2002). Angiotensinogen, the AT_1 receptor and the AT_2 receptor were increased in fetal kidneys after dexamethasone treatment. Although there was no difference in basal blood pressure between fetuses that had received dexamethasone and control animals, the glomerular filtration rate was reduced in response to angiotensin II in the dexamethasone-treated group (Moritz *et al.*, 2002).

Development of the heart and its biochemistry are also programmed by prenatal dexamethasone (Bian *et al.*, 1993; Langdown *et al.*, 2001a,b), as is the sympathetic innervation of some organs (Navarro *et al.*, 1989). These effects may be arterial-bed specific, notably with regard to endothelin-1 sensitivity (Docherty et al., 2001).

Muscle and fat

Exposure to antenatal dexamethasone in rats is also associated with programming of fat and muscle metabolism (Cleasby et al., 2003a). There is tissue-specific programming of GR expression; GR is down-regulated in soleus muscle, but elevated in visceral adipose tissue. Elevated GR expression in visceral adipose tissue in the presence of circulating hypercorticosteronaemia suggests increased glucocorticoid action in visceral fat. This may contribute to both adipose and hepatic insulin resistance. These changes in GR expression do not appear to be the result of metabolic derangement in the adult animal, correction of the hypercorticosteronaemia and insulin sensitization were not sufficient to normalize the programmed changes in GR (Cleasby et al., 2003b).

Adipose Factors and Programming: an Emerging Area?

Leptin

Leptin, an adipose gene product that signals both centrally and peripherally, where it plays a role in insulin sensitivity, is present in the circulation of human and porcine fetuses from mid-gestation (Jaquet et al., 1998; Chen et al., 2000), and in adipose tissue of human fetuses by 20 weeks' gestation (Lepercq et al., 2001). Additionally, mRNA for leptin and leptin receptors have been detected in the fetal tissues of many other species (Yuen et al., 1999; Hoggard et al., 2000; Lepercq et al., 2001; Mostyn et al., 2001; Thomas et al., 2001). In the human fetus, circulating leptin levels increase towards term, associated with a significant increase in body fat after 34 weeks of gestation (Jaquet et al., 1998; Geary et al., 1999; Cetin et al., 2000), and in fetal sheep, leptin mRNA increases in adipose tissue with increasing gestational age (Yuen et al., 1999). Intriguingly, leptin concentrations in human fetal cord blood correlate directly with body weight and adiposity at birth (Koistinen et al., 1997; Schubring et al., 1997; Jaquet et al., 1998; Ong et al., 1999; Lepercq et al., 2001), indicating a potential role linking fetal growth and metabolic programming.

In rats, antenatal treatment of the pregnant mother with dexamethasone reduces fetal plasma and placental levels of leptin, while maternal plasma leptin levels remain unchanged or increase (Sugden et al., 2001; Smith and Waddell, 2002). Additionally, dexamethasone reduces placental expression of the leptin receptor isoform Ob-Rb, which mediates leptin action (Smith and Waddell, 2002), while levels of the isoform ObR-S (the proposed transport form of the receptor) are modestly increased (Sugden et al., 2001). In contrast, in the sheep, exogenous cortisol or dexamethasone administration directly to the fetus increases plasma leptin concentrations, albeit transiently (Forhead et al., 2002; Mostyn et al., 2003). The differences between these studies may reflect the route of glucocorticoid administration, species, fetal body fat levels and/or maternal nutrient intake. Crucially, to separate cause from consequence, the effect of perinatal leptin 'replacement' upon the adult metabolic phenotype in low birthweight models remains to be determined.

Adiponectin

Adiponectin (acrp30, adipoQ) is an abundant, adipose-specific protein which is secreted into the blood. Deficiency of adiponectin, which is negatively associated with fat mass (Hu *et al.*, 1996) and positively associated with insulin sensitivity (Weyer *et al.*, 2001), may mediate obesity-related resistance to insulin. Lower plasma adiponectin levels appear to predict the later occurrence of type 2 diabetes (Lindsay *et al.*, 2002). The predictive effect of adiponectin on the development of type 2 diabetes seems independent of the degree of obesity (Vozarova *et al.*, 2002). Adiponectin is strikingly regulated by hormones and other factors during postnatal development (Combs *et al.*, 2003). Any role of adiponectin during prenatal development and in programming models is unexplored but, given the emerging biology of the adipocyte and its important role in some programming phenomena (Cleasby *et al.*, 2003a), is likely to be of interest.

Programming of the Brain: the Hypothalamic–Pituitary–Adrenal (HPA) Axis

Studies in animal models indicate that the HPA axis is an important target for glucocorticoid programming. The HPA axis is controlled by a negative feedback system in which glucocorticoids released by the adrenals interact with glucocorticoid receptors in the pituitary, hypothalamus and hippocampus. Overactivity at any point along the pathway should result in negative feedback to decrease the amount of corticotrophin-releasing hormone (CRH), and thus decrease the synthesis and release of glucocorticoids.

Prenatal dexamethasone exposure or 11β-HSD-2 inhibition permanently increases basal plasma corticosterone levels in adult rats (Levitt *et al.*, 1996; Welberg *et al.*, 2000). The resultant hypercorticosteronaemia with altered feedback may contribute directly to the observed hypertension and hyperglycaemia, particularly with the associated increase in hepatic glucocorticoid sensitivity. In sheep, exposure to betamethasone *in utero* alters HPA responsiveness in the offspring at up to 1 year of age. The outcomes varied according to the time of gestation at which the synthetic glucocorticoid was administered, and whether it was administered to the mother or the fetus (Sloboda *et al.*, 2002b). Maternal administration of betamethasone resulted in offspring with significantly elevated stimulated and basal cortisol levels, whereas betamethasone administration to the fetus resulted in attenuated ACTH responses to CRH + arginine vasopressin (AVP) when compared with control animals (Sloboda *et al.*, 2002b). Intriguingly, maternal undernutrition in rodents (Langley-Evans *et al.*, 1996b) or sheep

(Hawkins et al., 2000) also affects adult HPA axis function, suggesting that HPA programming may be a common outcome of prenatal environmental challenge, perhaps acting in part via alterations in placental 11β-HSD-2 activity, which is reduced by maternal dietary constraint (Langley-Evans et al., 1996a; Bertram et al., 2001).

Further evidence for the importance of the timing of exposure in determining the long-term effects of glucocorticoid programming comes from recent studies in guinea-pigs. These animals have a relative glucocorticoid resistance because of a mutant GR gene (Keightley and Fuller, 1994); prenatal glucocorticoid exposure therefore has smaller effects on the HPA axis in offspring (Dean et al., 2001; Liu et al., 2001). In males, short-term exposure to dexamethasone (2 days) leads to significantly elevated basal plasma cortisol levels, whereas repeated doses reduced basal and stimulated plasma cortisol levels in adults. In contrast, juvenile females exposed for 2 days have reduced HPA responses to stress, whereas adult females exposed to repeated antenatal doses of dexamethasone have higher plasma cortisol levels in the follicular and early luteal phases.

A single study of the effects of glucocorticoid programming in primates showed that the offspring of mothers treated with dexamethasone during late pregnancy had elevated basal and stress-stimulated cortisol levels and a 30% reduction in hippocampal size (Uno et al., 1994). These studies in guinea-pigs and primates indicate that exposure to excess glucocorticoids in utero can programme HPA axis function in species that produce neuroanatomically mature young.

Programming offspring behaviour

Overexposure to glucocorticoids in utero, as a result of either prenatal dexamethasone administration or 11β-HSD inhibition, leads to alterations in adult behaviour and may programme 'behavioural inhibition', and reduced coping under conditions of stress. Administration of dexamethasone to rats for all 3 weeks of gestation, or only in the last week, reduces ambulation and rearing in the open field in adult animals (Welberg et al., 2001), although another study did not find this (Holson et al., 1995). These studies employed subtly different timings of exposure, again suggesting that very specific time windows exist for the effects of prenatal treatments. Additionally, late gestation administration of dexamethasone alters exploration on an elevated plus-maze and reduces immobility both in the acquisition and the retrieval phase of a forced-swim test, implying impaired coping and a reduced capacity for acquisition, consolidation and/or retrieval of information under stressful circumstances (Welberg et al., 2001). This suggests that fetal glucocorticoid exposure, especially during the last week of gestation, may programme 'behavioural inhibition' (Fig. 16.3) and reduced coping in aversive situations later in life. Intriguingly, inhibition of 11β-HSD, which is most highly expressed in mid-gestation, produces a phenotype intermediate between continuous and final-week dexamethasone exposure (Welberg et al., 2000).

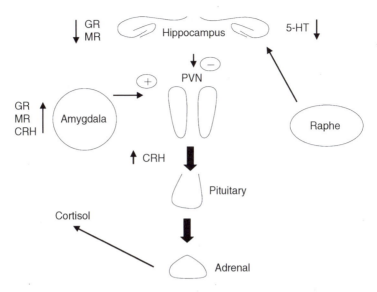

Fig. 16.3. Schematic diagram of the likely molecular mechanisms underpinning glucocorticoid programming of the hippocampus. In the rat, prenatal exposure to dexamethasone leads to an increase in presynaptic serotonin (5-HT) re-uptake in the raphe–hippocampal innervation. 5-HT is key to the maintenance of glucocorticoid receptor (GR) and mineralocorticoid receptor (MR) expression in fetal and adult hippocampal neurons. Reduction in hippocampal 5-HT, acting via specific 5-HT receptors, probably of the 5-HT$_7$ subtype, will alter the second and third messenger cascades, which impact on tissue-specific alternate promoters/first exons of the GR gene. Reduced GR and MR feedback in the hippocampus resulting from the reduction in GR and MR, leads to hypothalamus–pituitary–adrenal (HPA) activation. Conversely, GR and MR are permanently upregulated in the amygdala along with the increased amygdala corticotrophin-releasing hormone (CRH), which is presumed to underpin the 'anxiety-like' behaviour seen in this model. The amygdala, in turn, stimulates the HPA axis, and thus the increased GR and MR may amplify the effects of hippocampal desensitization. PVN, paraventricular nucleus.

Prenatal glucocorticoid exposure also affects the developing dopaminergic system (Diaz *et al.*, 1995, 1997a,b), with clear implications for proposed developmental contributions to schizo-affective, attention-deficit hyperactivity and extrapyramidal disorders.

Structural effects of antenatal glucocorticoids on the CNS

Exposure to glucocorticoids may alter brain structure (Matthews, 2000). Studies in young and aged animals and humans have demonstrated that stress and increased glucocorticoid concentrations can lead to changes in hippocampal structure (Bremner *et al.*, 1995; Sheline *et al.*, 1996; Stein *et al.*, 1997; Sapolsky, 1999). In rhesus monkeys, treatment with antenatal dexamethasone caused a dose-dependent neuronal degeneration of hippocampal neurons and reduced hippocampal volume in the fetuses, which persisted at 20 months of age (Uno et al., 1990). Fetuses receiving multiple lower-dose injections showed more severe damage than those receiving a single large injection (Uno et al., 1990). Human and animal studies have demonstrated that altered hippocampal structure may be associated with a number of consequences for memory and behaviour (Bremner et al., 1995; Sheline et al., 1996; Stein et al., 1997).

In mice, prenatal treatment with prednisolone appears to lead to delayed motor development, offspring having delayed eye opening, and delayed development of lifting, walking and gripping skills (Gandelman and Rosenthal, 1981). In rhesus monkeys, prenatal dexamethasone was not associated with delayed motor development (Uno et al., 1994). In sheep, betamethasone exposure in utero is associated with delayed myelination in those areas of the brain undergoing active myelination at the time of exposure, such as the optic nerve (Dunlop et al., 1997), with unknown consequences.

CNS programming mechanisms

The brain is clearly important as a target for glucocorticoid programming; however, the mechanisms of the programming effects appear to differ depending on the timing of the exposure, and are species specific. As with other tissues, changes in tissue receptor levels and in pre-receptor glucocorticoid metabolism may underpin these effects. In the rat, while both long- and short-term exposure to prenatal dexamethasone result in adults with elevated basal corticosterone levels, the underlying mechanisms differ depending on the timing of exposure. Exposure to dexamethasone during the last third of pregnancy reduces MR and GR levels in the hippocampus and increases CRH mRNA in the hypothalamic paraventricular nucleus (PVN) (Welberg et al., 2001). In contrast, dexamethasone throughout gestation does not alter hippocampal GR or MR, but increases receptor expression in the amygdala, a structure that stimulates the HPA axis (Levitt et al., 1996; Welberg et al., 2001). Thus in the rat, late-gestational dexamethasone exposure may permanently alter the 'set point' of the HPA axis at the level of the hippocampus, reducing feedback sensitivity, whereas continuous exposure may increase forward drive of the HPA axis through the amygdala. Thus, distinct neural mechanisms underlie the common outcome of altered HPA axis activity following prenatal glucocorticoid exposure.

The behavioural changes observed in prenatal glucocorticoid-exposed offspring may be associated with altered functioning of the amygdala, a structure involved in the expression of fear and anxiety. Intra-amygdala administration of corticotrophin-releasing hormone (CRH) is anxiogenic (Dunn and Berridge, 1990). Prenatal dexamethasone or 11β-HSD inhibition increase CRH mRNA levels specifically in the central nucleus of the amygdala, a key locus for the effects of the neuropeptide on the expression of fear and anxiety (Welberg et al., 2000, 2001). Indeed, corticosteroids facilitate CRH mRNA expression in this nucleus (Hsu et al., 1998) and increase GR and/or MR in the amygdala (Welberg et al., 2000, 2001). The amygdala stimulates the HPA axis, thus an elevated corticosteroid signal in the amygdala consequent on the hypercorticosteronaemia in the adult offspring of dexamethasone-treated dams, may produce the increased CRH levels in adulthood (Fig. 16.3). A direct relationship between brain corticosteroid receptor levels and anxiety-like behaviour is supported by the phenotype of transgenic mice with disrupted GR expression in the brain, which show markedly reduced anxiety behaviours (Tronche *et al.*, 1999). Intriguingly, the mechanisms by which the behavioural changes of glucocorticoid programming are effected appear to differ, depending on the timing of dexamethasone exposure, although the resultant HPA and behavioural phenotypes are similar. As discussed, although animals exposed to dexamethasone during the whole of pregnancy and those exposed only during the last week both have elevated basal glucocorticoid levels, the central changes are distinct (Welberg and Seckl, 2001). Dexamethasone exposure during the last week of gestation increases CRI I mRNA in the PVN and reduces GR and MR levels in the hippocampus (Welberg *et al.*, 2001), whereas exposure throughout gestation does not alter hippocampal GR or MR, but increases the expression of these receptors in the amygdala (Levitt *et al.*, 1996; Welberg *et al.*, 2001).

How might such mechanistically distinct effects come about with glucocorticoid exposure at different times during development? It seems reasonable to propose that programming may only happen at critical times during organ development. Thus, glucocorticoid exposure in the last days of gestation in the rat can target CNS regions actively developing, such as the hippocampus, but not those yet to develop or those already in their final state. The long and complex pre- and postnatal ontogeny of the brain makes it a prime target for programming. The complex patterns of expression of the key candidate genes, GR, MR and the 11β-HSDs, in the brain may underlie this (Diaz *et al.*, 1998; Matthews, 1998). While the details of brain ontogeny patterns are species-specific, the broad impression of tissues protected from, or allowing timed exposure to, glucocorticoids appears a tenable interpretation of these exquisite patterns of gene expression. Clearly exogenous (or endogenous) steroids can only have developmental effects on specific target genes and systems during their individual ontogenic windows of susceptibility.

Possible Common Final Mechanisms

Insulin-like growth factors (IGFs)

Considerable data suggest an important role for IGFs in the determination of placental and fetal growth (Jones and Clemmons, 1995). The IGFs are detectable in many fetal tissues from the first trimester, and IGF concentrations in the fetal circulation increase during pregnancy. An extensive series of null mutant knock-out mice has been used to document the roles played by many components of this system and the related insulin receptor system in fetal growth and organ development. Both IGF-I and IGF-II are essential for fetal growth; birthweights of IGF-I and IGF-II null mice are reduced by 40% when compared with their wild-type littermates. IGF-II is a paternally expressed gene in mammals, which is also essential for placental growth (Wood, 1995; D'Ercole *et al.*,

1996). Recent studies have suggested that the IGF-II gene may be important in regulating the placental supply of, and fetal demand for, maternal nutrients to the mammalian fetus (Constancia *et al.*, 2002). IGF-I is required for prenatal maturation and postnatal growth, and the type I IGF receptor mediates most of the actions of IGF-I and IGF-II on growth. Inactivation of the IGF-I receptor results in severe growth retardation (45% of normal birthweight).

IGF-I, IGF-II, both IGF receptors and several IGFBPs are regulated by glucocorticoids in fetal and adult tissues *in vivo* and *in vitro* (Luo *et al.*, 1990; Price *et al.*, 1992; Li *et al.*, 1993, 2002; Cheung *et al.*, 1994; Miell *et al.*, 1994; Delany and Canalis, 1995; Conover *et al.*, 1996; Mouhieddine *et al.*, 1996; Bach *et al.*, 1997). Such regulation is complex and highly developmentally- and tissue-specific (Li *et al.*, 1996; Forhead *et al.*, 2000). Offspring IGFs are also affected by maternal nutrition in rats (Woodall *et al.*, 1996) and in humans (Barker *et al.*, 1993a), and thus provide a putative pathway for maternal and feto-placental genetic, epigenetic and environmental factors (including 11β-HSD and glucocorticoids) to determine development and programming. Importantly, hepatic production of the binding protein (IGFBP-1), which neutralizes the action of IGF-I, is markedly induced in late-gestation fetuses by maternal dexamethasone (Price *et al.*, 1992). The IGFBP-1 gene is glucocorticoid-responsive (Goswami *et al.*, 1994) and transgenic mice overexpressing IGFBP-1 show low birthweight and adult hyperglycaemia (Rajkumar *et al.*, 1995). Moreover, GRs interact with the liver-enriched transcription factor hepatic nuclear factor-1 (HNF-1), in regulating IGFBP-1 and other genes (Suh and Rechler, 1997), and HNF-1 is mutated in some forms of diabetes (Yamagata *et al.*, 1996).

Molecular Mechanisms of Glucocorticoid Programming

Indications of the molecular mechanisms by which early life environmental factors may programme offspring physiology come from the studies of the processes underpinning postnatal environmental programming of the HPA axis in the 'neonatal handling' paradigm (Levine, 1957, 1962; Meaney *et al.*, 1988, 1996). In this model, 15 minutes of daily handling of rat pups during the first 2 weeks of life (Meaney *et al.*, 1988) permanently increases GR density in the hippocampus and prefrontal cortex, but not in other brain regions. This increase in receptor density potentiates the HPA axis sensitivity to glucocorticoid negative feedback and results in lower plasma glucocorticoid levels throughout life, a state compatible with a good adjustment to environmental stress (Meaney *et al.*, 1989, 1992). Neonatal glucocorticoid exposure may have similar effects (Catalani *et al.*, 1993). The neonatal handling model appears to be of physiological relevance, since handling enhances maternal care-related behaviours and natural variation in such maternal behaviour correlates similarly with the offspring HPA physiology and hippocampal GR expression (Liu *et al.*, 1997). The long-term manifestations of some prenatal programming can be substantially modified by the immediate postnatal environment (Maccari *et al.*, 1995), suggesting that distinct 'windows' occur, and showing that apparently similar early life events may produce different responses depending upon their degree, duration, developmental timing or sequence. Again, the implications for human epidemiology are that distinct offspring pathophysiologies may be determined merely by the timing and severity of the stimulus/stress involved.

Neuronal pathways and mechanisms

In recent years, the precise pathways involved in neonatal handling programming have been dissected. Handling acts via ascending serotonergic (5-HT) pathways from the midbrain raphe nuclei to the hippocampus (Smythe *et al.*, 1994). Activation of 5-HT induces GR gene expression in fetal hippocampal neurons *in vitro* (Mitchell *et al.*, 1990) and in neonatal (O'Donnell *et al.*, 1994) and adult hippocampal neurons *in vivo* (Yau *et al.*, 1997). The 'handling' induction of 5-HT requires thyroid hormones that are elevated by the stimulus. Consistent with this, administration of dexamethasone to fetal guinea-pigs leads to an elevation of fetal thyroid hormone and an upregulation of hippocampal GR mRNA (Dean and Matthews, 1999). At the hippocampal neuronal membrane, some recent findings implicate the ketanserin-sensitive 5-HT$_7$ receptor subtype, which is positively coupled to cAMP generation, in the handling effects (Meaney *et al.*, 2000). *In vitro*, 5-HT stimulation of GR expression in hippocampal neurons is blocked by ketanserin and mimicked by cAMP analogues (Mitchell *et al.*, 1990, 1992). 5-HT$_7$ receptors appear to play a key role in this action (Laplante *et al.*, 2002). *In vivo*, handling also stimulates cAMP generation in the hippocampus (Diorio *et al.*, 1996). The next step appears to involve stimulation of cAMP-associated and other transcription factors, most notably NGFI-A and AP-2 (Meaney *et al.*, 2000). NGFI-A and AP-2 may bind to the GR gene promoter (Encio and Detera-Wadleigh, 1991).

The GR gene: a programming target

The GR gene expression is regulated in a complex tissue-specific manner. Although GRs are expressed in all cells, the level of expression and receptor regulation vary considerably between tissues, and even within a tissue (Herman *et al.*, 1989). Transgenic mice with a reduction of 30–50% in tissue levels of GR have major neuroendocrine, metabolic and immunological abnormalities (Pepin *et al.*, 1992; King *et al.*, 1995). The level of expression of GR is thus critical for cell function. As discussed, there is much evidence to suggest that GR gene transcription can be programmed in a tissue-specific manner by perinatal events. The GR promoter is extremely complex, with multiple tissue-specific alternate untranslated first exons in rats (McCormick *et al.*, 2000) and mice (Cole *et al.*, 1995), most within a transcriptionally active 'CpG island'. All these mRNA species give rise to the same receptor protein, as only exons 2–9 encode the protein. The alternate untranslated first exons are spliced on to the common translated sequence beginning at exon 2. In the rat, two of the alternate exons are present in all tissues which have been studied; however, others are tissue specific (McCormick *et al.*, 2000). This permits considerable complexity of tissue-specific variation in the control of GR expression and, potentially, programming (Fig. 16.4).

The tissue-specific first exon usage appears to be altered by perinatal environment manipulations (McCormick *et al.*, 2000). Indeed, handling permanently programmes increased expression of only one of the six alternate first exons (exon 1_7) utilized in the hippocampus (McCormick *et al.*, 2000). Exon 1_7 contains sites appropriate to bind the very third messenger/intermediate early gene transcription factors (AP-2, NGF1-A) induced by neonatal manipulation (Meaney *et al.*, 2000). In contrast, prenatal dexamethasone exposure, which increases hepatic GR expression, decreased the proportion of hepatic GR mRNA containing the predominant exon (exon 1_{10}), suggesting an increase in a minor exon 1 variant (McCormick *et al.*, 2000). Such tissue specificity of promoter usage may help explain why prenatal dexamethasone programmes increased adult GR expression in the periportal zone of the liver and in the amygdala, but reduced GR expression in the hippocampus, and unchanged expression in many other brain regions and tissues.

Intriguingly, the apparent congruence between the effects of prenatal and postnatal environmental manipulations upon the adult HPA axis appears to reflect distinct underlying processes. Prenatal dexamethasone exposure permanently alters developing monoaminergic systems. Prenatal treatment decreases brain 5-HT levels and advances the expression of the neuronal 5-HT transporter, which functions as a re-uptake site, removing 5-HT from the synapse and thus attenuating its action, including that in the hippocampus (Slotkin *et al.*, 1996; Muneoka *et al.*, 1997). In the postnatal handling model, animals in the non-handled group have decreased hippocampal 5-HT turnover. It appears that distinct mechanisms operating at different times of development can produce apparently similar permanent alterations in phenotype, in this case increased HPA axis activity.

The next crucial questions ask how discrete late prenatal/early postnatal events can permanently alter gene expression. Intriguing recent data have explored this in terms of chromatin. Some evidence is emerging for selective methylation/demethylation of specific promoters of the GR gene. Preliminary

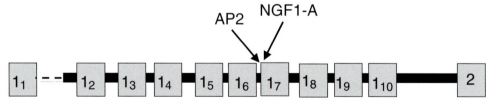

Fig. 16.4. Schematic diagram of the rat glucocorticoid receptor (GR) gene, which has multiple, untranslated tissue-specific first exons, allowing tissue-specific effects. There are eight translated exons (2–9), and over 10 untranslated first exons (here 1_1, 1_2, etc.), most of which lie within a transcriptionally active 'CpG island'. All mRNA transcripts produce the same protein but the levels of expression of the mRNAs containing the different exons 1, differ in a tissue-specific manner. Prenatal manipulations may alter the expression of specific promoters in specific tissues, allowing tissue-specific changes in GR density in response to an environmental challenge.

data suggest that the NGFI-A site around exon 1_7 is subject to differential and permanent methylation/demethylation in association with variations in maternal care (Weaver *et al.*, 2002). Moreover, GR itself appears under some circumstances to mediate differential demethylation of target gene promoters, at least in liver-derived cells. The demethylation persists after steroid withdrawal. During development, such target promoter demethylation occurs before birth and may fine-tune the promoter to 'remember' regulatory events occurring during development (Thomassin *et al.*, 2001).

Glucocorticoid Programming in Humans?

From the above it appears clear that exposure to glucocorticoids antenatally has an effect on birthweight in animal models and in humans, and may have effects on blood pressure, glucose tolerance and the HPA axis. What relevance might this have to human physiology?

Glucocorticoid treatment during pregnancy reduces birthweight (French *et al.*, 1999; Bloom *et al.*, 2001), but there is little evidence concerning the longer-term effects of glucocorticoids *in utero*. 11β-HSD-2 substrates, such as cortisol and prednisolone, would be anticipated to have little effect; however, glucocorticoids such as dexamethasone are commonly exploited because of their effect on the fetus. Substituted glucocorticoids such as dexamethasone and betamethasone, which are poor substrates for 11β-HSD-2, are most commonly used to treat fetuses at risk of preterm delivery, which may occur in up to 10% of pregnancies. There is no doubt that such synthetic glucocorticoids enhance lung maturation and reduce mortality in preterm infants (Crowley, 2000). Additionally, a single course of prenatal corticosteroid is associated with a significant reduction in the incidence of intraventricular haemorrhage and a trend toward less neurodevelopmental disability (Crowley, 2000). However, a recent survey of British obstetric departments showed that 98% were prescribing repeated courses of antenatal glucocorticoids (Brocklehurst *et al.*, 1999). Corticosteroid injections may be repeated four or more times in threatened preterm labour between 24 and 34 weeks of gestation. There is little evidence for the safety and efficacy of such a regime (Whitelaw and Thoresen, 2000). In addition, women at risk of bearing fetuses at risk of congenital adrenal hyperplasia often receive low-dose dexamethasone from the first trimester to suppress fetal adrenal androgen overproduction. Birthweight in such infants has been reported as normal (Forest *et al.*, 1993; Mercado *et al.*, 1995); however, it must be remembered that programming effects of antenatal glucocorticoids are seen in animal models in the absence of any reduction in birthweight (Moss *et al.*, 2001).

Antenatal glucocorticoid administration has also been linked with higher blood pressure in adolescence (Doyle *et al.*, 2000), although this study is complicated by the powerful effects of differential growth rates around puberty on blood pressure.

A number of studies aimed at establishing the long-term neurological and developmental effects of antenatal glucocorticoid exposure have been complicated by the fact that most of the children studied were born before term and were therefore already at risk of delayed neurological development. In a group of 6-year-old children, antenatal glucocorticoid exposure was associated with subtle effects on neurologic function, including reduced visual closure and visual memory (MacArthur et al., 1982). Children exposed to dexamethasone in early pregnancy because they were at risk of congenital adrenal hyperplasia, and who were born at term, showed increased emotionality, unsociability, avoidance and behavioural problems (Trautman et al., 1995). Furthermore, a recent study has shown that multiple doses of antenatal glucocorticoids, given to women at risk of preterm delivery, were associated with reduced head circumference in the offspring (French et al., 1999). There were also significant effects on behaviour: three or more courses of glucocorticoids were associated with an increased risk of externalizing behaviour problems, distractibility and inattention (French et al., 1998).

As in other animals, the human HPA axis appears to be programmed by the early life environment. Higher plasma and urinary glucocorticoid levels are found in children and adults who were of lower birthweight (Clark et al., 1996; Phillips et al., 1998). This appears to occur in disparate populations (Phillips et al., 2000) and may precede overt adult disease (Levitt et al., 2000), at least in a socially disadvantaged South African population. Additionally, adult HPA responses to ACTH stimulation are exaggerated in those of low birthweight (Levitt et al., 2000; Reynolds et al., 2001), reflecting the stress-axis biology elucidated in animal models. Furthermore, this HPA activation is associated with higher blood pressure, insulin resistance, glucose intolerance and hyperlipidaemia (Reynolds et al., 2001). Finally, the human GR gene promoter has multiple alternate untranslated first exons (R. Reynolds and K.E. Chapman, unpublished observations), analogous to those found in the rat and mouse. Whether these are the subjects of early life regulation, and the molecular mechanisms by which this is achieved, remain to be determined.

Thus in humans, as in rodents, prenatal glucocorticoid overexposure appears to programme an adverse adult cardiovascular, metabolic, neuroendocrine and behavioural phenotype. Whether this is an unusual or a common mechanism to explain the link between low birthweight/size at birth and adult disorders is the subject of ongoing studies.

References

Adamson, S.L. and Kingdom, J. (1999) Antenatal betamethasone and fetoplacental blood flow. Lancet 354, 255–256.

Albiston, A.L., Obeyesekere, V.R., Smith, R.E. and Krozowski, Z.S. (1994) Cloning and tissue distribution of the human 11 beta-hydroxysteroid dehydrogenase type 2 enzyme. Molecular and Cellular Endocrinology 105, R11–17.

Alfaidy, N., Gupta, S., DeMarco, C., Caniggia, I. and Challis, J.R. (2002) Oxygen regulation of placental 11 beta-hydroxysteroid dehydrogenase 2: physiological and pathological implications. Journal of Clinical Endocrinology and Metabolism 87, 4797–4805.

Arai, Y. and Gorski, R.A. (1968) Critical exposure time for androgenization of the developing hypothalamus in the female rat. Endocrinology 82, 1010–1014.

Bach, L.A., Leeding, K.S. and Leng, S.L. (1997) Regulation of IGF-binding protein-6 by dexamethasone and IGFs in PC12 rat phaeochromocytoma cells. *Journal of Endocrinology* 155, 225–232.

Baggia, S., Albrecht, E.D. and Pepe, G.J. (1990) Regulation of 11 beta-hydroxysteroid dehydrogenase activity in the baboon placenta by estrogen. *Endocrinology* 126, 2742–2748.

Baird, J., Osmond, C., MacGregor, A., Snieder, H., Hales, C.N. and Phillips, D.I. (2001) Testing the fetal origins hypothesis in twins: the Birmingham twin study. *Diabetologia* 44, 33–39.

Barker, D.J.P. (1991) *Fetal and Infant Origins of Adult Disease*. BMJ Publishing Group, London.

Barker, D.J.P. (1994) *Mothers, Babies and Disease in Later Life*. BMJ Publishing Group, London.

Barker, D.J., Bull, A.R., Osmond, C. and Simmonds, S.J. (1990) Fetal and placental size and risk of hypertension in adult life. *British Medical Journal* 301, 259–262.

Barker, D.J., Gluckman, P.D., Godfrey, K.M., Harding, J.E., Owens, J.A. and Robinson, J.S. (1993a) Fetal nutrition and cardiovascular disease in adult life [Comment]. *Lancet* 341, 938–941.

Barker, D.J., Hales, C.N., Fall, C.H., Osmond, C., Phipps, K. and Clark, P.M. (1993b) Type 2 (non-insulin-dependent) diabetes mellitus, hypertension and hyperlipidaemia (syndrome X): relation to reduced fetal growth. *Diabetologia* 36, 62–67.

Bavdekar, A., Yajnik, C.S., Fall, C.H., Bapat, S., Pandit, A.N., Deshpande, V., Bhave, S., Kellingray, S.D. and Joglekar, C. (1999) Insulin resistance syndrome in 8-year-old Indian children: small at birth, big at 8 years, or both? *Diabetes* 48, 2422–2429.

Beitins, I.Z., Bayard, F., Ances, I.G., Kowarski, A. and Migeon, C.J. (1973) The metabolic clearance rate, blood production, interconversion and transplacental passage of cortisol and cortisone in pregnancy near term. *Pediatric Research* 7, 509–519.

Benediktsson, R., Lindsay, R.S., Noble, J., Seckl, J.R. and Edwards, C.R. (1993) Glucocorticoid exposure *in utero*: new model for adult hypertension [Comment]. *Lancet* 341, 339–341.

Benediktsson, R., Brennand, J., Tibi, L., Calder, A.A., Seckl, J.R. and Edwards, C.R. (1995) Fetal osteocalcin levels are related to placental 11 beta-hydroxysteroid dehydrogenase activity in humans. *Clinical Endocrinology* 42, 551–555.

Benediktsson, R., Calder, A.A., Edwards, C.R. and Seckl, J.R. (1997) Placental 11 beta-hydroxysteroid dehydrogenase: a key regulator of fetal glucocorticoid exposure. *Clinical Endocrinology* 46, 161–166.

Berry, L.M., Polk, D.H., Ikegami, M., Jobe, A.H., Padbury, J.F. and Ervin, M.G. (1997) Preterm newborn lamb renal and cardiovascular responses after fetal or maternal antenatal betamethasone. *American Journal of Physiology* 272, R1972–R1979.

Bertram, C., Trowern, A.R., Copin, N., Jackson, A.A. and Whorwood, C.B. (2001) The maternal diet during pregnancy programs altered expression of the glucocorticoid receptor and type 2 11beta-hydroxysteroid dehydrogenase: potential molecular mechanisms underlying the programming of hypertension *in utero*. *Endocrinology* 142, 2841–2853.

Bian, X.P., Seidler, F.J. and Slotkin, T.A. (1992) Promotional role for glucocorticoids in the development of intracellular signalling: enhanced cardiac and renal adenylate cyclase reactivity to beta-adrenergic and non-adrenergic stimuli after low-dose fetal dexamethasone exposure. *Journal of Developmental Physiology* 17, 289–297.

Bian, X., Seidler, F.J. and Slotkin, T.A. (1993) Fetal dexamethasone exposure interferes with establishment of cardiac noradrenergic innervation and sympathetic activity. *Teratology* 47, 109–117.

Blondeau, B., Lesage, J., Czernichow, P., Dupouy, J.P. and Breant, B. (2001) Gluco-corticoids impair fetal beta-cell development in rats. *American Journal of Physiology – Endocrinology and Metabolism* 281, E592–E599.

Bloom, S.L., Sheffield, J.S., McIntire, D.D. and Leveno, K.J. (2001) Antenatal dexamethasone and decreased birth weight. *Obstetrics and Gynecology* 97, 485–490.

Bremner, J.D., Randall, P., Scott, T.M., Bronen, R.A., Seibyl, J.P., Southwick, S.M., Delaney, R.C., McCarthy, G., Charney, D.S. and Innis, R.B. (1995) MRI-based measurement of hippocampal volume in patients with combat-related posttraumatic stress disorder. *American Journal of Psychiatry* 152, 973–981.

Brocklehurst, P., Gates, S., McKenzie-McHarg, K., Alfirevic, Z. and Chamberlain, G. (1999) Are we prescribing multiple courses of antenatal corticosteroids? A survey of practice in the UK. *British Journal of Obstetrics and Gynaecology* 106, 977–979.

Brown, R.W., Diaz, R., Robson, A.C., Kotelevtsev, Y.V., Mullins, J.J., Kaufman, M.H. and Seckl, J.R. (1996a) The ontogeny of 11 beta-hydroxysteroid dehydrogenase type 2 and mineralocorticoid receptor gene expression reveal intricate control of glucocorticoid action in development. *Endocrinology* 137, 794–797.

Brown, R.W., Chapman, K.E., Kotelevtsev, Y., Yau, J.L., Lindsay, R.S., Brett, L., Leckie, C., Murad, P., Lyons, V., Mullins, J.J., Edwards, C.R. and Seckl, J.R. (1996b) Cloning and production of antisera to human placental 11 beta-hydroxysteroid dehydrogenase type 2. *Biochemical Journal* 313, 1007–1017.

Catalani, A., Marinelli, M., Scaccianoce, S., Nicolai, R., Muscolo, L.A., Porcu, A., Koranyi, L., Piazza, P.V. and Angelucci, L. (1993) Progeny of mothers drinking corticosterone during lactation has lower stress-induced corticosterone secretion and better cognitive performance. *Brain Research* 624, 209–215.

Celsi, G., Kistner, A., Eklof, A.C., Ceccatelli, S., Aizman, R. and Jacobson, S.H. (1997) Inhibition of renal growth by prenatal dexamethasone and the programming of blood pressure in the offspring. *Journal of the American Society of Nephrology* 8, A1360.

Cetin, I., Morpurgo, P.S., Radaelli, T., Taricco, E., Cortelazzi, D., Bellotti, M., Pardi, G. and Beck-Peccoz, P. (2000) Fetal plasma leptin concentrations: relationship with different intrauterine growth patterns from 19 weeks to term. *Pediatric Research* 48, 646–651.

Chen, X., Lin, J., Hausman, D.B., Martin, R.J., Dean, R.G. and Hausman, G.J. (2000) Alterations in fetal adipose tissue leptin expression correlate with the development of adipose tissue. *Biology of the Neonate* 78, 41–47.

Cheung, P.T., Wu, J., Banach, W. and Chernausek, S.D. (1994) Glucocorticoid regulation of an insulin-like growth factor-binding protein-4 protease produced by a rat neuronal cell line. *Endocrinology* 135, 1328–1335.

Clark, P.M., Hindmarsh, P.C., Shiell, A.W., Law, C.M., Honour, J.W. and Barker, D.J. (1996) Size at birth and adrenocortical function in childhood. *Clinical Endocrinology* 45, 721–726.

Clarke, K.A., Ward, J.W., Forhead, A.J., Giussani, D.A. and Fowden, A.L. (2002) Regulation of 11beta-hydroxysteroid dehydrogenase type 2 activity in ovine placenta by fetal cortisol. *Journal of Endocrinology* 172, 527–534.

Cleasby, M., Kelly, P.A., Walker, B.R. and Seckl, J.R. (2003a) Programming of rat muscle and fat metabolism by *in utero* over-exposure to glucocorticoids. *Endocrinology* 144, 999–1007.

Cleasby, M., Livingstone, D.E., Nyirenda, M., Seckl, J.R. and Walker, B.R. (2003b) Is programming of glucocorticoid receptor expression by glucocorticoids in the rat secondary to metabolic derangement in adulthood? *European Journal of Endocrinology* 148, 129–138.

Cole, T.J., Blendy, J.A., Monaghan, A.P., Schmid, W., Aguzzi, A. and Schutz, G. (1995) Molecular genetic analysis of glucocorticoid signaling during mouse development. *Steroids* 60, 93–96.

Combs, T.P., Berg, A.H., Rajala, M.W., Klebanov, S., Iyengar, P., Jimenez-Chillaron, J.C., Patti, M.E., Klein, S.L., Weinstein, R.S. and Scherer, P.E. (2003) Sexual differentiation, pregnancy, calorie restriction, and aging affect the adipocyte-specific secretory protein adiponectin. *Diabetes* 52, 268–276.

Conover, C.A., Lee, P.D.K., Riggs, B.L. and Powell, D.R. (1996) Insulin-like growth factor-binding protein-1 expression in cultured human bone cells: regulation by insulin and glucocorticoid. *Endocrinology* 137, 3295–3301.

Constancia, M., Hemberger, M., Hughes, J., Dean, W., Ferguson-Smith, A., Fundele, R., Stewart, F., Kelsey, G., Fowden, A., Sibley, C. and Reik, W. (2002) Placental-specific IGF-II is a major modulator of placental and fetal growth. *Nature* 417, 945–948.

Crowley, P. (2000) Prophylactic corticosteroids for preterm birth. *Cochrane Database of Systematic Reviews*: CD000065.

Curhan, G.C., Chertow, G.M., Willett, W.C., Spiegelman, D., Colditz, G.A., Manson, J.E., Speizer, F.E. and Stampfer, M.J. (1996a) Birth weight and adult hypertension and obesity in women. *Circulation* 94, 1310–1315.

Curhan, G.C., Willett, W.C., Rimm, E.B., Spiegelman, D., Ascherio, A.L. and Stampfer, M.J. (1996b) Birth weight and adult hypertension, diabetes mellitus, and obesity in US men. *Circulation* 94, 3246–3250.

Dave-Sharma, S., Wilson, R.C., Harbison, M.D., Newfield, R., Azar, M.R., Krozowski, Z.S., Funder, J.W., Shackleton, C.H., Bradlow, H.L., Wei, J.Q., Hertecant, J., Moran, A., Neiberger, R.E., Balfe, J.W., Fattah, A., Daneman, D., Akkurt, H.I., De Santis, C. and New, M.I. (1998) Examination of genotype and phenotype relationships in 14 patients with apparent mineralocorticoid excess. *Journal of Clinical Endocrinology and Metabolism* 83, 2244–2254.

Davis, E.C., Popper, P. and Gorski, R.A. (1996) The role of apoptosis in sexual differentiation of the rat sexually dimorphic nucleus of the preoptic area. *Brain Research* 734, 10–18.

Dean, F. and Matthews, S.G. (1999) Maternal dexamethasone treatment in late gestation alters glucocorticoid and mineralocorticoid receptor mRNA in the fetal guinea pig brain. *Brain Research* 846, 253–259.

Dean, F., Yu, C., Lingas, R.I. and Matthews, S.G. (2001) Prenatal glucocorticoid modifies hypothalamo-pituitary–adrenal regulation in prepubertal guinea pigs. *Neuroendocrinology* 73, 194–202.

Delany, A.M. and Canalis, E. (1995) Transcriptional repression of insulin-like growth factor I by glucocorticoids in rat bone cells. *Endocrinology* 136, 4776–4781.

D'Ercole, A.J., Ye, P. and Gutierrez-Ospina, G. (1996) Use of transgenic mice for understanding the physiology of insulin-like growth factors. *Hormone Research* 45, 5–7.

Diaz, R., Ogren, S.O., Blum, M. and Fuxe, K. (1995) Prenatal corticosterone increases spontaneous and D-amphetamine induced locomotor activity and brain dopamine metabolism in prepubertal male and female rats. *Neuroscience* 66, 467–473.

Diaz, R., Fuxe, K. and Ogren, S.O. (1997a) Prenatal corticosterone treatment induces long-term changes in spontaneous and apomorphine-mediated motor activity in male and female rats. *Neuroscience* 81, 129–140.

Diaz, R., Sokoloff, P. and Fuxe, K. (1997b) Codistribution of the dopamine D3 receptor and glucocorticoid receptor mRNAs during striatal prenatal development in the rat. *Neuroscience Letters* 227, 119–122.

Diaz, R., Brown, R.W. and Seckl, J.R. (1998) Distinct ontogeny of glucocorticoid and mineralocorticoid receptor and 11beta-hydroxysteroid dehydrogenase types I and II mRNAs in the fetal rat brain suggest a complex control of glucocorticoid actions. *Journal of Neuroscience* 18, 2570–2580.

Diorio, J., Francis, D., Walker, M., Steverman, A. and Meaney, M.J. (1996) Postnatal handling induces changes in the hippocampal expression of cyclic nucleotide-dependent response element binding proteins in the rat. *Society of Neuroscience Abstracts* 22, 486–487.

Docherty, C.C., Kalmar-Nagy, J., Engelen, M., Koenen, S.V., Nijland, M., Kuc, R.E., Davenport, A.P. and Nathanielsz, P.W. (2001) Effect of *in vivo* fetal infusion of dexamethasone at 0.75 GA on fetal ovine resistance artery responses to ET-1. *American Journal of Physiology – Regulatory Integrative and Comparative Physiology* 281 R261–R268.

Dodic, M., May, C.N., Wintour, E.M. and Coghlan, J.P. (1998) An early prenatal exposure to excess glucocorticoid leads to hypertensive offspring in sheep. *Clinical Science* 94, 149–155.

Dodic, M., Abouantoun, T., O'Connor, A., Wintour, E.M. and Moritz, K.M. (2002a) Programming effects of short prenatal exposure to dexamethasone in sheep. *Hypertension* 40, 729–734.

Dodic, M., Hantzis, V., Duncan, J., Rees, S., Koukoulas, I., Johnson, K., Wintour, E.M. and Moritz, K. (2002b) Programming effects of short prenatal exposure to cortisol. *FASEB Journal* 16, 1017–1026.

Doyle, L.W., Ford, G.W., Davis, N.M. and Callanan, C. (2000) Antenatal corticosteroid therapy and blood pressure at 14 years of age in preterm children. *Clinical Science* 98, 137–142.

Dunger, D.B., Ong, K.K., Huxtable, S.J., Sherriff, A., Woods, K.A., Ahmed, M.L., Golding, J., Pembrey, M.E., Ring, S., Bennett, S.T. and Todd, J.A. (1998) Association of the INS VNTR with size at birth. ALSPAC Study Team. Avon Longitudinal Study of Pregnancy and Childhood. *Nature Genetics* 19, 98–100.

Dunlop, S.A., Archer, M.A., Quinlivan, J.A., Beazley, L.D. and Newnham, J.P. (1997) Repeated prenatal corticosteroids delay myelination in the ovine central nervous system. *Journal of Maternal–Fetal Medicine* 6, 309–313.

Dunn, A.J. and Berridge, C.W. (1990) Physiological and behavioral responses to corticotropin-releasing factor administration: is CRF a mediator of anxiety or stress responses? *Brain Research – Brain Research Reviews* 15, 71–100.

Edwards, C.R., Benediktsson, R., Lindsay, R.S. and Seckl, J.R. (1993) Dysfunction of placental glucocorticoid barrier: link between fetal environment and adult hypertension? *Lancet* 341, 355–357.

Encio, I.J. and Detera-Wadleigh, S.D. (1991) The genomic structure of the human glucocorticoid receptor. *Journal of Biological Chemistry* 266, 7182–7188.

Eriksson, J.G., Forsen, T., Tuomilehto, J., Winter, P.D., Osmond, C. and Barker, D.J. (1999) Catch-up growth in childhood and death from coronary heart disease: longitudinal study. *British Medical Journal* 318, 427–431.

Fall, C.H., Pandit, A.N., Law, C.M., Yajnik, C.S., Clark, P.M., Breier, B., Osmond, C., Shiell, A.W., Gluckman, P.D. and Barker, D.J. (1995) Size at birth and plasma insulin-like growth factor-1 concentrations. *Archives of Disease in Childhood* 73 287–293.

Forest, M.G., David, M. and Morel, Y. (1993) Prenatal diagnosis and treatment of 21-hydroxylase deficiency. *Journal of Steroid Biochemistry and Molecular Biology* 45, 75–82.

Forhead, A.J., Li, J., Saunders, J.C., Dauncey, M.J., Gilmour, R.S. and Fowden, A.L. (2000) Control of ovine hepatic growth hormone receptor and insulin-like growth factor I by thyroid hormones *in utero*. *American Journal of Physiology – Endocrinology and Metabolism* 278, E1166–1174.

Forhead, A.J., Thomas, L., Crabtree, J., Hoggard, N., Gardner, D.S., Giussani, D.A. and Fowden, A.L. (2002) Plasma leptin concentration in fetal sheep during late gestation: ontogeny and effect of glucocorticoids. *Endocrinology* 143, 1166–1173.

Forsen, T., Eriksson, J.G., Tuomilehto, J., Teramo, K., Osmond, C. and Barker, D.J. (1997) Mother's weight in pregnancy and coronary heart disease in a cohort of Finnish men: follow up study. *British Medical Journal* 315, 837–840.

Forsen, T., Eriksson, J., Tuomilehto, J., Reunanen, A., Osmond, C. and Barker, D. (2000) The fetal and childhood growth of persons who develop type 2 diabetes. *Annals of Internal Medicine* 133, 176–182.

Fowden, A.L., Mijovic, J. and Silver, M. (1993) The effects of cortisol on hepatic and renal gluconeogenic enzyme activities in the sheep fetus during late gestation. *Journal of Endocrinology* 137, 213–222.

Frayling, T.M. and Hattersley, A.T. (2001) The role of genetic susceptibility in the association of low birth weight with type 2 diabetes. *British Medical Bulletin* 60, 89–101.

Frayling, T.M., Hattersley, A.T., McCarthy, A., Holly, J., Mitchell, S., Gloyn, A.L., Owen, K., Davies, D., Davey-Smith, G. and Ben-Shlomo, Y. (2002) A putative functional polymorphism in the IGF-I gene: association studies with type 2 diabetes, adult height, glucose tolerance, and fetal growth in U.K. populations. *Diabetes* 51, 2313–2316.

French, N.P., Hagan, R., Evans, S., Godfrey, M. and Newnham, J.P. (1998) Repeated antenatal corticosteroids: behaviour outcomes in a regional population of very preterm infants. *Pediatric Research* 43, 214A (Abstract no. 1252).

French, N.P., Hagan, R., Evans, S.F., Godfrey, M. and Newnham, J.P. (1999) Repeated antenatal corticosteroids: size at birth and subsequent development. *American Journal of Obstetrics and Gynecology* 180, 114–121.

Gandelman, R. and Rosenthal, C. (1981) Deleterious effects of prenatal prednisolone exposure upon morphological and behavioral development of mice. *Teratology* 24, 293–301.

Garofano, A., Czernichow, P. and Breant, B. (1997) *In utero* undernutrition impairs rat beta-cell development. *Diabetologia* 40, 1231–1234.

Garofano, A., Czernichow, P. and Breant, B. (1998) Beta-cell mass and proliferation following late fetal and early postnatal malnutrition in the rat. *Diabetologia* 41, 1114–1120.

Gatford, K.L., Wintour, E.M., De Blasio, M.J., Owens, J.A. and Dodic, M. (2000) Differential timing for programming of glucose homoeostasis, sensitivity to insulin and blood pressure by *in utero* exposure to dexamethasone in sheep. *Clinical Science* 98, 553–560.

Geary, M., Herschkovitz, R., Pringle, P.J., Rodeck, C.H. and Hindmarsh, P.C. (1999) Ontogeny of serum leptin concentrations in the human. *Clinical Endocrinology* 51, 189–192.

Goland, R.S., Jozak, S., Warren, W.B., Conwell, I.M., Stark, R.I. and Tropper, P.J. (1993) Elevated levels of umbilical cord plasma corticotropin-releasing hormone in growth-retarded fetuses. *Journal of Clinical Endocrinology and Metabolism* 77, 1174–1179.

Goland, R.S., Tropper, P.J., Warren, W.B., Stark, R.I., Jozak, S.M. and Conwell, I.M. (1995) Concentrations of corticotrophin-releasing hormone in the umbilical-cord blood of pregnancies complicated by pre-eclampsia. *Reproduction, Fertility, and Development* 7, 1227–1230.

Goswami, R., Lacson, R., Yang, E., Sam, R. and Unterman, T. (1994) Functional analysis of glucocorticoid and insulin response sequences in the rat insulin-like growth factor-binding protein-1 promoter. *Endocrinology* 134, 736–743.

Gunberg, D.L. (1957) Some effects of exogenous corticosterone on pregnancy in the rat. *Anatomical Research* 129, 133–153.

Gustafsson, J.A., Mode, A., Norstedt, G. and Skett, P. (1983) Sex steroid induced changes in hepatic enzymes. *Annual Review of Physiology* 45, 51–60.

Hattersley, A.T., Beards, F., Ballantyne, E., Appleton, M., Harvey, R. and Ellard, S. (1998) Mutations in the glucokinase gene of the fetus result in reduced birth weight. *Nature Genetics* 19, 268–270.

Hawkins, P., Steyn, C., McGarrigle, H.H., Calder, N.A., Saito, T., Stratford, L.L., Noakes, D.E. and Hanson, M.A. (2000) Cardiovascular and hypothalamic–pituitary–adrenal axis development in late gestation fetal sheep and young lambs following modest maternal nutrient restriction in early gestation. *Reproduction, Fertility, and Development* 12, 443–456.

Herman, J.P., Patel, P.D., Akil, H. and Watson, S.J. (1989) Localization and regulation of glucocorticoid and mineralocorticoid receptor messenger RNAs in the hippocampal formation of the rat. *Molecular Endocrinology* 3, 1886–1894.

Hill, D.J. and Duvillie, B. (2000) Pancreatic development and adult diabetes. *Pediatric Research* 48, 269–274.

Hoggard, N., Hunter, L., Lea, R.G., Trayhurn, P. and Mercer, J.G. (2000) Ontogeny of the expression of leptin and its receptor in the murine fetus and placenta. *British Journal of Nutrition* 83, 317–326.

Holmes, M.C., Welberg, L.A. and Seckl, J.R. (2002) Early life programming of the brain by glucocorticoids. *5th International Congress of Neuroendocrinology*, Bristol, UK, September, p. S57.

Holson, R.R., Gough, B., Sullivan, P., Badger, T. and Sheehan, D.M. (1995) Prenatal dexamethasone or stress but not ACTH or corticosterone alter sexual behavior in male rats. *Neurotoxicology and Teratology* 17, 393–401.

Hsu, D.T., Chen, F.L., Takahashi, L.K. and Kalin, N.H. (1998) Rapid stress-induced elevations in corticotropin-releasing hormone mRNA in rat central amygdala nucleus and hypothalamic paraventricular nucleus: an *in situ* hybridization analysis. *Brain Research* 788, 305–310.

Hu, E., Liang, P. and Spiegelman, B.M. (1996) AdipoQ is a novel adipose-specific gene dysregulated in obesity. *Journal of Biological Chemistry* 271, 10697–10703.

Huff, R.A., Seidler, F.J. and Slotkin, T.A. (1991) Glucocorticoids regulate the ontogenetic transition of adrenergic receptor subtypes in rat liver. *Life Sciences* 48, 1059–1065.

Huxley, R., Neil, A. and Collins, R. (2002) Unravelling the fetal origins hypothesis: is there really an inverse association between birthweight and subsequent blood pressure? *Lancet* 360, 659–665.

Ikegami, M., Jobe, A.H., Newnham, J., Polk, D.H., Willet, K.E. and Sly, P. (1997) Repetitive prenatal glucocorticoids improve lung function and decrease growth in preterm lambs. *American Journal of Respiratory and Critical Care Medicine* 156, 178–184.

Irving, R.J., Belton, N.R., Elton, R.A. and Walker, B.R. (2000) Adult cardiovascular risk factors in premature babies. *Lancet* 355, 2135–2136.

Jamieson, P.M., Walker, B.R., Chapman, K.E., Andrew, R., Rossiter, S. and Seckl, J.R. (2000) 11 beta-hydroxysteroid dehydrogenase type 1 is a predominant 11 beta-reductase in the intact perfused rat liver. *Journal of Endocrinology* 165, 685–692.

Jaquet, D., Leger, J., Levy-Marchal, C., Oury, J.F. and Czernichow, P. (1998) Ontogeny of leptin in human fetuses and newborns: effect of intrauterine growth retardation on serum leptin concentrations. *Journal of Clinical Endocrinology and Metabolism* 83, 1243–1246.

Jensen, E.C., Gallaher, B.W., Breier, B.H. and Harding, J.E. (2002) The effect of a chronic maternal cortisol infusion on the late-gestation fetal sheep. *Journal of Endocrinology* 174, 27–36.

Jones, J.I. and Clemmons, D.R. (1995) Insulin-like growth factors and their binding proteins: biological actions. *Endocrine Reviews* 16, 3–34.

Kari, M.A., Hallman, M., Eronen, M., Teramo, K., Virtanen, M., Koivisto, M. and Ikonen, R.S. (1994) Prenatal dexamethasone treatment in conjunction with rescue therapy of human surfactant: a randomized placebo-controlled multicenter study. *Pediatrics* 93, 730–736.

Keightley, M.C. and Fuller, P.J. (1994) Unique sequences in the guinea pig glucocorticoid receptor induce constitutive transactivation and decrease steroid sensitivity. *Molecular Endocrinology* 8(6), 731.

King, L.B., Vacchio, M.S., Dixon, K., Hunziker, R., Margulies, D.H. and Ashwell, J.D. (1995) A targeted glucocorticoid receptor antisense transgene increases thymocyte apoptosis and alters thymocyte development. *Immunity* 3, 647–656.

Koenen, S.V., Mecenas, C.A., Smith, G.S., Jenkins, S. and Nathanielsz, P.W. (2002) Effects of maternal betamethasone administration on fetal and maternal blood pressure and heart rate in the baboon at 0.7 of gestation. *American Journal of Obstetrics and Gynecology* 186, 812–817.

Koistinen, H.A., Koivisto, V.A., Andersson, S., Karonen, S.L., Kontula, K., Oksanen, L. and Teramo, K.A. (1997) Leptin concentration in cord blood correlates with intrauterine growth. *Journal of Clinical Endocrinology and Metabolism* 82, 3328–3330.

Kotelevtsev, Y., Holmes, M.C., Burchell, A., Houston, P.M., Schmoll, D., Jamieson, P., Best, R., Brown, R., Edwards, C.R., Seckl, J.R. and Mullins, J.J. (1997) 11beta-hydroxysteroid dehydrogenase type 1 knockout mice show attenuated glucocorticoid-inducible responses and resist hyperglycemia on obesity or stress. *Proceedings of the National Academy of Sciences USA* 94, 14924–14929.

Kotelevtsev, Y., Brown, R.W., Fleming, S., Kenyon, C., Edwards, C.R., Seckl, J.R. and Mullins, J.J. (1999) Hypertension in mice lacking 11beta-hydroxysteroid dehydrogenase type 2. *Journal of Clinical Investigation* 103, 683–689.

Langdown, M.L., Holness, M.J. and Sugden, M.C. (2001a) Early growth retardation induced by excessive exposure to glucocorticoids *in utero* selectively increases cardiac GLUT1 protein expression and Akt/protein kinase B activity in adulthood. *Journal of Endocrinology* 169, 11–22.

Langdown, M.L., Smith, N.D., Sugden, M.C. and Holness, M.J. (2001b) Excessive glucocorticoid exposure during late intrauterine development modulates the expression of cardiac uncoupling proteins in adult hypertensive male offspring. *Pflugers Archiv – European Journal of Physiology* 442, 248–255.

Langley-Evans, S.C. (1997) Hypertension induced by foetal exposure to a maternal low-protein diet, in the rat, is prevented by pharmacological blockade of maternal glucocorticoid synthesis. *Journal of Hypertension* 15, 537–544.

Langley-Evans, S.C., Phillips, G.J., Benediktsson, R., Gardner, D.S., Edwards, C.R., Jackson, A.A. and Seckl, J.R. (1996a) Protein intake in pregnancy, placental glucocorticoid metabolism and the programming of hypertension in the rat. *Placenta* 17, 169–172.

Langley-Evans, S.C., Gardner, D.S. and Jackson, A.A. (1996b) Maternal protein restriction influences the programming of the rat hypothalamic–pituitary–adrenal axis. *Journal of Nutrition* 126, 1578–1585.

Laplante, P., Diorio, J. and Meaney, M.J. (2002) Serotonin regulates hippocampal glucocorticoid receptor expression via a 5-HT7 receptor. *Brain Research. Developmental Brain Research* 139, 199–203.

Law, C.M., Shiell, A.W., Newsome, C.A., Syddall, H.E., Shinebourne, E.A., Fayers, P.M., Martyn, C.N. and de Swiet, M. (2002) Fetal, infant, and childhood growth and adult blood pressure: a longitudinal study from birth to 22 years of age. *Circulation* 105, 1088–1092.

Leon, D.A., Koupilova, I., Lithell, H.O., Berglund, L., Mohsen, R., Vagero, D., Lithell, U.B. and McKeigue, P.M. (1996) Failure to realise growth potential *in utero* and adult obesity in relation to blood pressure in 50 year old Swedish men. *British Medical Journal* 312, 401–406.

Lepercq, J., Challier, J.C., Guerre-Millo, M., Cauzac, M., Vidal, H. and Hauguel-de Mouzon, S. (2001) Prenatal leptin production: evidence that fetal adipose tissue produces leptin. *Journal of Clinical Endocrinology and Metabolism* 86, 2409–2413.

Lesage, J., Blondeau, B., Grino, M., Breant, B. and Dupouy, J.P. (2001) Maternal undernutrition during late gestation induces fetal overexposure to glucocorticoids and intrauterine growth retardation, and disturbs the hypothalamo-pituitary–adrenal axis in the newborn rat. *Endocrinology* 142, 1692–1702.

Levine, R.S., Hennekens, C.H. and Jesse, M.J. (1994) Blood pressure in prospective population based cohort of newborn and infant twins. *British Medical Journal* 308, 298–302.

Levine, S. (1957) Infantile experience and resistance to physiological stress. *Science* 126, 405–406.

Levine, S. (1962) Plasma free corticosteroid responses to electric shock in rats stimulated in infancy. *Science* 135, 795–796.

Levitt, N.S., Lindsay, R.S., Holmes, M.C. and Seckl, J.R. (1996) Dexamethasone in the last week of pregnancy attenuates hippocampal glucocorticoid receptor gene expression and elevates blood pressure in the adult offspring in the rat. *Neuroendocrinology* 64, 412–418.

Levitt, N.S., Lambert, E.V., Woods, D., Hales, C.N., Andrew, R. and Seckl, J.R. (2000) Impaired glucose tolerance and elevated blood pressure in low birth weight, nonobese, young South African adults: early programming of cortisol axis. *Journal of Clinical Endocrinology and Metabolism* 85, 4611–4618.

Li, J., Saunders, J.C., Gilmour, R.S., Silver, M. and Fowden, A.L. (1993) Insulin-like growth factor-II messenger ribonucleic acid expression in fetal tissues of the sheep during late gestation: effects of cortisol. *Endocrinology* 132, 2083–2089.

Li, J., Owens, J.A., Owens, P.C., Saunders, J.C., Fowden, A.L. and Gilmour, R.S. (1996) The ontogeny of hepatic growth hormone receptor and insulin-like growth factor I gene expression in the sheep fetus during late gestation: developmental regulation by cortisol. *Endocrinology* 137, 1650–1657.

Li, J., Forhead, A.J., Dauncey, M.J., Gilmour, R.S. and Fowden, A.L. (2002) Control of growth hormone receptor and insulin-like growth factor-I expression by cortisol in ovine fetal skeletal muscle. *Journal of Physiology* 541, 581–589.

Lindsay, R.S., Lindsay, R.M., Edwards, C.R. and Seckl, J.R. (1996a) Inhibition of 11-beta-hydroxysteroid dehydrogenase in pregnant rats and the programming of blood pressure in the offspring. *Hypertension* 27, 1200–1204.

Lindsay, R.S., Lindsay, R.M., Waddell, B.J. and Seckl, J.R. (1996b) Prenatal gluco-corticoid exposure leads to offspring hyperglycaemia in the rat: studies with the 11 beta-hydroxysteroid dehydrogenase inhibitor carbenoxolone. *Diabetologia* 39, 1299–1305.

Lindsay, R.S., Funahashi, T., Hanson, R.L., Matsuzawa, Y., Tanaka, S., Tataranni, P.A., Knowler, W.C. and Krakoff, J. (2002) Adiponectin and development of type 2 diabetes in the Pima Indian population. *Lancet* 360, 57–58.

Lithell, H.O., McKeigue, P.M., Berglund, L., Mohsen, R., Lithell, U.B. and Leon, D.A. (1996) Relation of size at birth to non-insulin dependent diabetes and insulin concentrations in men aged 50–60 years. *British Medical Journal* 312, 406–410.

Liu, D., Diorio, J., Tannenbaum, B., Caldji, C., Francis, D., Freedman, A., Sharma, S., Pearson, D., Plotsky, P.M. and Meaney, M.J. (1997) Maternal care, hippocampal glucocorticoid receptors, and hypothalamic–pituitary–adrenal responses to stress. *Science* 277, 1659–1662.

Liu, L., Li, A. and Matthews, S.G. (2001) Maternal glucocorticoid treatment programs HPA regulation in adult offspring: sex-specific effects. *American Journal of Physiology – Endocrinology and Metabolism* 280, E729–E739.

Luo, J., Reid, R.E. and Murphy, L.J. (1990) Dexamethasone increases hepatic insulin-like growth factor binding protein-1 (IGFBP-1) mRNA and serum IGFBP-1 concentrations in the rat. *Endocrinology* 127, 1456–1462.

MacArthur, B.A., Howie, R.N., Dezoete, J.A. and Elkins, J. (1982) School progress and cognitive development of 6-year-old children whose mothers were treated antenatally with betamethasone. *Pediatrics* 70, 99–105.

Maccari, S., Piazza, P.V., Kabbaj, M., Barbazanges, A., Simon, H. and Le Moal, M. (1995) Adoption reverses the long-term impairment in glucocorticoid feedback induced by prenatal stress. *Journal of Neuroscience* 15, 110–116.

Matthews, S.G. (1998) Dynamic changes in glucocorticoid and mineralocorticoid receptor mRNA in the developing guinea pig brain. *Brain Research. Developmental Brain Research* 107, 123–132.

Matthews, S.G. (2000) Antenatal glucocorticoids and programming of the developing CNS. *Pediatric Research* 47, 291–300.

McCormick, J.A., Lyons, V., Jacobson, M.D., Noble, J., Diorio, J., Nyirenda, M., Weaver, S., Ester, W., Yau, J.L., Meaney, M.J., Seckl, J.R. and Chapman, K.E. (2000) 5′-heterogeneity of glucocorticoid receptor messenger RNA is tissue specific: differential regulation of variant transcripts by early-life events. *Molecular Endocrinology* 14, 506–517.

McEvoy, R.C. and Hegre, O.D. (1976) Foetal rat pancreas in organ culture: effects of media supplementation with various steroid hormones on the acinar and islet components. *Differentiation* 6, 105–111.

McTernan, C.L., Draper, N., Nicholson, H., Chalder, S.M., Driver, P., Hewison, M., Kilby, M.D. and Stewart, P.M. (2001) Reduced placental 11beta-hydroxysteroid dehydrogenase type 2 mRNA levels in human pregnancies complicated by intra-uterine growth restriction: an analysis of possible mechanisms. *Journal of Clinical Endocrinology and Metabolism* 86, 4979–4983.

Meaney, M.J., Aitken, D.H., van Berkel, C., Bhatnagar, S. and Sapolsky, R.M. (1988) Effect of neonatal handling on age-related impairments associated with the hippocampus. *Science* 239, 766–768.

Meaney, M.J., Aitken, D.H., Viau, V., Sharma, S. and Sarrieau, A. (1989) Neonatal handling alters adrenocortical negative feedback sensitivity and hippocampal type II glucocorticoid receptor binding in the rat. *Neuroendocrinology* 50, 597–604.

Meaney, M.J., Aitken, D.H., Sharma, S. and Viau, V. (1992) Basal ACTH, corticosterone and corticosterone-binding globulin levels over the diurnal cycle, and age-related changes in hippocampal type I and type II corticosteroid receptor binding capacity in young and aged, handled and nonhandled rats. *Neuroendocrinology* 55, 204–213.

Meaney, M.J., Diorio, J., Francis, D., Widdowson, J., LaPlante, P., Caldji, C., Sharma, S., Seckl, J.R. and Plotsky, P.M. (1996) Early environmental regulation of forebrain glucocorticoid receptor gene expression: implications for adrenocortical responses to stress. *Developmental Neuroscience* 18, 49–72.

Meaney, M.J., Diorio, J., Francis, D., Weaver, S., Yau, J., Chapman, K. and Seckl, J.R. (2000) Postnatal handling increases the expression of cAMP-inducible transcription factors in the rat hippocampus: the effects of thyroid hormones and serotonin. *Journal of Neuroscience* 20, 3926–3935.

Mercado, A.B., Wilson, R.C., Cheng, K.C., Wei, J.Q. and New, M.I. (1995) Prenatal treatment and diagnosis of congenital adrenal hyperplasia owing to steroid 21-hydroxylase deficiency. *Journal of Clinical Endocrinology and Metabolism* 80, 2014–2020.

Miell, J.P., Buchanan, C.R., Norman, M.R., Maheshwari, H.C. and Blum, W.F. (1994) The evolution of changes in immunoreactive serum insulin-like growth factors (IGFs), IGF-binding proteins, circulating growth hormone (CH) and GH-binding protein as a result of short-term dexamethasone treatment. *Journal of Endocrinology* 142, 547–554.

Mitchell, J.B., Rowe, W., Boksa, P. and Meaney, M.J. (1990) Serotonin regulates type II corticosteroid receptor binding in hippocampal cell cultures. *Journal of Neuroscience* 10, 1745–1752.

Mitchell, J.B., Betito, K., Rowe, W., Boksa, P. and Meaney, M.J. (1992) Serotonergic regulation of type II corticosteroid receptor binding in hippocampal cell cultures: evidence for the importance of serotonin-induced changes in cAMP levels. *Neuroscience* 48, 631–639.

Moore, V.M., Miller, A.G., Boulton, T.J., Cockington, R.A., Craig, I.H., Magarey, A.M. and Robinson, J.S. (1996) Placental weight, birth measurements, and blood pressure at age 8 years. *Archives of Disease in Childhood* 74, 538–541.

Moritz, K.M., Johnson, K., Douglas-Denton, R., Wintour, E.M. and Dodic, M. (2002) Maternal glucocorticoid treatment programs alterations in the renin–angiotensin system of the ovine fetal kidney. *Endocrinology* 143, 4455–4463.

Moss, T.J., Sloboda, D.M., Gurrin, L.C., Harding, R., Challis, J.R. and Newnham, J.P. (2001) Programming effects in sheep of prenatal growth restriction and gluco-corticoid exposure. *American Journal of Physiology – Regulatory Integrative and Comparative Physiology* 281, R960–R970.

Mostyn, A., Keisler, D.H., Webb, R., Stephenson, T. and Symonds, M.E. (2001) The role of leptin in the transition from fetus to neonate. *Proceedings of the Nutrition Society* 60, 187–194.

Mostyn, A., Pearce, S., Budge, H., Elmes, M., Forhead, A.J., Fowden, A.L., Stephenson, T. and Symonds, M.E. (2003) Influence of cortisol on adipose tissue development in the fetal sheep during late gestation. *Journal of Endocrinology* 176, 23–30.

Mouhieddine, O.B., Cazals, V., Kuto, E., Le Bouc, Y. and Clement, A. (1996) Glucocorticoid-induced growth arrest of lung alveolar epithelial cells is ssociated with increased production of insulin-like growth factor binding protein-2. *Endocrinology* 137, 287–295.

Muneoka, K., Mikuni, M., Ogawa, T., Kitera, K., Kamei, K., Takigawa, M. and Takahashi, K. (1997) Prenatal dexamethasone exposure alters brain monoamine metabolism and adrenocortical response in rat offspring. *American Journal of Physiology* 273, R1669–R1675.

Murphy, V.E., Zakar, T., Smith, R., Giles, W.B., Gibson, P.G. and Clifton, V.L. (2002) Reduced 11beta-hydroxysteroid dehydrogenase type 2 activity is associated with decreased birth weight centile in pregnancies complicated by asthma. *Journal of Clinical Endocrinology and Metabolism* 87, 1660–1668.

Navarro, H.A., Kudlacz, E.M., Eylers, J.P. and Slotkin, T.A. (1989) Prenatal dexamethasone administration disrupts the pattern of cellular development in rat lung. *Teratology* 40, 433–438.

Newnham, J.P. and Moss, T.J. (2001) Antenatal glucocorticoids and growth: single versus multiple doses in animal and human studies. *Seminars in Neonatology* 6, 285–292.

Newnham, J.P., Evans, S.F., Godfrey, M., Huang, W., Ikegami, M. and Jobe, A. (1999) Maternal, but not fetal, administration of corticosteroids restricts fetal growth. *Journal of Maternal–Fetal Medicine* 8, 81–87.

Nyirenda, M.J. and Seckl, J.R. (1998) Intrauterine events and the programming of adulthood disease: the role of fetal glucocorticoid exposure. *International Journal of Molecular Medicine* 2, 607–614.

Nyirenda, M.J., Lindsay, R.S., Kenyon, C.J., Burchell, A. and Seckl, J.R. (1998) Glucocorticoid exposure in late gestation permanently programs rat hepatic phosphoenolpyruvate carboxykinase and glucocorticoid receptor expression and causes glucose intolerance in adult offspring. *Journal of Clinical Investigation* 15, 2174–2181.

O'Donnell, D., Larocque, S., Seckl, J.R. and Meaney, M.J. (1994) Postnatal handling alters glucocorticoid, but not mineralocorticoid messenger RNA expression in the hippocampus of adult rats. *Brain Research. Molecular Brain Research* 26, 242–248.

Ong, K.K., Ahmed, M.L., Sherriff, A., Woods, K.A., Watts, A., Golding, J. and Dunger, D.B. (1999) Cord blood leptin is associated with size at birth and predicts infancy weight gain in humans. ALSPAC Study Team. Avon Longitudinal Study of Pregnancy and Childhood. *Journal of Clinical Endocrinology and Metabolism* 84, 1145–1148.

Osmond, C., Barker, D.J., Winter, P.D., Fall, C.H. and Simmonds, S.J. (1993) Early growth and death from cardiovascular disease in women. *British Medical Journal* 307, 1519–1524.

Pepin, M.C., Pothier, F. and Barden, N. (1992) Impaired type II glucocorticoid-receptor function in mice bearing antisense RNA transgene. *Nature* 355, 725–728.

Phillips, D.I., Barker, D.J., Fall, C.H., Seckl, J.R., Whorwood, C.B., Wood, P.J. and Walker, B.R. (1998) Elevated plasma cortisol concentrations: a link between low birth weight and the insulin resistance syndrome? *Journal of Clinical Endocrinology and Metabolism* 83, 757–760.

Phillips, D.I., Walker, B.R., Reynolds, R.M., Flanagan, D.E., Wood, P.J., Osmond, C., Barker, D.J. and Whorwood, C.B. (2000) Low birth weight predicts elevated plasma cortisol concentrations in adults from 3 populations. *Hypertension* 35, 1301–1306.

Price, W.A., Stiles, A.D., Moats-Staats, B.M. and D'Ercole, A.J. (1992) Gene expression of insulin-like growth factors (IGFs), the type 1 IGF receptor, and IGF-binding proteins in dexamethasone-induced fetal growth retardation. *Endocrinology* 130, 1424–1432.

Rajkumar, K., Barron, D., Lewitt, M.S. and Murphy, L.J. (1995) Growth retardation and hyperglycemia in insulin-like growth factor binding protein-1 transgenic mice. *Endocrinology* 136, 4029–4034.

Rall, L., Pictet, R., Githens, S. and Rutter, W.J. (1977) Glucocorticoids modulate the *in vitro* development of the embryonic rat pancreas. *Journal of Cell Biology* 75, 398–409.

Reinisch, J.M., Simon, N.G., Karow, W.G. and Gandelman, R. (1978) Prenatal exposure to prednisone in humans and animals retards intrauterine growth. *Science* 202, 436–438.

Reynolds, R.M., Walker, B.R., Syddall, H.E., Andrew, R., Wood, P.J., Whorwood, C.B. and Phillips, D.I. (2001) Altered control of cortisol secretion in adult men with low birth weight and cardiovascular risk factors. *Journal of Clinical Endocrinology and Metabolism* 86, 245–250.

Rich-Edwards, J.W., Stampfer, M.J., Manson, J.E., Rosner, B., Hankinson, S.E., Colditz, G.A., Willett, W.C. and Hennekens, C.H. (1997) Birth weight and risk of cardiovascular disease in a cohort of women followed up since 1976. *British Medical Journal* 315, 396–400.

Rogerson, F.M., Kayes, K. and White, P.C. (1996) No correlation in human placenta between activity or mRNA for the K (type 2) isozyme of 11beta-hydroxysteroid dehydrogenase and fetal or placental weight. *Tenth International Congress of Endocrinology Abstracts* P1–231, 193.

Rogerson, F.M., Kayes, K.M. and White, P.C. (1997) Variation in placental type 2 11beta-hydroxysteroid dehydrogenase activity is not related to birth weight or placental weight. *Molecular and Cellular Endocrinology* 128, 103–109.

Rosella, G., Zajac, J.D., Kaczmarczyk, S.J., Andrikopoulos, S. and Proietto, J. (1993) Impaired suppression of gluconeogenesis induced by overexpression of a noninsulin-responsive phosphoenolpyruvate carboxykinase gene. *Molecular Endocrinology* 7, 1456–1462.

Saegusa, H., Nakagawa, Y., Liu, Y.J. and Ohzeki, T. (1999) Influence of placental 11beta-hydroxysteroid dehydrogenase (11beta-HSD) inhibition on glucose metabolism and 11beta-HSD regulation in adult offspring of rats. *Metabolism: Clinical and Experimental* 48, 1584–1588.

Sapolsky, R.M. (1999) Glucocorticoids, stress, and their adverse neurological effects: relevance to aging. *Experimental Gerontology* 34, 721–732.

Schubring, C., Kiess, W., Englaro, P., Rascher, W., Dotsch, J., Hanitsch, S., Attanasio, A. and Blum, W.F. (1997) Levels of leptin in maternal serum, amniotic fluid, and arterial and venous cord blood: relation to neonatal and placental weight. *Journal of Clinical Endocrinology and Metabolism* 82, 1480–1483.

Seckl, J.R. (1994) Glucocorticoids and small babies. *Quarterly Journal of Medicine* 87, 259–262.

Seckl, J.R. (1998) Physiologic programming of the fetus. *Clinics in Perinatology* 25, 939–962, vii.

Seckl, J.R. and Chapman, K.E. (1997) Medical and physiological aspects of the 11beta-hydroxysteroid dehydrogenase system. *European Journal of Biochemistry* 249, 361–364.

Shams, M., Kilby, M.D., Somerset, D.A., Howie, A.J., Gupta, A., Wood, P.J., Afnan, M. and Stewart, P.M. (1998) 11Beta-hydroxysteroid dehydrogenase type 2 in human pregnancy and reduced expression in intrauterine growth restriction. *Human Reproduction* 13, 799–804.

Sharma, S., Jhala, U.S., Johnson, T., Ferreri, K., Leonard, J. and Montminy, M. (1997) Hormonal regulation of an islet-specific enhancer in the pancreatic homeobox gene STF-1. *Molecular and Cellular Biology* 17, 2598–2604.

Sheline, Y.I., Wang, P.W., Gado, M.H., Csernansky, J.G. and Vannier, M.W. (1996) Hippocampal atrophy in recurrent major depression. *Proceedings of the National Academy of Sciences of the USA* 93, 3908–3913.

Simerly, R.B. (2002) Wired for reproduction: organization and development of sexually dimorphic circuits in the mammalian forebrain. *Annual Review of Neuroscience* 25, 507–536.

Sloboda, D.M., Newnham, J.P. and Challis, J.R.G. (2002a) Repeated maternal glucocorticoid administration and the developing liver in fetal sheep. *Journal of Endocrinology* 175, 535–543.

Sloboda, D.M., Moss, T.J., Gurrin, L.C., Newnham, J.P. and Challis, J.R. (2002b) The effect of prenatal betamethasone administration on postnatal ovine hypothalamic–pituitary–adrenal function. *Journal of Endocrinology* 172, 71–81.

Slotkin, T.A., Barnes, G.A., McCook, E.C. and Seidler, F.J. (1996) Programming of brainstem serotonin transporter development by prenatal glucocorticoids. *Brain Research. Developmental Brain Research* 93, 155–161.

Smith, J.T. and Waddell, B.J. (2002) Leptin receptor expression in the rat placenta: changes in Ob-Ra, Ob-Rb, and Ob-Re with gestational age and suppression by glucocorticoids. *Biology of Reproduction* 67, 1204–1210.

Smythe, J.W., Rowe, W.B. and Meaney, M.J. (1994) Neonatal handling alters serotonin (5-HT) turnover and 5-HT2 receptor binding in selected brain regions: relationship to the handling effect on glucocorticoid receptor expression. *Brain Research. Developmental Brain Research* 80, 183–189.

Stein, M.B., Koverola, C., Hanna, C., Torchia, M.G. and McClarty, B. (1997) Hippocampal volume in women victimized by childhood sexual abuse. *Psychological Medicine* 27, 951–959.

Stewart, P.M., Murry, B.A. and Mason, J.I. (1994) Type 2 11 beta-hydroxysteroid dehydrogenase in human fetal tissues. *Journal of Clinical Endocrinology and Metabolism* 78, 1529–1532.

Stewart, P.M., Rogerson, F.M. and Mason, J.I. (1995) Type 2 11 beta-hydroxysteroid dehydrogenase messenger ribonucleic acid and activity in human placenta and fetal membranes: its relationship to birth weight and putative role in fetal adrenal steroidogenesis. *Journal of Clinical Endocrinology and Metabolism* 80, 885–890.

Sugden, M.C., Langdown, M.L., Munns, M.J. and Holness, M.J. (2001) Maternal glucocorticoid treatment modulates placental leptin and leptin receptor expression and materno-fetal leptin physiology during late pregnancy, and elicits hypertension associated with hyperleptinaemia in the early-growth-retarded adult offspring. *European Journal of Endocrinology* 145, 529–539.

Suh, D.S. and Rechler, M.M. (1997) Hepatocyte nuclear factor 1 and the glucocorticoid receptor synergistically activate transcription of the rat insulin-like growth factor binding protein-1 gene. *Molecular Endocrinology* 11, 1822–1831.

Sun, K., Yang, K. and Challis, J.R. (1997) Differential expression of 11 beta-hydroxysteroid dehydrogenase types 1 and 2 in human placenta and fetal membranes. *Journal of Clinical Endocrinology and Metabolism* 82, 300–305.

Tangalakis, K., Lumbers, E.R., Moritz, K.M., Towstoless, M.K. and Wintour, E.M. (1992) Effect of cortisol on blood pressure and vascular reactivity in the ovine fetus. *Experimental Physiology* 77, 709–717.

Thomas, L., Wallace, J.M., Aitken, R.P., Mercer, J.G., Trayhurn, P. and Hoggard, N. (2001) Circulating leptin during ovine pregnancy in relation to maternal nutrition, body composition and pregnancy outcome. *Journal of Endocrinology* 169, 465–476.

Thomassin, H., Flavin, M., Espinas, M.L. and Grange, T. (2001) Glucocorticoid-induced DNA demethylation and gene memory during development. *EMBO Journal* 20, 1974–1983.

Trautman, P.D., Meyer-Bahlburg, H.F., Postelnek, J. and New, M.I. (1995) Effects of early prenatal dexamethasone on the cognitive and behavioral development of young children: results of a pilot study. *Psychoneuroendocrinology* 20, 439–449.

Tronche, F., Kellendonk, C., Kretz, O., Gass, P., Anlag, K., Orban, P.C., Bock, R., Klein, R. and Schutz, G. (1999) Disruption of the glucocorticoid receptor gene in the nervous system results in reduced anxiety. *Nature Genetics* 23, 99–103.

Uno, H., Lohmiller, L., Thieme, C., Kemnitz, J.W., Engle, M.J., Roecker, E.B. and Farrell, P.M. (1990) Brain damage induced by prenatal exposure to dexamethasone in fetal rhesus macaques. I. Hippocampus. *Brain Research. Developmental Brain Research* 53, 157–167.

Uno, H., Eisele, S., Sakai, A., Shelton, S., Baker, E., DeJesus, O. and Holden, J. (1994) Neurotoxicity of glucocorticoids in the primate brain. *Hormones and Behavior* 28, 336–348.

Vaessen, N., Heutink, P., Janssen, J.A., Witteman, J.C.M., Testers, L., Hofman, A., Lamberts, S.W.J., Oostra, B.A., Pols, H.A.P., Valera, A., Pujol, A., Pelegrin, M. and Bosch, F. (1994) Transgenic mice overexpressing phosphoenolpyruvate carboxy-kinase develop non-insulin-dependent diabetes mellitus. *Proceedings of the National Academy of Sciences USA* 91, 9151–9154.

Van Duijn, C.M. (2001) A polymorphism in the gene for IGF-I: functional properties and risk for type 2 diabetes and myocardial infarction. *Diabetes* 50, 637–642.

Voice, M.W., Seckl, J.R., Edwards, C.R. and Chapman, K.E. (1996) 11 beta-hydroxysteroid dehydrogenase type 1 expression in 2S FAZA hepatoma cells is hormonally regulated: a model system for the study of hepatic glucocorticoid metabolism. *Biochemical Journal* 317, 621–625.

Vozarova, B., Stefan, N., Lindsay, R.S., Krakoff, J., Knowler, W.C., Funahashi, T., Matsuzawa, Y., Stumvoll, M., Weyer, C. and Tataranni, P.A. (2002) Low plasma adiponectin concentrations do not predict weight gain in humans. *Diabetes* 51, 2964–2967.

Waddell, B.J. and Atkinson, H.C. (1994) Production rate, metabolic clearance rate and uterine extraction of corticosterone during rat pregnancy. *Journal of Endocrinology* 143, 183–190.

Waddell, B.J., Benediktsson, R., Brown, R.W. and Seckl, J.R. (1998) Tissue-specific messenger ribonucleic acid expression of 11beta-hydroxysteroid dehydrogenase types 1 and 2 and the glucocorticoid receptor within rat placenta suggests exquisite local control of glucocorticoid action. *Endocrinology* 139, 1517–1523.

Wallace, E.M. and Baker, L.S. (1999) Effect of antenatal betamethasone administration on placental vascular resistance. *Lancet* 353, 1404–1407.

Ward, R.M. (1994) Pharmacologic enhancement of fetal lung maturation. *Clinics in Perinatology* 21, 523–542.

Weaver, I.C.G., Szyf, M. and Meaney, M.J. (2002) From maternal care to gene expression: DNA methylation and the maternal programming of stress responses. *Endocrine Research* 28, 699.

Welberg, L.A. and Seckl, J.R. (2001) Prenatal stress, glucocorticoids and the programming of the brain. *Journal of Neuroendocrinology* 13, 113–128.

Welberg, L.A., Seckl, J.R. and Holmes, M.C. (2000) Inhibition of 11beta-hydroxysteroid dehydrogenase, the foeto-placental barrier to maternal glucocorticoids, permanently programs amygdala GR mRNA expression and anxiety-like behaviour in the offspring. *European Journal of Neuroscience* 12, 1047–1054.

Welberg, L.A., Seckl, J.R. and Holmes, M.C. (2001) Prenatal glucocorticoid programming of brain corticosteroid receptors and corticotrophin-releasing hormone: possible implications for behaviour. *Neuroscience* 104, 71–79.

Weyer, C., Funahashi, T., Tanaka, S., Hotta, K., Matsuzawa, Y., Pratley, R.E. and Tataranni, P.A. (2001) Hypoadiponectinemia in obesity and type 2 diabetes: close association with insulin resistance and hyperinsulinemia. *Journal of Clinical Endocrinology and Metabolism* 86, 1930–1935.

Whitelaw, A. and Thoresen, M. (2000) Antenatal steroids and the developing brain. *Archives of Disease in Childhood Fetal and Neonatal Edition* 83, F154–F157.

Whorwood, C.B., Franklyn, J.A., Sheppard, M.C. and Stewart, P.M. (1992) Tissue localization of 11 beta-hydroxysteroid dehydrogenase and its relationship to the glucocorticoid receptor. *Journal of Steroid Biochemistry and Molecular Biology* 41, 21–28.

Wijnberger, L.D.E., Bilardo, C.M., Hecher, K., Stigter, R.H. and Visser, G.H.A. (1999) Antenatal betamethasone and fetoplacental blood flow. *Lancet* 354, 255–256.

Wood, T.L. (1995) Gene-targeting and transgenic approaches to IGF and IGF binding protein function. *American Journal of Physiology* 269, E613–E622.

Woodall, S.M., Breier, B.H., Johnston, B.M. and Gluckman, P.D. (1996) A model of intrauterine growth retardation caused by chronic maternal undernutrition in the rat: effects on the somatotrophic axis and postnatal growth. *Journal of Endocrinology* 150, 231–242.

Yajnik, C.S., Fall, C.H., Vaidya, U., Pandit, A.N., Bavdekar, A., Bhat, D.S., Osmond, C., Hales, C.N. and Barker, D.J. (1995) Fetal growth and glucose and insulin metabolism in four-year-old Indian children. *Diabetic Medicine* 12, 330–336.

Yamagata, K., Oda, N., Kaisaki, P.J., Menzel, S., Furuta, H., Vaxillaire, M., Southam, L., Cox, R.D., Lathrop, G.M., Boriraj, V.V., Chen, X., Cox, N.J., Oda, Y., Yano, H., Le Beau, M.M., Yamada, S., Nishigori, H., Takeda, J., Fajans, S.S., Hattersley, A.T., Iwasaki, N., Hansen, T., Pedersen, O., Polonsky, K.S., Bell, G.I. *et al.* (1996) Mutations in the hepatocyte nuclear factor-1alpha gene in maturity-onset diabetes of the young (MODY3). *Nature* 384, 455–458.

Yang, K., Matthews, S.G. and Challis, J.R. (1995) Developmental and glucocorticoid regulation of pituitary 11 beta-hydroxysteroid dehydrogenase 1 gene expression in the ovine fetus and lamb. *Journal of Molecular Endocrinology* 14, 109–116.

Yau, J.L., Noble, J. and Seckl, J.R. (1997) Site-specific regulation of corticosteroid and serotonin receptor subtype gene expression in the rat hippocampus following 3,4-methylenedioxymethamphetamine: role of corticosterone and serotonin. *Neuroscience* 78, 111–121.

Yuen, B.S., McMillen, I.C., Symonds, M.E. and Owens, P.C. (1999) Abundance of leptin mRNA in fetal adipose tissue is related to fetal body weight. *Journal of Endocrinology* 163, R11–14 [republished from *Journal of Endocrinology* 1999; 163(1), R1–4].

Index

Note: Page numbers in **bold** refer to figures in the text; those in *italics* refer to tables and boxed material.

abdominal circumference
    at birth 119
    see also waist–hip ratio
Aborigines 252
acidaemia 68
activin-βB 174
adaptive responses, fetal 9–10
adenosine 65–66
adipogenesis 224–226
adipoinsular axis 224–226
adiponectin 393
adipose factors 392–393
adipose tissue
    glucocorticoid receptors 392
    insulin action 175
    insulin sensitivity 182, 212, 215
adiposity, adult 92–93, 205–206
    and cardiovascular disease risk 96
    indicators 195–196
    and postnatal nutrition 216–219
    see also overweight/obesity
adolescence
    blood pressure 401
    immune function 318–327
adrenal glands 64
    blood flow 57
    congenital hyperplasia 401, 402

adrenaline 64
aeroallergens 264–267, 289
Africa *164*
African-Americans 252, 277–278
ageing 138, 250
agouti locus 341
agouti-related protein 225
albumin:creatinine ratio, urinary 252
albumin excretion, urinary 252–253
allergens, prenatal exposure 264–267
allergic diseases 314–315
    and breastfeeding 278–280
    childhood environmental factors
      288–291
    childhood infections 282–288
    fetal origins 291–292
    genetic factors 263–264
    and infant intestinal flora 282
    known and putative determinants
      260
    maternal infections 276–277
    maternal nutrition 270–276
    maternal smoking 267–270
    maternal stress 277–278
    prenatal allergen exposure 264–267
    prevalence 259–261, 263–264
    prevention 289, *290*

419

altitude, pregnancy 75–77
amino acids 38–40, 138–140
    feto-placental 35–36
    and insulin secretion 175
    pancreatic development 177–179,
        180–181, 187
    transport across placenta 34
ammonium, culture media 336
amygdala **395**, 396, 400
anabolic hormones 26
anaemia 140
    maternal 34–35
androgens 9, 383
Angelmann syndrome 336
angiotensin-converting enzyme 148
angiotensin II 23, 65, 244
angiotensin II receptors 145, 148, **149**,
        391
angiotensin receptor antagonists 244
angiotensinogen 391
antibiotic use in pregnancy 276
antioxidants 270
antipyretic use in pregnancy 276
anxiety 396–397
AP-2 transcription factor 399
apoptosis 176–177, **178**, 180, 186–187,
        223
apparent mineralocorticoid excess (AME)
        143, 387
arginine vasopressin 65
asphyxia, birth 71–74
assisted reproduction 23, 336–337
    large offspring syndrome 335–337
    low birthweight and birth defects
        334–335
asthma
    birthweight/gestational age 271,
        272–273
    breastfeeding 278–280
    childhood infections 282–288,
        283–288
    environmental factors *260*,
        288–291
    and infant intestinal flora 282
    maternal infections in pregnancy
        276–277
    maternal nutrition in pregnancy
        270–276
    maternal during pregnancy 280–282,
        384, 389
    maternal smoking 267–270

    maternal stress in pregnancy
        277–278
    prevalence 259–261
    prevention 289, *290*
    serum IgE levels 261
atherosclerosis 137–138
Atole 202
atopy
    defined 261
    genetic factors 263–264
    prevalence 259–261
    see also allergic diseases
autoantibody production 314
Aymara Indians 76

baboon 385
BCG vaccination 288, *313*
Beckwith–Weidemann Syndrome (BWS)
        336
behavioural changes 394–395, 396–397
β-adrenoceptor antagonists 64–65
β-adrenoceptors 64–65
β-alanine 187
β-cells 40, 41, 42, 172, 215, 391
    differentiation 172–174
    function 174–175
    mass 160, 175–176, 182, 183,
        184–187, 223
betaine 340, 341
betamethasone treatment 145, 385, 390,
        393, 401
birth, fetal asphyxia/hypoxia 56, 58,
        71–74
birth defects 39, 334–335
birth order *284–286*
birthweight 16
    adjustment for adult adiposity
        205–206
    and adult obesity 198–203, 212–214
    and adult overweight/obesity
        197–207
    assessment errors 117–118
    assisted reproduction 334–335
    and blood pressure
        adjustment for current body size
        117
        meta-analyses 108–118
        role of measurement error
        117–118
        twin studies 115–117

and cardiovascular disease 6, 16, 88–96, 106, 381–382
 cohort studies 89–99, 106
 ecological and migrant studies 88–89
 future research 100–101
 public health implications 120–123
 significance of correlation 99–100
and childhood allergic diseases 271–276
and cholesterol metabolism 119–120
and fetal glucocorticoid exposure 384, 401
and glucose tolerance 162
in high altitude pregnancies 75–77
and maternal nutrition 4–6, **7**, 37, 120–121
and maternal size 23
as proxy for fetal health 99–100
and renal development 249–250
socio-economic factors 75–76
trends in 122
blastocyst culture 334–335, 344
blastocyst development 42
blood pressure 15
 and birthweight 249, 249–250, 382
  confounding factors 114–115
  meta-analyses 108–118
  public health implications 120–123
  twin studies 115–117
 fetal in hypoxaemia **69**
 gender differences 253–254
 and glucocorticoid exposure 143–145, 213–214, 385, 388, 391, 401
 high-altitude populations 77
 impact of risk factor modification 121–123
 and maternal body weight 38
 and maternal stress 240
 and maternal undernutrition 6, 41–42, 118–119, 241–248
 global 130–133, 216
 protein restriction 133–140, 214–215, 240, 337–338, 342
 and renal function 241–248
blood vessel development, pancreas 177–179
body fat 218, **219**
 at birth 28

children 162
 determination of 195–196
 maternal 38
 see also overweight/obesity; waist–hip ratio
body mass index (BMI) 92–93, 195–196
 and birthweight 197–203
 in birthweight:disease associations 117, 205–206
 childhood 98
 and glucose tolerance 159
 WHO classification *196*
 see also overweight/obesity
body proportions at birth 6, 30–32, 164, 292, 326
Bolivia 75–76
bradycardia, fetal 56, 61, **62–63**, 77
brain
 blood flow 56–58
 development 13
 glucocorticoid programming 384, 393–397
 growth 32, 136
 structural changes 395–396
'brain sparing' 136, 164
brainstem, fetal 57
breastfeeding
 and adult body weight 205, 207
 and allergic disease 278–280
 and immune function 320
bronchial hyper-responsiveness 261, 271
bumetanide-sensitive Na-K-Cl cotransporter 248

Caesarean section 282
calcium 41, 141
calorie intake
 maternal 179–180, 183–184, 185
 postnatal 217–219, 224, 226
cancer 340
carbenoxolone (CBX) 144, 249, 387, 388, 390
carbohydrate, maternal diet 37–38
carbohydrate metabolism 182, 215–216, 223
cardiac output, fetal *see* combined ventricular output
cardiovascular disease 6, 16, 320–321, 340

cardiovascular disease *continued*
   and birthweight 16, 381–382
      cohort studies 89–99, 106
      ecological and migrant studies
        88–89
      future research 100–101
      meta-analysis 108–118
      public health implications 120–123
      significance of correlation 99–100
   and maternal undernutrition
      118–119
   and postnatal growth 96–99, 381
   risk factor modification in adulthood
      121–122, **123**
cardiovascular system, fetal
   response to hypoxaemia 55–60
      mechanisms 60–67
      modification by chronic hypoxia
      67–74
carotid body function 66
carotid chemoreflex 61–63
carunclectomy 142, 236
catabolic hormones 26
'catch-up' growth 96–99, 206, 214, 217,
   381
catecholamines 64–65, 68
causative relationships 106–108,
   114–115
Cebu Longitudinal Health and Nutrition
   Study (CLHNS) 315–325
   antibody response to typhoid
      vaccination 319–320
   associations between immune
      measures 322–323
   data analysis 317, *318*
   IgE levels 322
   immune function measures 316–317
   leptin levels 323–325
   participants and protocol 315–316
   prenatal and postnatal influences on
      immune function 318–319
   thymopoietin concentration 321–322
cell culture, pancreatic cells 180
cell cycle 176
cell division 3
   methyl groups 338–339
central nervous system programming
   393–397, 400
cerebrovascular disease *90–91*, 92, 93,
   95
chicken embryo 56, 57–58

Childhood Asthma Prevention Study
   270–271
China 122–123, 167
cholesterol levels 119–120, 121, 123, 165
choline, dietary 340
chorioamnionitis 276
cigarette smoking 88, 121, 267–270
circulation, redistribution 31, 55–58,
   63–65, 68–71, 164
clonal selection 12
Clostridium difficile 282
coat colour 40, 341
cobalt, dietary 340, 343
coconut oil 140
cohort studies
   birthweight and adult body weight
      198–201
   birthweight and cardiovascular
      disease 89–99, 106
   blood pressure 118–119
   maternal nutritional supplements
      201–203
   retrospective 101
   type 2 diabetes 158–162
colostrum 280
combined ventricular output (CVO),
   redistribution 31, 55–58, 63–65,
   68–71
concanavalin *313*
conceptual period, maternal nutrition
   28–29, 42–43, 337–338
coping behaviour 394–395
cord-blood mononuclear cells (CBMC)
   264–267, 270
corticosterone 386
corticotrophin-releasing hormone (CRH)
   277, 389, 396–397
cortisol 143, 277, 385, 390, 391,
   392–393
   metabolism 386
   and tissue hormone receptors
      370–373
'couch potato' syndrome 221–223
cow serum 344
C-peptide 165
CRH *see* corticotrophin-releasing
   hormone
critical periods 3–4, 42–43, 136–137
   kidney development 243–244, 246
   pancreas development 171,
      181–182

rat pregnancy 136–137
crocodilians, sex determination 2
cysteine, synthesis 139, 339–340
cytokines
    in atopic disease 261–267
    β-cell sensitivity 186–187, 215
    in breastmilk 280

delayed-type hypersensitivity (DTH) *313*
demethylation 345–346
Denmark 165–166
developing countries 141
    fetal growth 315
    Philippines CLHNS study 315–325
    'westernization' 122–123, 164–165,
        216–217
dexamethasone treatment 385, 388, 390
    and blood pressure 42, 143–145,
        249, 391
    central nervous system programming
        393–397, 400
    fat and muscle metabolism 392
    and food intake 249
    and offspring adiposity 213–214
    and plasma leptin 392–393
    use in preterm delivery risk 401
diabetes mellitus
    type 1 181, 186–187, 252
    type 2 10, 252, 341, 393
        evidence of programming
            157–162, 181–184
        future research perspectives
            166–167
        mechanisms of programming
            163–166
diarrhoeal disease, infant 320, 322, 326
diet
    methyl deficient 340–343
    nutrient balance 37–38, 240
    'westernization' 216–217
    see also maternal protein restriction;
        maternal undernutrition; postnatal
        nutrition
Diet and Nutrition Survey, Britain 131
dietary supplements 120–121, 201–203,
    346
diethylstilbestrol (DES) 8
'diseases of affluence' 220
DNA methylation 38–39, 40, 139, 333,
    334

and disease 340–341
    methyl group metabolism 338–340
    and nutritional deficiencies 340,
        341–343
    and nutritional supplementation 346
    role in programming embryo
        343–346
    variability in fetal tissue 345
DNA methyltransferases 338–339,
    345–346
dopaminergic system 395
ductus venosus 59
dust mite exposure
    infant 289
    maternal 265–267
Dutch Hunger Winter 16, 23, 25, 33, 41
    causes 199
    offspring blood pressure 38, 118
    offspring body weight 199–201,
        212–213
    offspring cholesterol levels 120
    offspring glucose tolerance 166

ecological studies, cardiovascular disease
    88–89, 106, 118–119
eczema, atopic *266*
    and breastfeeding 278–280
    and childhood infections 282–288
    prevalence 259–260
embryo culture
    fetal overgrowth following 335–337
    methyl cycle activity 344
    variability of abnormal fetal
        development 344–345
    zygote donor diet 336–337
endocrine disruptors 8–9
endocrine status, maternal 143–145
endothelium–endocrine interactions
    177–179
end-stage renal disease (ESRD) 252
energy intake, excess 141
environmental factors 8–9, 14–15
    and allergic diseases *260*, 288–291
environmental hypotheses 382, **383**
epidemiological studies 16, 381–382
    birthweight and cardiovascular
        disease 88–96
    distinguishing causation from
        association 106–108, 114–115
Estonia 282

Ethiopia 291
ethnic differences 252, 277–278
Eubacterium 282
evolutionary advantage 9–10, 288
Exendin-4 184
experimental models
    birthweight and adult obesity
        198–203, 212–214
    birthweight and blood cholesterol
        120
    immune function programming 312
    large animal species 142
    maternal nutrition 22, 27–28,
        130–141, 235–236
    rodents 130–141
    type 1 diabetes 186–187
    type 2 diabetes 181–184

Falashas 10
family size 283–288
famine 6, 16, 23, 41, 101
    offspring blood pressure 38, 118
    offspring body weight 198–201,
        212–213
    offspring cholesterol levels 120
    offspring glucose tolerance 166
fat intake
    childhood/adulthood 121–122,
        217–218, **219**
    maternal 140, 141, 236, 240
fat metabolism 392
fat pad mass 218, **219**
fats
    polyunsaturated 270
    saturated 140
fear 396–397
femoral vasoconstriction 61, 63, 66,
        68–71, 72–74
fetal growth
    and body proportions 30–32
    and childhood atopy 271–276
    and fetal nutrition 26
    high altitude pregnancies 75–77
    and maternal nutrition 4–6, 24–32,
        135–136
    trajectory 28–30
    see also intrauterine growth
        retardation; small for gestational
        age
fetal insulin hypothesis 162–163

fetal metabolic substrates 26–28, 32,
        34–36
fetal nutrition 24–26
fetal origins of adult disease (FOAD)
        hypothesis
    human evidence 16, 88–96
    origins 105–106
fetal overgrowth 335–336
fetal undernutrition
    and blood pressure 240–241
    models 216, 235–236
    and renal disease 250–253
    and renal structure and function
        236–240
    see also maternal protein restriction;
        maternal undernutrition
feto-placental metabolism 35–36
fibroblast growth factor (FGF) 174
Finland 94, 95, 98–99
Flk-1 expression 179
folate 38–40, 341, 342
folate cycle **339**, 340
follicle stimulating hormone (FSH) 336
food intake
    excess 141
    global restriction 130–133, 216, 240,
        249
    see also famine
food intolerance 289
Fresco 202
functional capacity concept 10–12

Gambia 323
gender differences 162, 183
    hypertension 253–254
    immune programming 321, 322, 327
    insulin resistance in young adults
        162
genetic factors 382, **383**
    atopic disease 263–264
    insulin resistance 163
    overweight/obesity 224–225
Germany 291
gestational age
    and atopic diseases 271, *272–273*
    cardiovascular response to
        hypoxaemia 56
    and immune function 312–314
gestational stage 41–43, 213, 246
global undernutrition 130–133, 216, 240

glomerular filtration rate (GFR) 237, 239, **243**, 244
glomerular hypertrophy 239
glomerular number 236–239, 244–246, **247**, 249–250
    determination of 237
glomerulosclerosis 241, 250, 253
glucocorticoid receptor (GR) gene 147, 399–401
glucocorticoid receptors (GRs) 383–384
    adipose tissue 392
    brain 223, 396–397, 398–399
    kidney 215
    muscle 392
glucocorticoids
    fetal 'barriers' 386–387
    fetal exposure 213–214, 370–373, 383–384, 401–402
    and birthweight 384
    and blood pressure 143–149, 213–214, 248–249, 384, 385, 388, 391
    and brain development 384, 393–397
    and glucose homeostasis 385
    liver function 389–391
    and maternal undernutrition 213–214
    molecular mechanisms 398–401
    and pancreas development 391
    timing of exposure 385
    postnatal 147–149
glucose consumption, placenta 34–35
glucose metabolism 181–184, 385, 390–391
glucose tolerance 158–162, 181–184, 215
glucose transporter 1 (GLUT1) gene 341
glucose transporters 34, 174–175, 182
glutamine–glutamate cycle 35
glycine 35–36, 38, 138–139, 342
glycine–serine cycle 35–36, 38–39
glycogen synthase 161
granulocyte macrophage colony stimulating factor (GM-CSF) 261
growth *see* fetal growth; postnatal growth
growth curves
    fetal 28–30
    postnatal 203–204, 206, 381
growth factors 174
growth hormone 36–37, 216

growth hormone–insulin-like growth factor (GH–IGF) axis 370–373
Guatemala, INCAP Longitudinal Study 202–203
Guinea-Bassau 288, 314
guinea-pigs 22, 28, 33, 56, 212
    glucocorticoid programming 394
    maternal undernutrition 132, 133
    pancreatic development 171
gut endoderm 172

handling, neonatal 398–399, 400
hay fever 283, 283–288
head size 6, 31, 106, 164, 314, 326
heart:fetal weight ratio 336, **337**
heart, fetal
    development and prenatal glucocorticoid exposure 391–392
    growth 32
    sympathetic innervation 61
heart rate
    and fetal hypoxaemia 55–56, **69**, 77
    neural control 61–63
hedgehog gene family 172
Helsinki cohort study 94, 95, 98–99, 204
hepatic nuclear factor-1 (HNF-1) 398
Hertfordshire cohort study 97, 106, 158–160
heterochromatin 338
high altitude, pregnancy 75–77
hippocampus 384, 395–397, 398, 400
Homeostasis Model Assessment (HOMA) scale 162
homocysteine 139–140, 337–342
homocysteine-betaine methyl transferase 340
homosexuality 9
hormone disruptors 8–9
'horse racing' 204
house dust mite exposure
    infant 289
    maternal 265–267
household income 322, 326
HPA axis *see* hypothalamic–pituitary–adrenal (HPA) axis
human embryonic stem cells (hESC) 346
human imprinting syndromes 336
11β-hydroxysteroid dehydrogenase (11β-HSD) 5, 143–146, 213–214, 248–249, 384, 385–389, 390, 393

hygiene hypothesis 283, 287, 314–315
hypercaloric diet 217–219, 224, 226
hypercorticosteronaemia 393
hyperfiltration 239
hyperglycaemia 34, 385, 390
hyperinsulinaemia 225, 385, 390
hyperleptinaemia 225
hyperlipidaemia 41, 183–184
hyperphagia 217, 218, 221–222
hypertension
    renal mechanisms 241–248
    risk factor modification in adulthood
        121–123
    see also blood pressure
hypoglycaemia 34, 68
hypothalamic–pituitary–adrenal (HPA)
        axis 29, 41–42, 213–214, 223,
        383–387, 398–399, 402
hypothalamus 224–225
hypoxaemia, fetal 9, 31, 55
    cardiovascular response 55–60
        mechanisms 60–67
        modulation by chronic hypoxia
        67–74
    chronic at high altitude 75–77

Iceland 94
IGF2 gene 344
immune function programming
    current perspectives 325–327
    evidence for 311–315
    health implications 327
    Philippines study 315–325
    prenatal allergen exposure 264–267
    transgeneration effects 2–3
    vaccination responses 316, 319–321,
        323
immunoglobulin E (IgE) levels 314, 317,
        319, 322–325
    in atopic disease 261, 280
imprinted genes 343–344
'imprinting' 2
imprinting syndromes 336
INCAP Longitudinal Study, Guatemala
        202
India 122–123, 162, 166, 167, 216–217
infant mortality
    and cardiovascular disease risk 88,
        106
    high altitude 77

infant weight
    and glucose tolerance 158–159
    see also birthweight
infections
    childhood 282–288, 314–315, 320,
        322, 326
    maternal during pregnancy 276–277
    morbidity/mortality 327
insulin 26
    action 174–175, 182
    fetal insulin hypothesis 162–163
    and leptin 225–226
    secretion 160, 175, 180, 181–184
insulin-like growth factor binding proteins
        (IGFBPs) 398
insulin-like growth factors (IGFs) 37, 174,
        176–177, **178**, 216, 391,
        397–398
insulin receptors 175, 182, 215
insulin receptor substrates (IRS) 175, 226
insulin resistance 138, 181–184,
        217–218, 341
    children and young adults 161–162
    development 160–161
    obesity-related 393
    pregnancy 36
insulin secretion 217–218
    in pregnancy 185–186
insulin sensitivity 182, 212, 215
insults and stimuli 4–9
    timing of in pregnancy 41–43, 213,
        246
intelligence tests 201
interferon-γ (IFN-γ) 261–262, 264–265,
        270
interleukin-1β 186–187, 215
interleukin-2 (IL-2) 270
interleukin-3 (IL-3) 261
interleukin-4 (IL-4) 261–262, 270, 276,
        280
interleukin-5 (IL-5) 261, **262**, 280
interleukin-6 (IL-6) 212, 261, **262**
interleukin-12 (IL-12) 262
interleukin-13 (IL-13) 280
International Study of Asthma and
        Allergies in Childhood (ISAAC)
        259
intersex 8
intestinal flora, infant 282
intrauterine growth retardation (IUGR)
        developing world 315

high altitude 75–77
and immune function 312–314, 315
see also birthweight; fetal growth;
small for gestational age
intrauterine milieu, metabolic 185
Inuit 291
iron 40, 140
islets of Langerhans 172, 175–177,
179–181
cell culture 180
cell differentiation 172–174
vascularization 177–179
Italy 165
IUGR *see* intrauterine growth retardation

Janus kinase (JAK)-2 225
Jewish migrants 10

ketones 27–28, 32
kidneys 10, 11, 12, 13
angiotensin II receptors 148, **149**
development 214–215, 243–244,
246
and birthweight 249–250
function 237, 239–240
and hypertension 241–248
glucocorticoid receptors 215
renin–angiotensin system 243, 244,
245, 253, 391
structure 136–137, 236–241
see also renal disease

labour 56, 58
fetal hypoxia 71–74
lactate 32, 35
lactobacilli 282
lactogen, placental 36–37
Lamarckian theory 3
large animals
as models of programming 142
see also pigs; sheep
large offspring syndrome (LOS) 335–337
Leipzig 291
Leningrad, Siege of 118, 120, 198–199
leptin 183–184, 217–218, **219**, 323–325,
327, 392–393
and insulin 225
resistance 225–226

signalling 184, 224–226, 392
life span 138, 214
lifestyle factors *160*, 291
liver
blood flow in fetal hypoxaemia
59–60
carbohydrate metabolism 182, 223
glucocorticoid programming
389–391
maternal protein restriction 215–216,
337, 342
llama fetus 68, 71
locomotor activity 221–222, 224
Lorenz, Konrad 2
losartan 244
low-density lipoprotein (LDL) cholesterol
121, 138–139
Lucas, Alan 2
lungs 10, 11, 14, 215
lymphoid tissues 314

macronutrient balance 37–38, 240
macrosomic infants 96, 335–337
magnesium 40
malaria parasites 276
male reproductive development 8
MAP-kinase pathway 225
maternal constraint 23–24, 26
maternal–fetal interface, cytokine
expression 262–263
maternal nutrition, dietary excess 141
maternal protein restriction 6, 214
and adult obesity 212–214
and blood pressure 39, 133–140,
145–149, 214–215, 240,
241–248, 337–338
and DNA methylation 337–338, 342
and fetal growth 135–136
and 11β-HSD 145–146, 387
liver development and function
215–216, 337, 342
pancreatic development 175–181,
186–187
pre-implantation embryonic
development 337–338, 342
and renal disease 250–252
and renal structure/development
136–137, 236–240
timing in pregnancy 41, 246
maternal size 23

maternal undernutrition 4–7, 37–41
    and atopic disease 270–276
    biological plausibility as programming
        stimulus 23–24
    and birthweight 120–121
    and blood pressure 118–119
    experimental models 130–141,
        235–236
    and fetal body proportions 30–32
    global 130–133, 216, 240
    HPA axis function 393–394
    human versus animals 27–28
    large offspring syndrome 336–337
    macronutrient balance 37–38, 240
    and muscle development 160–161
    periconceptual period 28–29, 42–43,
        337–338
    and placental size 32–34
    specific nutrients 140–141
    timing in pregnancy 3–4, 28–29,
        41–43, 136–137, 213, 246
    see also maternal protein restriction
measles infection 287, 314
meta-analyses 108–158
metabolic adaptations 9–10
metabolic substrates 26–28, 32, 34–36
metabolic syndrome 159, 219–223, 385
methionine 38, 39, 40, 187
    dietary deficiency 139–140
    dietary excess 38, 339–340,
        341–342
methionine cycle **339**, 340
methionine–homocysteine metabolism
    139–140
methionine synthase 343
methyl-deficient diet 340–341, 342–343
methylene tetrahydrofolate **36**, 38–39
methyl groups 338–340, 344
N^5-methyltetrahydrofolate (MTHF) 340,
    341
methyltransferases 338–339
mice
    agouti locus 341
    coat colour 40
    11β-HSD-2 gene silencing 388
    immune function programming 312
    imprinted genes 344
    prenatal glucocorticoids 396
micronutrients 38–41, 140–141, 214,
    236
microsphere technique 56, 59

migrants 10, 88–89, 166
milk, unpasteurized 282
mineral nutrition 41
mineralocorticoid receptors (MRs) 383,
    396–397
miscarriage 39, 341
motor development 396
multiple regression models 205–206
Munich 291
muscle
    development 160–161
    metabolism 175, 182, 225, 226,
        392
Mycobacterium leprae 263
Mycobacterium tuberculosis 287–288
myocardial circulation 57–58

L-NAME (NG-nitro-L-arginine methyl
    ester) 67
National Health and Nutrition
    Examination Survey III
    (NHANES III) 278
Nauruan islanders 164–165
neonatal handling model 398–399, 400
nephrectomy, unilateral 245–246
nephrogenesis 243–244, 246
nephron number 12, 136–137, 237–238,
    241, **242**, 244–246, 253
neural tube defects 39, 341
neuroendocrine regulatory systems 223
Neurogenin-3 gene 172–174
neurological development 384, 393–397,
    396, 401–402
neuropeptide Y (NPY) 6, 63–64, 225
NGFI-A transcription factor 399
niacin 40
nitric oxide 66–67, 72–74, 77–78, 133,
    186–187, 388
nitric oxide clamp technique 67, 72–74
nitric oxide synthase, inducible (iNOS)
    176
nitrogen metabolism 336–337
NG-nitro-L-arginine methyl ester *see*
    L-NAME
noradrenaline 63–64, 64, 68
Notch pathway 172–174
nutritional deficiencies 2–3, 139–140,
    340, 342–343
nutritional supplementation 120–121,
    201–203, 346

obesity *see* overweight/obesity
OB-Rb receptor 225
observational data, limitations 87–88
obstetric complications 39, 281–282
oestrogen-like compounds 8
oestrogens 383
omega-6 fatty acids 270
oocytes, *in vitro* maturation 334–335
oral contraceptives 8
organs
    development 3–4, 164
    functional capacity 10–12
    size 31
    see also named organs
osteocalcin 386–387
ovarian stimulation 334, 335–336, 336
overweight/obesity 16
    adipogenesis 224–226
    and birthweight 197–207
    and breastfeeding 205, 207
    children 162, 203–204
    endocrine and metabolic mechanisms
        223–224
    experimental evidence for
        programming 212–214
    genetic factors 224–225
    global prevalence 196–197
    indicators of 195–196
    and postnatal nutrition 221–223
    sedentary behaviour 221–223
    thrifty phenotype hypothesis
        164–166, 221–222
    WHO classification *196*
oxidative metabolic substrates 26–28, 32,
    34–35
oxidative processes 137–138
oxygen deprivation *see* hypoxaemia, fetal
ozone 291

Pacific region 164–165
pancreas
    adaptation in pregnancy 185–186
    β-cells 40, 41, 42, 160, 172–176,
        184–187, 223, 391
    development 158, 160, 171–174
    and low protein diet 138, 175–181,
        186–187, 215, 391
    function 41, 42, 138
    functional capacity 10–11
    leptin receptors 184

transgenerational progamming
    184–186
pancreatic cells, culture 180
Papua New Guinea 164
paracetamol 276
paraventricular nucleus (PVN) 223, 396
Pdx-1 expression 174, 179, 184
PEPCK (phosphoenol-pyruvate
    carboxykinase) 182, 223,
    389–390
periconceptual nutrition 28–29, 42–43,
    337–338
perinatal mortality 71
peripheral blood mononuclear cells
    (PBMC) 264–267
peripheral vascular resistance 56, 57, **58**,
    61, 63–64, 68–74
pertussis immunization 287
phentolamine 65
Philippines, Cebu Longitudinal Health
    and Nutrition Study 315–325
phosphatidylinositol 3-kinase (PI3K) 175,
    215, 223, 226
phosphoenol-pyruvate carboxykinase
    (PEPCK) 182, 223, 389–390
phosphorus 40
Physicians Health Study 341
phytohaemagglutinin *313*
phyto-oestrogens 8
pigs 31, 142, 236, 249
Pima Indians 163, 252
placenta
    endocrinology 36–37
    11β-HSD-2 143–146, 248–249,
        385–389
    metabolism 34–36
    size/weight 32–34, 135, 216
    transport capacity 34, 37
    vascular resistance 34, 388–389
placental function 27
    nutritional regulation 32–37
    and pancreatic development 184,
        185–186
    variation between species 27–28
placenta praevia 281
placentation 132
platelet activating factor 267–268
platelet-derived growth factor (PDGF)
    174
pokeweed nitrogen (PWM) *313*
pollen exposure 265

pollutants 265–267, 288–291
ponderal index at birth 6, **7**, 31, 98, 106,
        162, 203
postnatal environment 398–399, 400,
        402
    and atopic disease *260*, 288–291
    and immune function development
        325–327
postnatal growth 24, 106
    and adult body weight 203
    and cardiovascular disease 96–99
    'catch-up' 206, 217, 381
    and immune system development
        322
    and maternal nutritional
        supplementation 202–203
    patterns of 203–204, 206, 381
    and type 2 diabetes 158–159,
        181–182
postnatal nutrition
    and adult body weight 216–219, 226
    and immune function 312
prednisolone 384
pre-eclampsia 26, 39, 341, 384, 388–389
pregnancy
    asthma 280–282
    at high altitude 75–77
    complications 39, 281–282
    maternal–fetal interface 262–263
    nutritional supplementation 201–203
    pancreatic adaptation 185–186
    timing of programming insults/stimuli
        3–4, 28–29, 41–43, 136–137,
        213, 246
Preston cohort study 106, 158–160, 382
preterm births 267–268, 271, *272–273*,
        281, 381, 384, 401–402
primates, non-human 56, 57, 312, 385,
        395–396
priming 264–267
progesterone 42, 389
programming
    concept 2, 382, **383**
    critical periods 3–4, 42–43, 136–137,
        171, 181–182, 243–244, 246
    demonstration of principle 2–3
    human evidence 6–7, 16, 23,
        158–162, 401–402
    and maternal nutrition 37–41, *see
        also* maternal protein restriction;
        maternal undernutrition

origins of hypothesis 105–106
    and physiological function 10–15
    survival advantage 9–10, 288
    transgenerational effects 2–3,
        184–186
propanolol 64–65
protein, excess dietary 141
protein kinase B (PKB) 223
protein restriction *see* maternal protein
        restriction
proximal tubules 236–237
psychosocial stress, maternal 277–278
public health issues
    birthweight and cardiovascular
        disease risk 120–123
    immune programming 327
    overweight/obesity 206, 222–223
    postnatal nutrition and metabolic
        disease 218–219
purine synthesis 39

race 252, 277–278
rats
    critical developmental periods
        136–137
    fetal glucocorticoid exposure 385,
        390, 391, 392, 396
    11β-HSD-2 activity 143–146, 389
    kidney structure and function
        136–137, 236–240, 243–248
    maternal nutrition 133–140,
        337–338
    neonatal handling paradigm
        398–399, 400
    pancreatic development 171–174
Raven's Progressive Matrices 201
regression analysis 205–206
    adjustment for current body size
        117
renal disease
    and fetal undernutrition 250–253
    gender differences 253–254
renal failure, chronic 252
renin–angiotensin system (RAS) 141,
        147–149, 214–215
    intrarenal 243, 244, **245**, 253, 391
replicative senescence 3
reproductive development 8–9
respiratory tract infections, maternal 276
retinoic acid 241

retroperitoneal fat pad 218, **219**
Reykjavik Study 94
rhesus monkey 56, 57, 395–396
rhinitis, allergic *266*, 280
riboflavin 40
rodents
    maternal undernutrition 133–140,
       216, 337–338
    muscle development 161
    see also guinea-pigs; mice; rats

S-adenosyl homocysteine (SAH) 339,
    341–342, 343, 344
S-adenosyl methionine (SAM) 40,
    338–340, 344
S-adenosyl methionine (SAM):*S*-adenosyl
    homocysteine (SAH) ratio 139,
    341–342, 343, 344
salt intake 236, 241, 253
saturated fatty acids 140
sciatic nerve section 63
Second World War famine 6, 16, 23, 25,
    33, 38, 41, 118, 166, 198–201,
    212–213
sedentary behaviour 221–223
senescence, replicative 3
serine 35–36
serine–glycine cycle 35–36, 38–39
serine kinases 175
serotonin (5-HT) **395**, 399, 400
serotype c-specific polysaccharide antigen
    (SpA) *313*
serum, embryo culture 344
sex dependent responses 183
sex determination, crocodilians 2
sex differences *see* gender differences
sex steroids 383
sexual behaviour, human 9
sexual development 8–9
sheep
    assisted reproduction 335–336
    critical periods of development 3
    fetal glucocorticoid exposure 385,
       390, 391, 392–393
    fetal growth trajectory 28–30
    fetal hypoxaemia 55–56, 68–71
    maternal nutrition 27–29, 42–43,
       337
    as model of programming 142
    placental metabolism 34–35

placental weight 33
renal development 243
Sheffield study 97, 106
signal transducers and activators or
    transcription (STAT) 225–226
Simpson–Golabi–Behmel syndrome 336
skinfold thickness, maternal 38
skin-prick test positivity 268, 279, 283
small for gestational age (SGA) 312–314,
    318–319, 325–327
    see also fetal growth
smoking 88, 121, 267–270
snacking 217
social class 201
social mobility 89
socio-economic factors
    atopic disease 278, 279
    and birthweight 75–76
    immune function 322
    maternal protein intake 134
    and obesity 219–220
sodium intake 141, 236, 241, 253
sodium nitroprusside 67
sodium transporters 248
soleus muscle 392
South America, Bolivia 75–77
spermidine 339
spermine 339
Sprague–Dawley rat 239, 244
8-SPT (8-*p*-(sulphophenyl)-theophylline)
    66
starch intake 240
stature, adult 205
stem cells 346
stress
    coping behaviour 394–395
    maternal 224, 240, 277–278
stroke *90–91*, 92, 93, 95
subscapular:triceps skinfolds ratio *199*
sugar intake 6, **7**, 240
8-*p*-(sulphophenyl)-theophylline *see*
    8-SPT
sulphydryl group 187
superovulation 334
suppressors of cytokine signalling (SOCS)
    225–226
Sweden 93–94, 95, 282
sympathetic nervous system 63–64
syndrome of apparent mineralocorticoid
    excess (AME) 143, 387
syndrome 'X' *see* metabolic syndrome

synthetic oviductal fluid 344
system A amino transporter 34
systematic overviews (meta-analyses)
    108–118

tachypnoea, newborn 281
taurine 40, 177–179, 180–181, 187, 215,
    339–340
T cells 312, *313*, 316
    activation 261–264
    allergen exposure *in utero* 264–267
    Th1/Th2 cytokine expression
        261–264, 276, 288
teratogens 9
testosterone 2, 9, 383
tetrahydrofolate (THF) 38–39
thalidomide 9
thiamin 40
thiazide-sensitive Na–Cl cotransporter
    248
thinness at birth 160, 162
threonine 138
thrifty genotype 220
thrifty phenotype 9–10, 97, 163–166,
    183, 217–222
thymopoietin 316–317, *319*, 321–322,
    324
thymus 314, 316
thyroid hormones 26, 399
Tibet 76
transcription factors 174, 398, 399
transforming growth factors 174
transgenerational programming 2–3,
    184–186
transit-time flowmetry 57
transposable elements 343
triglycerides 159, 165
tumour necrosis factor-α (TNF-α) 212,
    224, 261
tumour necrosis factor-β (TNF-β) 261,
    262
twin studies
    birthweight and adult BMI 197
    birthweight and blood pressure
        115–117, 381
    birthweight and cardiovascular
        disease 101
    type 2 diabetes 165–166
typhoid fever vaccination 316, 319–321,
    322–323

UK 97, 106, 158–160
    maternal nutrition 130–131, 134,
        141
umbilical blood flow 59–60
umbilical cord compression 71–72, **73**
uninephrectomy 245–246
urea, plasma 336, **337**
urea synthesis 35
Ureaplasma urealyticum 276
urticaria *266*
uterine artery ligation 184, 212
uterine blood flow 26
uterine horn ligation 132, 237
uterine infections 276
utero-placental embolization 247
utero-placental insufficiency 184,
    185–186
USA
    birthweight and cardiovascular
        disease 93, 95, 382
    National Collaborative Perinatal
        Project 101

vaccination
    and atopic disease 287–288
    responses to *313*, 316, 319–321,
        322–323
vaginitis 276
vascular development, pancreas
    177–179
vascular endothelial growth factor (VEGF)
    174, 178–179
vascular resistance
    fetal in hypoxaemia 56, 57, **58**, 61,
        63, 66, 68–74
    placenta 34, 388–389
vasopressin 68
vegans 130–131
vegetarians 130–131
vinclozolin 8
vitamins 40–41, 236, 241
    vitamin A 241
    vitamin B₆ 341
    vitamin B₁₂ 340, 341, 342–343
    vitamin C 40–41
    vitamin E 267, 270

waist–hip ratio (WHR) 16, 196, 197, 199,
    201

weight gain, postnatal 97–99, 320
Western diet 216–217, 270
westernization 122–123, 164–165,
    216–217, 219–220
wheezing illness *266*, 267–268
    and breastfeeding 279
    and childhood infections 283–287
    environmental factors 289–291
    and maternal infections in pregnancy
      276–277

and prenatal smoking exposure
    267–270
preterm birth 271, *272–273*
prevalence 259–260
Wistar–Kyoto rat 239
World Health Organization (WHO) *196*,
    219

zinc-deficient diet 2–3

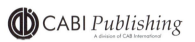
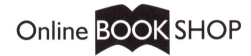

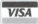

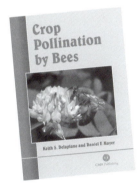
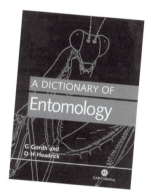
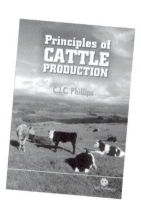
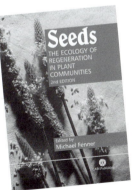